Introduction to
Diagnostic Microbiology

Introduction to
Diagnostic
Microbiology

Elmer W. Koneman, MD
Section Chief
Microbiology Laboratory
Department of Pathology
Veterans Affairs Hospital
Professor of Pathology
University of Colorado School of Medicine
Denver, Colorado

Stephen D. Allen, MD
Professor of Pathology and Laboratory Medicine
Indiana University School of Medicine
Director
Division of Clinical Microbiology
Indiana University Hospitals
Clinical Microbiologist
Wishard Memorial Hospital
Roudebush Veterans Affairs Hospital
Indianapolis, Indiana

William M. Janda, PhD
Associate Professor of Pathology
Associate Director
Clinical Microbiology Laboratory
University of Illinois College of Medicine
 at Chicago
Chicago, Illinois

Paul C. Schreckenberger, PhD
Assistant Professor of Pathology
Director
Clinical Microbiology Laboratory
University of Illinois College of Medicine
 at Chicago
Chicago, Illinois

Washington C. Winn, Jr, MD
Professor of Pathology
University of Vermont College of Medicine
Director
Clinical Microbiology Laboratory
Medical Center Hospital of Vermont
Burlington, Vermont

J.B. LIPPINCOTT COMPANY
Philadelphia

Acquisitions Editor: Richard Winters
Sponsoring Editor: Jody Schott
Associate Managing Editor: Grace R. Caputo
Indexer: Sandi Schroeder
Designer: Doug Smock
Cover Designer: Louis Fuiano
Production Manager: Caren Erlichman
Production Coordinator: Sharon McCarthy
Compositor: Circle Graphics
Printer/Binder: Courier/Westford
Color Insert Printer: Princeton Polychrome Press

6 5 4 3 2

Library of Congress Cataloging-in-Publication Data

Introduction to diagnostic microbiology / Elmer W. Koneman [et al.].
    p. cm.
   Includes bibliographical references and index.
   ISBN 0-397-51215-5
   1. Diagnostic microbiology.   I. Koneman, Elmer W.
QR67.I58   1994
616'.01–dc20

          93-35744
          CIP

Every effort has been made to ensure drug selections and dosages are in accordance with current recommendations and practice. Because of ongoing research, changes in government regulations, and the constant flow of information on drug therapy, reactions, and interactions, the reader is cautioned to check the package insert for each drug for indications, dosages, warnings, and precautions, particularly if the drug is new or infrequently used.

Preface

The volume of relevant information in diagnostic microbiology has reached such levels that most entry-level students are unable to assimilate it in the time allotted in most course curricula. For fear of leaving something out, authors of scientific texts attempt to include as much information as possible, resulting in treatises that increase dramatically in size from one edition to the next. Not only have many texts become so large that they are impossible to carry in a knapsack, they also include information that exceeds the needs of new students in certain training programs. This problem of too much material is exemplified by the common practice—of students and faculty alike—of highlighting with special pens the information in comprehensive textbooks that they consider to be essential.

Therefore, we perceived the need for a text in diagnostic microbiology designed for use by entry-level students, particularly those enrolled in associate degree/medical laboratory technician programs. *Introduction to Diagnostic Microbiology* might also serve as a valuable resource for information needed by individuals who plan to sit for certification or board examinations.

The focus of *Introduction to Diagnostic Microbiology* is on the clinical microbiology laboratory practices and policies necessary to recover and identify the more important agents of infectious diseases. Although select identification tables have been included in this text when necessary to present the comparative cultural and biochemical characteristics of the more important microbes, it is not intended as a detailed cookbook bench manual. Rather, *concepts* are emphasized to encourage the development of a fundamental understanding of clinical microbiology. In striving for succinctness, much of the information included in comprehensive microbiology texts must be reduced. However, frequent reference is made to other resources where the student can find additional information beyond that included in *Introduction to Diagnostic Microbiology*.

Chapter 1 covers techniques for the collection and direct gross and microscopic examination of clinical specimens, culture techniques, approaches to the presumptive and definitive identification of isolates, and basic information on quality assurance, risk management, and laboratory safety. Many of the tasks described are in the domain of work performed by laboratory technicians.

Chapters 2 through 11, covering the various families and genera of gram-negative and gram-positive bacteria, have the common feature of highlighting the important species within each group. Specifically presented are culture media required for optimal recovery, cultural and biochemical characteristics of the scores of bacteria included in these chapters, and practical approaches to their identification to the level appropriate for clinical purposes. Quick-screening methods for rapid presumptive identification of the important microbes within each genus and species and the use of packaged kit identification systems are also featured.

Chapter 12, on antimicrobial susceptibility testing, highlights the various disk diffusion and broth dilution methods used to determine various "drug/bug" profiles.

Although the amount of space devoted here to the subspecialty disciplines of mycobacteriology, mycoplasma/ureaplasma, spirochetes, mycology, parasitology, and virology (Chapters 13 to 18) has been reduced from that found in more encyclopedic texts and monographs, the material included is more than adequate for beginning students to assimilate in the amount of time provided in most curricula. Specifically, sufficient information is included in *Introduction to Diagnostic Microbiology* so that students can formulate a clear picture in their minds of the key characteristics by which the more important microbes can be identified when detected in or recovered from clinical specimens. For example, several composite photographs and illustrated tables have been included for the identification of the important fungal and viral agents that cause infectious diseases. The short chapters on mycoplasma/ureaplasma and the spirochetes focus primarily on the serologic techniques required to make a diagnosis. A brief concluding chapter (Chapter 19) addresses some of the new nonculture technologies, such as various techniques that provide rapid direct detection of microbes or molecular components thereof in biologic specimens.

In a time when the trend is toward sprawling, comprehensive texts, *Introduction to Diagnostic Microbiology* provides beginning students in microbiology with the essentials of a massive amount of old and new information, narrated as succinctly as possible in a single manageable volume.

ELMER W. KONEMAN, MD
STEPHEN D. ALLEN, MD
WILLIAM M. JANDA, PhD
PAUL C. SCHRECKENBERGER, PhD
WASHINGTON C. WINN, JR, MD

Contents

Color Plates

1

Laboratory and Clinical Diagnosis of Infectious Diseases

1

CLASSIFICATION AND IDENTIFICATION OF BACTERIA

Although the entry-level microbiologist may not be required to know in detail the attributes of the vast array of microbes that can infect humans, certain rules pertaining to microbial taxonomy and nomenclature should nevertheless be appreciated. Taxonomy, classification, identification, speciation, and nomenclature are terms that must be understood because they are often used incorrectly in the medical literature.

Taxonomy is the branch of biology concerned with the classification of living organisms. *Classification* is the systematic division of organisms into related groups based on similar characteristics and includes *species* as the smallest and most definitive level of division. Although phylum or division, subphylum, class, subclass, order, suborder, and superfamily are descending orders of taxonomic groups (taxa) within the higher plant and animal kingdoms, family, tribe, genus, and species are the levels most commonly used for the Protista (a third major branch of microorganisms that include algae, fungi, protozoa, and bacteria).

Speciation is done only once at the time the type strain of a microorganism is classified (although it may from time to time be reclassified). *Identification*, in contrast to speciation, is the process by which an unknown microorganism is confirmed as belonging to a previously established taxa.

Nomenclature is the assignments of names to the taxonomic groups following international rules:

1. There is only one correct name for an organism.

2. Names that cause error or confusion should be rejected.
3. All names are in Latin regardless of origin.
   a. The first work (*genus*) is capitalized.
   b. The second word (*species* or epithet) is not capitalized.
   c. Both words are underlined or italicized when appearing in print.
4. The correct name of a species or higher taxonomic designation is determined by valid publication, legitimacy of the name with regard to nomenclature rules, and priority of publication.

A bacterial species is a collection of strains that share many common characteristics. Strains are descendants of a pure culture isolate; the type strain represents the permanent example of the species and carries the reference name. The species name often reflects a morphologic feature or biochemical characteristic of the microorganism or may commemorate a famous person or place. All species are assigned to a genus, which is usually morphologically and biochemically well defined; there is often subjectivity among microbiologists, however, as to exactly what constitutes a genus and species. Genera are, in turn, assigned to tribes and families, each of which have general morphologic, physiologic, and biochemical features. By current convention, family names have the suffix *-aceae* (eg, Enterobacteriaceae); tribe names end in *-eae* (eg, Proteae).

Because phenotypes may change or additional biochemical characterizations may be discovered that preclude an organism from retaining a previous designation, name changes will continue to occur, much to the consternation of microbiologists and practitioners. The current focus on genetic determinants, based on DNA homology and relatedness studies, would, however, allow a more stable taxonomy in which future name changes will be less frequent.

A proper set of characteristics have been established for each microorganism to establish that it belongs to a given species. Thus, in the clinical laboratory, identifications are made based on the following characteristics:

- Gram stain morphology
- Cellular morphology
- Motility
- Presence or absence of spores
- Growth characteristics
  - Rapidity
  - Morphology in solid and liquid culture media
  - Optimal atmospheric conditions and temperature of incubation
- Colonial features
- Differential biochemical reactions
- Serologic tests, including direct detection of antigens, as well as serum antibodies
- Metabolic products, such as long-chain fatty acid analysis by gas–liquid chromatography
- Nucleic acid homology studies

It is in applying these criteria that microorganisms are classified within the taxa previously discussed and a final genus and species name is derived. It is the primary role of the clinical microbiologist to provide physicians with timely and accurate identifications of microorganisms recovered from clinical specimens and to provide information on the relative susceptibility of pathogenic strains to antimicrobial agents. Physicians use this information as a guide in the selection of appropriate treatment, to monitor therapy and to evaluate the course of illness. The intent of this textbook is to help clinical microbiologists fulfill this role.

THE ROLE OF THE CLINICAL MICROBIOLOGIST

The clinical microbiologist's role is to examine and culture specimens for microorganisms, to make accurate species identification of important isolates, and to perform antibiotic susceptibility tests when indicated. The information received from these tasks will assist physicians in the diagnosis and treatment of infectious diseases. Microbiology data are also valuable in monitoring the course of antibiotic therapy and in providing epidemiologic information for defining common sources of infection.

Cultures from one or more anatomic sites may be indicated, depending on the findings of medical history and physical examination. An appropriate specimen for culture must be collected and a transport container selected that will maintain the viability of any pathogenic organisms during transit. The specimen container must be properly labeled with the patient's name, location, date and time of collection, and source of specimen. This information along with the physician's orders must be transcribed to a laboratory request form or entered into a computer data file. Ideally the request form should include essential clinical findings, a working diagnosis, and any information that may require laboratory personnel to apply other than routine procedures to recover uncommon or particularly fastidious microorganisms. Physicians should either call the laboratory or indicate on the laboratory request slip if an infectious disease caused by less commonly encountered or fastidious microorganisms is suspected.

The laboratory may not have available or routinely use certain culture media required for the optimum recovery of certain fastidious or slow-growing microorganisms. For example, the recovery of bacterial species belonging to the genera *Brucella*, *Pasteurella*, *Moraxella*, *Haemophilus*, *Neisseria*, *Leptospira*, *Vibrio*, *Campylobacter*, and *Legionella*, among others, may require special culture media or alternate techniques. The request form and specimen are then sent to the laboratory for processing and analysis. Even within the subspecialized areas of mycobacteriology, mycology, and virology, it is helpful for laboratory personnel to know more exactly which fungal or viral disease is suspected in any given case because special culture media, incubation temperatures, or analytical techniques may be necessary.

Once the specimen is received in the laboratory, the information on the request form is entered into a computer file or log book. The specimens are examined visually, and, depending on the physician's order and the nature of the specimen, wet mounts and smears may be prepared and stained for microscopic examination. Observations may or may not be immediately reported to the physician, depending on the definitiveness of the results. Timely information may often be used to establish a presumptive diagnosis and to institute a specific course of therapy.

Specimens that require definitive identification of potentially pathogenic microbes are processed further. One or more culture media are selected, or, in the case of suspected viral diseases, appropriate cell lines are chosen, to be inoculated with a portion of the specimen. All agar plates are streaked for colony isolation; then plates, broths, and cell cultures are placed in an incubator with appropriate temperature and environmental conditions to maximize the growth and replication of microbes. After a specified period of incubation, the cultures are examined both visually and microscopically. Presumptive microbial identifications can often be made. A final report is issued if a definitive answer can be given; if not, the report should be delayed while subcultures and additional test procedures are performed to identify the organisms.

BASIC CONCEPTS OF INFECTIOUS DISEASE

To establish a working clinical diagnosis, the physician must be aware of the various manifestations of infectious disease and order appropriate radiographic and laboratory procedures to supplement the medical history and physical findings. These responsibilities are of consequence because infectious diseases account for about 125,000 deaths annually in the United States, representing the fourth most common cause of death after heart disease (650,000), cancer (375,000), and cerebrovascular conditions (389,000). These deaths exceed all accidental deaths (100,000), suicides (25,000), homicides (19,000), and cirrhosis (31,000).[15] It is estimated that over 5 million patients admitted to US hospitals have infections (about 3 million of which are community acquired and 2 million of which are hospital acquired).

Koch's Postulates

Near the close of the 19th century, Robert Koch proposed the following postulates, which are a se-

ries of criteria that must be met before a given agent can be accepted as the cause of a given infectious disease:

1. The microorganism must be present in every case of the infectious disease.
2. The microorganism can be isolated in pure culture.
3. Inoculation of the pure culture into animals produces a similar disease.
4. The same species of microorganism must be recovered from the diseased animal.

Thus, once the genus and species of a microorganism have been determined and it has been accepted as an agent of an infectious disease, it is possible to study in detail the host response to invasion by the virulent microbe and to determine a course of therapy that will eradicate the agent and lead to healing. The terms *infection* and *disease* are not necessarily synonymous. Infection is narrowly defined as the presence of microorganisms in a host; disease is a process of abnormal morbidity in which reactive responses are observable in the host. Whether an infectious disease occurs in the presence of an organism depends on the relationship among the host's resistance, the organism's virulence, and sometimes the effects of prophylactic therapy. To establish an infectious disease, an organism must (1) reach the host and find a portal of entry; (2) overcome the host defenses; (3) invade and proliferate in the host tissues and produce toxins or other virulence factors; and (4) be capable of resisting host defenses. Organisms may reach the host by exogenous routes (inhalation, ingestion, direct contact, or inoculation) or endogenous routes (following breaks in natural barriers, change in virulence of "normal flora," or changes in host defense mechanisms).

Definition of Terms

The following terms are essential to an understanding of the infectious disease process:

Infection—invasion and multiplication of microorganisms in or on a host (a disease process may or may not be present)
Infectious disease—an infection in which there is functional or structural harm or both to the host accompanied by signs and symptoms. In some instances, overt signs and symptoms may be lacking, requiring indirect evidence of infection,

such as a rise in serum antibody titer or a cellular immune response (eg, skin test).

Opportunistic infectious disease — an infection in a compromised host by infectious agents that do not cause disease in normal hosts

Acute suppurative or purulent infection — an infection in which pus is formed. Pus is liquid material with a specific gravity exceeding 1.013 that contains large numbers of segmented neutrophils, the hallmarks of acute inflammation. Cell death (necrosis) of tissue is commonly found.

Chronic infection — a long-standing infection in which the cellular response includes predominantly mononuclear inflammatory cells (lymphocytes, plasma cells, and monocytes)

Granulomatous infection — a type of infection in which granulomas are formed. A granuloma can be most simply defined as focal collections of large macrophages or histiocytes that have an increased capacity for phagocytosis and digestion of foreign particles ("activated"). These cells are also called "epithelioid' cells because they have some resemblance to squamous epithelial cells. Several macrophages often aggregate to form multinucleated giant cells. In certain granulomas a particular type of necrosis, called "caseous necrosis," may be found in which the tissue has a cheeselike consistency. The presence of multinucleated giant cells and caseous necrosis is characteristic of tuberculosis but may also be found in certain other infections.

Inflammation — a morbid process or abnormal alteration of tissues or organs caused by injury or tissue destruction that produces local signs and symptoms (pain, heat, swelling), which may also affect the whole body (systemic effects). Inflammation may or may not result from infections.

Cellulitis — a diffuse purulent inflammation, especially of loose subcutaneous connective tissue in which the exudate spreads between layers of the involved tissues

Abscess — a localized collection of segmented neutrophils producing a walled-off area of suppurative inflammation. Abscesses may be infectious or sterile (devoid of viable organisms), showing destruction of tissue at the site of pus formation.

Commensalism — a relationship in which a microorganism lives on or within a host such that neither derives benefit or harm. This relationship is also called *colonization*.

Symbiosis — a relationship in which a microorganism lives on or within a host such that both

derive mutual advantage or benefit. Such an organism is also referred to as an opportunist or a saprophyte, depending on the symbiotic relationship.

Parasitism — a relationship in which a microorganism lives on or within a host and gains benefit at the expense of the host

Saprophytism — a relationship in which a microorganism lives on dead organic matter. Saprobes are generally not pathogenic to humans except in cases of immunosuppression or chronic debilitating disease, when superinfections may occur.

Pathogen — a microorganism capable of causing an infectious disease. An opportunistic pathogen is one that most commonly causes infectious disease only in an immunosuppressed host.

Virulence — the degree of pathogenicity and extent to which a microorganism can cause damage to the infected host

SIGNS AND SYMPTOMS OF INFECTION

Signs and symptoms of infection may be generalized or systemic or may be focal or localized to a given organ or organ system. Early Greek and Roman physicians recognized four cardinal features of inflammation: *dolor* (pain), *calor* (heat), *rubor* (redness), and *tumor* (swelling).

Localized redness and heat and the production of a swelling or tumorous mass can generally be observed, either visually if present on the external surfaces or by radiography or other noninvasive techniques (eg, echography, computed tomography, magnetic resonance imaging). If nerve endings are irritated or stretched by the expanding mass, pain may be experienced either in the immediate area or in adjacent or distant sites through complementary efferent pathways (known as "referred" pain). The presence of a draining sinus and the excretion of a purulent exudate are also indications of a local inflammatory or infectious process. Any of these signs and symptoms should direct the physician to collect material for direct microscopic examination and culture.

In the acute phase of infection, the patient may experience fever (often high grade and spiking), chills, flushing (vasodilation), and an increase in pulse rate. Patients with subacute or chronic infections may present with minimal or vague symptoms — intermittent low-grade fever, weight loss, or fatigability and lassitude. Toxic reactions to bacterial products may produce eczematous or hemorrhagic skin reactions or a variety of neuromuscular, cardiorespiratory, or gastrointestinal signs and symptoms, which are initial indicators of an underlying infectious disease.

Radiographic manifestations of infectious disease include pulmonary infiltrates, fibrous thickening of cavity linings, the presence of gas and swelling in soft tissues, and radiopaque masses and accumulation of fluid within body cavities and organs.

Laboratory values suggesting an infectious disease in patients with minimal or early symptoms include an elevation in the erythrocyte sedimentation rate, peripheral blood leukocytosis or monocytosis, and alterations in the types and levels of plasma proteins. Elevation in IgG or the presence of certain reactants, such as C-reactive protein, or the production of type-specific antibodies may also indicate infection.

COLLECTION OF SPECIMENS FOR CULTURE   most important

It is well established that the proper collection of a specimen for culture is possibly the most important step in the ultimate confirmation that a microorganism is responsible for the infectious disease process. A poorly collected specimen not only may result in failure to recover important microorganisms but also may lead to incorrect or even harmful therapy if treatment is directed toward a commensal or contaminant. The following are fundamental considerations in the collection of specimens:

1. The specimen must be material from the actual infection site and must be collected with a minimum of contamination from adjacent tissues, organs, or secretions. For example, contamination of sputum or lower respiratory tract specimens with oropharyngeal secretions must be minimized. Failure to culture the depths of a wound or draining sinus without touching the adjacent skin, inadequate cleansing of a woman of the periurethral tissue and perineum before collecting a clean-catch urine sample, contamination of an endometrial sample with vaginal secretions, and failure to reach deep abscesses with aspirating needles or cannulas are other examples that may lead to misleading laboratory results.

2. Optimal times and total numbers of specimens for collection must be established for the best chance of recovery of causative microorganisms. In general, blood samples for culture should be drawn as soon after a fever spike as possible when the concentration of microorganisms is highest. At least two sets of blood cultures per bacteremic episode are recommended. Routine throat, sputum, urine, stool, and wound cultures should be limited to one per 24- to 72-hour period. First-morning deep cough sputum specimens and first-void morning urine samples should be collected for the diagnosis of pulmonary and urinary tract infections, respectively, when the bacteria are in highest concentration. Twenty-four-hour collections of sputum and urine are discouraged because of the chance for contamination and overgrowth of commensal bacteria.

3. A sufficient quantity of specimen must be obtained to perform the culture techniques requested. Guidelines should be established for each specimen type outlining what constitutes a sufficient volume of material for culture, depending on the site of infection. All too frequently 0.5 mL or less of material may be submitted, which is too little to satisfy requests for bacterial, fungal, mycobacterial, and viral cultures. Making available separate vials of appropriate transport media for the recovery of each of these groups of microbes, with instructions that at least 1 mL of material be collected per vial will maximize the chance for recovery of each infective agent.

4. Appropriate collection devices, specimen containers, and culture media must be used to ensure optimal recovery of microorganisms.

   Swabs are commonly used for obtaining many types of cultures; they are, however, generally inferior to other methods for collecting specimens, and their use should be discouraged as much as possible. If swabs are used, certain precautions should be taken. Several types are available, varying in the absorptive material used as the tip and in the construction of the shaft. Cotton and rayon have high absorption capacities, a useful property when recovering organisms that are in low concentration in the specimen. Because of residual fatty acids on cotton fibers that may inhibit some strains of fastidious bacteria, rayon, calcium alginate, Dacron, or polyester tips are often preferred. Specimens should not be allowed to remain in contact with the swab any longer than necessary.

Swabs should be placed in a transport medium or moist container to prevent drying and death of bacteria. Swabs and transport media are usually contained within a plastic jacket. One commonly used tube, Culturette (Becton Dickinson Microbiology Systems, Cockeysville, MD), illustrated in Figure 1-1, includes a swab and Stuart transport medium in a glass vial that can be broken to provide moisture during transport after reinserting the inoculated swab. Several collection systems are available for the recovery of anaerobes from clinical specimens. In general, the use of swabs for collection of specimens for recovery of anaerobic bacteria has been discouraged and aspiration of loculated fluid or abscess material with a needle and syringe has been recommended. The commercially available anaerobic systems are essentially of three types: tubes or vials, swabs in plastic holders, and clear plastic pouches or bags (Table 1-1).

Becton Dickinson Microbiology Systems has several anaerobic transport containers available. The BD Anaerobic Specimen Collector is commonly used (Fig. 1-2). The swab is attached to a plunger handle that can be pushed to the bottom of the tube after obtaining the specimen. The BD Anaerobic Culturette system includes a swab within a plastic holder also containing a gas-generating vial. After the sample is obtained with the swab, it is returned to the plastic holder and sealed. Then the gas-generating vial is crushed, producing an anaerobic environment. The BD Bio-Bag and the Difco Pouch System (Difco Laboratories, Detroit, MI) are plastic bags sufficiently large to hold Petri dishes containing prereduced culture media and a gas-generating packet or ampule. After the specimen is collected and the plates are inoculated following standard techniques,

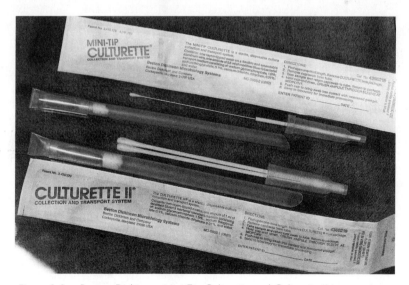

Figure 1-1. Becton Dickinson Mini-Tip Culturette and Culturette II transport systems are shown here. Each system consists of a plastic tube containing a rayon-tipped swab. At the end of the tube is a glass-lined ampule containing 0.5 mL of modified Stuart's bacterial transport medium. After the swab is inoculated with the specimen, it is placed into the tube, and the glass in the ampule is broken by squeezing between the thumb and forefinger, releasing the medium to provide moisture for the tip of the swab. The handle of the swab is attached to the cap, which makes a tight seal when the swab is fully extended into the tube. The two-swab Culturette II system is designed for use when both culture and an additional procedure are required, such as obtaining throat cultures, both for direct antigen testing and culture in the event the direct test is negative.

Table 1-1
Transport Containers for Anaerobic Specimens

CONTAINER	RATIONALE OR DESCRIPTION	PRODUCT
Syringe and needle for aspiration	Fresh exudate or liquid specimens can be transported to the laboratory after bubbles are carefully expelled from the syringe and the tip of the needle is inserted into a sterile stopper. This procedure is valid only if the specimen can be transported to the laboratory without delay. This practice is under question because of the chance of human immunodeficiency virus transmission from needle stick injury.	Standard equipment from several commercial laboratory supply companies
Tube or vial	Tube or vial contains semi-solid holding medium, an atmosphere of 5% CO_2, a reducing agent, and reazurin indicator to give visual indication of anaerobiosis. The tube is used primarily for insertion of swab specimens; the vials are used for inoculation of liquid specimens.	Port-A-Cul System, Becton Dickinson Microbiology Systems, Cockeysville, MD Anaerobic Transport Medium, Anaerobe Systems, San Jose, CA Anaport and Anatube, Scott Laboratories, Fiskeville, RI
Swab/plastic jacket system	Plastic tube or jacket is fitted with a swab and contains either Cary-Blair, Amies transport, or prereduced (PRAS) medium. The Culturette System also includes a vial or chamber separated by a membrane that contains chemicals resulting in generation of CO_2, catalysts, and desiccants to "scavenger" any residual O_2 that may get into the system.	Anaerobic Culturette System, Becton Dickinson Microbiology Systems, Cockeysville, MD PRAS Anaerobic Transport System, Remel Inc., Lenexa, KS
Bio-bag or plastic pouch	Transparent plastic bag containing a CO_2-generating system, palladium catalyst cups, and an anaerobic indicator. The bag is sufficiently large to enclose an inoculated Petri dish containing prereduced media, or a biochemical identification microtube tray such as for performing Minitek tests. Bag or pouch is sealed after inoculated plates have been inserted and the CO_2-generating system is activated. The advantage of these systems is that the plates can be directly observed through the thin, clear plastic of the bag for visualization of early growth of colonies.	Pouch System, Difco Laboratories, Detroit, MI Bio-Bag, Becton Dickinson Microbiology Systems, Cockeysville, MD

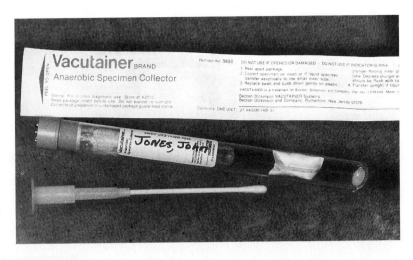

Figure 1-2. Becton Dickinson's Anaerobic Specimen Collector. The system consists of a sealed, gassed, oxygen-free outer glass tube within which is contained an inner glass vial fixed within the rubber stopper. The inoculated swab is placed into the inner glass tube, and the plunger is depressed, detaching the inner tube from the rubber stopper into the lower portion of the outer tube so that the tip of the swab is exposed to the oxygen-free atmosphere during transport. A redox indicator is contained in the bottom of the outer tube to indicate contamination with oxygen.

the plates are placed in the bag or pouch, which is then sealed. Then the ampule is crushed, releasing CO_2 and reducing agents. The Difco Pouch System has an "oxygen scavenger system" with a reserve capacity to bind any residual oxygen, even that which may diffuse through a pinhole leak in the bag. An indicator strip is included to offer visual proof that an anaerobic environment has been achieved within the bag. The BD Bio-Bag also includes a CO_2-generating system, a palladium catalyst cup, and an anaerobic indicator system. Both bags are translucent, allowing easy, direct visualization of any growth that may occur on the plates. Bio-Bag systems are also available to produce CO_2-rich and microaerophilic environments for the recovery of *Neisseria gonorrhoeae* and *Campylobacter jejuni*, respectively.

5. Whenever possible, cultures should be obtained before the administration of antibiotics. This practice is particularly recommended for the recovery of organisms that are usually highly susceptible to antibiotics, such as β-hemolytic streptococci from throat specimens, *Neisseria gonorrhoeae* from genitourinary samples, or *Haemophilus influenzae* and *Neisseria meningitidis* from cerebrospinal fluid. Administration of antibiotics does not, however, necessarily preclude recovery of other microorganisms from clinical specimens, and therefore specimens should not be rejected on the basis of this criterion alone.

6. The culture container must be properly labeled. For the microbiologist to use proper culture techniques and provide the physician with accurate and compete information, each culture container must have a legible label, with the following minimum information:

Name
ID
Source
Doctor
Date and hour

The patient's full name should be used. The identification number may be the hospital number, clinic, or office number, the home address, or the social security number, depending on the circumstances. The physician's name or office title is necessary should consultation or early reporting be required.

Methods of Specimen Collection From Various Body Sites

Throat Swab Specimens

The proper method for obtaining a throat swab specimen is shown in Figure 1-3. A bright light from over the shoulder of the specimen collector should be focused into the oral cavity so that the swab can be guided to the posterior pharynx. The patient is instructed to tilt his or her head back and breathe deeply. The tongue is gently depressed with a tongue blade to visualize the tonsillar fossae and posterior pharynx. The swab is extended between the tonsillar pillars and behind the uvula. Care should be taken not to touch the lateral walls of the buccal cavity or the tongue to minimize contamination with commensal bacteria. Having

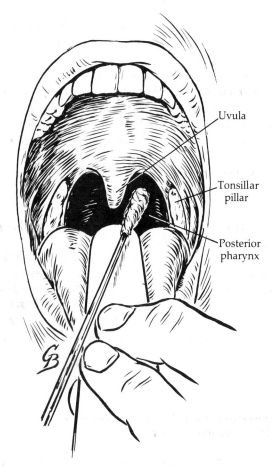

Uvula

Tonsillar
pillar

Posterior
pharynx

Figure 1-3. Throat culture technique. The patient is asked to open the mouth widely and phonate an "ah." The tongue is gently depressed with a tongue blade and a swab guided over the tongue into the posterior pharynx. The mucosa behind the uvula and between the tonsillar pillars is swabbed with a gentle back-and-forth sweeping motion.

the patient phonate a long "ah" serves to lift the uvula and helps prevent gagging. The tonsillar areas and the posterior pharynx should be firmly rubbed with the swab. Any purulent exudate should also be sampled. After collection, the swab should be placed immediately into a sterile tube or other suitable container for transport to the laboratory.

Nasopharyngeal Specimens

Nasopharyngeal specimens are obtained under direct vision using over-the-shoulder illumination. With the thumb of one hand, gently elevate the tip of the nose. Moisten the tip of a small flexible wire nasopharyngeal swab with sterile water or saline

and gently insert it into one of the nares. Guide the swab backward and upward along the nasal septum until a distinct give of resistance indicates that the posterior pharynx has been reached. Gently remove the swab. If, while guiding the swab, undue resistance is met, attempt the procedure through the opposite naris.

Sputum Specimens

Inability to adequately prevent contamination by oral secretions and difficulty in obtaining secretions representative of the lower respiratory tract significantly compromise the diagnostic utility of coughed and expectorated sputum samples for culture. Having the patient brush his or her teeth and gargle with water immediately before obtaining the sputum specimen reduces the number of contaminating oropharyngeal bacteria. The use of proprietary mouthwashes or gargles, which may contain antibacterial substances, should be avoided.

Early morning sputum samples, which contain pooled overnight secretions in which pathogenic bacteria are more likely to be concentrated, should be collected. Twenty-four-hour collections should be discouraged since there is a greater likelihood of contamination and because bacterial pathogens that may be in high concentration in one sample may become diluted with the addition of subsequent, more watery specimens. When sputum production is scant, induction with nebulized saline may produce a specimen more representative of the lower respiratory tract (avoid using "saline for injection" preparations that may contain antibacterial substances.[38]

Transtracheal aspiration, bronchial washing, and bronchoalveolar lavage are other techniques for obtaining respiratory specimens. A description of these techniques, however, is beyond the scope of this book and can be found elsewhere.[28]

Upper Gastrointestinal Tract Specimens

Gastric specimens for culture are only rarely obtained and are limited to those few situations in which a diagnosis may not be possible by other means. The bacterial agents of acute toxic food poisoning may be recovered from vomitus material. Gastric biopsies are being performed with increasing frequency to detect *Helicobacter* (*Campylobacter*) *pylori*.[31,32,42] Aspirations of duodenal contents may be helpful in making the diagnosis of giardiasis and strongyloidiasis when repeated stool examinations have failed to uncover the causative organisms. The use of the commercial "string test" (Enterotest, HEDECO, Palo Alto, CA) is an alternative to passing a gastric tube. The Enterotest is a capsule containing a tightly wound string. Before the capsule is swallowed, the string is unraveled for a short distance and the end taped to the cheek. In 30 to 60 minutes, when the capsule has reached the upper duodenum, the string is carefully removed and any mucus adhering to the strand is milked onto the surface of a glass slide for direct microscopic examination.

Fecal Specimens

The collection of diarrheal stools is not difficult. In cases of diarrhea, stool specimens should be collected in clean (not necessarily sterile), wide-mouthed containers that can be covered with a tight-fitting lid. Contamination with urine should be avoided.

In some instances, collection of a rectal swab rather than stool specimens may be necessary, particularly in neonates or in severely debilitated adults. Because certain strains of *Shigella* species are susceptible to cooling and drying, rectal swabs may be more effective in recovering these organisms. McFarland and colleagues[33] have demonstrated that rectal swabs may be more effective than stool specimens in recovering *Clostridium difficile* in hospitalized patients, presumably because delays in transport or specimen processing are circumvented.

Urine Specimens

Except for the urethral mucosa, which harbors a microflora, the normal urinary tract is usually devoid of bacteria.[25] Since an indigenous flora is present in the male and female urethras and on the periurethral mucosa and skin, urine can easily become contaminated with bacteria from the vaginal canal or perineum. The interpretation of urine culture isolates is presented later in this chapter.

MIDSTREAM COLLECTION TECHNIQUE.   Urine samples are most commonly collected by obtaining the midstream flow by the clean-catch technique. Urine collection from women by the clean-catch technique requires supervision by a nurse for best results.[29] The periurethral area and perineum are first cleansed with two or three gauze pads saturated with soapy water, using a forward to back motion, followed by a rinse with sterile saline or water. The labia should be held apart during voiding and the first few milliliters of urine passed into a bedpan or toilet bowl to flush out bacteria from the urethra. The midstream portion of urine is then collected in a sterile, wide-mouthed container that can be covered with a tightly fitted lid. Preservative systems are available to maintain bacterial counts if a delay in transit is anticipated.[17,24]

CATHETER COLLECTION TECHNIQUE.   Catheterization for the expressed purpose of obtaining a urine specimen should be avoided if possible because of the high risk of introducing nosocomial infections. Catheterization should be restricted to those patients who are unable to produce a midstream sample, and it should be performed with meticulous attention to aseptic technique. The first several milliliters of urine from the catheter should be discarded to wash out any organisms that may have lodged in the catheter tip during transit through the urethra. Urine samples can be obtained from an indwelling catheter using a No. 28 needle and syringe. The area where the needle puncture is to be made must be disinfected. Urine can be aspirated. Foley catheter tips are unsuitable for culture because they are invariably contaminated with urethral organisms.

Genital Tract Specimens

MALES.   Exudate may be expressed from the urethral orifice by gently "milking" the penis; if material is not readily obtained, the tip of a narrow-diameter cotton, rayon, or Dacron swab on a plastic or aluminum shaft may be inserted 3 to 4 cm into the anterior urethra. The swab should be left in place for a few seconds to allow the fibers to become saturated with the exudate. If a culture for chlamydia is being obtained, the swab should be rotated 360 degrees to dislodge some of the epithelial cells. A 12-hour water fast and the collection of mucin threads from the first early morning urine sample for Gram staining may establish the diagnosis in occasional asymptomatic males who have negative urethral smears and cultures.[17] If intracellular gram-negative diplococci are still not seen, the possibility of nongonococcal urethritis secondary to *Chlamydia trachomatis* must be considered.

FEMALES. In females with signs and symptoms of acute genital infection, samples are most commonly obtained from the uterine cervix and the urethra. Cervical specimens are obtained with the aid of a speculum. A swab with a plastic shaft and a Dacron or polyester tip is recommended. The tip of the swab is inserted a few millimeters past the cervical os, rotated firmly to obtain both exudate and cervical cells, and removed, taking care not to touch the lateral walls of the vaginal canal. Urethral samples may be obtained by milking the urethra and collecting the discharge or, if no discharge is observed, by inserting a small urogenital swab into the urethra and leaving it in place for a few seconds to saturate the fibers with exudate.

Blood Specimens

Every precaution should be taken to eliminate contaminated blood samples for cultures. In many laboratories, a quality assurance threshold is set at less than 3% of blood samples that can be contaminated. To reduce the chance of contaminating organisms from the skin the venipuncture site should ideally be prepared as follows: (1) wash with green soap; (2) rinse with sterile water; (3) apply 1% to 2% tincture of iodine or povidone-iodine and allow to dry for 1 or 2 minutes; and (4) remove the iodine with a 70% alcohol wash. In practice, the green soap wash is usually omitted; the combined use of iodine compound and alcohol to disinfect the venipuncture site is, however, essential. If the site must again be palpated after the iodine and alcohol preparation, the finger must be disinfected or a sterile glove must be worn.

Blood samples are commonly obtained by using a needle and syringe (Fig. 1-4). A closed system, consisting of a vacuum bottle and double-needle collection tube, is also used in many institutions.

NUMBER AND TIMING. Most investigators agree that routinely obtaining blood samples for more than three blood cultures within 24 hours does not result in a significant increase in positive results.[3,39] Samples for blood cultures should be drawn before the use of systemic antimicrobial agents if possible. Obtaining the blood sample 30 minutes before a temperature spike is ideal because the highest concentration of organisms is circulating at that time. Since the temperature spike is usually unpredictable, however, an educated guess must suffice in most cases when timing blood sampling. In acute febrile illnesses (eg, meningitis, bacterial pneumonia) when immediate empiric antibiotic therapy may be necessary, or for patients with infectious diseases (eg, osteomyelitis, suppurative arthritis) who are to undergo emergency surgery, two separate samples should be drawn immediately in tandem, from opposite arms. If the origin of a fever syndrome is unknown, two blood samples can initially be drawn with an interval of 45 to 60 minutes. In cases of acute infective endocarditis, three blood samples from three separate venipuncture sites should be drawn during the first 1 to 2 hours of evaluation and then therapy begun. In cases of suspected subacute bacterial endocarditis, three blood samples should be obtained on the first day, spacing venipuncture at least 30 minutes apart. If these samples are negative on culture, two more sets are obtained on a subsequent day.

VOLUME. Sufficient blood should be drawn to inoculate at least two bottles; one is to be incubated

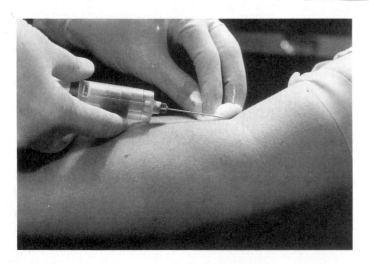

Figure 1-4. Venipuncture technique for blood culture using a sterile needle and syringe. A tourniquet is applied to the upper arm above the venipuncture site to distend the antecubital veins. The site has previously been prepared with tincture of iodine and alcohol. The blood is removed with the syringe and needle and injected into an appropriate blood culture bottle. To reduce the chance of skin contamination, it is recommended that a second syringe be used to draw the blood to be cultured. Rubber gloves must be worn during this procedure.

anaerobically, the other vented through a cotton-plugged needle to allow atmospheric air to enter. At least 10 mL of blood per draw is required[3]; the percentage yield of positive cultures drops significantly if less is obtained.[39] In infants and children who have a lower total blood volume, 1 to 5 mL of blood usually suffices for each culture. Blood for culture should be added to culture broth in a ratio of 1:5 or 1:10 to dilute any inherent antibiotics or other antibacterial substances.

CULTURE MEDIUM. Most commercially available blood culture media (tryptic or trypticase-soy, supplemented peptone broth, brain-heart infusion, Columbia broth, and *Brucella* broth are commonly used) contain the anticoagulant sodium polyanetholsulfonate (SPS) in concentrations varying from 0.025% to 0.05%. In addition to its anticoagulant properties (anticoagulation is a desired effect because certain bacteria do not survive well within the clot where phagocytosis by neutrophils and macrophages remains active), SPS inactivates neutrophils and certain antibiotics (eg, streptomycin, kanamycin, gentamicin, and polymyxin) and precipitates fibrinogen, β-lipoproteins, β1C globulin, and other components of serum complement.

LYSIS CENTRIFUGATION BLOOD CULTURE SYSTEM. The Isolator system (formerly the DuPont Isolator, currently marketed by Wampole Laboratories, Cranbury, NJ) is widely accepted as a blood culture method for improving the recovery of many microorganisms in suspected cases of septicemia, particularly fungemia.[7,9,26] The Isolator is a special tube that contains saponin, a chemical that lyses both the red and the white blood cells. After 7.5 to 10 mL of blood is added to the tube, the contents are thoroughly mixed by inverting the tube several times so that the lysis reaction can be completed. The tube is then placed into an angle centrifuge and spun at 3000 rpm for 15 minutes to concentrate any microorganisms that may be present. After centrifugation, the sediment is aspirated to remove the sedimented organisms and subcultured to appropriate recovery culture media.

SPECIMEN TRANSPORT

The primary objectives in the transport of diagnostic specimens, whether within the hospital or clinic or externally by mail to a distant reference laboratory, is to maintain the samples as near to their original state as possible. Containers with tightly fitting lids should be used to minimize transmission of infection to specimen handlers. Adverse environmental conditions, such as exposure to extremes of heat and cold, rapid changes in pressure (during air transport), or excessive drying should be avoided.

If prolonged delay is expected before the specimen can be processed (eg, more than 4 days), it is generally preferable to freeze the specimen at 70°C. A 20°C freezer may be used (it must be nondefrosting) if the periods of storage are brief.

Sputum samples that have been collected primarily for recovery of mycobacteria and fungi may be shipped without further treatment if collected in sterile propylene or polyethylene containers. To avoid breakage during transport, glass containers should not be used.

Most fluid specimens, particularly urine samples, should be transported to the laboratory as quickly as possible. In a hospital setting, a maximum 2-hour time limit between collection and delivery of specimens to the laboratory is recommended.[1,21] This time limit poses a problem for specimens collected in physicians' offices. Urine transport containers containing a small amount of boric acid may be used if rapid transport is not possible. A holding or transport medium can be used for most other specimens, following the manufacturer's instructions. Stuart, Amies, and Carey-Blair transport media are most frequently used. Sodium borate solution can be recommended as a preservative for shipping specimens suspected of containing mycobacteria to distant laboratories.[40] Sucrose-phosphate-glutamate is a good transport buffer medium for recovery of certain viruses, such as herpesvirus.

All microbiology specimens to be transported through the US mail must be packaged under strict regulations specified by the Public Health Service. A complete list of etiologic agents that are included under these regulations is available on request from the Centers for Disease Control (CDC) and is accompanied by a presentation of several recommended standard procedures published by the National Committee for Clinical Laboratory Standards.[35]

Specimens must be packaged to withstand shocks or pressure changes that may occur during handling and cause the contents to leak. A leaking container not only predisposes the specimen to potential contamination but may also expose mail handlers or personnel at the receiving site to pathogenic microorganisms. Figure 1-5 illustrates the proper technique for packaging and labeling etiologic agents. The primary container (test tube, vial) must be fitted with a watertight cap and surrounded by sufficient packing material to absorb the fluid contents should a leak occur. In turn, this container is placed in a secondary container, preferably constructed of metal, fitted with a screw-cap lid. The primary and secondary containers are then enclosed in an outer shipping carton constructed of corrugated fiberboard, cardboard, or styrofoam.

Dry ice is considered a hazardous material. A shipping carton containing dry ice as a refrigerant for a specimen must be marked, "Dry Ice Frozen Medical Specimen." Packaging should be done so that CO_2 can escape, preventing a buildup of pressure that could rupture the container. The dry ice should be placed outside the secondary container along with shock-absorbent material in such a manner that the secondary container does not become loose inside the outer container as the dry ice sublimates.

In addition to the address label, the outer container must also have the etiologic agents/biomedical material label (with its red logo against a white background) affixed as well as a notice to the carrier (Fig. 1-6).

SPECIMEN HANDLING IN THE LABORATORY

Specimen Receipt and Preliminary Observations

In most clinical laboratories, a special area is designated for the receipt of culture specimens. Because of the increasing possibility that laboratory per-

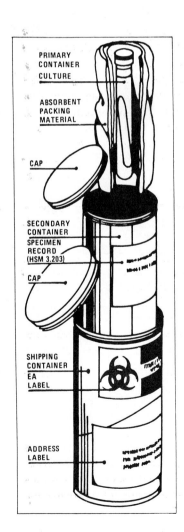

PRIMARY CONTAINER CULTURE

ABSORBENT PACKING MATERIAL

CAP

SECONDARY CONTAINER SPECIMEN RECORD (HSM 3.203)

CAP

SHIPPING CONTAINER EA LABEL

ADDRESS LABEL

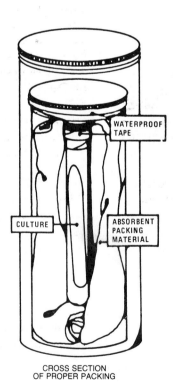

WATERPROOF TAPE

CULTURE

ABSORBENT PACKING MATERIAL

CROSS SECTION OF PROPER PACKING

Figure 1-5. Proper technique for packaging of biologically hazardous materials. (CDC laboratory manual. DHEW publication No. [CDC] 74-8272. Atlanta, Centers for Disease Control, 1974.)

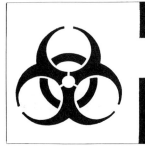

ETIOLOGIC AGENTS

BIOMEDICAL MATERIAL

IN CASE OF DAMAGE
OR LEAKAGE
NOTIFY: DIRECTOR, CDC
ATLANTA, GEORGIA
404/633.5313

NOTICE TO CARRIER

This package contains LESS THAN 50 ml of AN ETI-OLOGIC AGENT, N. O. S., is packaged and labeled in accordance with the U.S. Public Health Service Interstate Quarantine Regulations (42 CFR, Section 72.25(c), (1) and (4), and MEETS ALL REQUIREMENTS FOR SHIPMENT BY MAIL AND ON PASSENGER AIRCRAFT.

This shipment is EXEMPTED FROM ATA RESTRICTED ARTICLES TARIFF 6-D (see General Requirements 386 ([d] [1]) and from DOT HAZARDOUS MATERIALS REGULATIONS (see 49 CRF, Section 173, 386 [d] [3]). SHIPPER'S CERTIFICATES, SHIPPING PAPERS, AND OTHER DOCUMENTATION OR LABELING ARE NOT REQUIRED.

Date   Signature of Shipper

CENTERS FOR DISEASE CONTROL
ATLANTA, GEORGIA 30333

Figure 1-6. Required label for outer container for specimen transport.

sonnel may incur a laboratory-acquired infection from specimens potentially contaminated with pathogenic microbes, bacteria, or viruses, initial observations and handling should be performed under a laminar-flow hood. Personnel should wear protective clothing as appropriate—laboratory coats, rubber gloves, and, in some instances, surgical masks. Previously, these precautions were taken only for specimens carrying hazard labels; because it is not possible to determine if a patient may be harboring a transmittable disease, or if a given sample may contain a highly contagious pathogen, it is prudent to practice special care when handling all specimens.

Specimen Processing

The processing of specimens includes (1) the entry of essential data into a log book or computer termi-

nal, (2) visual examination and determination of whether all criteria for acceptance are met (see next section for criteria for rejection), and (3) the microscopic examination of direct mounts or stained smears to make a presumptive diagnosis if applicable.

Criteria for Specimen Rejection

Criteria for rejection of unsuitable specimens for culture must be established in all laboratories. Rejection criteria should be clearly listed in the ward manual, and in-service classes to instruct hospital personnel in the importance of submitting relevant specimens for culture should be conducted on a regular basis. The following specimen types or culture requests should appear on the reject list and not be processed further:

- Any specimen received in formalin. The only exception might be large specimens in which the time of exposure to formalin is short (less than 1 hour). In these instances, the tissue should be bisected with a sterile knife or scissors and an innermost portion sampled for culture.
- Twenty-four-hour sputum collections. It is difficult to prevent contamination, and individual collections containing a high concentration of microorganisms will be diluted out by subsequent, less-concentrated sampling.
- Smears of secretions from uterine cervix, vaginal canal, or anus for Gram stain detection of *Neisseria gonorrhoeae*
- A single swab submitted for multiple requests, for example, "aerobes, anaerobes, fungus and TB"
- Submission in an improper, nonsterile, or obviously contaminated container in which portions of the specimen have leaked out. Any leaking container having a biohazard label should be handled with extreme care.
- Culture plates that are overgrown or dried out. One exception might be a culture plate obtained for the recovery of one of the pathogenic fungi (see Chapter 14). At times, one of the slower-growing pathogenic fungi will still grow on top of bacteria or another mold. Consultation with the physician may be in order.
- Specimens that are obviously contaminated as evidenced by the presence of foreign materials such as barium, colored dyes, or oily chemicals
- The following specimens are not acceptable for anaerobic culture:

- Gastric washings
- Midstream urine
- Prostatic secretions collected transurethrally
- Feces (except for the recovery of *Clostridium* species associated with gastrointestinal disease—*C. difficile*, *C. perfringens*, *C. septicum*)
- Ileostomy or colostomy swabs
- Throat, nose, or other oropharyngeal specimens (except specimens obtained from deep tissue during oral surgery)
- Superficial skin
- Environmental cultures

The names of other specimen types may also appear on rejection lists. When a specimen is to be rejected, the person who submitted the specimen should be contacted and made aware of the nature of the problem. As a rule, every effort should be made not to reject specimens that are difficult to collect, such as cerebrospinal fluid, bronchial washings, and so on. Cultures should be set up on these specimens following routine procedures or using special media to recover a particular suspected pathogen. In such instances, the decision can be made afterward whether to report the results; and, if the results are reported, the condition of the specimen should be indicated, transferring to the requesting physician the responsibility to apply the data in light of the clinical history, physical examination, and results of other laboratory determinations.

MICROSCOPIC EXAMINATION

The reasons for microscopic examination of clinical materials have been emphasized by several authors.[4,5,21,22] First, the number and percentage of segmented neutrophils that are present usually indicate the magnitude and type of inflammatory response. Second, the quality of the specimens can be validated and the observation of bacteria, mycelial elements, yeast forms, parasitic structures, or viral inclusions may provide sufficient information to render an immediate presumptive diagnosis leading to specific therapy. Third, direct microscopic examination may also give immediate presumptive evidence that species of anaerobic bacteria are present.

Direct Gram stains of clinical material may also be used to determine whether a specimen is representative of the site of infection. This technique has

Table 1-2
Barlett's Grading System for Assessing the Quality of Sputum Samples

	GRADE
Number of neutrophils/10× low-power field	
<10	0
10–25	+1
>25	+2
Presence of mucus	+1
Number of epithelial cells/10× low-power field	
10–25	−1
>25	−2
Total	

Average the number of epithelial cells and neutrophils in about 20 or 30 separate 10× microscope fields and then calculate the total. A final score of 0 or less indicates lack of active inflammation or contamination with saliva. Repeat sputum specimens should be requested.

been applied to the evaluation of sputum samples. Based on the relative numbers of squamous epithelial cells and segmented neutrophils in direct Gram stains of sputum samples, Bartlett[2] has devised a grading system for evaluating sputum samples (Table 1-2).

Negative numbers are assigned to a smear when squamous epithelial cells are observed, indicating contamination with oropharyngeal secretions (saliva). Positive numbers are assigned for the presence of segmented neutrophils, indicating the presence of active infection. The magnitude of these negative and positive designations depends on the relative numbers of epithelial cells and segmented neutrophils, as shown in the outline of Bartlett's grading system. A final score of 0 or less indicates either lack of inflammatory response or presence of significant salivary contamination, thus invalidating the specimen.

Stain Techniques in Microbiology

A number of techniques may be used in the direct microscopic examination of clinical specimens, either to demonstrate the presence of microorganisms or to observe certain biochemical, physiologic, or serologic characteristics. The techniques more commonly used in clinical microbiology laboratories are outlined in Table 1-3. Because the

Table 1-3
Techniques for Direct Examination of Unstained Specimens

METHODS AND MATERIALS	PURPOSE	TECHNIQUES
Saline mount Sodium chloride, 0.85% (aqueous) Glass microscope slides, 3 × 1-inch Coverslips Paraffin-petrolatum mixture (Vaspar)	To determine biologic activity of microorganisms, including motility or reactions to certain chemicals or serologic reactivity in specific antisera. The latter includes the quellung (capsular swelling) reaction used to identify different capsular types of *Streptococcus pneumoniae* and *Haemophilus influenzae*.	Disperse a small quantity of the specimen to be examined into a drop of saline on a microscope slide. Overlay a coverslip and examine directly with a 40× or 100× (oil immersion) objective of the microscope, closing the iris diaphragm to reduce the amount of transmitted light. To prevent drying, ring the coverslip with a small amount of paraffin-petrolatum before overlaying the specimen drop on the slide.
Hanging-drop procedure Hanging-drop glass slide (This is a thick glass slide with a central concave well.) Coverslip Physiologic saline or water Paraffin-petrolatum mixture	The hanging-drop mount serves the same purpose as the saline mount, except there is less distortion from the weight of the coverslip and a deeper field of focus into the drop can be achieved. This technique is generally used for studying the motility of bacteria.	A small amount of paraffin-petrolatum mixture is placed around the lip of the well on the undersurface of the hanging-drop slide. Cells from a bacterial colony to be examined are placed in the center of the coverslip, into a small drop of saline or water. The slide is inverted and pressed over the coverslip, guiding the drop of bacterial suspension into the center of the well. The slide is carefully brought to an upright position for direct examination under the microscope.
Iodine mount Lugol's iodine solution: Iodine crystals, 5 g Potassium iodide, 10 g Distilled water, 100 mL Dissolve KI in water and add iodine crystals slowly until dissolved. Filter and store in tightly stoppered bottle. Dilute 1:5 with water before use. Microscope slides, 3 × 1-inch Coverslips	Iodine mounts are usually used in parallel with saline mounts when examining feces or other materials for intestinal protozoa or helminth ova. The iodine stains the nuclei and intracytoplasmic organelles so that they are more easily seen. Iodine mounts cannot be used to the exclusion of saline mounts because iodine paralyzes the motility of bacteria and protozoan trophozoites.	A small amount of fecal matter or other material is mixed in a drop of the iodine solution on a microscope slide. This is mixed to form an even suspension, and a coverslip is placed over the drop. The mount is then examined directly under a microscope. If this is to be delayed or if a semipermanent preparation for future study is desired, the edges of the coverslip can be sealed with the paraffin-petrolatum mixture.
Potassium hydroxide (KOH) mount Potassium hydroxide, 10% (aqueous) Microscope slides, 3 × 1-inch Coverslips	The KOH mount is used to aid in detecting fungus elements in thick mucoid material or in specimens containing keratinous material, such as skin scales, nails, or hair. The KOH dissolves the background keratin, unmasking the fungus elements to make them more apparent.	Suspend fragments of skin scales, nails, or hair in a drop of 10% KOH. Add coverslip over the drop and let sit at room temperature for about a half hour. The mount may be gently heated in the flame of a Bunsen burner to accelerate the clearing process. Do not boil. Examine under a microscope for fungal hyphae or spores.

(continued)

Table 1-3 (continued)

METHODS AND MATERIALS	PURPOSE	TECHNIQUES
India ink preparation India Ink (Pelikan brand) or Nigrosin (granular)* Microscope slides, 3 × 1-inch Coverslips	India ink or Nigrosin preparations are used for the direct microscopic examination of the capsules of many microorganisms. The fine granules of the india ink or Nigrosin give a semiopaque background against which the clear capsules can be easily seen. This technique is particularly useful in visualizing the large capsules of *Cryptococcus neoformans* in cerebrospinal fluid, sputum, and other secretions.	Centrifuge the cerebrospinal fluid or other fluid specimens lightly to concentrate any microorganisms in the sediment. Emulsify a small quantity of the sediment into a drop of india ink or Nigrosin on a microscope slide and overlay with a coverslip. Do not make the contrast emulsion too thick, or the transmitted light may be completely blocked. Examine the mount directly under a microscope, using the 10× objective for screening and the 40× objective for confirmation of suspicious encapsulated microorganisms.
Darkfield examination Compound microscope equipped with a darkfield condenser Microscope slides, 3 × 1-inch Coverslips Physiologic saline Applicator sticks or curet Paraffin-petrolatum mixture	Darkfield examinations are used to visualize certain delicate microorganisms that are invisible by brightfield optics and stain only with great difficulty. This method is particularly useful in demonstrating spirochetes from suspicious syphilitic chancres for *Treponema pallidum*.	The secretion to be examined is obtained from the patient. In the case of a chancre, the top crust is scraped away with a scalpel blade and a small quantity of serous material is placed on a microscope slide. Ring a coverslip with paraffin-petrolatum mixture and place over the drop of material. Examine the mount directly under a microscope fitted with a darkfield condenser with a 40× or 100× objective. Spirochetes will appear as motile, bright "corkscrews" against a black background.
Neufeld's quellung reaction Homologous anticapsular serum Physiologic saline Microscope slides, 3 × 1-inch Coverslips	When species of encapsulated bacteria are brought into contact with serum containing homologous anticapsular antibody, their capsules undergo a change in refractive index to produce "swelling" that is visible by microscopic examination. This serologic procedure is useful in identifying the various types of *Streptococcus pneumoniae* and *Haemophilus influenzae* in biologic fluids or in cultures.	A loopful of material, such as emulsified sputum, body fluid, or broth culture, is spread over a 1-cm area in two places on opposite ends of a microscope slide. A loopful of specific anticapsular typing serum is spread over the area of one of the dried preparations; the opposite area is overlaid with a loopful of saline to serve as a control. Each area is overlaid with a coverslip and examined under the 100× (oil immersion) objective of the microscope. Organisms showing a positive reaction appear surrounded with a ground-glass, refractile halo because of capsular swelling. Compare the test preparation with the saline control, where no capsular swelling occurs.

*Available from Harleco Co., Philadelphia, PA

refractive index of bacteria and other microorganisms is similar to that of the mounting medium, bacteria are not visible when examined by bright-field illumination and stains are generally required to visualize bacteria adequately and demonstrate the fine detail of internal structures. A full description of dyes and stains commonly used in the microbiology laboratory, their chemical formulas, components, and purposes can be found elsewhere.[28] A brief summary of some of the more commonly used stains follows.

Gram Stain

Crystal violet (gentian violet) serves as the primary stain, binding to the bacterial cell wall after treatment with a weak solution of iodine, which serves as the mordant to bind the dye. Some bacterial species, because of the chemical nature of their cell walls, have the ability to retain the crystal violet even after treatment with an organic decolorizer, such as a mixture of equal parts of 95% ethyl alcohol and acetone. Dye-retaining bacteria appear blue-black when observed under the microscope and are called gram-positive (Color Plate 1-1*A* through *F*). Certain bacteria lose the crystal violet primary stain when treated with the decolorizer, presumably because of the high lipid content of their cell wall. These decolonized bacteria then pick up the safranin counterstain and appear red when observed under the microscope and are called gram-negative (see Color Plates 1-1*G* and *H* and 1-2*A*).

Acid-Fast Stains

Mycobacteria cell walls have a high lipid and wax content that resists staining; once stained, however, the bacterial cells resist decolorization by strong organic solvents such as acid alcohol. For this reason, these bacteria are known as acid-fast. Special treatment is required for the primary stain, carbolfuchsin, to penetrate the waxy material of the acid-fast bacilli. Heat is used in the conventional Ziehl-Neelsen technique. After the carbolfuchsin is overlaid on the surface of the smear to be stained, the flame of a Bunsen burner is passed back and forth beneath the slide. The smear is heated to steaming, stopping short of boiling. The Kinyoun modification of the acid-fast stain is called the "cold method" because a surface-active detergent, such as Tergitol, is used rather than heat treatment. Acid-fast bacilli appear red against a blue green background when viewed microscopically (see Color Plate 1-2*B*).

The fluorochrome dyes auramine and rhodamine can also be used to demonstrate acid-fast bacilli. When viewed by fluorescence microscopy, the bacterial cells appear yellow against a dark background when potassium permanganate is used as a counterstain. Use of the fluorescence procedure facilitates the screening of smears, particularly when a 25× objective is being used. This objective provides magnification low enough to scan wide microscopic fields, yet sufficiently high to see the points of yellow light emanating from the fluorescing bacterial cells (see Color Plate 1-2*C*). Higher magnification can be used to confirm suspicious objects observed with a 25× lens.

Acridine Orange Stain

The acridine orange fluorescent stain is used to detect bacteria in smears prepared from fluids and exudates in which bacteria are expected to be in low concentration (1000 to 10,000 colony-forming units per milliliter) or are trapped within a heavy aggregate of background debris, making them difficult to visualize by conventional staining procedures.[30] The stain detects both living and dead bacteria but does not indicate whether they are gram-negative or gram-positive. Once bacteria have been detected using the acridine orange stain, Gram stain must be used to determine their differential staining characteristics (see Color Plate 1-2*D*).

Toluidine Blue and Methylene Blue Stains

Toluidine blue, a stain closely related to azure A and methylene blue, is being used more frequently in the staining of lung biopsy imprints and respiratory secretions for the rapid detection of *Pneumocystis carinii*. Methylene blue stains should be performed on cerebrospinal fluid sediments along with Gram stains. The gram-negative staining bacterial cells of *Haemophilus influenzae* and *Neisseria meningitidis* often do not stand out against the red-staining background in Gram stains; with the use of methylene blue, the bacterial cells are deep blue and easier to detect against the light-gray staining background (see Color Plate 1-2*E*).

Calcofluor White Stain

Calcofluor white, a colorless dye used in industry to whiten textiles and paper, has two properties that make it useful in microbiology: (1) binding to 1-3,1-4 polysaccharides (specifically cellulose and chitin), and (2) fluorescence when exposed to long-wavelength ultraviolet and short-wavelength visible light (see Color Plate 1-2F). Because the cell walls of fungi and plants are rich in chitin, calcofluor white is a valuable fluorochrome stain for the rapid detection of fungi in wet mounts, smears, and tissue sections. The stain has been most useful in detecting yeast cells, hyphae, and pseudohyphae in skin and mucous membrane scrapings.

Silver Stains

Certain bacteria, namely, the spirochetes (including the recently recognized agent of Lyme disease, *Borrelia burgdorferi*) and the small bacillary organisms associated with cat-scratch disease, are not readily stained by conventional methods. The silver stain has been used to observe these organisms in tissue sections. Darkfield microscopy has also been used to identify *Treponema pallidum*, the etiologic agent of syphilis, and other nontreponemal spirochetes, such as *Leptospira* species.

A Wright-Giemsa stain may be effective in staining intracellular organisms in a variety of smear preparations. One common use is in the demonstration of the intracellular yeast cells of *Histoplasma capsulatum*, particularly in bone marrow smears and less commonly in peripheral blood smears (see Color Plate 1-2G). The periodic acid–Schiff (PAS) stain, having an avidity for reacting with the polysaccharide-rich cell walls of fungi, is also commonly used for demonstrating fungal elements in histologic tissue sections. The stain may be helpful in identifying fungal elements in touch preparations of infected tissues or, as shown in Color Plate 1-2H, in material obtained from abscesses and cavities harboring "fungus balls."

The use of one or more of these stains in providing presumptive diagnoses of infectious diseases in the direct examination of culture specimens is outlined in Table 1-4.

PROCESSING OF CULTURES

After a specimen for culture has been received in the microbiology laboratory, the following key decisions must be made to recover and identify microorganisms that may be present:

1. Select primary culture media appropriate for the particular specimen type.
2. Determine the temperature and atmosphere of incubation to recover all organisms of potential significance.
3. Determine which of the isolates recovered on primary media require further characterization.
4. Determine whether antimicrobial susceptibility tests are required once the identification of the organism is known.

Selection of Primary Culture Media

From among the several hundred culture media commercially available, in addition to numerous "private" formulations that have been reported in the medical literature, only a small number is required for daily use. Agar plates are commonly used. Inoculation of broth media for primary recovery of organisms should be limited to only those specimens, such as body fluids, needle biopsy specimens, or deep tissue aspirations, in which recovery of only a few organisms in low concentration may be significant. It has been common practice in most laboratories to inoculate thioglycolate broth with most clinical specimens to recover hidden anaerobes. This practice should be questioned because the results may be difficult to interpret if the specimen had not been collected and transported under strictly anaerobic conditions. Considerable extra work can be involved in making final identifications of broth-only isolates, which in the great majority of cases have little clinical relevance.

It is presently recommended that only enriched, prereduced CDC or other suitable anaerobe blood agar plates be used for the recovery of anaerobes from most clinical specimens. If thioglycolate broth is used, growth after several days of incubation, in the presence of no growth or the appearance of only an isolated colony on agar media, should probably be interpreted as minimal or rare and thus costly subcultures for biochemical characterization should not be performed. Gram stain of a drop of the broth isolate usually serves as a reliable guide for correlation with culture findings and determination if further analysis of the organism is necessary.

Media may be selective or nonselective. Nonselective media are free of inhibitors and support

Table 1-4
Diagnosis of Infectious Disease by Direct Examination of Culture Specimens

SPECIMEN	SUSPECTED DISEASE	LABORATORY PROCEDURE	POSITIVE FINDINGS
Throat culture	Diphtheria	Gram stain	Delicate pleomorphic gram-positive bacilli in Chinese letter arrangement
		Methylene blue stain	Light-blue—staining bacilli with prominent metachromatic granules
	Acute streptococcal pharyngitis	Direct fluorescent antibody technique (after 4 to 6 hours incubation in Todd-Hewett broth)	Fluorescent cocci in chains; use positive and negative controls with each stain
Oropharyngeal ulcers	Vincent's disease	Gram stain	Presence of gram-negative bacilli and thin, spiral-shaped bacilli
Sputum Transtracheal aspirates Bronchial washings	Bacterial pneumonia	Gram stain	Variety of bacterial types; *Streptococcus pneumoniae* with capsules particularly diagnostic
	Tuberculosis Pulmonary mycosis	Acid-fast stain Gram stain, Wright-Giemsa stain or Gram-Weigert stain Calcofluor white	Acid-fast bacilli Budding yeasts, pseudohyphae, true hyphae, or fruiting bodies
Cutaneous wounds or purulent drainage from subcutaneous sinuses	Bacterial cellulitis	Gram stain	Variety of bacterial types; suspect anaerobic species
	Gas gangrene (myonecrosis)	Gram stain	Gram-positive bacilli suspicious for *Clostridium perfringens*; spores usually not seen
	Actinomycotic mycetoma	Direct saline mount Gram stain or modified acid-fast stain	"Sulfur granules" Delicate, branching gram-positive filaments; *Nocardia* species may be weakly acid fast
	Eumycotic mycetoma	Direct saline mount Gram stain or lactophenol cotton blue mount	White, grayish, or black grains True hyphae with focal swellings or chlamydospores
Cerebrospinal fluid	Bacterial meningitis	Gram stain	Small gram-negative pleomorphic bacillic (*Haemophilus* species) Gram-negative diplococci (*Neisseria meningitidis*) Gram-positive diplococci (*Streptococcus pneumoniae*)

(continued)

Table 1-4 (continued)

SPECIMEN	SUSPECTED DISEASE	LABORATORY PROCEDURE	POSITIVE FINDINGS
		Methylene blue stain	Bacterial forms that stain blue-black
		Acridine orange stain	Bacterial forms that glow brilliant orange under ultraviolet illumination
		Quellung reaction (type-specific antisera)	Swelling and ground-glass appearance of bacterial capsules
	Cryptococcal meningitis	India ink or Nigrosin mount	Encapsulated yeast cells with buds attached by thin thread
	Listeriosis	Gram stain Hanging-drop mount	Delicate gram-positive bacilli Bacteria with tumbling motility
Urine	Yeast infection	Gram stain or Wright-Giemsa stain	Pseudohyphae or budding yeasts
	Bacterial infection	Gram stain	Variety of bacterial types
	Leptospirosis	Darkfield examination	Loosely coiled motile spirochetes
Purulent urethral or cervical discharge	Gonorrhea	Gram stain	Intracellular gram-negative diplococci
	Chlamydial infection	Direct fluorescent antibody stain of smear	Elementary bodies
Purulent vaginal discharge	Yeast infection	Direct mount or Gram stain	Pseudohyphae or budding yeasts
	Trichomonas infection	Direct mount	Flagellates with darting motility
	Gardnerella vaginalis	Pap stain or Gram stain Measure pH of vaginal secretions	"Clue cells" or pH of vaginal secretions > 5.5
Penile or vulvar ulcer (chancre)	Primary syphilis	Darkfield mount of chancre secretion	Tightly coiled motile spirochetes
	Chancroid	Gram stain of ulcer secretion or aspirate of inguinal bubo	Intracellular and extracellular small gram-negative bacilli
Eye	Purulent conjunctivitis	Gram stain	Variety of bacterial species

(continued)

Table 1-4 (continued)

SPECIMEN	SUSPECTED DISEASE	LABORATORY PROCEDURE	POSITIVE FINDINGS
	Trachoma	Giemsa stain of corneal scrapings	Intracellular perinuclear inclusion clusters
Feces	Purulent enterocolitis	Gram stain	Neutrophils and aggregates of staphylococci
	Cholera	Direct mount of alkaline peptone water enrichment	Bacilli with characteristic darting motility; no neutrophils
	Parasitic disease	Direct saline or iodine mounts Examine purged specimens	Adult parasites or parasite fragments; protozoa or ova
Skin scraping, nail fragments, or plucked hairs	Dermatophytosis	10% KOH mount	Delicate hyphae or clusters of spores
	Taenia versicolor	10% KOH mount or lactophenol cotton blue mount	Hyphae and spores resembling spaghetti and meatballs
Blood	Relapsing fever (*Borrelia*)	Wright or Giemsa stain Darkfield examination	Spirochetes with typical morphology
	Blood parasites: malaria, trypanosomiasis, filariasis	Wright or Giemsa stain Direct examination of anticoagulated blood for the presence of microfilaria	Intracellular parasites (malaria, babesia) Extracellular forms: trypanosomes or microfilaria

anaerobes no CO_2

the growth of most microorganisms encountered in clinical laboratories. Five percent sheep blood agar is the most commonly used nonselective medium and is included in the battery of primary isolation media for virtually every clinical specimen. Horse blood is preferred for the recovery of *Haemophilus influenzae* because it has no inhibitory effects on bacterial growth and is a rich source of factor X. Blood agar can be made selective by adding one or more antibiotics or certain chemicals. Kanamycin and vancomycin are added to blood agar (KV agar) used to recover anaerobic gram-negative bacilli (eg, *Bacteroides* species); a combination of four or five antibiotics (bacitracin, novobiocin, colistin, cephalothin, polymyxin B, and others) is added to blood agar Campy-BAP to permit the recovery of *Campylobacter jejuni* from the heavy concentration of mixed flora in stool specimens. Colistin and nalidixic acid (CNA) or phenylethyl alcohol (PEA) can be added to blood agar to inhibit the growth of gram-negative bacteria in contaminated specimens, thus enhancing the recovery of gram-positive organisms. MacConkey agar is the selective culture medium most commonly used to inhibit gram-positive organisms. Bile salts and crystal violet are the active inhibitors. Eosin Y and methylene blue are the inhibitors used in eosin methylene blue (EMB) agar.

Enrichment broth is used to recover pathogenic organisms from specimens, such as feces, in which there is a heavy concentration of commensal organisms. For example, *Escherichia coli* and other "enteric" commensals are held in a prolonged lag phase of growth by the inhibitors in the enrichment broth, allowing the relatively few pathogens to enter an uninhibited log phase of growth and to better compete for survival.

The routine media used in a microbiology laboratory and a list of organisms that will not be recovered unless specifically requested should be published in a laboratory newsletter or manual. Physicians will then know for which infectious disease syndromes they will need to inform the laboratory that the anticipated causative organism is not covered by the culture media routinely used.

Techniques for Transfer and Culturing of Clinical Specimens

Once a specimen has "passed" the various criteria for rejection and has been accepted for culture, appropriate portions must be transferred to the various culture media described earlier. This activity is also usually performed in a designated part of the laboratory known as the "streak-out" area. The transfer of all specimens to culture media should be performed under a biologic safety cabinet or laminar flow hood where there is a glass or plastic shield protecting the neck and face of the user. Although it is the policy in most hospitals to tag with a special biohazard label all potentially infectious specimens, it is not possible to screen completely all such samples. Therefore, the best policy is to handle all specimens as if they were highly infectious. Personnel should be required to wear rubber gloves when handling most specimens; the wearing of a surgical mask is optional but usually unnecessary.

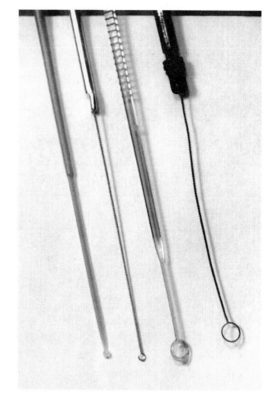

Figure 1-7. Bacteriology loops for inoculation and transfer of bacterial cultures. The two loops to the left (plastic and wire construction, respectively) are calibrated to deliver 0.001 mL of fluid for performing semiquantitative colony counts. The plastic and the wire loops to the right are calibrated to deliver 0.01 mL of fluid.

Techniques for Culturing of Specimens

The equipment required for the primary inoculation of specimens is relatively simple. A nichrome, platinum, or currently commercially available plastic inoculating loop can be recommended (Fig. 1-7). The surface of agar media in Petri plates may be inoculated with the specimen by several methods, one of which is shown in Figure 1-8. The primary inoculation can be made with a loop, swab, or other suitable device. Once the primary inoculum is made, a loop or straight wire can be used to spread the material into the four quadrants of the plate, as illustrated in Figures 1-8 and 1-9. The inoculum is successively streaked with a back-and-forth motion into each quadrant by turning the plate at 90-degree angles.

The streaking technique used for inoculation of

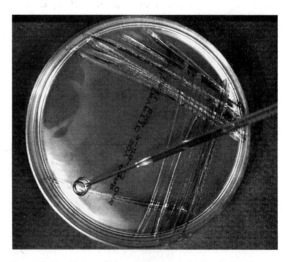

Figure 1-8. The surface of this agar plate is being inoculated with an inoculating loop. Actual inoculation is accomplished by streaking the agar surface with a back-and-forth sweeping motion of the loop, following the pattern of streaking shown in Figure 1-9.

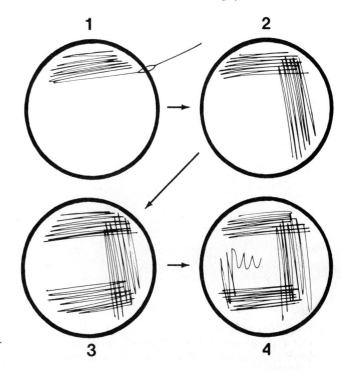

Figure 1-9. Streaking pattern for inoculating culture plates for isolation of bacterial colonies.

agar media for semiquantitative colony counts is shown in Figure 1-10. Nonferrous (nichrome or platinum) inoculating loops, calibrated to contain either 0.01 or 0.001 mL of fluid, are immersed into an uncentrifuged urine sample. The loop is then carefully removed and the entire volume delivered to the surface of an agar plate by making a single streak across the center. The inoculum is spread evenly at right angles to the primary streak; then the plate is turned 90 degrees and the inoculum is spread to cover the entire surface. After 18 to 24 hours of incubation, the number of bacteria in urine samples is estimated by counting the number of colonies that appear on the surface of the media. As illustrated in Figure 1-11, greater than 100 colonies can be counted, indicating a concentration of greater than 100,000 colony-forming units per milliliter.

Media in tubes may be liquid, semisolid (0.3% to 0.5% agar), or solid (1% to 2% agar). Semisolid

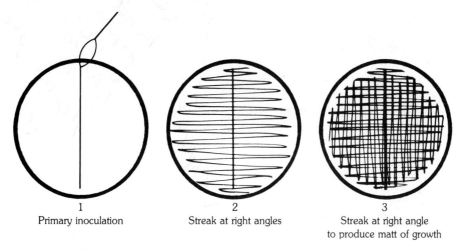

Figure 1-10. Streaking pattern for inoculating media for semiquantitative bacterial colony counts.

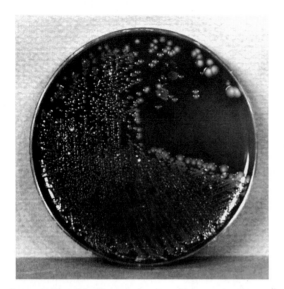

Figure 1-11. Blood agar plate on which are growing well over 100 colonies after being streaked with a 0.001-mL loop (see Fig. 1-7) for semiquantitative colony count. At this dilution, 100 colonies per plate is equivalent to a colony count of 100,000 colony-forming units (CFU) per milliliter, a cutoff that is commonly used, above which the chance for a urinary tract infection is high. The plate in this photograph would be reported out as "greater than 10^5 CFU/mL."

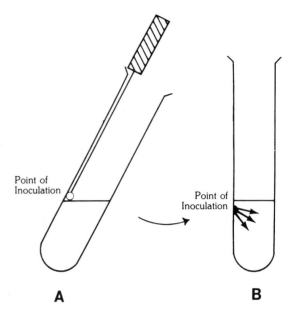

Figure 1-12. Technique for inoculating a tube of broth medium. (*A*) Slant and inoculate side of the tube as shown. (*B*) Replace the tube upright. This submerges the inoculation site under the surface.

agar is suitable for motility testing. Broth media in a tube can be inoculated by the method shown in Figure 1-12. The tube should be tipped at an angle of about 30 degrees and an inoculating loop touched to the inner surface of the glass, just above the point where the surface of the agar makes an acute angle. When the culture tube is returned to its upright position, the area of inoculation is submerged beneath the surface.

Slants of agar medium are inoculated by first stabbing the depth of the agar, followed by streaking the slant from bottom to top with an S motion as the inoculating wire is removed (Fig. 1-13). When inoculating semisolid tubed agar for motility testing, it is important that the inoculating wire be removed along the exact same track used to stab the medium. A fanning motion can result in a growth pattern along the stab line that may be falsely interpreted as bacterial motility.

Body fluids, such as those obtained from thoracentesis and paracentesis, should first be allowed to settle and then aliquots of the sediment centrifuged to further concentrate any bacteria that are present. Cerebrospinal fluid specimens, particularly for the recovery of *Cryptococcus neoformans*, should be centrifuged and portions of the sediment transferred to appropriate culture media; or, preferably, the fluid should be passed through a 0.45-μm microbiologic filter to trap any of the larger yeast cells that may be present.

Microorganisms differ in their optimal temperatures of incubation. Most are incubated at 35°C; the growth of most organisms is enhanced by an atmosphere of 5% to 10% CO_2. If only an ambient air, non-CO_2 incubator is available, the culture tubes and plates can be placed in a candle extinction jar and the entire assembly placed in the incubator. Humidity control within the incubator is also important. Most organisms grow maximally when the humidity is 70% or greater, and culture media tend to deteriorate more rapidly when undue drying or desiccation is allowed.

INTERPRETATION OF CULTURES

Interpretation of primary cultures after 24 to 48 hours of incubation requires considerable skill. From initial observations, the microbiologist must

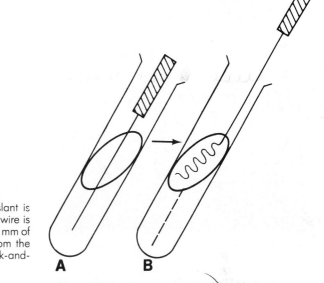

Figure 1-13. Technique for inoculating an agar slant is performed with a straight inoculating wire. (*A*) The wire is first stabbed into the deep of the tube to within 2 to 3 mm of the glass bottom. (*B*) After the wire is removed from the deep, it is streaked over the agar surface with a back-and-forth "S" motion.

assess the colonial growth and decide whether additional procedures are required. This assessment is made by noting the characteristics and relative number of each type of colony recovered on agar media; by determining the purity, Gram stain reaction, and morphology of the bacteria in each type of colony; and by observing changes in the media surrounding the colonies, which reflect specific metabolic activities of the bacteria recovered.

Gross Colony Characteristics

Assessment of gross colony characteristics is usually performed by visually inspecting growth on the surface of agar plates. Inspection of cultures is carried out by holding the plate in one hand and observing the surface of the agar for the presence of bacterial growth (Fig. 1-14). During examination, plates should be tilted in various directions under bright, direct illumination so that light is reflected from various angles. The use of a hand lens or a dissecting microscope to assist in the detection of tiny or immature colonies and to better observe their characteristics is recommended (Fig. 1-15). Blood agar plates should also be examined when transilluminated by bright light from behind the plate to detect hemolytic reactions in the agar (Fig. 1-16). Figure 1-17 illustrates various colony types and the terms used to describe them.

Gram Stain Examination *+ morph.*

Smears are prepared by touching with the tip of an inoculating wire or loop the surface of a well-isolated colony growing on the surface of an agar plate (Fig. 1-18). The inoculum is then emulsified in a drop of water or physiologic saline on the surface of a glass slide (Fig. 1-19). This preparation is allowed to dry and then heat fixed and stained

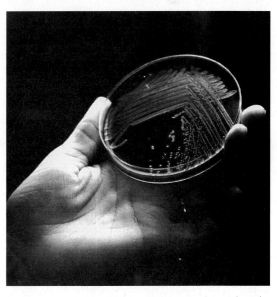

Figure 1-14. Technique for examining a plate culture by reflected light. *colony morph*

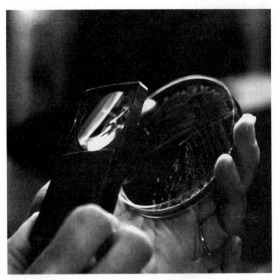

Figure 1-15. Technique for examining a plate culture using a hand lens.

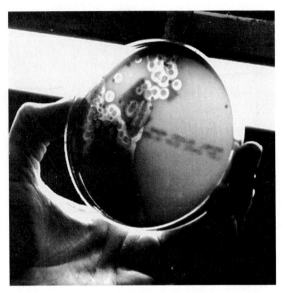

Figure 1-16. Technique for examining a plate culture using transmitted light. This technique is most useful in studying the hemolytic patterns of colonies on blood agar.

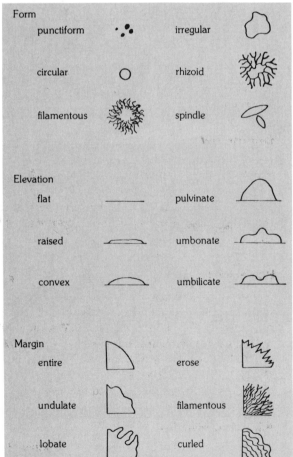

Form		
punctiform		irregular
circular		rhizoid
filamentous		spindle

Elevation		
flat		pulvinate
raised		umbonate
convex		umbilicate

Margin		
entire		erose
undulate		filamentous
lobate		curled

[handwritten annotations] size

motility
growth chara.
1. Time
2. temp.

color of agar
hemolytic reaction
Alpha
Beta
gama

pigment.

Alpha prime
incomplete hemol.
w/ B in zone of
complete hemol.

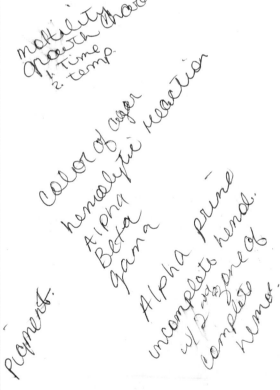

Figure 1-17. Terms used to describe gross colony morphology.

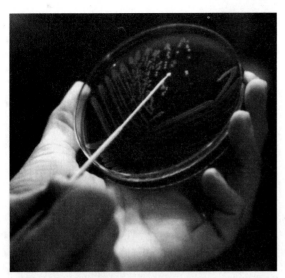

Figure 1-18. Technique for picking an isolated bacterial colony using a straight inoculating wire.

with the Gram technique or other appropriate stain. The stained smear should be examined microscopically using an oil immersion objective. With the Gram stain, in addition to the color reactions assumed by the bacterial cells (gram-positive bacteria appear blue; gram-negative bacteria appear red or pink), other characteristics are helpful in making a preliminary identification of isolates include size and shape of the bacterial cells, arrangement of the bacterial cells, and presence or lack of specific structures or organelles (eg, spores,

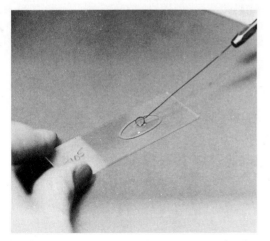

Figure 1-19. Technique for preparing a smear for Gram staining. A portion of the bacterial colony to be studied is sampled with an inoculating loop or needle and emulsified in a drop of water or saline on a 3 × 1-inch glass microscopic slide.

metachromatic granules, swollen bodies). Representative photomicrographs of Gram stains are illustrated in Color Plate 1-1.

PRELIMINARY IDENTIFICATION BASED ON METABOLIC CHARACTERISTICS

Direct Biochemical Procedures for Making Preliminary Bacterial Identifications

Certain preliminary observations or direct rapid tests can be performed on select colonies. In many cases, an isolate can be identified to the level that is clinically useful based on these assessments alone. For example, the lactose-utilizing properties of gram-negative bacilli can be directly evaluated from MacConkey agar by observing the red pigmentation of the colonies; hydrogen sulfide production may be detected on *Salmonella-Shigella* (SS) agar by observing colonies with black centers; and lysine decarboxylase activity should be suspected in the presence of clear or black colonies surrounded by a red halo on xylose lysine deoxycholate (XLD) agar. These tests are briefly described in subsequent chapters in this text and elsewhere.[28]

Catalase Test

Observe for the rapid effervescence produced on addition of a drop of 3% hydrogen peroxide to a portion of the test colony transferred to the surface of a glass slide (see Chapter 8). The catalase test is commonly used to differentiate staphylococci (positive) from streptococci (negative).

false + RBC's from plate.

Bile Solubility Test *presumptive*

Streptococcus pneumoniae cells lyse in a 10% solution of sodium deoxycholate. In the plate test, one or two drops of 10% sodium deoxycholate are added to the colonies growing on the surface of an agar plate. Disappearance of the colonies is looked for after 15 minutes of incubation. Alternately, the tube test can be performed as described in Chapter 9.

Slide Coagulase Test

A colony suspected of being a *Staphylococcus* species is emulsified in a drop of rabbit plasma on a glass

*vs.   Staph aureus (+)
Staph species (-)*

[handwritten margin notes: drop H2O some clump ⇒ have to back up by tube]

slide. Bacterial clumping within 2 minutes indicates the presence of bound coagulase and constitutes a positive test result (see Chapter 8). Several commercial systems are available for performing the coagulase test,[2,8] many of which have been favorably evaluated by Berke and Tilton.[6]

[handwritten: tube - @ up to 4 hrs.]

Direct Spot Indole Test

A small portion of the colony to be tested is transferred from a nonselective medium such as blood or chocolate agar to a strip of filter paper that has been saturated with Kovac's reagent or *p*-dimethylaminocinnamaldehyde (PACA) solution. The immediate development of a red color using Kovac's reagent indicates the presence of indole and a positive test result. PACA is more sensitive than Kovac's reagent; a positive test reaction is shown by display of a rapid blue color (see Chapter 2). *[handwritten: e. coli presumptive.]*

Cytochrome Oxidase Test

A portion of the colony to be tested is smeared on the reagent-impregnated area of an oxidase test strip. The immediate development of a blue color indicates cytochrome oxidase activity and a positive test result (see Chapter 2). *[handwritten: non-fermenting non-glucose bacteria pseudomonas nisseria branhalla. ect.]*

PYR Substrate

Bosley and associates[8] have described the use of L-pyrrolidonyl-naphthylamide (PYR) substrate for the rapid identification of enterococci. After 4 hours of incubation following heavy inoculation of the substrate with a liquid suspension of the unknown organism prepared from a primary isolation plate, the production of a red color after adding N,N-methyl-aminocinnamaldehyde reagent is indicative of group D enterococci (see Chapter 9). *[handwritten: mug.]*

BACTERIAL SPECIES IDENTIFICATION AND SELECTION OF DIFFERENTIAL IDENTIFICATION CHARACTERISTICS

The final identification of an unknown bacterium to genus and species levels is usually accomplished by testing for certain enzyme systems that are unique to each species. In the laboratory, these enzyme systems are detected by inoculating a small portion of a well-isolated bacterial colony into a series of culture media containing specific substrates and chemical indicators that detect pH changes or the presence of specific byproducts. The clinical microbiologist must select appropriate sets of differential characteristics that allow for the identification of each group of bacteria. A guide to the selection process can be found elsewhere.[28]

Reporting of Results

Reports of microbiology culture results should be issued as soon as useful information becomes available. Positive Gram stain results on smears prepared from clinical materials or the observations made from direct antigen detection procedures should be telephoned immediately to the physician or ward. Microbiologists must be familiar with state statutes governing their responsibility for handling reportable diseases. Most state public health laboratories have a "Report of a Communicable Disease" card that lists reportable diseases.

INFECTIONS OF SPECIFIC ORGAN SYSTEMS

Having carried out all of the activities described previously concerning the collection, delivery, processing, analysis, and reporting of clinical specimens submitted for culture, the etiologic agents of infectious diseases can usually be clearly identified and appropriate therapy instituted based on this information. Details of the clinical presentations for various microorganisms and specific methods for recovery from common body sites are reviewed briefly in later chapters in this text and elsewhere.[28] Only a brief summary is included here.

Infections of the Upper Respiratory Tract

Acute pharyngitis is the most common infection of the upper respiratory tract, caused by streptococci, mycoplasma, viruses, or *Clostridium diphtheriae*.

Diphtheria is primarily an infection of children, occurring in sporadic outbreaks, although adults may become infected, particularly those in lower socioeconomic groups. The thick, blue-white or gray diphtheritic membrane that covers an edematous posterior pharynx can usually be differentiated from the fire-red throat of a patient with acute streptococcal pharyngitis. Streptococcal pharyngitis may also be accompanied by scarlatiniform rash.[18]

Pharyngitis Caused by Group A, β-Hemolytic Streptococci

Recovery and identification of group A streptococci in throat swabs is accomplished by inoculating a 5% sheep blood agar plate for organism isolation and making two or three stabs through the inoculation areas to amplify the effect of the oxygen labile hemolysins. After 18 to 24 hours of incubation, the plate is examined for the presence of β-hemolytic colonies. Those colonies determined to be streptococci by Gram-staining and catalase testing can then be definitively identified by further tests as discussed in Chapter 9. Direct detection of streptococcal antigen on throat swabs has become accepted practice in many clinic and laboratory settings.[27,36] All direct detection methods require extraction of the group A streptococcal antigen from the swab after collection and before detection. The original method for extraction of group-specific polysaccharide antigens of β-hemolytic streptococci was the use of nitrous acid.[14] Acid-extraction techniques and subsequent detection methods provide results within 10 to 15 minutes.[30,34] Evaluations of the kit systems available as of 1985 and 1987 were reviewed by Campos and Charilaou[10] and Facklam,[15] respectively.

The recovery and identification of miscellaneous pathogens from throat cultures, such as *Corynebacterium diphtheriae*, *Bordetella pertussis*, *Neisseria gonorrhoeae*, and viral agents of pharyngitis, including adenoviruses, Epstein-Barr virus, and group A coxsackieviruses, are discussed in Chapters 10, 3, 7, and 16, respectively. Local health departments should be consulted instructions on recovery and identification of *C. diphtheriae* in suspected cases. For the recovery of *B. pertussis* from patients suspected of having whooping cough, a portion of nasopharyngeal washings should be streaked with an inoculating loop at the bedside to the agar surface of a plate of Bordet-Gengou potato infusion agar[20] or Regan and Lowe agar.[37] Inoculated plates are immediately placed into a CO_2-enriched environment at 35°C.

Infections of the Oral Cavity

Bacteria, fungi, and viruses commonly cause a variety of infections of the oral cavity. In fact, a specimen labeled "buccal mucosa," "tongue," "gums," or "inner lip" should alert microbiologists that the cause may be a microorganism other than bacteria. If the clinical history reveals a long-standing, non-healing mucosal ulcer in the oral cavity, the possibility of the cutaneous extension of a systemic fungal disease must be considered. An immediate diagnosis of histoplasmosis or blastomycosis may be possible by observing typical yeast forms in direct saline or potassium hydroxide mounts of material scraped from the base or margins of the ulcer. Tissue biopsy for histologic study and direct examination of exudative material may be required.

Infections of the Lower Respiratory Tract

Infections of the lower respiratory tract may involve the trachea and bronchial tree (tracheitis, bronchitis, and bronchiolitis) and the lung tissue (alveolitis and pneumonia). Presenting symptoms usually include cough and varying degrees of sputum production. Fever may or may not be present in lower respiratory tract infections. Chest pain may be diffuse, vague, and constant or localized and intermittent, accentuated by deep respiration if pleuritis is present. Shortness of breath and dyspnea usually indicate involvement of the terminal bronchioles and alveoli in a more diffuse pneumonitic process. Physical signs pointing to lower respiratory tract infection include rales and rhonchi, diminished breath sounds, and localized dullness to percussion in cases of lobar pneumonia.

Because so many species of bacteria can be found as normal flora or commensals in the respiratory tract, establishing the bacterial etiology of acute and chronic bronchitis can also be difficult (Table 1-5). The recovery of *Streptococcus pneumoniae*, *Klebsiella pneumoniae*, *Haemophilus influenzae*, and *Moraxella* (*Branhamella*) *catarrhalis* as the predominant microorganisms from respiratory secretions, particularly when these organisms are also recovered from concomitant blood samples, supports their role in the development of acute pneumonia. Induced sputum samples, collected after inhalation of nebulized saline, may be required

Table 1-5
Commensal Flora and Pathogenic Bacteria in the Respiratory Tract

COMMENSAL FLORA	POTENTIAL PATHOGENS	RECOMMENDED ISOLATION MEDIA
α-Streptococci	Group A, β-hemolytic streptococci	5% sheep blood agar, with or without trimethoprim-sulfamethoxazole
S. mutans		
S. salivarius	Streptococcus pneumoniae	
S. pneumoniae	Klebsiella pneumoniae and other Enterobacteriaceae	5% sheep blood agar and MacConkey (or eosin methylene blue) agar
β-Streptococci other than group A	Pseudomonas aeruginosa	
Staphylococci	Neisseria gonorrhoeae and N. meningitidis	Modified Thayer-Martin (MTM)
S. aureus		
S. epidermidis		
Haemophilus species	S. aureus	Horse blood with colistin and nalidixic acid (CNA)
Neisseria species	Haemophilus influenzae type b and nontypeable H. influenzae	
Branhamella species		
Corynebacterium species ("diphtheroids")	Corynebacterium diphtheriae	Loeffler or Pai slant and serum-tellurite agar
	Moraxella catarrhalis	
Escherichia coli and other Enterobacteriaceae	Capnocytophaga species	5% sheep blood or chocolate agar
Anaerobes	Bordetella pertussis	Bordet-Gengou potato agar or Regan and Lowe medium
	Mycobacterium species	Löwenstein-Jensen (LJ) egg medium or Middlebrook 7H11
	Legionella pneumophila and other legionellae	Charcoal yeast extract (CYE) agar

to increase the yield of detection of certain organisms, particularly *Pneumocystis carinii*.

Infections of the Gastrointestinal Tract

Upper Gastrointestinal Tract Infections

Upper gastrointestinal signs and symptoms of infection include anorexia, a feeling of nausea, occasionally overt vomiting, and upper abdominal pain. The pain may be generalized if the stomach and upper duodenum are diffusely inflamed (as may occur in cases of viral gastritis) or localized to specific areas in the upper abdomen or referred to regions of the back if the stomach wall is affected. The bacterium *Helicobacter pylori* (formerly *Campylobacter pylori*) has been associated with gastritis and peptic ulcer disease.[31,32,42] The organism has the unique biochemical property of rapidly and avidly hydrolyzing urea and releasing ammonium

ions. The acute and often fulminant gastritis accompanied by generalized weakness and vomiting, experienced after ingesting food heavily contaminated with organisms such as *Staphylococcus aureus*, *Salmonella* species, *Clostridium perfringens*, and *Bacillus cereus*, does not result from direct bacterial invasion of the stomach wall; rather, it comes from the emetic action of preformed neurotoxins on the central autonomic nervous system. The more protracted and vague symptoms of upper abdominal bloating, belching, or increased flatulence may be caused by infections of the duodenum and upper ileum by parasitic organisms such as *Giardia lamblia* and *Strongyloides stercoralis*.

Lower Gastrointestinal Tract Infections

The most common presenting symptom pointing to an infection of the lower intestinal tract is diarrhea. The diarrhea may be accompanied by cramping abdominal pain of varying degrees of severity. *Dysentery* is a term used to describe the condition in which diarrhea is accompanied by cramping abdominal pain and *tenesmus* (painful straining when passing the stool). Dysentery results from "enteroinvasive" microorganisms that penetrate through the mucosa and cause inflammation of the intestinal wall. At the opposite end of the spectrum are the nonpainful, profusely watery diarrheal syndromes caused by *Vibrio cholerae* and other noninvasive "enterotoxigenic" bacteria that produce *Vibrio*-like toxins.

The bacterial species most commonly encountered are *Salmonella* species and *Shigella* species, *Campylobacter jejuni*, *Vibrio species* (particularly *Vibrio cholerae*) and certain halophilic, non–*V. cholerae* vibrios (particularly prevalent in the southeastern Gulf Coast regions and acquired from contact with or ingestion of fish and animal handlers), *Yersinia enterocolitica*, *Aeromonas* species, and *Plesiomonas* species. The recovery of pathogenic strains of *Escherichia coli* in cases of diarrhea may be significant, particularly serogroup 0157:H7, the cause of hemorrhagic colitis. The culture recovery and identification of these enteric pathogens is presented in more detail in Chapters 2 and 4.

Infections of the Urinary Tract

The urinary tract is divided into two major divisions—upper (the kidneys, renal pelves, and ureters) and lower (urinary bladder and urethra). Upper urinary tract infections are most commonly ascending; that is, they originate in the urinary bladder and ascend through the ureters to the kidneys. Upper urinary tract infections may result from hematogenous spread of bacteria into the glomeruli and renal cortex in patients with septicemia. Microfocal abscesses or acute suppurative pyelonephritis are common manifestations. The cardinal clinical manifestations of upper urinary tract infections are fever (often with chills) and flank pain. Most lower urinary tract infections involve the urinary bladder, with potential spread to the prostate gland in males and to the urethra (acute urethral syndrome) in females. Frequent and painful urination of small amounts of turbid urine and suprapubic heaviness or pain are the usual clinical features. Elderly persons may harbor asymptomatic urinary tract infections that are recognized only because the urine may appear cloudy or because segmented neutrophils and an increased concentration of bacteria are observed microscopically.

For the recovery of urinary pathogens, both selective and nonselective media are required. A combination of 5% sheep blood agar and MacConkey agar is usually sufficient for the recovery of the most common uropathogens. Uropathogenic strains of *Escherichia coli*, *Klebsiella* species, *Enterobacter* species, and *Proteus* species cause most urinary tract infections; *Pseudomonas aeruginosa*, *Acinetobacter* species, and *Enterococcus* species are other agents that may be less commonly recovered. The recovery of coagulase-negative staphylococci (except for *S. saprophyticus*), diphtheroid bacilli, lactobacilli, and α-hemolytic streptococci is usually considered of little significance.

Infections of the Genital Tract

A purulent urethral discharge appearing some days after sexual exposure to an infected partner is the classic presenting symptom of acute genital gonorrhea in the male. The traditional approach to diagnosis is to examine a Gram-stained preparation of the smear for the presence of intracellular gram-negative, kidney bean–shaped diplococci. A water fast and culture of mucin strands following prostate massage may be necessary to diagnose gonorrhea in asymptomatic patients.[16] Although the presenting symptom in females may also be a urethral discharge, clinical features are usually more complex, and varying degrees of exudative cervicitis, vaginitis, salpingitis, and pelvic inflammatory disease may be present. Examining a Gram-stained smear of cervical or urethral exudate alone is not sufficient to establish the diagnosis in the female, since the cell morphology and staining characteristics of other bacterial species mimic the gonococcus; rather, the recovery of *Neisseria gonorrhoeae* in culture is necessary. The incidence of *Chlamydia trachomatis* equals or even exceeds that of *N. gonorrhoeae* as a cause of acute suppurative genital infections.[19,41] The signs and symptoms of the two diseases are often indistinguishable from one another, and culture and direct detection techniques are required.

Herpes simplex virus type 2 infections, most frequently manifesting as painful and often ulcerating vesicular lesions with an erythematous base on the glans penis, vulva, perineum, buttocks, or cervix, syphilis, chancroid (caused by *Haemophilus ducreyi*), lymphogranuloma venereum (caused by certain *C. trachomatis* serotypes), and granuloma inguinale (caused by the difficult to isolate bacterium *Calymmatobacterium granulomatis*) are other genital infections that may be encountered. *Trichomonas vaginalis* classically produces a copious, frothy yellow or yellow-green discharge that collects in the posterior vaginal fornix. The discharge in candidiasis is typically more thick and curdlike, and the vaginal mucosa tends to be erythematous. Both of these infections can be diagnosed by observing the characteristic microscopic forms—the motile trophozoites of *T. vaginalis* and the budding yeast and pseudohyphal forms of *Candida* species—in direct wet mount preparations. A condition known as bacterial vaginosis, characterized by production of a malodorous vaginal discharge, is caused by *Gardnerella vaginalis* and *Mobiluncus* species, probably in concert with anaerobic bacteria. Observing dense aggregates of bacterial cells on desquamated epithelial cells ("clue" cells) provides a "clue" to the diagnosis.

Infections of the Central Nervous System

Patients with early acute meningitis may experience an influenza-like syndrome—sore and stiff neck, headache, low-grade fever, and lethargy. Various degrees of confusion, agitation, disorientation, or coma may be observed. A positive Brudzinski sign (resistance to passive neck flexion) and Kernig sign (inability to extend the leg when the thigh is flexed at a 90-degree angle with the trunk) are signs of meningeal irritation.

In cases of acute bacterial meningitis, cerebrospinal fluid cell counts may range between 500 and 20,000 segmented neutrophils per milliliter. In tuberculous or viral meningitis, lymphocyte counts between 200 and 2000 cells/µL may be seen. In bacterial meningitis, the cerebrospinal fluid glucose value is decreased (relative to blood glucose levels), and the cerebrospinal fluid protein value is elevated. In acute viral meningitis, the white blood cell count is generally below 500 cells/µL and mononuclear cells predominate. Group B streptococci and *Escherichia coli* are the organisms most often recovered in cases of neonatal meningitis; *Haemophilus influenzae* is the most common cause of acute bacterial meningitis in the 6-month to 5-year age group. *Neisseria meningitidis* and *Streptococcus pneumoniae* are most commonly recovered

from adults; *Listeria monocytogenes, Klebsiella pneumoniae, Serratia* species, *Pseudomonas* species, *Staphylococcus aureus,* and miscellaneous anaerobic bacteria are recovered less frequently. *Cryptococcus neoformans* is in particular recovered from patients with the acquired immunodeficiency syndrome.

Viral meningoencephalitis is seasonal: enteroviruses and arboviruses are the agents most commonly recovered in summer and early fall, and mumps virus and lymphocytic choriomeningitis virus are found in winter and spring. Herpes simplex virus infections have no seasonal patterns.

Examining stained smears of cerebrospinal fluid sediment and performing direct antigen detection tests may be helpful both in establishing a presumptive diagnosis and in providing guidelines for the selection of culture media. Microorganisms can often be detected in Gram-stained or methylene blue–stained cerebrospinal fluid smears if they are present in concentrations of 10,000 cells/mL or more. It is recommended that both Gram-stained and methylene blue–stained smears be prepared in parallel. Gram-negative organisms are often better observed in the methylene blue–stained smear because the deep-blue–staining cells are easier to differentiate from the background debris. Safranin stains the background red in Gram stain, tending to obscure any pink-staining bacteria.

Wounds and Abscesses

The accumulation of pus, either within an abscess or exuding from a sinus tract or from a mucocutaneous surface, is one of the cardinal indicators of local sepsis. Varying degrees of redness, pain, and swelling may also be present. Exogenous wound infections include those associated with traumatic injury—wounds or decubitus ulcers, animal or human bites, burns, or foreign bodies in the skin or mucous membranes. Endogenous wounds and abscesses may be associated with appendicitis, cholecystitis, cellulitis, dental infections, osteomyelitis, empyema, septic arthritis, sinusitis, or many other internal infections.

Because wounds may be contaminated with commensal flora commonly inhabiting the skin and mucous membranes, both selective and enriched nonselective media should be used to recover both eugonic and fastidious bacterial species. As mentioned earlier, the use of a swab should be discouraged, particularly for the recovery of anaerobic bacteria.

Eye, Ear, and Sinus Infections

[handwritten: mim of 3 days bld. Thyro-glicate EmB. Chocol.]

Suppurative material from the conjunctiva of an infected eye should be collected from the cul-de-sac or the inner canthus. A direct Gram stain of the material obtained should be prepared to determine the type of bacteria present. If trachoma is suspected, conjunctival scrapings should be smeared onto a glass microscope slide, air dried, and fixed in absolute methanol. *Chlamydia* enzyme-linked antigen detection systems are now available using fluorescent-tagged monoclonal antibodies. The presence of the characteristic elementary bodies of *C. trachomatis* indicates a positive test. The sensitivity of these techniques is about 95%, and the answers can be available within 1 hour. Since *Haemophilus influenzae* and other *Haemophilus* species commonly cause conjunctivitis, either chocolate agar or *Haemophilus* isolation media should be used.

Cultures of the external auditory canal generally do not reflect the bacterial cause of otitis media unless the tympanic membrane has recently ruptured. Tympanic membrane aspiration is rarely performed for obtaining material for culture. On occasion, cultures of the posterior pharynx may reveal the organisms causing otitis media. Cultures from the maxillary, frontal, or other sinuses should be collected by the syringe aspiration technique and cultures set up for recovery of both aerobic and anaerobic bacteria. Polymicrobial infection, usually including several species of anaerobic bacteria, is often found in cases of chronic sinusitis.

Infections of the Blood: Bacteremia and Septicemia

Bacteremia is the term used to describe the presence of circulating microorganisms in the blood; septicemia is a clinical syndrome characterized by fever, chills, malaise, tachycardia, hyperventilation, and toxicity or prostration that results when the circulating bacteria multiply at a rate that exceeds removal by phagocytes. "Failure to thrive" may indicate chronic septicemia in infants.

The important factors that must be decided by laboratory directors include the type of collection, number and timing of blood samples, the volume of blood to be cultured, the amount and composition of the culture medium, when and how frequently to subculture, and the interpretation of results. These items are reviewed by Bartlett,[2] Reller and coworkers,[39] and Washington.[42] In brief, at least two sets of blood samples per bacteremic episode, each consisting of at least 10 mL of blood, should be obtained. Blood culture bottles should be incubated at 35°C and examined visually for evidence of growth (hemolysis, gas production, or turbidity) during the first 6 to 18 hours after collection. Several semiautomated and automated blood culture systems are commercially available that read bottles on frequencies as short as 10 minutes. Most of these systems rely on the detection of the CO_2 produced by the metabolizing bacteria. Information can be obtained from the several manufacturers who have products on the market.

TISSUE SAMPLES FOR CULTURE

Tissue samples for culture should be delivered promptly to the laboratory in sterile gauze or in a suitably capped, sterile container. Formalinized specimens are not suitable for culture unless the exposure time has been short and the culture can be obtained from a central portion of the tissue not exposed to formalin. Bone marrow cultures may be helpful in establishing the diagnosis of infectious granulomatous diseases such as brucellosis, histoplasmosis, and tuberculosis. Using the Isolator System to process the bone marrow samples may be helpful in improving the recovery of bacteria, particularly if the infections are caused by intracellular organisms.

ANTIBIOTIC SUSCEPTIBILITY TESTING

Decisions must be made whether to perform antibiotic susceptibility tests on organisms recovered from clinical specimens. Not all isolates should be tested, even if physicians have made the usual request for "culture and sensitivities." Antibiograms should not be performed on bacterial species with known patterns of susceptibility and resistance. The procedures and practices for antimicrobial susceptibility testing are reviewed in Chapter 12.

[handwritten notes at bottom: — Contaminated + growth — recomened ab's therapy sepept in againg. ↑ — frctious for Ab'c Therapy cardemia. No Sensitivity → — not cost effective]

LABORATORY MANAGEMENT AND OPERATIONS PRACTICES

Quality Assurance: Definition and Applications

The quality of care provided for patients is the main focus of administrative and regulatory practices. In fact, medical care facilities are now required to have in effect an ongoing system to evaluate the quality of medical care being provided, designated by the term *quality assurance*. Although the criteria for assessing when patient care is of high or acceptable quality is somewhat vague, current quality assurance practices are designed to provide some objectivity to the process.

Quality assurance is a concept and process that implies that certain standards of performance can be delineated in each practice situation and that a set of monitors can be established to measure how close to an accepted norm a given activity might come. Assessments of quality have been addressed for many years by medical audit and peer review committees, the members of whom make direct observations of medical practice in their locale. Persons serving on these committees have struggled with assessments of outcomes, either based on hard data related to morbidity, mortality, and disability statistics or, more subjectively, based on judgments whether adverse reactions or progression of disease could have been averted. Quality assurance, therefore, has emerged as an objective approach to measurement of the level of care being provided in reference to previously accepted criteria and standards and, when necessary, to the mechanisms to improve it.

The practice of quality assurance requires that monitors be set up to evaluate certain procedures and practices. The following monitors have been used in microbiology laboratories where quality assurance practices have been implemented:

- Blood culture utilization: With what frequency are single sets being received?
- With what frequency are blood samples contaminated with skin flora?
- How often are clean-voided urine samples contaminated?
- Culture utilization: How frequently are more than three blood samples per 24 hours, more than three fecal specimens for parasites, or duplicate samples of all types being received in the laboratory?

Threshold levels of performance for each of these monitors must be established by the microbiology staff, in conjunction with the infectious disease service and perhaps with the approval of the quality assurance committee. For example, the following threshold levels have been set for the previously listed monitors: (1) 5% or less of blood samples should be single sets; (2) 3% or less of blood samples should contain contaminating skin flora; (3) 10% or less of urine samples should have colony counts in the range of 100 to 10,000 (an indicator of contamination); and (4) more than three blood samples in 24 hours, more than three stool specimens for parasite examination, and duplicate sample requests should occur no more than 2% of the time. Several additional monitors have been published by Bartlett.[5]

Risk Management

Many hospitals and clinics have established formal risk management offices, fully funded and staffed, to help reduce to a minimum the chances for accidents or high-risk practices to potentially cause harm to both employees and patients.[49] Working in conjunction with the quality assurance committee, a risk manager is assigned to investigate cases in which quality management falls below the established thresholds or situations in which employees and patients may be at undue risk. Although the major focus of risk management is directed to patient care, the clinical laboratory personnel participate in seeing that all operations are in compliance with the overall practices and policies. If equipment or instruments are damaged because of fire or electrical accidents, or if personnel are injured or contract serious laboratory-acquired infections, work flow may be disrupted with a delay in producing laboratory results. Thus, for the most part, laboratory risk management is related to implementing and monitoring laboratory safety practices, directed more to employees than to patients. Liability for injury clearly rests with the employer, even though the negligence leading to the injury is that of a fellow worker.[28] This is why risk managers of the future will be so insistent on conducting safety-oriented education courses and seeing that all rules and regulations of laboratory safety are implemented.

Laboratory Safety

Although it is the legal responsibility of hospital and laboratory managers to provide for a safe working environment, employees must also bear the responsibilities to adhere to safety standards outlined in the laboratory safety manual, to bring to the attention of the supervisor any hazards or potential hazards that may be encountered during work activities, and to seek immediate medical attention for any possible job-related injury.[23] One person in the laboratory should be designated the safety officer whose duties are to see that safety standards and guidelines are written and published, that employees are informed of these standards through regularly scheduled laboratory safety courses and in-service briefings, and that a system is in place to monitor compliance. The safety officer will work closely with the hospital risk manager to reconcile and correct any breaches of conduct or any irregularities discovered.

Universal Precautions

Certain safety practices should be routinely implemented in microbiology laboratories. All laboratories must practice universal precautions.[11] All blood and body fluids from all patients must be handled as infectious material, assuming that all patients harbor infectious pathogens. All specimens of blood and body fluids should be put in a well-constructed container with a secure lid to prevent leaking during transport. Gloves should be worn when processing blood and body fluid specimens; a mask with glasses or goggles should be made available for personnel who must handle blood or body fluids that are expected to splatter. Laboratory work surfaces should be decontaminated with an appropriate chemical germicide after a spill of blood or other body fluids and when work activities are completed. All contaminated materials used in laboratory tests should be autoclaved before reprocessing or be placed in bags and disposed of in accordance with institutional policies. All persons should wash their hands after completing laboratory activities and should remove protective clothing before leaving the laboratory. The CDC and Occupational Safety and Health Administration recommendations have also been established for follow-up for persons exposed to hepatitis B and human immunodeficiency virus; these recommendations are available in the safety office of all medical care facilities.[12]

General Safety Rules and Regulations

Laboratory workers are advised not to take unnecessary risks. Carelessness, negligence, and unsafe practices may result in serious injuries, not only to the individual but also to coworkers and patients.

Each laboratory worker should consult the safety manual and determine the rules and practices for the following activities:

- Centrifugation
- Disposal of needles and chipped or broken glassware
- Electrical safety
- Corridor cautions
- Lifting precautions to minimize back injury
- Handling of contaminated specimens and spills
- Handling of toxic and radioactive wastes
- Handling and storage of volatile and flammable chemicals and toxic reagents
- Fire prevention and what to do in case of a fire

Details of practices and procedures within each of these activities can be found elsewhere.[28]

Quality Control

In a narrow sense, quality control has consisted of an ongoing, systematic assessment of work to ensure that the final product conforms, to an acceptable degree, to previously established tolerance limits of precision and accuracy. Quality of work performed must continue as before; laboratory directors and supervisors must now realize that quality control is only one facet in the larger arenas of quality assurance and risk management.

In a broad sense, quality control in microbiology is more an art than a science. It involves intangible items such as common sense, good judgment, and constant attention to detail. Programs should be organized with well-defined objectives in mind. In the end, high-level laboratory performance requires an alert, interested and well-motivated laboratory staff. Emphasis is shifting to some extent away from rigorous point-by-point details of in-laboratory quality control to a broader assessment of quality assurance in patient care. It may be more important to ensure that timely reports are made available to physicians and maximally used to direct patient care, rather than worrying whether, for example, a daily indole reaction is in control.

Components of a Quality Control Program

At the onset, a quality control coordinator must be selected. The duties of the coordinator must be clearly established and appropriate authority conferred to the extent that problems can be efficiently handled when they arise. The College of American Pathologists has established the various components of a quality control program. Included is detailed information concerning several of the components of a standard quality control program: (1) rules and regulations governing the proficiency testing program, participation in which is required of all accredited laboratories; (2) guidelines for developing a procedure manual; (3) guidelines for establishing schedules for preventive maintenance and the monitoring of all laboratory equipment; (4) guidelines for the monitoring of culture media, reagents, and supplies; (5) methods for calculating personnel needs based on the application of workload recording data; and (6) the requirements for laboratory space. Lack of adequate space is, in fact, among the most frequent deficiencies cited by College of American Pathologists laboratory inspectors (see Elin and associates[13] for practical guidelines).

REFERENCES

1. Bartlett RC. A plea for clinical relevance in microbiology. Am J Clin Pathol 1974;61:867–872.
2. Bartlett RC. Medical microbiology: quality cost and clinical relevance. New York, John Wiley & Sons, 1974.
3. Bartlett RC, Ellner PD, Washington JA II. Cumitech 1: blood cultures. Sherris JC, coordinating ed. Washington, DC, American Society for Microbiology, 1974.
4. Bartlett RC. Cost containment in microbiology. Clin Lab Med 1985;5:761–791.
5. Bartlett RC. Leadership for quality. ASM News 1991;57:15–21.
6. Berke A, Tilton RC. Evaluation of rapid coagulase methods for the identification of *Staphylococcus aureus*. J Clin Microbiol 1985;23:916–919.
7. Bille J, Edson RS, Roberts GD. Clinical evaluation of the lysis-centrifugation blood culture system for the detection of fungemia and comparison with a conventional biphasic broth blood culture system. J Clin Microbiol 1984;19:126–128.
8. Bosley GS, Facklam RR, Grossman D. Rapid identification of enterococci. J Clin Microbiol 1983; 18:1275–1277.
9. Brannon P, Kiehn TE. Large scale clinical comparison of the lysis centrifugation and radiometer systems for blood culture. J Clin Microbiol 1985; 22:951–954.
10. Campos JM, Charilaou CC. Evaluation of Detect-A-Strep and the culturette ten-minute strep ID kits for detection of group A streptococcal antigen in oropharyngeal swabs from children. J Clin Microbiol 1985;22:145–148.
11. Centers for Disease Control. Guidelines for prevention of transmission of human immunodeficiency virus and hepatitis B virus to health-care and public-safety workers. MMWR 1989;38:1–37.
12. Centers for Disease Control. Public health service statement on management of occupational exposure to human immunodeficiency virus, including considerations regarding ziduvudine postexposure use. MMWR 1990;39:1.
13. Elin RJ, Robertson EA, Sever GA. Workload, space and personnel of microbiology laboratories in teaching hospitals. Am J Clin Pathol 1984;82: 78–84.
14. El Kholy A, Wannamaker LW, Krause RM. Simple extraction procedure for serological grouping of beta-hemolytic streptococci. Appl Microbiol 1974;28:836–839.
15. Facklam RR. Specificity study of kits for detection of group A streptococci directly from throat swabs. J Clin Microbiol 1987;25:504–508.
16. Gersh I, Karsh H, Koneman EW. Asymptomatic chronic gonorrhoea in a male patient. Rocky Mt Med J 1976;73:36–40.
17. Goodman LJ, Kaplan RL, Landou W, et al. A urine preservative system to maintain bacterial counts: a laboratory and clinical evaluation. Clin Pediatr 1985;24:383–386.
18. Gwaltney JM Jr. Pharyngitis. In: Mandell GL, Douglas RG Jr, Bennett JE, eds. Principles and practice of infectious diseases. 3rd ed. New York, Churchill Livingstone, 1990:493–498.
19. Holmes KK. The *Chlamydia* epidemic. JAMA 1981;245:1718–1723.
20. Hoppe JE. Methods for isolation of *Bordetella pertussis* from patients with whooping cough. Eur J Clin Microbiol Infect Dis 1988;7:616–620.
21. Isenberg HD, Washington JA, Doern G, Amsterdam D. Collection, handling and processing of specimens. In: Balows A, ed. Manual of clinical microbiology. 5th ed. Washington, DC, American Society for Microbiology, 1991:15–28.
22. Jacobson JT, Burke JP, Jacobson JA. Ordering pat-

terns, collection, transport and screening of sputum cultures in a community hospital. Infect Cont 1981;2:307–311.

23. James AN. Legal realities and practical applications in laboratory safety management. Lab Med 1988;19:84–87.

24. Jewkes FE, McMaster DJ, Napier WA, et al. Home collection of urine specimens—boric acid bottles or Dipslides? Arch Dis Child 1990;65:286–289.

25. Kaye E. Antibacterial activity of human urine. J Clin Invest 1968;42:2374–2390.

26. Kellogg JA, Manzella JP, McConville JH. Clinical laboratory comparison of the 10-ml Isolator blood culture system with BACTEC radiometric blood culture media. J Clin Microbiol 1984;20:618–623.

27. Kellogg JA. Suitability of throat culture procedures for detection of group A streptococci and as reference standards for evaluation of streptococcal antigen detection kits. J Clin Microbiol 1990; 28:165–169.

28. Koneman EW, Allen SD, Janda WM, Schreckenberger PG, Winn WC Jr. The color atlas and textbook of diagnostic microbiology. Philadelphia, JB Lippincott, 1992.

29. Kunin CM. Detection, prevention and management of urinary tract infections: a manual for the physician, nurse and allied health worker, 2nd ed. Philadelphia, Lea & Febiger, 1974.

30. Lauer BA, Reller LB, Mirrett S. Comparisons of acridine orange and Gram stains for detection of microorganisms in cerebrospinal fluid and other clinical specimens. J Clin Microbiol 1981;14: 201–205.

31. Lee A, Hazell SL. *Campylobacter pylori* in health and disease: an ecological perspective. Microbial Ecol Health Dis 1988;1:1–16.

32. Marshall BJ, Warren JR. Unidentified curved bacilli in the stomach of patients with gastritis and peptic ulceration. Lancet 1984;1:1311–1315.

33. McFarland LV, Coyle MB, Kremer WH, Staff WE. Rectal swab cultures for *Clostridium difficile* surveillance studies. J Clin Microbiol 1987;25: 2241–2242.

34. Miceika BG, Vitous AS, Thompson KD. Detection of Group A streptococcal antigen directly from throat swabs with a ten-minute latex agglutination test. J Clin Microbiol 1985;21:467–469.

35. National Committee for Clinical Laboratory Standards (NCCLS). Standard procedures for the handling and transport of diagnostic specimens and etiologic agents. Villanova, PA, NCCLS, 1980.

36. Otero JR, Reyes S, Noriega AR. Rapid diagnosis of group A streptococcal antigen extracted directly from swabs by an enzymatic procedure and used to detect pharyngitis. J Clin Microbiol 1983;18: 318–326, 1983.

37. Regan J, Lowe F. Enrichment medium for the isolation of *Bordetella*. J Clin Microbiol 1977;6: 303–309.

38. Rein MF, Mandell GL. Bacterial killing by bacteriostatic saline solutions: potential for diagnostic error. N Engl J Med 1973;289:794–795.

39. Reller LB, Murray PR, MacLowry JD. Cumitech 1A: blood cultures II. Washington, DC, American Society for Microbiology, 1982.

40. Richards P, Rathbun K. Medical risk management: preventive strategies for heath care providers. Rockville, MD, Aspen Press, 1983

41. Schachter J, Grossman M. *Chlamydia* infections. Annu Rev Med 1981;32:45–61.

42. Taylor DE, Hargreaves JA, Lai-King NG, et al. Isolation and characterization of *Campylobacter pyloridis* from gastric biopsies. Am J Clin Pathol 1987;87:49–54.

2

The Enterobacteriaceae

The Enterobacteriaceae are widely dispersed in nature and are found in soil and water, on plants, and, as the family name indicates, within the intestinal tracts of humans and animals.

Members of the Enterobacteriaceae may be incriminated in virtually any type of infectious disease and recovered from any specimen received in the laboratory. Immunocompromised or debilitated patients are highly susceptible to hospital-acquired infections, either after colonization with environmental strains or following invasive procedures, such as catheterization, bronchoscopy, colposcopy, or surgical biopsies in which mucous membranes are traumatized or transected.

CHARACTERISTICS FOR PRESUMPTIVE IDENTIFICATION

What are the initial clues that an unknown isolate recovered from a clinical specimen may belong to the Enterobacteriaceae? In specimens other than feces, a Gram-stained preparation may reveal gram-negative bacillary or coccobacillary cells, ranging from 0.5 to 2 μm wide to 2 to 4 μm long. Species differentiation, however, cannot be made only on the basis of Gram stain morphology.

Characteristic colonial morphology of an organism growing on solid media may provide a second clue. Typically, members of the Enterobacteriaceae produce relatively large, dull gray, dry, or mucoid colonies on sheep blood agar, the latter suggesting encapsulated strains of *Klebsiella pneumoniae* (Color Plate 2-1*A* and *B*). Hemolysis on blood agar is variable and indistinctive. Colonies appearing as a thin film or as waves (a phenomenon known as *swarming*) suggest that the organism is motile and probably a *Proteus* species (see Color Plate 2-1*C* and *D*). Colonies that appear red on MacConkey agar or have a green sheen on eosin methylene blue (EMB) agar (Color Plate 2-2) indicate that the organism is capable of forming acid from lactose in the medium.

Differentiation of the Enterobacteriaceae, however, is based primarily on the presence or absence of different enzymes coded by the genetic material of the bacterial chromosome. These enzymes direct the metabolism of bacteria along one of several pathways that can be detected by special media used in in vitro culture techniques. Substrates on which these enzymes can react are incorporated into the culture medium together with an indicator that can detect either the utilization of the substrate or the presence of specific metabolic products. By selecting a series of media that measure different metabolic characteristics of the microorganisms to be tested, a biochemical profile can be determined for making a species identification.

Screening Characteristics

Definitive identification of the members of the Enterobacteriaceae may require a battery of biochemical tests. Considerable time and possible misidentification can be avoided if a few preliminary observations are made to ensure that the organism being tested belongs to this group. If the organism is a gram-negative organism of another group, it may be necessary to use a different set of characteristics than that commonly used for the identification of the Enterobacteriaceae. With few exceptions, all members of the Enterobacteriaceae demonstrate the following characteristics:

- Glucose is fermented (see Color Plate 2-1*E* and *F*).
- Cytochrome oxidase is negative (see Color Plate 2-1*H*).
- Nitrate is reduced to nitrite (see Color Plate 2-1*G*).

Carbohydrate Utilization

All Enterobacteriaceae ferment carbohydrates to produce energy. By definition, fermentation is an oxidation-reduction metabolic process that takes place in an anaerobic environment, and, instead of oxygen, an organic substrate serves as the final hydrogen (electron) acceptor. In bacteriologic test systems, this process is detected by observing color changes in *p*H indicators as acid products are formed from carbohydrate fermentation. Acidification of a test medium may occur through the degradation of carbohydrates by pathways other than fermentation, or there may be ingredients other than carbohydrates in some media that result in acid end products. Although most bacteria that utilize carbohydrates are facultative anaerobes, the utilization may not always be under strictly anaerobic conditions, as is observed in the production of acid products by bacterial colonies growing on the surface of agar media.

Cytochrome Oxidase Activity

Any organism that displays cytochrome oxidase activity is excluded from the Enterobacteriaceae. The test is commonly performed by one of two methods: (1) the direct plate technique, in which two or three drops of reagent are added directly to isolated bacterial colonies growing on plate medium, or (2) the indirect paper strip procedure, in which either a few drops of the reagent are added to a filter paper strip or commercial disks or strips impregnated with dried reagent are used. In either method, a loopful of suspected bacteria is smeared into the reagent zone of the filter paper. Bacterial colonies having cytochrome oxidase activity develop a deep blue color at the inoculation site within 10 seconds (see Color Plate 2-1*H*). The developing color reaction must be interpreted within 10 to 20 seconds because many organisms, including selected members of the Enterobacteriaceae, may produce delayed false-positive reactions. Platinum inoculating loops or wires should be used, instead of those made from stainless steel or nichrome, for transferring bacteria to the oxidase reagent because trace amounts of iron oxide on the flamed surface of stainless steel may produce false-positive reactions. Alternatively, a wooden applicator stick or cotton swab can be used to transfer bacterial colonies to the reagent strip. Both oxidase-positive and oxidase-negative control organisms should be tested if there is difficulty in interpreting the cytochrome oxidase reaction (see Color Plate 2-1*H*).

Nitrate Reduction

All Enterobacteriaceae, with the exception of certain biotypes of *Pantoea (Enterobacter) agglomerans* and certain species of *Serratia* and *Yersinia* reduce nitrate to nitrite. Because a variable period of incubation (3 to 24 hours depending on the system used) is required to perform the nitrate reduction test, it is not commonly used to prescreen unknown bacterial isolates. Rather, the test is used in most laboratories either to confirm the correct classification of an unknown microorganism or as an aid in determining the identification of bacterial species.

Any basal medium that supports the growth of the organism and contains a 0.1% concentration of potassium nitrate (KNO_3) is suitable for performing this test. Nitrate broth and nitrate agar in a slant are the media forms most commonly used in clinical laboratories. The medium is inoculated with a loopful of the test organism isolated in pure culture on agar medium and incubated at 35°C for 18 to 24 hours. At the end of incubation, 1 mL each of reagents A (α-naphthylamine) and B (sulfanilic acid) are added to the test medium, in that order. The development of a red color within 30 seconds indicates the presence of nitrites and represents a positive reaction for nitrate reduction (see Color Plate 2-1*G*). If no color develops after adding the test reagents, this may indicate either that nitrates have not been reduced (a true negative reaction) or that they have been reduced to products other than nitrites, such as ammonia or molecular nitrogen. Since the test reagents detect only nitrites, it is necessary to add a small quantity of zinc dust to all negative reactions. Zinc ions reduce nitrates to nitrites, and the development of a red color after adding zinc dust indicates the presence of residual nitrates and confirms a true negative reaction. No color change after the addition of zinc indicates that nitrate has been reduced all the way to ammonia or nitrogen gas and confirms a positive reaction. The red compound that forms from the reaction of the reduced nitrate and reagents is relatively unstable, and the color tends to fade; thus readings should be made soon after the reagents are added (see Color Plate 2-1*G*).

CULTURE MEDIA USED FOR DETECTION OF CARBOHYDRATE FERMENTATION

A variety of different liquid or agar media can be used to measure the ability of a test organism to fermentatively utilize carbohydrates. The principle of carbohydrate fermentation is based on Pasteur's studies of bacteria and yeasts, written more than 100 years ago, which state that the action of many species of microorganisms on a carbohydrate substrate results in acidification of the medium. A typical basal fermentation medium includes a tryptic hydrolysate of casein as a source of carbon and nitrogen, sodium chloride as an osmotic stabilizer, and phenol red indicator, which turns yellow when the *p*H of the medium drops below 6.8. The carbohydrate to be tested, such as glucose, is filter sterilized and added aseptically to the basal medium to a final concentration of 0.5% to 1%. Plate 2-1*F* illustrates acid fermentation in purple broth medium.

Use of Kligler Iron Agar and Triple Sugar Iron Agar

In practice, microorganisms that are incapable of fermenting glucose are commonly detected by observing the reactions they produce when growing on Kligler iron agar (KIA) or triple sugar iron (TSI) agar. An alkaline-slant/alkaline-butt (no change) reaction (Fig. 2-1) on either of these media indicates a lack of acid production and an inability of the test organism to ferment the glucose and other carbohydrates present. This reaction alone is sufficient to exclude an organism from the Enterobacteriaceae.

KIA and TSI media include four protein derivatives—beef extract, yeast extract, peptone, and proteose peptone; therefore, they are nutritionally very rich. The lack of inhibitors permits the growth of all but the most fastidious bacterial species (excluding the obligate anaerobes). For this reason, KIA and TSI agar can be used only when testing a

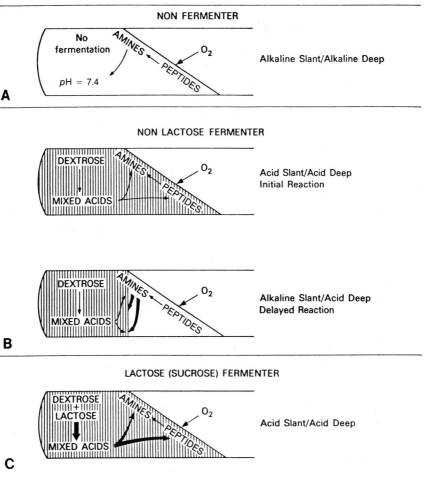

Figure 2-1. The three general types of reactions produced by bacteria growing on Kligler iron agar. (*A*) Nonfermentative bacilli that are unable to produce acids from the fermentation of glucose or lactose; there is no change in the media (*represented by white*). (*B*) Initial acidification of both the deep and the slant of the medium (*vertical lines*) by bacteria that ferment glucose, but the slant reverts back to an alkaline pH as alkaline amines are formed from the oxidative decarboxylation of peptides (derived from protein in the medium) near the surface. (*C*) Complete permanent acidification of both the deep and the slant of the tube by lactose-fermenting bacteria.

bacterial species selected from a single colony recovered on primary or selective agar plates. Glucose and lactose (and sucrose in TSI medium) are evenly distributed throughout both the slant and deep portion of the tube. Lactose, however, is present in a concentration 10 times that of glucose (similarly, the ratio of sucrose to glucose is 10:1 in TSI medium). This 10:1 ratio is important to the understanding of the biochemical principles discussed later. Ferrous sulfate as a hydrogen sulfide detector is somewhat less sensitive than other ferric or ferrous salts; therefore, there may be discrepancies in the hydrogen sulfide readings between KIA and TSI and other test media. The phenol red indicator is yellow below a pH of 6.8. Because the pH of the uninoculated medium is buffered at 7.4, relatively small quantities of acid production result in a visible color change.

Biochemical Principles

The biochemical principles underlying the reactions observed in KIA or TSI agar are illustrated in Figure 2-1. Note that the molten agar is allowed to solidify in a slant. This configuration results in essentially two reaction chambers within the same tube. The *slant* portion, exposed throughout its surface to atmospheric oxygen, is aerobic; the lower portion, called the *butt* or the *deep*, is protected from the air and is relatively anaerobic. It is important, when preparing the media, that the slant and the deep be kept equal in length, about 1.5 inches or 3 cm each, so that this two-chamber effect is preserved.

KIA and TSI tubes are inoculated with a long, straight wire. The well-isolated test colony recovered from an agar plate is touched with the end of the inoculating needle, which is then stabbed into the deep of the tube, extending to within 3 to 5 mm of the bottom of the tube. When the inoculating wire is removed from the deep of the tube, the slant surface is streaked with a back-and-forth motion. Inoculated tubes are placed into an incubator at 35°C for 18 to 24 hours. The color photographs shown in Color Plates 2-1E and 3-1A reveal the following reactions:

- Alkaline slant/alkaline deep (K/K)
  - No carbohydrate fermentation. This is characteristic of nonfermentative bacteria such as *Pseudomonas aeruginosa*.

- Alkaline slant/acid deep (K/A)
  - Glucose fermented; lactose (or sucrose for TSI medium) not fermented. This is characteristic of non–lactose-fermenting bacteria such as *Shigella* species.
- Alkaline slant/acid (black) deep (K/A/H$_2$S)
  - Glucose fermented; lactose not fermented, hydrogen sulfide produced. This is characteristic of non–lactose-fermenting, hydrogen sulfide–producing bacteria such as *Salmonella* species, *Citrobacter* species, and *Proteus* species.
- Acid slant/acid deep (A/A)
  - Glucose and lactose (or sucrose with TSI) fermented. This is characteristic of lactose-fermenting coliforms such as *Escherichia coli* and the *Klebsiella-Enterobacter* species.

If an organism can be excluded from the Enterobacteriaceae before an extended battery of biochemical tests is set up, considerable time and labor will be saved. It is recommended that either a KIA or a TSI slant be set up on all isolates suspected of being one of the Enterobacteriaceae at the time that differential test media or kit systems are set up. Even if an organism is a fermenter and is suspected of being one of the Enterobacteriaceae, a cytochrome oxidase test should be performed to exclude organisms belonging to other genera of fermenting bacteria, such as *Aeromonas*, *Plesiomonas*, *Vibrio*, and *Pasteurella* species, that are oxidase-positive.

SELECTION OF PRIMARY ISOLATION MEDIA

For the recovery of the Enterobacteriaceae from clinical specimens that potentially harbor mixed bacteria, three general types of media are available: (1) nonselective media for primary isolation (eg, blood agar); (2) selective or differential agars (eg, MacConkey and Hektoen enteric agars); and (3) enrichment broths. Tables 2-1 and 2-2 compare different media commonly used in clinical practice. The formulas are complex and include ingredients that not only inhibit the growth of certain bacterial species (selective) but also detect several biochemical characteristics that are important in making a preliminary identification of the microorganisms present in the specimen (differential).

(text continues on page 48)

Table 2-1
Selective Differential Media for Recovery of Enterobacteriaceae

MEDIUM	FORMULATION		PURPOSE AND DIFFERENTIAL INGREDIENTS	REACTIONS AND INTERPRETATION
MacConkey agar (Color Plate 2-2A and B)	Peptone	17 g	MacConkey agar is a differential plating medium for the selection and recovery of the Enterobacteriaceae and related enteric gram-negative bacilli.	Typical strong lactose fermenters, such as species of *Escherichia, Klebsiella*, and *Enterobacter*, produce red colonies surrounded by a zone of precipitated bile.
	Polypeptone	3 g		
	Lactose	10 g		
	Bile salts	1.5 g		
	Sodium chloride	5 g	The bile salts and crystal violet inhibit the growth of gram-positive bacteria and some fastidious gram-negative bacteria.	Slow or weak lactose fermenters, such as *Citrobacter, Providencia, Serratia*, and *Hafnia*, may appear colorless after 24 hours or slightly pink in 24 to 48 hours.
	Agar	13.5 g		
	Neutral red	0.03 g		
	Crystal violet	0.001 g		
	Distilled water to	1 L		
	Final pH = 7.1		Lactose is the sole carbohydrate. Lactose-fermenting bacteria produce colonies that are varying shades of red, owing to the conversion of the neutral red indicator dye (red below pH 6.8) from the production of mixed acids. Colonies of non–lactose-fermenting bacteria appear colorless or transparent.	Species of *Proteus, Edwardsiella, Salmonella*, and *Shigella*, with rare exceptions, produce colorless or transparent colonies. Representative colonies, showing these various reactions, are shown in Color Plate 2-2.
Eosin methylene blue (EMB) agar (Color Plate 2-2 C through F)	Peptone	10 g	EMB agar is a differential plating medium that can be used in place of MacConkey agar in the isolation and detection of the Enterobacteriaceae or related coliform bacilli from specimens with mixed bacteria.	Typical strong lactose-fermenting colonies, notably *Escherichia coli*, produce colonies that are green-black with a metallic sheen.
	Lactose	5 g		
	Sucrose*	5 g		
	Dipotassium, PO$_4$	2 g		Weak fermenters, including *Klebsiella, Enterobacter, Serratia*, and *Hafnia*, produce purple colonies within 24 to 48 hours.
	Agar	13.5 g		
	Eosin y	0.4 g		
	Methylene blue	0.065 g	The aniline dyes (eosin and methylene blue) inhibit gram-positive and fastidious gram-negative bacteria. They combine to form a precipitate at acid pH, thus also serving as indicators of acid production.	Non–lactose fermenters, including *Proteus, Salmonella*, and *Shigella*, produce transparent colonies.
	Distilled water to	1 L		
	Final pH = 7.2			*Yersinia enterocolitica*, a non-lactose, sucrose fermenter, produces transparent colonies on Levine EMB and purple to black colonies on the modified formula.
			Levine EMB, with only lactose, gives reactions more in parallel with MacConkey agar; the modified formula also detects sucrose fermenters.	See Color Plate 2-2.

*Modified Holt-Harris Teague formula. Sucrose is not contained in Levine EMB agar.

Table 2-2
Highly Selective Media for Recovery of Enterobacteriaceae From Gastrointestinal Specimens

MEDIUM	FORMULATION		PURPOSE AND DIFFERENTIAL INGREDIENTS	REACTIONS AND INTERPRETATION
Salmonella-Shigella (SS) agar	Beef extract	5 g	SS agar is highly selective medium formulated to inhibit the growth of most coliform organisms and permit the growth of species of *Salmonella* and *Shigella* from environmental and clinical specimens. The high bile salts concentration and sodium citrate inhibit all gram-positive bacteria and many gram-negative organisms, including coliforms. Lactose is the sole carbohydrate, and neutral red is the indicator for acid detection. Sodium thiosulfate is a source of sulfur. Any bacteria that produce hydrogen sulfide gas are detected by the black precipitate formed with ferric citrate (relatively insensitive). High selectivity of SS agar permits use of heavy inoculum.	Any lactose-fermenting colonies that appear are colored red by the neutral red. Rare strains of *Salmonella arizonae* are lactose fermenting, and colonies may simulate *Escherichia coli.* Growth of species of *Salmonella* is uninhibited, and colonies appear colorless with black centers owing to hydrogen sulfide gas production. Species of *Shigella* show varying inhibition and colorless colonies with no blackening. Motile strains of *Proteus* that appear on SS agar do not swarm.
	Peptone	5 g		
	Lactose	10 g		
	Bile salts	8.5 g		
	Sodium citrate	8.5 g		
	Sodium thiosulfate	8.5 g		
	Ferric citrate	1 g		
	Agar	12.5 g		
	Neutral red	0.025 g		
	Brilliant green	0.033 g		
	Distilled water to	1 L		
	Final pH = 7.4			
Hektoen enteric (HE) agar (Color Plate 2-3*E* and *F*)	Peptone	12 g	HE agar is a recent formulation devised as a direct plating medium for fecal specimens to increase the yield of species of *Salmonella* and *Shigella* from the heavy numbers of normal flora. The high bile salt concentration inhibits growth of all gram-positive bacteria and retards the growth of many strains of coliforms. Acids may be produced from the carbohydrates, and acid fuchsin reacting with thymol blue produces a yellow color when the pH is lowered. Sodium thiosulfate is a sulfur source, and hydrogen sulfide gas is detected by ferric ammonium citrate (relatively sensitive).	Rapid lactose fermenters (such as *Escherichia coli*) are moderately inhibited and produce bright orange to salmon pink colonies. *Salmonella* colonies are blue-green, typically with black centers from hydrogen sulfide gas. *Shigella* appear more green than *Salmonella*, with the color fading to the periphery of the colony. *Proteus* strains are somewhat inhibited; colonies that develop are small, transparent, and more glistening or watery in appearance than species of *Salmonella* or *Shigella*. See Color Plate 2-3.
	Yeast extract	3 g		
	Bile salts	9 g		
	Lactose	12 g		
	Sucrose	12 g		
	Salicin	2 g		
	Sodium chloride	5 g		
	Sodium thiosulfate	5 g		
	Ferric ammonium citrate	1.5 g		
	Acid fuchsin	0.1 g		
	Thymol blue	0.04 g		
	Agar	14 g		
	Distilled water to	1 L		
	Final pH = 7.6			

(continued)

Table 2-2 (continued)

MEDIUM	FORMULATION		PURPOSE AND DIFFERENTIAL INGREDIENTS	REACTIONS AND INTERPRETATION
Xylose lysine deoxycholate (XLD) agar (Color Plate 2-3A through D)	Xylose	3.5 g	XLD agar is less inhibitory to growth of coliform bacilli than HE agar and was designed to detect shigellae in feces after enrichment in gram-negative broth.	Organisms such as *Escherichia coli* and *Klebsiella-Enterobacter* species may utilize more than one carbohydrate and produce bright yellow colonies. Colonies of many species of *Proteus* are also yellow.
	Lysine	5 g		
	Lactose	7.5 g		
	Sucrose	7.5 g		
	Sodium chloride	5 g	Bile salts in relatively low concentration make this medium less selective than the other two included in this chart.	Most species of *Salmonella* produce red colonies, most with black centers from hydrogen sulfide gas.
	Yeast extract	3 g		
	Phenol red	0.08 g		
	Agar	13.5 g	Three carbohydrates are available for acid production, and phenol red is the pH indicator.	*Shigella*, *Providencia*, and many *Proteus* species utilize none of the carbohydrates and produce translucent colonies.
	Sodium deoxycholate	2.5 g		
	Sodium thiosulfate	6.8 g		
	Ferric ammonium citrate	0.8 g	Lysine-positive organisms, such as most *Salmonella* species, produce initial yellow colonies from xylose utilization and delayed red colonies from lysine decarboxylation.	*Citrobacter* colonies are yellow with black centers; many *Proteus* species are yellow or translucent with black centers; *Salmonella* species are red with black centers. See Color Plate 2-3.
	Distilled water to	1 L		
	Final pH = 7.4		Hydrogen sulfide detection system is similar to that of HE agar.	

Selective Isolation Media

In 1905 MacConkey first described a selective differential medium (neutral red-bile salt agar) that he used to isolate gram-negative enteric bacilli from specimens containing mixtures of bacterial species. He incorporated lactose and the indicator neutral red into this medium to provide a visual means for detecting lactose utilization by the test organism. At that time, all non–spore-forming, gram-negative bacilli were still referred to as enteric organisms; microbiologists had, however, recognized that certain species were more pathogenic to humans than others. The carbohydrate-utilization patterns of several species of bacteria were already known by the turn of the century, and the fermentation of lactose in particular was recognized as an important marker for differentiating certain enteric pathogens. Holt-Harris and Teague,[14] in 1916, described a medium with eosin and methylene blue as indicators for differentiating between lactose-fermenting and non–lactose-fermenting colonies. Sucrose was included in the medium to detect those members of the coliform group that ferment sucrose more readily than lactose.

MacConkey and EMB agars are only moderately inhibitory and are designed primarily to prevent growth of gram-positive bacteria from mixed cultures. Many species of fastidious gram-negative organisms are inhibited as well; all Enterobacteriaceae, however, grow well. Table 2-1 compares the formulas, inhibitory ingredients, and key differential characteristics for MacConkey and EMB agars.

Deciding whether to use MacConkey or EMB agar is largely a matter of personal preference, since bacterial species that utilize lactose can be differentiated on both. MacConkey agar contains neutral red as the pH indicator, and, as a result, lactose-utilizing colonies appear pink from the production of mixed acids (see Color Plates 2-2A and B). Strong acid-producing bacteria, such as *Escherichia coli*, form deep red colonies. Weaker acid-producing bacteria form light pink colonies or colonies that are clear at the periphery and have pink centers. On EMB agar, strong acid-producing bacteria form colonies that have a metallic sheen (see Color Plate 2-2*C* and *D*). The appearance of the sheen, due to precipitation of dye in the colonies, is highly suggestive of *E. coli*, although other strong acid producers, such as *Yersinia enterocolitica*, may have a similar appearance.

Highly Selective Isolation Media Used Primarily for Gastrointestinal Specimens

Media are made highly selective by the addition of a variety of inhibitors to their formulas, generally in higher concentrations than in MacConkey and EMB agars. These media are used primarily to inhibit the growth of *Escherichia coli* and other "coliforms" but allow *Salmonella* species and *Shigella* species to grow out from stool specimens.

A number of the selective media formulated for use in clinical laboratories are discussed here. The most commonly used—*Salmonella-Shigella* (SS) agar, xylose lysine deoxycholate (XLD) agar, and hektoen enteric (HE) agar—are considered in greater detail in Table 2-2. Bile salts are added to selective media because other species of enteric bacilli, including some of the more fastidious strains of *Shigella*, grow poorly or not at all. SS and HE agars contain relatively high concentrations of bile salts and are well adapted for recovering *Salmonella* species from specimens heavily contaminated with other coliform bacilli. Because of its inhibitory effect on the recovery of certain strains of *Shigella* species, the routine use of SS agar as a single selective medium for isolation of enteric pathogens from stool specimens is not recommended.

XLD agar contains lactose, sucrose, and xylose; thus, microorganisms that ferment these carbohydrates form yellow colonies (Color Plate 2-3*A*). Bacteria incapable of fermenting these carbohydrates do not produce acids and form colorless colonies (see Color Plate 2-3*B*). Organisms that produce hydrogen sulfide form black pigment beginning in the center of the colonies (see Color Plate 2-3*C*). XLD agar also contains lysine. This is important because many species of *Salmonella* ferment xylose and therefore initially produce yellow colonies on XLD, but because these same species also decarboxylate lysine, the colonies revert to pink after the small amount of xylose in the medium is used up. Lactose and sucrose, added in

excess, prevent lysine-positive coliforms from similarly reverting. Because the decarboxylation of lysine results in the formation of strongly alkaline amines, a light pink halo may appear around the colonies on XLD agar (see Color Plate 2-3*C*). Black colonies without a pink halo are more suggestive of a hydrogen sulfide–producing strain of *Proteus* species (see Color Plate 2-3*D*).

The carbohydrates in HE agar are lactose, sucrose, and salicin. Microorganisms capable of fermenting these carbohydrates also form yellow colonies (see Color Plate 2-3*E*); asaccharolytic strains produce colonies that are translucent or light green (see Color Plate 2-3*F*). Lactose- and sucrose-negative bacteria that acidify salicin may produce orange colonies. HE agar also contains ferric salts; thus hydrogen sulfide–producing colonies appear black.

Enrichment Media

An enrichment medium is used to enhance the growth of certain bacterial species while inhibiting the development of unwanted microorganisms. Enrichment media are most commonly used in clinical laboratories for the recovery of *Salmonella* and *Shigella* species from fecal specimens. Enrichment media work on the principle that *E. coli* and other gram-negative organisms, which constitute the normal fecal flora, are maintained in a prolonged *lag* phase by the inhibitory chemicals in the broth. *Salmonella* and *Shigella* species are far less inhibited, enter into a *logarithmic* phase of growth, and are more readily recovered from fecal samples. After several hours, however, the enrichment media no longer suppress the growth of *E. coli* and other enteric organisms that will ultimately overgrow the culture. Thus, for maximal recovery of *Salmonella* and *Shigella* species from fecal samples, it is recommended that the enrichment broth be subcultured within 8 hours.

The two most commonly used enrichment media are selenite broth and gram-negative (GN) broth. Selenite broth is more inhibitory to the growth of *E. coli* and other enteric gram-negative bacilli than is GN broth. Thus, selenite broth is best adapted for the recovery of *Salmonella* or *Shigella* species from heavily contaminated specimens, such as feces or sewage. GN broth is used with greater frequency in clinical laboratories because it is less inhibitory to the growth of many of the more fastidious strains of *Shigella* species. Enrichment of fecal specimens in GN broth for 4 to 6 hours and then subculturing to HE or XLD agar is the optimal technique for the recovery of *Shigella* species in suspected cases of bacillary dysentery. The formulas and salient characteristics of these two enrichment media are summarized in Table 2-3.

Guidelines for Choosing Selective Isolation Media

For specimens other than feces or rectal swabs, a combination of MacConkey or EMB agar and

a blood agar is usually sufficient. Media with greater inhibitory properties are not routinely required because the concentration of commensal flora or contaminating organisms is relatively low in most nonenteric specimens. Subculturing to a more inhibitory medium can be done in instances in which it appears necessary.

For fecal specimens or rectal swabs, it is necessary to select only one medium from each of the groups listed in Tables 2-1 and 2-2. The following approach is suggested:

1. Inoculate the specimen directly to a MacConkey or EMB agar plate for primary isolation of all species of enteric gram-negative bacilli.

Table 2-3
Enrichment Broths for Recovery of Enterobacteriaceae

BROTH	FORMULATION		PURPOSE AND DIFFERENTIAL INGREDIENTS	REACTIONS AND INTERPRETATION
Selenite broth	Peptone	5 g	Selenite F broth is recommended for the isolation of salmonellae from specimens such as feces, urine, or sewage that have heavy concentrations of mixed bacteria. Sodium selenite is inhibitory to *Escherichia coli* and other coliform bacilli, including many strains of *Shigella*. The medium functions best under anaerobic conditions, and a pour depth of at least 2 inches is recommended.	Within a few hours after inoculation with the specimen, the broth becomes cloudy. Because coliforms or other intestinal flora may overgrow the pathogens within a few hours, subculture to *Salmonella–Shigella* (SS) agar or bismuth sulfite is recommended within 8 to 12 hours. Overheating of the broth during preparation may produce a visible precipitate, making it unsatisfactory for use.
	Lactose	4 g		
	Sodium selenite	4 g		
	Sodium phosphate	10 g		
	Distilled water to	1 L		
	Final pH = 7.0			
Gram-negative (GN) broth	Polypeptone peptone	20 g	Because of the relatively low concentration of deoxycholate, GN broth is less inhibitory to *Escherichia coli* and other coliforms. Most strains of *Shigella* grow well. The deoxycholate and citrate are inhibitory to gram-positive bacteria. The increased concentration of mannitol over glucose limits the growth of *Proteus* species, nonetheless encouraging growth of *Salmonella* and *Shigella* species, both of which are capable of fermenting mannitol.	GN broth is designed for the recovery of *Salmonella* species and *Shigella* species when they are in small numbers in fecal specimens. The broth may become cloudy within 4 to 6 hours of inoculation, and subculture to HE agar or XLD agar within that time is recommended.
	Glucose	1 g		
	D-mannitol	2 g		
	Sodium citrate	5 g		
	Sodium deoxycholate	0.5 g		
	Dipotassium phosphate	4 g		
	Monopotassium phosphate	1.5 g		
	Sodium chloride	5 g		
	Distilled water to	1 L		
	Final pH = 7.0			

2. Directly inoculate either an XLD or an HE agar plate for the selective screening of *Salmonella* species and *Shigella* species.

3. Enrich a small portion of the specimen by heavily inoculating either selenite or GN broth. If selenite is used, subculture to HE agar within 8 to 12 hours; if GN is used, subculture within 4 hours.

4. Incubate all plate cultures at 35°C for 24 to 48 hours. Select suspicious colonies for definitive biochemical or serologic testing.

DIFFERENTIAL IDENTIFICATION CHARACTERISTICS

Although a preliminary identification of the Enterobacteriaceae is possible based on colonial characteristics and biochemical reactions on primary isolation media, further species identification requires the determination of additional phenotypic characteristics that reflect the genetic code and unique identity of the organism being tested. Following is a list of differential tests that are widely used in clinical laboratories to measure those metabolic characteristics by which all but a few rare or atypical species of the Enterobacteriaceae can be identified:

- Carbohydrate utilization (discussed previously)
- Indole production
- Methyl red
- Voges-Proskauer test (production of acetylmethyl carbinol)
- Citrate utilization
- Urease production
- Decarboxylation of lysine, ornithine, and arginine
- Phenylalanine deaminase production
- Hydrogen sulfide production
- Motility

Indole Production

Indole is one of the degradation products from the metabolism of the amino acid tryptophan. Bacteria that possess the enzyme tryptophanase are capable of cleaving tryptophan, thus producing indole, pyruvic acid, and ammonia. Indole can be detected in tryptophan test medium by observing the development of a red color after adding a solution containing *p*-dimethylaminobenzaldehyde (eg, Ehrlich's or Kovac's reagent). The biochemistry and details of the indole test are schematically illustrated in Figure 2-2.

Methyl Red Test

Bacteria that follow primarily the mixed acid fermentation route often produce sufficient acid to maintain a *p*H below 4.4 (the acid color breakpoint of the methyl red indicator). The methyl red test provides a valuable characteristic for identifying bacterial species that produce strong acids from glucose. The test is performed by inoculating methyl red–Voges-Proskauer broth with a pure culture of the test organism. After incubation for 48 to 72 hours, 5 drops of the methyl red reagent are added directly to the broth. The development of a red color on the surface of the medium indicates a positive test. Because this test, as originally described, requires 48 to 72 hours of incubation before a valid result can be obtained, an amount of time unacceptable to most clinical microbiology laboratories, the methyl red test is not commonly performed in most laboratories.

Voges-Proskauer Test

The Voges-Proskauer test is used to detect the formation of acetylmethyl carbinol (acetoin) as a product of glucose fermentation. Acetoin is formed as a product of an alternate pathway of glucose fermentation that is utilized by only certain species of Enterobacteriaceae. Acetoin can be detected in methyl red–Voges-Proskauer broth medium by observing the development of a red color after adding a solution of 5% α-naphthol followed by 40% potassium hydroxide. The tube is shaken gently and then allowed to remain undisturbed for 10 to 15 minutes before the reaction is read. Bacteria that utilize this pathway, such as certain strains within the *Klebsiella-Enterobacter-Serratia-Hafnia* group, produce only small quantities of mixed acids that may be insufficient to lower the *p*H of the methyl red medium enough to produce a color change. For this reason, most species of the Enterobacteriaceae that are Voges-Proskauer–posi-

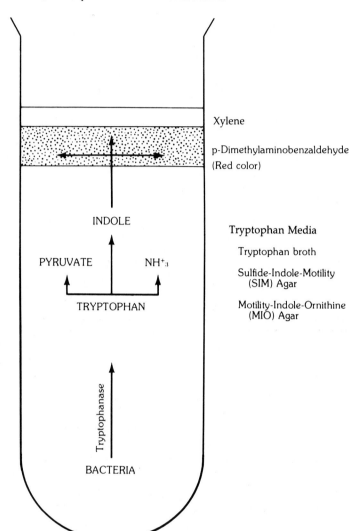

Xylene

p-Dimethylaminobenzaldehyde
(Red color)

INDOLE

Tryptophan Media

Tryptophan broth

Sulfide-Indole-Motility
(SIM) Agar

Motility-Indole-Ornithine
(MIO) Agar

PYRUVATE NH_3^+

TRYPTOPHAN

Tryptophanase

BACTERIA

Figure 2-2. Formation of indole by tryptophanase-producing bacteria growing on a culture medium containing tryptophan. Indole is one of the immediate degradation products (in addition to pyruvic acid and ammonia) resulting from the deamination of tryptophan. Indole can be extracted from the aqueous phase of the medium by chloroform and detected by the addition of Ehrlich's reagent (dimethylaminobenzaldehyde).

tive, with rare exceptions, are methyl red–negative and vice versa.

Citrate Utilization

The principle of the citrate utilization test is to determine the ability of an organism to utilize sodium citrate as the sole source of carbon for metabolism and growth. To perform the test, a well-isolated colony is picked from the surface of a primary isolation medium and inoculated as a single streak on the slant surface of the citrate agar tube. The production of a blue color in the test medium after 24 hours of incubation at 35°C indicates the presence of alkaline products and a positive citrate utilization test result. Occa-

sionally, visible growth is detected along the streak line before conversion of the medium to a blue color. This visible growth also indicates a positive test result.

Urease Production

Microorganisms that possess the enzyme urease hydrolyze urea, releasing ammonia and producing a pink-red color change in the medium. The test is most commonly performed using a Christensen's urea agar slant. The surface of the agar slant is streaked with the test organism and allowed to incubate overnight at 35°C. A red color on the slant or throughout the medium indicates a positive test for urea hydrolysis.

Decarboxylation of Lysine, Ornithine, and Arginine

Many species of bacteria possess enzymes capable of decarboxylating specific amino acids in the test medium. The decarboxylase enzymes remove a molecule of CO_2 from an amino acid to form alkaline-reacting amines. The following are the amino acids most commonly tested and their amine degradation products:

Lysine → cadaverine
Ornithine → putrescine
Arginine → citrulline

A number of test systems have been described to measure this property, based on either detection of an alkaline pH shift in the test medium (Moeller test, used to test most Enterobacteriaceae) or direct measurement of the reaction products (Carlquist ninhydrin reaction, used primarily to detect the weak decarboxylase activity of many of the nonfermentative gram-negative bacilli and certain species of anaerobic bacteria). The test is performed by inoculating two tubes of Moeller decarboxylase medium, one containing the amino acid to be tested, the other to be used as a control tube devoid of amino acid. Both tubes are overlaid with sterile mineral oil to cover about 1 cm of the surface. The end point of the reaction is the production of an alkaline pH shift in the medium containing the amino acid and the development of a blue-purple color. The control tube turns yellow as a result of the fermentation of glucose in the medium and the absence of amino acid decarboxylation.

Phenylalanine Deaminase Production

This test is based on the principle that certain bacteria are capable of deaminating phenylalanine with the production of phenylpyruvic acid. The test is performed by inoculating the test organism onto the slant of phenylalanine test medium and incubating overnight at 35°C. The test is positive if a visible green color develops after the addition of 4 or 5 drops of 10% ferric chloride solution. The phenylalanine deaminase determination is useful in the initial differentiation of *Proteus*, *Morganella*, and *Providencia* species from other gram-negative bacilli. Only members of these genera, and a few relatively rare isolates of the *Enterobacter* group, possess the enzyme responsible for the oxidative deamination of phenylalanine.

Hydrogen Sulfide Production

The ability of certain bacterial species to liberate sulfur from sulfur-containing amino acids or other compounds in the form of hydrogen sulfide is an important characteristic for their identification. The media most commonly used for the detection of hydrogen sulfide and the sources of sulfur and the sulfide indicators are listed in Table 2-4.

Table 2-4
Media for the Detection of Hydrogen Sulfide (H₂S)

MEDIA	SULFUR SOURCE	H₂S INDICATOR
Bismuth sulfite	Peptones plus sulfite	Ferrous sulfate
Citrate sulfide agar	Sodium thiosulfate	Ferric ammonium citrate
Deoxycholate citrate agar	Peptones	Ferric citrate
Lysine iron agar	Sodium thiosulfate	Ferric ammonium citrate
Kligler iron agar	Sodium thiosulfate	Ferrous sulfate
Triple sugar iron agar	Sodium thiosulfate	Ferrous sulfate
Lead acetate agar	Sodium thiosulfate	Lead acetate
Salmonella–Shigella agar	Sodium thiosulfate	Ferric citrate
Sulfide indole motility medium	Sodium thiosulfate	Peptonized iron
Xylose lysine desoxycholate or Hektoen enteric	Sodium thiosulfate	Ferric ammonium citrate

The sequence of steps leading to the production and detection of hydrogen sulfide in a test system is believed to be as follows:

1. Release of sulfide from cysteine or thiosulfate by bacterial enzymatic action
2. Coupling of sulfide (S^{-2}) with a hydrogen ion (H^+) to form H_2S
3. Detection of hydrogen sulfide by iron, bismuth, or lead to produce insoluble, heavy metal sulfides that appear as a black precipitate

The capability of detecting hydrogen sulfide production in the different media results from alteration in one or more of these conditions. Hydrogen sulfide detected in one medium may not be detected in another, and it is necessary to know the test system used when interpreting identification charts. Ferrous sulfate, ferric ammonium citrate, and peptonized iron are the hydrogen sulfide–detecting compounds most commonly used in differential culture media. Lead acetate is the most sensitive indicator and should be used whenever bacteria that produce only trace amounts of hydrogen sulfide are tested. The test is performed by draping a lead acetate–impregnated filter paper strip under the cap of a culture tube of KIA medium; the chemical cannot be added to the culture medium because it is toxic to many species of bacteria.

With all hydrogen sulfide detection systems, the end point is an insoluble, heavy metal sulfide, which produces a black precipitate in the medium or on the filter paper strip. Because hydrogen ions must be available for hydrogen sulfide formation, the blackening is first seen in test media where acid formation is maximum, that is, along the inoculation line, within the deeps of slanted agar media, or in the centers of colonies growing on agar surfaces.

Motility

Bacteria are motile by means of flagella, the number and location of which vary among the different species. Bacterial motility can be observed directly by placing a drop of culture broth medium on a microscope slide and viewing it under a microscope, a technique used primarily for detecting the motility of bacterial species that do not grow well in semisolid agar media. Motility media is semisolid, with agar concentrations of 0.4% or less, permitting the organisms to spread freely. The test is

performed by inoculating a small portion of the unknown colony into a motility agar tube with a straight needle and observing for a wave of turbidity emanating laterally from the stab line after several hours of incubation at 35°C if the organism is motile.

Of the Enterobacteriaceae, species of *Shigella* and *Klebsiella* are uniformly nonmotile. Most motile species of the Enterobacteriaceae can be detected at 35°C; *Yersinia enterocolitica*, in which flagellar proteins develop more rapidly at lower temperatures, is motile at 22°C (room temperature) but not at 35°C.

TAXONOMY OF THE ENTEROBACTERIACEAE

The application of new technologies to study the taxonomy of microorganisms has led to a rapid increase in the number of genera and species of bacteria that fit the general criteria for Enterobacteriaceae. In 1972, Edwards and Ewing[9] described 11 genera and 26 species belonging to the Enterobacteriaceae. In 1985, Farmer and associates[11] described 22 genera comprising 69 species and 29 enteric groups. In this chapter, 28 genera and 112 species, biogroups, and unnamed enteric groups of Enterobacteriaceae are described.

Systems of Nomenclature

Three approaches are used to name the various genera and species within the Enterobacteriaceae: (1) the nomenclature proposed by Ewing, using phenotypic subgroupings into eight tribes;[10] (2) the classification proposed by Brenner and colleagues, as published in the 1984 edition of *Bergey's Manual of Systematic Bacteriology*,[2] in which 14 major genera and 6 "additional" genera are defined, based primarily on DNA relatedness studies; and (3) the system published by Farmer and associates[11,12] at the Centers for Disease Control (CDC), in which the Enterobacteriaceae are subgrouped into 27 genera, 100 named species, subspecies, and biogroups, and 8 unnamed enteric groups based both on DNA relatedness studies and phenotypic characteristics derived from the study of hundreds of clinical isolates referred for identification. These three systems are outlined in Table 2-5. With a few

Table 2-5
Nomenclature for the Family Enterobacteriaceae

EWING: 1986	BERGEY: 1984	CDC: 1991
Tribe I: Escherichieae		
Genus I: *Escherichia*	Genus I: *Escherichia*	Genus: *Escherichia-Shigella*
1. *E. coli*	1. *E. coli*	E. coli
2. *E. blattae*	2. *E. blattae*	E. coli, inactive
3. *E. hermannii*	Species Incertae Sedis: *E. adecar-*	Shigella, O groups A, B, C
4. *E. vulneris*	*boxylata*	Shigella sonnei
5. *E. fergusonii*		E. fergusonii
		E. hermannii
Genus II: *Shigella*	Genus II: *Shigella*	E. vulneris
1. *S. dysenteriae*	1. *S. dysenteriae*	E. blattae
2. *S. flexneri*	2. *S. flexneri*	
3. *S. boydii*	3. *S. boydii*	
4. *S. sonnei*	4. *S. sonnei*	
Tribe II: Edwardsielleae		
Genus I: *Edwardsiella*	Genus X: *Edwardsiella*	Genus: *Edwardsiella*
1. *E. tarda*	1. *E. tarda*	E. tarda
2. *E. hoshinae*	2. *E. hoshinae*	E. tarda biogroup 1
3. *E. ictaluri*	3. *E. ictaluri*	E. hoshinae
		E. ictaluri
Tribe III: Salmonelleae		
Genus I: *Salmonella*	Genus III: *Salmonella*	Genus: *Salmonella*
1. *S. enterica* subsp. *enterica*	All salmonellae and arizonae form	Subgroup 1 strains
2. *S. enterica* subsp. *salamae*	one species composed of five sub-	Most serotypes
3a. *S. enterica* subsp. *arizonae*	groups each referred to as a "sub-	S. typhi
	genus." Selected serovars of the	S. choleraesuis
	subgenera are as follows:	S. paratyphi
		S. gallinarum
3b. *S. enterica* subsp. *diarizonae*	Subgenus I: typical *Salmonella*	S. pullorum
4. *S. enterica* subsp. *houtenae*	S. choleraesuis	Subgroup 2 strains
5. *S. enterica* subsp. *bongori*	S. hirschfeldii	S. salamae
	S. typhi	Subgroup 3a strains
	S. paratyphi-A	S. arizonae
	S. schottmuelleri	Subgroup 3b strains
	S. typhimurium	S. diarizonae
	S. enteritidis	Subgroup 4 strains
	S. gallinarum	S. houtenae
	Subgenus II: atypical *Salmonella*	Subgroup 5 strains
	S. salamae	S. bongori
	Subgenus III:	Subgroup 6 strains
	S. arizonae	S. choleraesuis subsp. *indica*
	Subgenus IV: atypical *Salmonella*	
	S. houtenae	
	Subgenus V: strains (positive) for dul-	
	citol, ONPG, and KCN	
	S. bongor	
Tribe IV: Citrobactereae		
Genus I: *Citrobacter*	Genus IV: *Citrobacter*	Genus: *Citrobacter*
1. *C. freundii*	1. *C. freundii*	C. freundii
2. *C. diversus*	2. *C. diversus*	C. diversus
3. *C. amalonaticus*	3. *C. amalonaticus*	C. amalonaticus
		C. amalonaticus biogroup 1

(continued)

Table 2-5 (continued)

EWING: 1986	BERGEY: 1984	CDC: 1991

Tribe V: Klebsielleae

Genus I: *Klebsiella*
1. *K. pneumoniae*
2. *K. ozaenae*
3. *K. oxytoca*
4. *K. rhinoscleromatis*
5. *K. planticola*
6. *K. terrigena*
7. *K. trevisanae*

Genus V: *Klebsiella*
1. *K. pneumoniae* subsp. *pneumoniae*
   K. pneumoniae subsp. *ozaenae*
   K. pneumoniae subsp. *rhinoscleromatis*
2. *K. oxytoca*
3. *K. terrigena*
4. *K. planticola*

Genus: *Klebsiella*
   K. pneumoniae
   K. oxytoca
   K. ornithinolytica
   K. planticola
   K. ozaenae
   K. rhinoscleromatis
   K. terrigena

Genus II: *Enterobacter*
1. *E. cloacae*
2. *E. aerogenes*
3. *E. agglomerans*
4. *E. sakazakii*
5. *E. gergoviae*
6. *E. amnigenus*
7. *E. intermedium*
8. *E. taylori*
9. *E. dissolvens*
10. *E. nimipressuralis*

Genus VI: *Enterobacter*
1. *E. cloacae*
2. *E. sakazakii*
3. *E. agglomerans*
4. *E. aerogenes*
5. *E. gergoviae*
6. *E. intermedium*
7. *E. amnigenus*
Note: Two other organisms listed under the genus *Erwinia* (*E. dissolvens* and *E. nimipressuralis*) belong to the genus *Enterobacter* on the basis of DNA relatedness. Both belong to the genus *Enterobacter* either as new species or as biogroups of *E. cloacae.*

Genus: *Enterobacter*
   E. aerogenes
   E. cloacae
   E. agglomerans
   E. gergoviae
   E. sakazakii
   E. taylorae
   E. aminigenus biogroup 1
   E. amnigenus biogroup 2
   E. intermedius
   E. asburiae
   E. cancerogenus
   E. dissolvens
   E. nimipressuralis

Genus III: *Hafnia*
1. *H. alvei*
2. *Hafnia* species
3. *Hafnia* species

Genus IX: *Hafnia*
1. *H. alvei*

Genus: *Hafnia*
   H. alvei
   H. alvei biogroup 1

Genus IV: *Serratia*
1. *S. marcescens*
2. *S. liquefaciens*
3. *S. rubidaea*
4. *S. fonticola*
5. *S. odorifera*
6. *S. ficaria*
7. *S. grimesii*
8. *S. plymuthica*
9. *S. proteamaculans*

Genus VIII: *Serratia*
1. *S. marcescens*
2. *S. liquefaciens*
3. *S. plymuthica*
4. *S. rubidaea*
5. *S. odorifera*
6. *S. ficaria*
Species Incertae Sedis: *S. fonticola*

Genus: *Serratia*
   S. marcescens
   S. marcescens biogroup 1
   S. liquefaciens group
   S. rubidaea
   S. oderifera biogroup 1
   S. oderifera biogroup 2
   S. plymuthica
   S. ficaria
   S. entomophila
   "*Serratia*" *fonticola*

Tribe VI: Proteeae

Genus I: *Proteus*
1. *P. vulgaris*
2. *P. mirabilis*
3. *P. penneri*
4. *P. myxofaciens*

Genus XI: *Proteus*
1. *P. vulgaris*
2. *P. mirabilis*
3. *P. myxofaciens*

Genus: *Proteus*
   P. mirabilis
   P. vulgaris
   P. penneri
   P. myxofaciens

Genus II: *Morganella*
1. *M. morganii*

Genus XIII: *Morganella*
1. *M. morganii*

Genus: *Morganella*
   M. morganii
   M. morganii biogroup 1

Genus III: *Providencia*
1. *P. alcalifaciens*
2. *P. stuartii*
3. *P. rettgeri*
4. *P. rustigianii*

Genus XII: *Providencia*
1. *P. alcalifaciens*
2. *P. stuartii*
3. *P. rettgeri*

Genus: *Providencia*
   P. rettgeri
   P. stuartii
   P. alcalifaciens
   P. rustigianii
   P. heimbachae

(continued)

Table 2-5 (continued)

EWING: 1986	BERGEY: 1984	CDC: 1991

Tribe VII: Yersinieae

Genus I: *Yersinia*
1. *Y. pseudotuberculosis*
2. *Y. pestis*
3. *Y. enterocolitica*
4. *Y. frederiksenii*
5. *Y. kristensenii*
6. *Y. intermedia*
7. *Y. ruckeri*
8. *Y. aldovae*

Genus XIV: *Yersinia*
1. *Y. pestis*
2. *Y. pseudotuberculosis*
3. *Y. enterocolitica*
4. *Y. intermedia*
5. *Y. frederiksenii*
6. *Y. kristensenii*
7. *Y. ruckeri*
Species Incertae Sedis: *Y. philomiragia*

Genus: *Yersinia*
Y. enterocolitica
Y. frederiksenii
Y. intermedia
Y. kristensenii
Y. rohdei
Y. pestis
Y. pseudotuberculosis
Y. aldovae
Y. bercovieri
Y. mollaretii
"*Yersinia*" *ruckeri*

Tribe VIII: Erwinieae (Plant Pathogens)

Genus I: *Erwinia*
1. *E. amylovora*
2. *E. carotovora*

Genus VII: *Erwinia*
1. *E. amylovora*
(15 additional species)
Species Incertae Sedis
E. cancerogena
E. carnegieana
E. dissolvens
E. nimipressuralis

Dr. Farmer believes that the concept of *Erwinia* as a separate genus is not useful in clinical microbiology because the "true *Erwinia* species" represented by *Erwinia amylovora* do not grow at 35° to 37°C and are inactive biochemically in the tests used to identify Enterobacteriaceae. "Enterobacter agglomerans group" is the name used by the CDC for a heterogeneous group of bacteria that have been reported as various species of *Erwinia* in the literature.

Other Genera (Farmer et al, 1991)

Genus *Budvicia*
Genus *Buttiauxella*
Genus *Cedecea*
Genus *Ewingella*
Genus *Kluyvera*
Genus *Koserella*
Genus *Leclercia*

Genus *Leminorella*
Genus *Moellerella*
Genus *Obesumbacterium*
Genus *Pragia*
Genus *Rahnella*
Genus *Tatumella*
Genus *Xenorhabdus*

Unnamed species:

Enteric group 58	Enteric group 68
Enteric group 59	Enteric group 69
Enteric group 60	Enteric group 90
Enteric group 63	
Enteric group 64	

exceptions, the classification of bacterial species within the three systems is similar. The approach used is a matter of personal preference according to specific applications.

Classification of Enterobacteriaceae by Tribes

The tribe concept provides both students and practitioners with a convenient method of grouping together the major genera within the family that share similar biochemical reactions and are of similar diagnostic importance. We believe it is important that practicing microbiologists maintain a base of knowledge that is firmly grounded in the morphology, physiology, and biochemistry of medically important bacteria. Furthermore, certain phenotypic patterns that allow easy subgrouping and clustering of related species must be committed to memory. This orientation is especially important if microbiologists use semiautomated and automated "packaged" systems with computer-assisted identification, because it serves as a quality control check to validate machine-generated information. Using the tribe concept as an approach to learning the Enterobacteriaceae serves these goals well and is the approach chosen for use in this text for teaching the key features of the established genera of the Enterobacteriaceae.

Key Identification Characteristics for the Most Common Species

Table 2-6 shows the key identification characteristics used in separating the established genera of the Enterobacteriaceae into seven tribes. Students should study this table and learn to categorize an unknown isolate into one of these tribes on the basis of reactions seen with these key tests. The following observations are made to assist students in identifying the most common species.

The members of the Escherichieae have the following key reactions: indole-positive, methyl red–positive, Voges-Proskauer–negative, and citrate-negative (the classic example of mixed acid fermenters). They are negative for all the other key biochemical tests—hydrogen sulfide, phenylalanine deaminase, and urea. Note from Table 2-6 that *Shigella* species are like *Escherichia* species except they are negative for CO_2 gas and motility.

The Edwardsielleae are like Escherichieae except for the property of being hydrogen sulfide–positive. Students may wish to think of *Edwardsiella tarda* as hydrogen sulfide–positive *E. coli*. Salmonelleae resemble Edwardsielleae except that they are indole-negative and citrate-positive. *Citrobacter freundii* is like *Salmonella* except for being lysine-negative. *C. diversus* differs from *C. freundii* by being hydrogen sulfide–negative and indole-positive.

The Klebsielleae are composed of the Voges-Proskauer–positive members of the Enterobacteriaceae. As shown in Table 2-6, most members of this tribe produced copious amounts of CO_2, so much so that the deep portion of KIA and TSI slants is often pushed halfway up the tube. *Klebsiella* species are nonmotile, and *Pantoea* is triple decarboxylase–negative (lysine-negative, arginine-negative, and ornithine-negative).

The Proteeae are separated from all others by virtue of being phenylalanine deaminase–positive, a feature unique to this tribe. The urea reaction for the species in the genus *Proteus* and *Morganella* as

well as one of the *Providencia* species (*P. rettgeri*) is strongly positive. Both species of *Proteus* listed in Table 2-6 are hydrogen sulfide–positive and exhibit swarming motility.

The Yersinieae represented here by the most commonly isolated species, *Y. enterocolitica*, are very similar to members of the Escherichieae except that *Y. enterocolitica* is usually urea-positive. Students may wish to think of *Y. enterocolitica* as urea-positive *E. coli*. The motility for *Y. enterocolitica* is negative at 36°C but positive at 22°C.

KEY FACTS TO REMEMBER

Hydrogen Sulfide–Positive
Edwardsiella tarda
Salmonella species
Citrobacter freundii
Proteus vulgaris
Proteus mirabilis

Voges-Proskauer–Positive
Klebsiella species
Enterobacter species
Hafnia species
Pantoea species
Serratia species

Phenylalanine Deaminase–Positive
Proteus species
Morganella species
Providencia species

Nonmotile at 36°C
Shigella species
Klebsiella species
Yersinia species

A brief summary of the cultural characteristics, the key biochemical reactions, and the infectious disease syndromes associated with the genera and species included within the several tribes of Enterobacteriaceae follows.

Tribe Escherichieae

The two genera within this tribe are *Escherichia* and *Shigella*, an association which on first inspection may not seem reasonable. *E. coli* characteristically ferments lactose; *Shigella* species do not. *E. coli* is generally biochemically active, compared with *Shigella* species, which tend to be inert. *E. coli* and *Shigella* species are, however, closely related genetically; in fact, all four species of *Shigella* and *E. coli* form a single species on the basis of DNA hybridiz-ation studies.[2] Because *Shigella* species are associ-ated with a specific disease spectrum (bacillary dys-entery) and since specific typing antisera for separating *E. coli* from *Shigella* are commercially available, *Shigella* species will continue to be classi-fied in a separate genus, at least for now. Students should note, however, that certain late lactose-fer-menting, nonmotile, and biochemically inactive strains of *E. coli* can be difficult to differentiate from *Shigella* species, and rare strains of *Shigella* species (*S. flexneri*) also can produce gas from the fermentation of glucose. Although the pathogenic spectrum of *E. coli* is much broader than that of *Shigella* species, toxigenic strains of *E. coli* can pro-duce dysentery-like diarrheal syndromes indis-tinguishable from shigellosis. Serologic testing may be required in some instances to differentiate certain closely related strains.

GENUS *ESCHERICHIA*. *E. coli* is the bacterial spe-cies most commonly recovered in the clinical labo-ratories and has been incriminated in infectious diseases involving virtually every human tissue and organ system. *E. coli* is one of the common organ-isms involved in gram-negative sepsis and endo-toxin-induced shock. Urinary tract and wound infections, pneumonia in immunosuppressed hos-pitalized patients, and meningitis in neonates are other common infections caused by *E. coli*.

Certain strains of *E. coli* can cause enteritis or gastroenteritis by four distinct mechanisms result-ing in four different clinical syndromes.

Enterotoxigenic strains (ETEC) form heat-labile and heat-stable enterotoxins that produce a se-cretory diarrhea ("traveler's diarrhea") similar to that of *Vibrio cholerae*.
Enteropathogenic strains (EPEC) cause diarrheal syndromes primarily in infants. The patho-genesis is unclear.
Enteroinvasive strains (EIEC) are capable of pene-trating the intestinal epithelial cells and produc-ing an inflammatory diarrhea similar to that caused by *Shigella* species. This strain can be suspected when observing blood, mucus, and segmented neutrophils in fecal smears.
Verotoxin-producing *E. coli* (VTEC), also known as *enterohemorrhagic E. coli* (EHEC), produces bloody diarrhea in humans, probably secondary to toxin damage of vascular endothelial cells. The clinical significance of VTEC was not known until 1982, when these organisms were associated with two conditions of previously un-known etiology: hemorrhagic colitis and hemo-lytic uremic syndrome.[21] A large portion of VTEC isolates have been found to belong to serotype 0157:H7.[21] The recovery of this se-rotype from stool is made simple by the fact that serotype 0157:H7 is sorbitol-negative. This property is the basis for a selective MacConkey agar that contains 1% D-sorbitol rather than lactose to differentiate sorbitol-negative *E. coli* strains (colonies appear colorless, similar to lac-tose-negative colonies on regular MacConkey agar). Suspected isolates should be confirmed with specific 0157:H7 antisera.

GENUS *SHIGELLA*. *Shigella* species can be sus-pected in cultures because they are non–lactose fermenters and tend to be biochemically inert. They typically do not produce gas from carbohy-drates, with the exception of certain biogroups of *S. flexneri* that are aerogenic. Rare strains of *S. sonnei* can slowly ferment lactose (2%) and su-crose (1%), and most strains can decarboxylate ornithine—characteristics not shared by other *Shigella* species.

Fever, watery diarrhea with cramping abdomi-nal pain, and generalized myalgias are the most common early symptoms suggesting shigellosis. Fluid and electrolyte losses may also be noted early in the illness owing to the action of enterotoxin on the intestinal epithelial cells. After 2 or 3 days, bowel movements become less frequent and the quantity of stool decreases, but the presence of bright red blood and mucus in the feces and the onset of tenesmus (straining at stool) indicate the dysenteric phase of illness, suggesting that bacte-rial penetration of the bowel has probably oc-curred. *Shigella* is the most communicable of the bacterial diarrheas. Humans serve as the natural host, and disease is transmitted by the fecal-oral route, with as few as 200 viable organisms being able to cause disease.

S. sonnei is the serotype most commonly associ-ated with diarrheal disease in the United States; symptoms, however, tend to be mild, and some patients may be asymptomatic. *S. dysenteriae* is the least commonly recovered species but is the most virulent serotype. *Shigella* infections should be sus-pected in community-wide outbreaks of diarrheal illness that disproportionately affect young chil-dren. Outbreaks can occur at any time of the year but are most common in the summer.

Table 2-6
Key Identification Characteristics for the Most Common Enterobacteriaceae

	KIA	GAS	H₂S	MR	VP	IND	CIT	PAD	URE	MOT	LYS	ARG	ORN	ONPG
Tribe I: Escherichieae														
Genus: *Escherichia*														
E. coli	A/A	+	−	+	−	+	−	−	−	+	+	−/+	+/−	+
Genus: *Shigella*														
Groups A, B, C	Alk/A	−	−	+	−	−/+	−	−	−	−	−	−	−	−
S. sonnei	Alk/A	−	−	+	−	−	−	−	−	−	−	−	+	+
Tribe II: Edwardsielleae														
Genus: *Edwardsiella*														
E. tarda	Alk/A	+	+	+	−	+	−	−	−	+	+	−	+	−
Tribe III: Salmonelleae														
Genus: *Salmonella*														
Salmonella	Alk/A	+	+	+	−	−	+	−	−	+	+	+/−	+	−
Tribe IV: Citrobactereae														
Genus: *Citrobacter*														
C. freundii	A/A; Alk/A	+	+	+	−	−	+	−	+/−	+	−	+/−	−/+	+
C. diversus	Alk/A	+	−	+	−	+	+	−	+/−	+	−	+/−	+	+
Tribe V: Klebsielleae														
Genus: *Klebsiella*														
K. pneumoniae	A/A	+	−	−	+	−	+	−	+	−	+	−	−	+
K. oxytoca	A/A	+	−	−	+	+	+	−	+	−	+	−	−	+,

	KIA	GAS	H₂S	MR	VP	IND	CIT	PAD	URE	MOT	LYS	ARG	ORN	ONPG
Genus: Enterobacter														
E. aerogenes	A/A	++	–	–	++	–	+	–	–	+	+	–	+	+
E. cloacae	A/A	++	–	–	++	–	+	–	+/–	+	–	+	+	+
Genus: Hafnia														
H. alvei	Alk/A	+	–	–/+	+	–	–	–	–	+	+	–	+	+
Genus: Pantoea														
P. agglomerans	A/A; Alk/A	–/+	–	–/+	+/–	–/+	+/–	–/+	–/+	+	–	–	–	+
Genus: Serratia														
S. marcescens	Alk/A	+	–	–/+	+	–	+	–	–	+	+	–	+	+

Tribe VI: Proteeae

	KIA	GAS	H₂S	MR	VP	IND	CIT	PAD	URE	MOT	LYS	ARG	ORN	ONPG
Genus: Proteus														
P. vulgaris	Alk/A	+/–	++	+	–	+	–/+	++	++	+*	–	–	–	–
P. mirabilis	Alk/A	+	++	+	+/–	–	+/–	++	++	+*	–	+	+	–
Genus: Morganella														
M. morganii	Alk/A	+	–	+	–	+	–	+	++	+	–	–	+	–
Genus: Providencia														
P. rettgeri	Alk/A	–	–	+	–	+	+	+++	+	+	–	–	–	–
P. stuartii	Alk/A	–	–	+	–	+	+	+++	–/+	+/–	–	–	–	?
P. alcalifaciens	Alk/A	+/–	–	+	–	+	+	+++	–	+	–	–	–	–

Tribe VII: Yersinieae

	KIA	GAS	H₂S	MR	VP	IND	CIT	PAD	URE	MOT	LYS	ARG	ORN	ONPG
Genus: Yersinia														
Y. enterocolitica	Alk/A	–	–	+	–	+/–	–	–	+/–	–†	–	–	+	+

KIA, Kligler's iron agar; H₂S, hydrogen sulfide; MR, methyl red; VP, Voges-Proskauer; IND, indole; CIT, citrate; PAD, phenylalanine deaminase; URE, urease; MOT, motility; LYS, lysine; ARG, arginine; ORN, ornithine; ONPG, ortho-nitrophenyl-β-D-galactopyranoside; ++, strong positive reaction; +, 90% or more strains positive; –, 90% or more strains negative; +/–, 50%–90% of strains positive; –/+, 50%–90% of strains negative; shaded areas indicate key reactions.

*Swarming motility demonstrated on noninhibitory media.

†Nonmotile at 36°C, motile at 22°C.

Tribe Edwardsielleae

The Edwardsielleae consists of one genus, *Edwardsiella*, which has three species; only one species, *E. tarda*, is of medical importance. The chief reservoirs in nature are reptiles (especially snakes, toads, and turtles) and freshwater fish.

A key feature of *E. tarda* is the production of abundant amounts of hydrogen sulfide. Except for this feature, the bacterium has biochemical properties similar to those of *Escherichia coli*. The organism also resembles some *Citrobacter* and *Salmonella* species by its production of hydrogen sulfide in TSI agar and its failure to utilize lactose. This failure to ferment lactose and many other carbohydrates is the basis for the species name *tarda*. *E. tarda* has been reported as the cause of a variety of extraintestinal infections, including wound infections resulting from trauma often related to aquatic accidents, liver abscesses, and bacteremias.

Tribe Salmonelleae

The Salmonelleae contain a single genus, *Salmonella*, and are named after the American microbiologist, D.E. Salmon. The salmonellae are the most complex of all the Enterobacteriaceae, with more than 2200 serotypes described in the Kauffman-White schema. In this schema, the salmonellae are grouped (A,B,C, etc) on the basis of somatic O antigens and subdivided into serotypes (1, 2, etc) by their flagellar H antigens (ie, A1, A2, B1, B2). Before July 1, 1983, three species of *Salmonella* were used to report positive results: *Salmonella choleraesuis*, *Salmonella typhi*, and *Salmonella enteritidis*. Most of the 2200 serotypes belonged to the last species, *S. enteritidis*. It is now accepted that all former species and subgroups of *Salmonella* and *Arizona* are all considered to be the same species but can be separated into six distinct subgroups (see Table 2-5). Accordingly, all organisms identified as *Salmonella* are now reported by genus and serotype, omitting reference to species:

Previous Nomenclature
Salmonella enteritidis serotype Enteritidis
Salmonella enteritidis serotype Typhimurium
Salmonella enteritidis serotype Heidelberg

Current Nomenclature
Salmonella serotype enteritidis
Salmonella serotype typhimurium
Salmonella serotype heidelberg

In day-to-day practice, unknown isolates from clinical specimens that are biochemically suggestive of *Salmonella* species continue to be subgrouped in most laboratories to confirm the identification. Subcultures of confirmed isolates are forwarded to public health laboratories, where serotype designations (eg, *Salmonella* serotype *typhimurium*) are made based on serologic reactions to O and H determinants.

Although most *Salmonella* serotypes cannot be distinguished by biochemical reactions, one serotype, *S. typhi*, possesses some unique biochemical characteristics that will allow it to be differentiated from other serotypes. First and foremost is the observation that strains of *S. typhi* produce only a trace amount of hydrogen sulfide, which is usually observed as a crescent-shaped wedge of black precipitate forming at the interface of the slant and butt in KIA or TSI media. Additionally, *S. typhi* strains are less active biochemically than the more common serotypes and specifically are negative in the following reactions: Simmon's citrate, ornithine decarboxylase, gas from glucose, fermentation of dulcitol, arabinose, rhamnose, mucate, and acetate utilization. Consequently, we believe that it is within the capabilities of most clinical laboratories to make a preliminary report of *S. typhi* or *Salmonella* species not *typhi* while the laboratory awaits specific serotype confirmation from the local public health laboratory.

Human *Salmonella* infections are most commonly caused by ingestion of food, water, or milk contaminated by human or animal excreta. About half of the salmonellosis epidemics are the result of contaminated poultry and poultry products. Historically, *S. typhimurium* has been the most frequently reported serotype and *S. enteritidis* the second most frequently reported serotype. Several *S. enteritidis* outbreaks occurring in the United States in 1990 were associated with shell eggs. The largest single source outbreak of salmonellosis in U.S. history occurred in Illinois and surrounding states in 1987[5] and was traced to a faulty valve in a major commercial milk supply firm.[6]

Tribe Citrobactereae

Included in the Citrobactereae are one genus—*Citrobacter*—and three species—*C. freundii*, *C. diversus*, and *C. amalonaticus*. The characteristics that suggest an isolate may belong to the genus

Citrobacter are given in Table 2-6. Typically, *C. freundii*, the type strain of the genus, is hydrogen sulfide–positive and indole-negative, while the reverse is true for the other species in the genus.

The key characteristics that differentiate *C. freundii* from salmonellae are growth in KCN (*Salmonella* species are negative), absence of lysine decarboxylase activity (*Salmonella* species are positive), and the hydrolysis of *ortho*-nitrophenol-β-D-galactopyranoside (ONPG) (*Salmonella* species are negative). *C. freundii* has been reported as a possible cause of diarrhea (although most fecal isolates do not appear to be associated with disease) and as a cause of isolated cases of extraintestinal infections. *C. diversus* has also been reported as a cause of meningitis and brain abscesses in neonates.

Tribe Klebsielleae

The Klebsielleae include four major genera—*Klebsiella, Enterobacter, Hafnia,* and *Serratia*—each of which includes several species that are overt and opportunistic pathogens in humans. A fifth genus, *Pantoea*, has been added to accommodate the reclassification of the organism formerly named *Enterobacter agglomerans* and now called *Pantoea agglomerans*. The key characteristics suggesting that an unknown isolate belongs to the Klebsielleae are given in Table 2-6. The biochemical differences between the major genera and species in the tribe are presented in Table 2-7.

GENUS *KLEBSIELLA*. *Klebsiella* species should be suspected when large colonies with a mucoid consistency are recovered on primary isolation plates. On MacConkey agar, the colonies typically appear large, mucoid, and red, with red pigment usually diffusing into the surrounding agar, indicating fermentation of lactose and acid production. Not all strains, however, are mucoid, and certain species of *Enterobacter* can closely simulate the *Klebsiella* species in screening tests. All *Klebsiella* species are nonmotile and most do not decarboxylate ornithine (*K. ornithinolytica* is ornithine-positive)—characteristics that are positive for most *Enterobacter* species. Many strains of *Klebsiella* hydrolyze urea slowly, producing a light pink color in the slant of Christensen's urea agar. Production of indole from tryptophan can be used to separate the two principal species. *K. pneumoniae* is indole-negative, and *K. oxytoca* is indole-positive.

Klebsiella pneumoniae is most frequently recovered from clinical specimens and can cause a classic form of primary pneumonia. *K. pneumoniae* is infrequently found in the oropharynx of normal persons (1% to 6% carrier rate); a prevalence as high as 20% may, however, occur in hospitalized patients.[20] This colonization may prove to be the source of lung infections that generally occur in patients with debilitating conditions such as alcoholism, diabetes mellitus, and chronic obstructive pulmonary disease. *K. pneumoniae* can also cause a variety of extrapulmonary infections, including enteritis and meningitis (in infants), urinary tract infections (in children and adults), and septicemia. Virtually all clinical strains demonstrate resistance to ampicillin and carbenicillin, a finding that can also be used to cross check the identification of *Klebsiella* species.

GENUS *ENTEROBACTER*. Because large amounts of gas are produced by many strains of the genus *Enterobacter*, for many years the type species was called *Aerobacter aerogenes*. The genus designation was changed to *Enterobacter* by Edwards and Ewing in 1962.

There are 11 species included in the genus *Enterobacter*. A recent development has been the removal of *E. agglomerans* and its placement in the genus *Pantoea*.[13] As a genus, *Enterobacter* has the general characteristics of the Klebsielleae but can be differentiated from most *Klebsiella* species because they are motile and ornithine-positive (see Table 2-7).

Enterobacter aerogenes and *E. cloacae* are the species most commonly encountered in clinical specimens. They are widely distributed in water, in sewage, in soil, and on vegetables. They are part of the commensal enteric flora and are not believed to cause diarrhea. They are also associated with a variety of opportunistic infections involving the urinary tract, respiratory tract, and cutaneous wounds and, on occasion, cause septicemia and meningitis.

Other species of *Enterobacter* may also be infrequently encountered. *E. sakazakii*, known as yellow-pigmented *E. cloacae*, has been found in several cases of neonatal meningitis and sepsis.[18] The bright yellow pigment (which is particularly intense if cultures are incubated at 25°C) and "tough" nature of the colonies are the initial clues that this organism is present.

Table 2-7
Differentiation of the Major Genera and Species Within the Tribe Klebsielleae

BIOCHEMICAL TEST	KLEBSIELLA		ENTEROBACTER		PANTOEA	HAFNIA	SERRATIA	
	K. pneumoniae	K. oxytoca	E. aerogenes	E. cloacae	P. agglomerans	H. alvei	S. marcescens	S. liquefaciens
Indole	−	+	−	−	V (20)	−	−	−
Motility	−	−	+	+	V (85)	V (85)	+	+
Lysine	+	+	+	−	−	+	+	+
Arginine	−	−	−	+	−	−	−	−
Ornithine	−	−	+	+	−	+	+	+
DNase (25°C)	−	−	−	−	−	−	+	V (85)
Gelatinase (22°C)	−	−	−	−	−	−	+	+
Fermentation of								
Lactose	+	+	+	+	V (40)	−	−	−
Sucrose	+	+	+	+	V (75)	−	+	+
Sorbitol	+	+	+	+	V (30)	−	+	+
Adonitol	+	+	+	V (25)	−	−	V (40)	−
Arabinose	+	+	+	+	+	+	−	+

+, 90% or more strains positive; −, 90% or more strains negative; V, 11%–89% of strains positive.

Enterobacter gergoviae, E. hormaechei, E. taylorae, E. amnigenus, and *E. asburiae* are other species less commonly recovered in clinical laboratories. They have been recovered from a variety of human sources, including blood, urine, wounds, respiratory tract, and feces.

GENUS *PANTOEA.* In the early 1970s, *P. agglomerans* (then called *Enterobacter agglomerans*) was responsible for a nationwide outbreak of septicemia caused by contaminated intravenous fluids. One clue to the recognition of this genus is the triple decarboxylase-negative reaction (lysine-negative, arginine-negative, and ornithine-negative) that separates *Pantoea* from other genera in the tribe Klebsielleae.

GENUS *HAFNIA. Hafnia alvei,* formerly *Enterobacter hafnia,* is the only species in the genus *Hafnia.* The biochemical characteristics are similar to those of *Enterobacter* species except that *H. alvei* does not produce acids from the following carbohydrates: lactose, sucrose, melibiose, raffinose, adonitol, sorbitol, dulcitol, and inositol (see Table 2-7). *H. alvei* can be distinguished from *Serratia* species because it does not produce lipase or deoxyribonuclease. Unlike other species of Enterobacteriaceae, this organism gives off a strong scent of human feces. The clinical significance of *H. alvei* is not well defined. Isolated cases of infection have been reported in which *H. alvei* has been recovered from wounds, abscesses, sputum, urine, blood, and other sites.

GENUS *SERRATIA. Serratia* species are unique among the Enterobacteriaceae in producing three hydrolytic enzymes: lipase, gelatinase, and DNAse. Resistance to colistin and cephalothin are additional distinguishing features. *Serratia marcescens* is the most important member of the genus *Serratia* and is often associated with a variety of human infections, particularly pneumonia and septicemia in patients with reticuloendothelial malignancies who are receiving chemotherapeutic agents. The species referred to as *S. liquefaciens* is now known to be not a single species but a collection of several DNA hybridization groups including species named *S. proteamaculans* and *S. grimesii.* Since the species that make up this hybridization group cannot be separated by currently used biochemical tests, it is suggested that members of this species be reported as "*Serratia liquefaciens* group." This group is dif-

ferentiated from *S. marcescens* by virtue of its ability to ferment L-arabinose (see Table 2-7).

Tribe Proteeae

The Proteeae comprise three genera: *Proteus, Morganella,* and *Providencia.* The characteristics suggesting that an organism belongs to this tribe are given in Table 2-6. The genus *Proteus* now includes four species: *P. vulgaris, P. mirabilis, P. myxofaciens,* and *P. penneri.* The organism previously designated *P. morganii* is now reassigned to the new genus *Morganella* as *M. morganii.* Five species of *Providencia* are now recognized: *P. alcalifaciens, P. stuartii, P. rettgeri,* and the newly described species *P. rustigianii* and *P. heimbachae.* The differential characteristics for the three genera in the Proteeae are included in Table 2-6.

GENUS *PROTEUS.* The genus *Proteus* is found in soil, water, and fecally contaminated materials. *Proteus* species exhibit the characteristic feature of swarming motility, which is observed on noninhibitory agar (eg, blood agar plate) as a wavelike spreading of the organism across the entire surface of the agar (see Color Plate 2-1*C*). Whenever swarming is observed, *Proteus* species should be suspected. *P. mirabilis* is the species most frequently recovered from humans, particularly as the causative agent of both urinary tract and wound infections. *P. vulgaris* is more commonly recovered from infected sites in immunosuppressed hosts, particularly those receiving prolonged regimens of antibiotics. *P. vulgaris* is indole-positive while *P. mirabilis* is indole-negative. Thus, by performing a rapid spot indole test on a characteristic swarming colony, a rapid presumptive identification of *P. mirabilis* or *P. vulgaris* can be made. The new species, *P. penneri* and *P. myxofaciens,* are also indole-negative but are rarely encountered in clinical laboratories. Therefore, for practical purposes, the recovery of an indole-negative *Proteus* species can be presumptively identified as *P. mirabilis.* Virtually all strains of *P. mirabilis* are sensitive to ampicillin and cephalosporins, while *P. vulgaris* is resistant; therefore, most patients with clinical infection, from whom an indole-negative *Proteus* species is recovered, can be treated with one of the broad-spectrum penicillins or cephalosporins. When *P. penneri* is suspected, a chloramphenicol susceptibility test should be performed for identification purposes. *P. penneri* is chloramphenicol resistant, while other indole-negative *Proteus* species are chloramphenicol susceptible. Documented human infections with *P. penneri* have been limited mainly to the urinary tract and wounds of the abdomen, groin, neck, and ankle.[17]

GENUS *MORGANELLA*. *M. morganii* is a cause of both urinary tract and wound infections and has been implicated as a cause of diarrhea. As shown in Table 2-6, the pattern of Simmons citrate–negative, hydrogen sulfide–negative, and ornithine decarboxylase–positive is characteristic of this genus.

GENUS *PROVIDENCIA*. All species of the genus *Providencia* deaminate phenylalanine, but only *P. rettgeri* consistently hydrolyzes urea. *Providencia* species have been reported to cause nosocomial urinary tract infections, however, infections of sites other than the urinary tract are uncommon. All species may be recovered from feces, but only *P. alcalifaciens* has been associated with diarrheal illness, usually in children.

Tribe Yersinieae

Three species of *Pasteurella*, including the causative agent of human plague, *P. pestis*, were formally assigned to a new genus, *Yersinia*, in the eighth edition of *Bergey's Manual*[2] and placed in the Enterobacteriaceae.

Although *Yersinia* species qualify biochemically for inclusion in the Enterobacteriaceae, the cells appear small and coccobacillary in Gram-stained smears and may be small and pinpoint on MacConkey agar, particularly for certain strains of *Y. pestis* and *Y. pseudotuberculosis*. Colonies tend to be pinpoint in size after 24 hours of incubation on sheep blood agar. Optimal growth occurs from 25°C to 32°C.

GENUS *YERSINIA*. *Yersinia* is the only genus in the Yersinieae. Three species, *Y. pestis*, *Y. pseudotuberculosis*, and *Y. enterocolitica*, were included when the genus was transferred to the Enterobacteriaceae. In 1980, three new species were proposed for strains that were former subgroups of *Y. enterocolitica*, namely, *Y. frederiksenii*, *Y. intermedia*, and *Y. kristensenii*.[3,4] Eleven species are now included in the genus *Yersinia*.

Y. pestis is endemic in various rodents, including rats and ground squirrels. Sporadic cases of human infection are reported annually in the United States, particularly in the Southwest.[19] The organism is transferred from rodent to rodent or from rodent to human by the rat flea. Three clinical forms of disease may occur: bubonic, pneumonic, and septicemic plague. Gram stains of bubo aspirates show gram-negative rods in about two thirds of cases, and Wright-Giemsa staining of peripheral blood smears often reveal the characteristic bipolar staining typical of *Yersinia*. The colonies are slow growing on ordinary media and are said to have the appearance of beaten cooper when viewed under the stereoscope. The reaction observed on TSI agar in 24 hours is similar to that seen with *Pasteurella* species (ie, weak acid production on the slant with little or no change in the butt).

Y. pseudotuberculosis is also endemic in a wide variety of animals, including fowl, and is responsible for mesenteric lymphadenitis, particularly in children who manifest a clinical disease simulating appendicitis. The major biochemical tests that differentiate *Y. pseudotuberculosis* from *Y. enterocolitica* are ornithine decarboxylase, sucrose, and sorbitol. *Y. pseudotuberculosis* is negative for all three, whereas *Y. enterocolitica* is positive.

Y. enterocolitica is widely distributed in lakes and reservoirs, and epizootic outbreaks of diarrhea, lymphadenopathy, pneumonia, and spontaneous abortions occur in various animals.[1] It is the most common species of *Yersinia* recovered from clinical specimens. It is associated with terminal ileitis, lymphadenitis, and acute enterocolitis, with secondary manifestations of erythema nodosum, polyarthritis, and, less commonly, septicemia.[8] *Y. enterocolitica* is more biochemically reactive at room temperature than at 37°C and has been recovered from contaminated units of donor blood after transfusion reactions, illustrating this organism's ability to grow at cold temperatures. Investigation of these cases has led to the conclusion that blood contamination resulted from asymptomatic *Y. enterocolitica* bacteremia in the blood donors at the time of donation.[7,15]

RECOVERY OF *YERSINIA* FROM CLINICAL SPECIMENS. The recovery of *Yersinia* species is low in most clinical laboratories. Most strains of *Y. enterocolitica* will grow on selective enteric agars and will appear as small, lactose-negative colonies on MacConkey and SS agars in 48 hours. In some laboratories, plates of MacConkey agar inoculated with stool specimens suspected of harboring *Yersinia* species are routinely incubated at room temperature. *Y. enterocolitica*, in particular, can best be recovered from stool specimens that are incubated at 25°C. Cold enrichment of highly contaminated specimens, such as feces, by incubating cultures at 4°C for 1 to 3 weeks in phosphate-buffered saline before subculture onto enteric media, also enhances the recovery of *Y. enterocolitica*. Superior recovery of *Y. enterocolitica* from stool has also been reported using cefsulodin irgasan novobiocin (CIN) agar.

Tribe Erwinieae

The Erwinieae are primarily pathogens in plants and only saprophytic in humans. Farmer[11] believes that the concept of *Erwinia* as a separate genus is not useful in clinical microbiology because "true *Erwinia* species" represented by *E. amylovora*, do not grow at 35° to 37°C and are inactive biochemically in the tests used to identify Enterobacteriaceae. "*Enterobacter agglomerans* group" (now assigned to the genus *Pantoea*) is the name used by the CDC for a heterogeneous group of bacteria that have been reported as various species of *Erwinia* in the literature.

Miscellaneous New Genera of Enterobacteriaceae

The identifying characteristics of several new genera of the Enterobacteriaceae have been officially recognized during the past decade. New genus and species designations have evolved from DNA hybridization studies and biochemical characterizations performed on atypical strains referred to the CDC and other reference laboratories for identification and classification. Many of these new genus names have been applied to bacterial strains that at one time were designated atypical enteric groups at the CDC. Several enteric groups remain unnamed but will probably achieve genus status in the future when a sufficient number of strains are gathered. These organisms will not be described here; rather, the reader is referred elsewhere.[16] In addition, the landmark report by Farmer and associates[11] summarizes all of the old and new genera of Enterobacteriaceae known as of January 1985.

QUICK SCREENING METHODS FOR RAPID IDENTIFICATION

Escherichia coli, the bacterial isolate most frequently recovered in clinical laboratories, is often presumptively identified if an oxidase-negative, lactose-fermenting, dry colony on MacConkey agar gives a positive spot indole reaction (when tested on a colony growing on noninhibitory media such as blood agar), particularly if the organism has been recovered in pure culture. The spot indole test is also used in many laboratories for rapid speciation of swarming *Proteus* from primary isolation plates. A rapid (2-minute) spot urease test has been described that can be used to separate possible stool pathogens that require further biochemical testing from the nonpathogenic *Proteus-Providencia-Morganella* group. The rapid catalase test (with 3% H_2O_2) can also be used for screening suspicious colonies on enteric media that mimic stool pathogens. Colonies of *Serratia, Proteus, Providencia,* or *Pseudomonas* are quickly eliminated because they produce vigorous catalase reactions, in contrast to salmonellae, which give weak to moderate reactions, or shigellae, which are negative and are therefore flagged for further work-up. Clearly, any of these approaches has validity in an era of cost containment and the desire to receive test results quickly.

CLASSIC IDENTIFICATION SYSTEMS

Systems for the identification and naming of microorganisms are either computer assisted or manual. Before discussing the derivation and applications of numerical coding systems, two manual bacterial identification schemes that are still in use will be reviewed: (1) the cross-hatch or checkerboard matrix, and (2) the branching or dichotomous flow charts.

Checkerboard Matrix

Tables 2-6 an 2-7 are examples of the checkerboard matrix. The signs and letters in the intersecting squares represent the typical reactions of the various bacterial species listed in one column to the biochemical tests listed in the opposing column. A reaction is generally considered positive if 90% or more of the strains are reactive, negative if 10% or less of the strains fail to produce a result, and variable if 11% to 89% of reactions are positive. The ability to determine both the positive and negative reactions for the various characteristics being measured in this type of identification system results in a high degree of diagnostic accuracy. The major disadvantage of the checkerboard matrix is the tedium involved in matching point-by-point the various reactions against those derived from the test media and constructing the patterns that best match with a specific genus, species, or biogroup.

Branching Flow Diagrams

During the 1960s, flow diagrams were designed to reduce the tedium of reading the checkerboard matrices and to facilitate the likely bacterial identification by tracing a series of positive and negative branch points in a dichotomous algorithm (Fig. 2-3). With the advent of automated instruments and packaged identification systems that rely on computer-assisted analyses of the various reactions of the characteristics being measured, flow diagrams are now used less frequently in clinical laboratories. One problem with flow diagrams has been the potential for inaccuracy if the reaction at a given branch point is either aberrant (ie, not typical for the species), misinterpreted, or the result of the reactions of a mixed culture. Many flow diagrams are constructed to repeat some species names at several junctures to accommodate reactions that may be less than 100% or in the variable category. This built-in protection does not always apply for reactions that are misinterpreted, either by an automated instrument's detection system or by the human eye.

NUMERICAL CODING SYSTEMS

The identification of the Enterobacteriaceae and many other families and groups of bacteria has been facilitated by the use of automated and packaged kit systems, by which organisms are identified with computer-assisted numerical codes. A numerical code is a system by which the several identify-ing characteristics of bacteria are translated into a sequence of numbers that represent one or more bacterial species. The fact that the identification of microorganisms is based on a series of positive and negative biochemical reactions makes computer programming easy since computer logic is also constructed on a sequence of positive and negative entries, using a binary numerical system. In binary logic there are only two numbers—0 (or off) and 1 (or on). As can quickly be surmised, the identification characteristics of microorganisms can be easily translated into binary numbers by assigning a 1 to all positive reactions and a 0 to all negative reactions. This approach can be illustrated using the sequence of characteristics in the API 20E strip (bioMérieux Vitek, Inc, Hazelwood, MO) as a point of reference and converting the positive and negative reactions into binary numbers (Table 2-8).

If the binary numbers shown in Table 2-8 are read from top to bottom and rearranged horizontally, the following 21-digit binary number is derived:

101010000111111011100

Although computers are constructed to receive 1/0 bits of data from which to calculate meaningful results, the human mind cannot efficiently manipulate binary logic; therefore, binary codes must be converted into simpler mathematical systems to become usable. Conversion of the two-digit (binary) system into an eight-digit (octal) system serves this purpose. To understand the conversion of binary into octal numbers, visualize a series of three light bulbs. By turning different lights on and off, a total of eight combinations is possible, each of which can be represented by one of eight numbers ranging from 0 to 7. If all lights are off (−), the combination − − − is equivalent to octal 0. If only the left bulb is turned on (+), the combination + − − is equivalent to octal 1. Octal 2 is represented by the binary pattern − + −, and octal 3 by the pattern + + −. The octal equivalents of the eight combinations of a three-digit binary number are shown in Table 2-9.

To illustrate how binary numbers longer than three digits can be converted into their octal equivalents, use the binary number that was derived from the API 20E reactions listed above:

101010000111111011100

Beginning to the right, because binary numbers

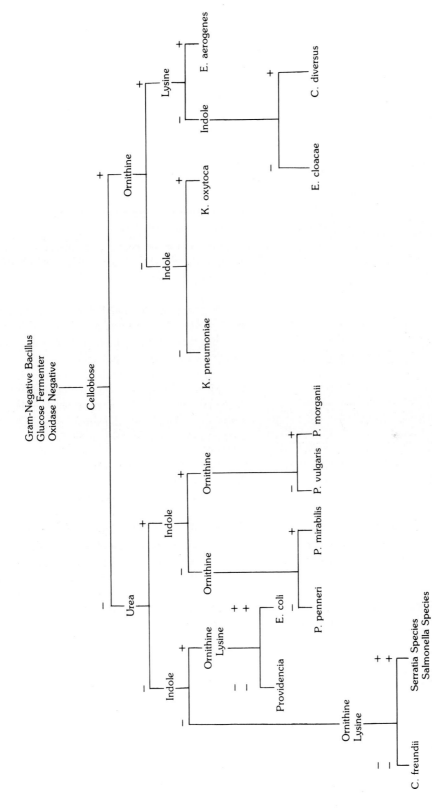

Figure 2-3. Flow diagram depicting the LOGIC system for biochemical identification of antibiotic-resistant Enterobacteriaceae isolates from urine. (Modified from Perry JD, Ford M, Hjersing N, Gould FK. Rapid conventional scheme for biochemical identification of antibiotic-resistant Enterobacteriaceae isolates from urine. J Clin Pathol 1988;41:1010–1012.)

Table 2-8
Binary Conversion of Reactions of Unknown Organism on API 20E Strip

CHARACTERISTIC	REACTION	BINARY CONVERSION
ONPG	+	1
Arginine	−	0
Lysine	+	1
Ornithine	−	0
Citrate	+	1
Hydrogen sulfide	−	0
Urease	−	0
Tryptophan deaminase	−	0
Indole	−	0
Voges-Proskauer	+	1
Gelatin	+	1
Glucose	+	1
Mannitol	+	1
Inositol	+	1
Sorbitol	+	1
Rhamnose	−	0
Sucrose	+	1
Melibiose	+	1
Amygdalin	+	1
Arabinose	−	0
Oxidase	−	0

Table 2-9
Octal Conversion of Binary Code

BINARY	CONVERSION FORMULA	OCTAL
− − −	0 + 0 + 0 =	0
+ − −	1 + 0 + 0 =	1
− + −	0 + 2 + 0 =	2
+ + −	1 + 2 + 0 =	3
− − +	0 + 0 + 4 =	4
+ − +	1 + 0 + 4 =	5
− + +	0 + 2 + 4 =	6
+ + +	1 + 2 + 4 =	7

are read from right to left, divide the binary numbers into subsets of three:

101 010 000 111 111 011 100

Now convert each three-digit subset into its octal equivalent using the formula given in Table 2-9.

The number 5207761 is far easier to remember and simpler to enter into a computer than the binary number 101010000111111011100.

A simpler way of remembering how to convert each binary triplet into its corresponding octal equivalent is to assign the following values: a value of 1 to a positive reaction for the first (left) test in each triplet, a value of 2 to a positive reaction for the second (center) test in each triplet, a value of 4 to a positive reaction for the third (right) test in each triplet, and a value of 0 to any negative reactions.

These octal derivatives are known as *biotype numbers*, that is, a numerical representative of a series of phenotypic characteristics expressed by and unique to a particular bacterial species. It is important that everyone using biotype numbers, particularly those who are teaching students, understand that each number in the octal system is representative of three biochemical characteristics and that the number itself represents a pattern of positive and negative reactions. There is great danger that modern microbiologists consider biotype numbers as magic figures that can be read from charts or put into computers to derive automatic organism identification, thus losing sight not only of the biochemical reactions that they represent but also of the biochemical principles on which the discipline of microbiology is based.

Reading the Octal Number in Numerical Code Registers

All manufacturers who have packaged identification kits on the market, and the designers of many manual systems as well, publish numerical code registers in which hundreds of biotype numbers are matched with one or more bacterial species that are unique for that number. For example, for the biotype number 5207761, derived from the API 20E set of reactions used in the previous example, the following species are listed in the API 20E Profile Index:

Serratia marcescens = acceptable identification
S. marcescens: 1/243
S. rubidaea: 1/2859

The message "acceptable identification" in the API Profile Index for biotype number 5207761 for *S. marcescens* indicates that *S. marcescens* can be reported. This assessment is based on a computer-derived calculation of the percent likelihood that

S. marcescens is the correct identification compared with all the other organisms entered into the data base.

PACKAGED KIT IDENTIFICATION SYSTEMS

It has now become almost standard practice in many clinical laboratories to use one or more available packaged systems for the identification of certain groups of microorganisms. Many of the systems have been in use for a decade or more, a sufficient time for most microbiologists to overcome the initial reluctance to give up the time-honored conventional methods. Improvements in kit design, the inclusion of alternate or additional substrates, and changes in reagents to improve the specificity and sensitivity of biochemical reactions have all served to correct inaccuracies in the initial systems. Extensive testing in diagnostic and research laboratories has demonstrated a 95% or greater agreement between most packaged identification systems and conventional methods in the identification of microorganisms. Thus, packaged systems have found wide acceptance in clinical laboratories for the following reasons:

1. Their accuracy has proved to be comparable to that of conventional identification systems.
2. Several of the systems have a long shelf life—6 months to 1 year—so that outdating of media, a problem particularly with conventional systems, is minimized.
3. The systems require only a minimum of space for storage and incubation.
4. Some of the systems are as easy or easier to use than conventional methods. Inoculation is simple, reactions are generally clear-cut within 24 hours, and the availability of computer-assisted file registers makes final identification easy and accurate.

Whether to use one of the packaged identification systems and which one to select is largely a matter of personal preference. The ease of inoculation, the ability to select only the characteristics to be measured, the manipulation required in adding reagents after incubation, and the availability of interpretive charts or numerical coding devices are the main items that potential users should consider before selecting a system. If strict attention is paid to the instructions provided by the manufacturer, essentially the same degree of accuracy and reliability of performance can be attained with minor differences in the sensitivity of individual tests.

Following is a brief discussion of the identification systems most commonly used in the clinical laboratory. The interested reader is requested to contact company representatives for demonstrations of individual products that may be of interest.

API 20E

The API 20E identification system (bioMérieux Vitek, Inc, Hazelwood, MO) has become the reference method against which the accuracy of other systems is compared. The system consists of a plastic strip with 20 miniaturized cupules containing dehydrated substrates and a plastic incubation chamber with a loosely fitting lid. Each cupule has a small hole at the top through which the bacterial suspension can be inoculated with a pipette. Bacterial action on the substrates produces color changes that are interpreted visually. The 20 characteristics that can be determined by the API 20E system make it among the largest test sets of the packaged kits. The system identifies a high percentage of bacterial species within 24 hours without the need to determine additional physiologic characteristics.[5]

Enterotube II

Of all the systems, Enterotube II (Becton Dickinson Microbiology Systems, Cockeysville, MD) is the easiest to inoculate. The Enterotube II is a pencil-shaped, self-contained, compartmented plastic tube containing 12 chambers of differential media from which 15 differential characteristics can be determined. An inoculating wire is positioned through the center of all the media chambers and extends out from each end of the tube. One end serves as the inoculating tip; the other as the handle. Both ends are covered with a screwcap when packaged. Inoculation is carried out by touching the inoculating tip to the surface of a well-isolated colony on an agar plate. The tube is held firmly while the inoculating wire is pulled through all of the chambers and then reinserted into the first four compartments. The caps are replaced, and the tube is incubated overnight at 35°C. The system takes up little space, and the risk of contamination is minimal. The color reactions are generally easy to interpret. The manufacturer provides a convenient computer coding and identification system (CCIS) that lists the possible bacterial identifications for the five-digit biotype numbers that are derived from the interpretation of color changes.

Micro-ID

Micro-ID (Organon Teknika, Durham, NC) is the ideal system for laboratories where identification of bacteria within 4 to 6 hours is desired. The Micro-ID consists of a molded styrene tray containing 15 reaction chambers and a hinged cover. Each reaction chamber has an opening at the top that serves as the port for inoculation of the test organism suspension. The first five chambers contain a substrate disk and a detection disk, while the remaining chambers contain only a single combination substrate/detection disk. The disks contain all of the substrate and detection reagents required to perform the biochemical tests included in the strip, with the exception of the Voges-Proskauer test, which requires the addition of 2 to 3 drops of 20% KOH. Inoculation of the system is relatively easy, and the units occupy little space during incubation or storage. Reactions are distinct and can be compared against a color guide. A profile register that lists the probable organism identification for the five-digit biotype numbers is supplied by the manufacturer, and computer comparisons can be made to search for the best fit.

Minitek

Minitek (Becton Dickinson Microbiology Systems, Cockeysville, MD) can be highly recommended to microbiologists who desire freedom of choice in the selection of the characteristics for identification. The manufacturer provides approximately 40 different reagent-impregnated disks to which a broth suspension of the organism to be tested is added. The disks can be selected in any combination desired by the user providing the user wide flexibility in identifying groups of microorganisms other than the Enterobacteriaceae; considerable success has been achieved in the identification of nonfermentative bacilli, anaerobes, and medically important yeasts. Generally, the color reactions are visibly distinct, and the use of a stack of color comparison cards makes interpretation relatively

easy. The manufacturer also supplies a Minicoder, a plastic grid device that permits quick classification of bacterial candidates with each biochemical profile selected.

Microtube Identification Systems

All microtube identification systems are based on the use of plastic microtiter trays (usually containing 96 wells), which are prefilled by the manufacturer with the substrates to be tested and are shipped either frozen or lyophilized. These systems are all inoculated in a comparable manner by first preparing a bacterial suspension that is diluted with sterile water and poured into a specially constructed plastic tray called the "seed tray." The seed trays come with a specially designed transfer lid containing inoculating prongs that are designed to hold a measured amount of bacterial suspension and are aligned to exactly fit into the microtiter substrate trays. To inoculate the trays, the transfer lid is first lowered into the bacterial suspension in the seed tray. The lid is then removed and immediately lowered into the corresponding wells of the substrate tray. The inoculum is pulled off the prongs by capillary action when they touch the media in the wells. The lid is removed and discarded and the substrate plate is covered and incubated overnight at 35°C.

The Biolog Microplate (Biolog, Inc, Hayward, CA), the Micro Media Systems FOX Panel (Micro Media Systems, Cleveland, OH), the MicroScan System (Baxter Diagnostics, Inc, West Sacramento, CA), the Sceptor System (Becton Dickinson Diagnostic Instrument Systems, Towson, MD), and the Sensititre System (Radiometer America, Inc, Westlake, OH) are all representative of microtiter plate technology. Company representatives should be contacted for detailed information on the use of these products.

SEMIAUTOMATED AND AUTOMATED IDENTIFICATION SYSTEMS

Automicrobic System

The Automicrobic System (AMS; bioMérieux Vitek, Inc, Hazelwood, MO) has found wide use in clinical microbiology laboratories and has generally been accepted as a reliable approach to the rapid identification of commonly encountered gram-negative bacilli. The basis of this system is disposable polystyrene cards that include 30 tiny reaction chambers, each of which contain biochemical substrates or dehydrated antibiotics. The entire system consists of three modules: (1) a filling module that automatically fills and seals the substrate cards with the test organism; (2) an incubation/reader module that can handle 30, 60, or 120 cards that are optically scanned by light transmission nephelometry on a 1-hour rotational basis; and (3) a computer module that records biochemical reactions and performs computer-assisted identification. Final reports are available after 6 to 18 hours of incubation.

AutoSCAN-W/A

The AutoSCAN-W/A (Baxter Diagnostics, Inc, West Sacramento, CA) is a fully automated instrument that incubates any combination of up to 96 conventional and Rapid MicroScan panels simultaneously, automatically adds reagents to conventional panels when required, reads and interprets panel results, and prints results, all without operator intervention. Rapid fluorescence panels in addition to the conventional MicroScan panels are available for use with the AutoSCAN-W/A. The rapid panels use fluorescently labeled compounds and require only a 2-hour incubation for bacterial identification. Each fluorescent substrate consists of a fluorophore, either methylumbelliferone (MEU) or 7-amino-4-methyl-coumarin (AMC) attached to a phosphate, sugar, or amino acid compound. Two types of reactions occur: fluorogenic and fluorometric. In fluorogenic reactions, a specific enzyme, if present in the bacterial suspension, cleaves the fluorescent compound releasing the fluorophore, which then fluoresces. For example:

L-alanine-AMC (nonfluorescent) $\xrightarrow[\text{aminopeptidase}]{\text{Alanine}}$ alanine + AMC (fluorescent)

Fluorometric reactions detect changes in pH such as occurs with carbohydrate fermentation. The resultant acid production causes a drop in pH and a decrease in fluorescence. In addition, eight fluorogenic rate reactions are used. These reactions measure the rate of release of the fluorophore and are used in differentiating phenotypically simi-

lar species. Results of the ID reactions are converted into 15-digit biocodes for interpretation by the computer.

Sensititre AutoIdentification System

The Sensititre Gram-Negative AutoIdentification System (Radiometer America, Inc, Westlake, OH) uses fluorescent technology to detect bacterial growth and enzyme activity. The system consists of 32 newly formulated biochemical tests including selected classic biochemical media reformulated to yield a fluorescent signal, along with newly developed fluorescent tests. Each biochemical test medium along with an appropriate fluorescent indicator is dried into the individual wells of the Sensititre plate. Each plate is designed to test three separate organisms. Because these are dried plates, they may be stored at room temperature. All AutoIdentification tests are read on the Sensititre AutoReader for the presence or absence of fluorescence. The results are transmitted to a computer for analysis and identification. Results may be read after 5 hours of incubation. If a satisfactory level of identification cannot be obtained at 5 hours, the plate may simply be reincubated and read after overnight incubation.

Summary

In summary, commercial manufacturers continue to provide new systems and modifications of existing systems for the identification of microorganisms. To pass Food and Drug Administration standards, all of these systems must perform with an accuracy equal to or better than reference methods. Therefore, each system can be used in clinical laboratories, but the choice depends on several variables, including volume of testing, experience of the technical staff, need for definitive identifications, and cost of operation. The Enterobacteriaceae, as a group, are rapidly expanding and, for the most part, are biochemically very active; therefore, they are well suited for processing by automated and semiautomated systems.

REFERENCES

1. Bottone EJ, ed. *Yersinia enterocolitica*. Boca Raton, FL, CRC Press, 1981.

2. Brenner DJ. Enterobacteriaceae. In: Krieg NR, Holt JG, eds. Bergey's manual of systematic bacteriology. Baltimore, Williams & Wilkins, 1984;1: 408–420.

3. Brenner DJ, Bercovier H, Ursing J, et al. *Yersinia intermedia*: a new species of Enterobacteriaceae composed of rhamnose-positive, melibiose-positive, raffinose-positive strains (formerly called *Yersinia enterocolitica* or *Yersinia enterocolitica*–like). Curr Microbiol 1980;4:207–212.

4. Brenner DJ, Ursing J, Bercovier H, et al. Deoxyribonucleic acid relatedness in *Yersinia enterocolitica* and *Yersinia enterocolitica*-like organisms. Curr Microbiol 1980;4:195–200.

5. Castillo CB, Bruckner DA. Comparative evaluation of the Eiken and API 20E systems and conventional methods for identification of members of the family Enterobacteriaceae. J Clin Microbiol 1984; 20:754–757.

6. Centers for Disease Control. Update: milkborne salmonellosis—Illinois. MMWR 1985;34:200.

7. Centers for Disease Control. Update: *Yersinia enterocolitica* bacteremia and endotoxin shock associated with red blood cell transfusions—United States, 1991. MMWR 1991;40:176–178.

8. Cover TL, Aber RC. Medical progress: *Yersinia enterocolitica*. N Engl J Med 1989;321:16–24.

9. Edwards PR, Ewing WH. Identification of Enterobacteriaceae. 3rd ed. Minneapolis, Burgess, 1972.

10. Ewing WH. Identification of Enterobacteriaceae. 4th ed. New York, Elsevier, 1986.

11. Farmer JJ III, Davis BR, Hickman-Brenner FW, et al. Biochemical identification of new species and biogroups of Enterobacteriaceae isolated from clinical specimens. J Clin Microbiol 1985;21: 46–76.

12. Farmer JJ, Kelley MT. Enterobacteriaceae. In: Ballows A, ed. Manual of clinical microbiology. 5th ed. Washington, DC, American Society of Microbiology, 1991:360–383.

13. Gavini F, Mergaert J, Beji A, et al. Transfer of *Enterobacter agglomerans* (Beijerinck 1988) Ewing and Fife 1972 to *Pantoea* gen. nov. as *Pantoea agglomerans* comb. nov. and description of *Pantoea dispersa* sp. nov. Int J Syst Bacteriol 1989;39: 337–345.

14. Holt-Harris JE, Teague O. A new culture medium for the isolation of *Bacillus typhosus* from stools. J Infect Dis 1916;18:596–600.

15. Jacobs J, Jamaer D, Vandeven J, et al. *Yersinia enterocolitica* in donor blood: a case report and review. J Clin Microbiol 1989;27:1119–1121.

16. Koneman EW, Allen SD, Janda WM, Schreckenberger PC, Winn WC, eds. Color atlas and textbook of diagnostic microbiology. 4th ed. Philadelphia, JB Lippincott, 1992:105–184.

17. Krajden S, Fuksa M, Petrea C, et al. Expanded clinical spectrum of infections caused by *Proteus penneri*. J Clin Microbiol 1987;25:578–579.

18. Muytjens HL, Zanen HC, Sonderkamp HJ, et al. Analysis of eight cases of neonatal meningitis and sepsis due to *Enterobacter sakazakii*. J Clin Microbiol 1983;18:115–120.

19. Reed WP, et al. Bubonic plague in the southwestern United States. Medicine 1970;49:465–486.

20. Reynolds HY. Pneumonia due to *Klebsiella* (Friedlander's pneumonia). In: Wyngaarden JB, Smith LH, eds. Cecil textbook of medicine. 16th ed. Philadelphia, WB Saunders, 1982:1430–1432.

21. Riley LW, Remis RS, Helgerson SD, et al. Hemorrhagic colitis associated with rare *Escherichia coli* serotypes. N Engl J Med 1983;308:681–685.

3

The Nonfermentative Gram-Negative Bacilli

The nonfermentative gram-negative bacilli are a group of aerobic, non–spore-forming, gram-negative bacilli that either do not utilize carbohydrates as a source of energy or degrade them through metabolic pathways other than fermentation. Within this group are several genera and species of bacteria with special growth requirements that are not discussed in this chapter. The dividing line between what is a "nonfermenter" and what may otherwise be designated a "fastidious," "unusual," or "miscellaneous" non–glucose-fermenting gram-negative bacillus (discussed in Chapter 6) is based more on convention than on well-defined genetic or phenotypic characteristics. The term *nonfermentative gram-negative bacilli* is used in this chapter to mean all aerobic gram-negative rods that show abundant growth within 24 hours on the surface of Kligler iron agar (KIA) or triple sugar iron (TSI) medium but neither grow in nor acidify the butt of these media.

The genera of nonfermenters to be discussed in this chapter include *Acidovorax, Acinetobacter, Agrobacterium, Alcaligenes, Bordetella, Chryseomonas, Comamonas, Flavimonas, Flavobacterium, Methylobacterium, Moraxella, Ochrobactrum, Oligella, Pseudomonas, Psychrobacter, Shewanella, Sphingobacterium, Sphingomonas, Weeksella, Stenotrophomonas,* and a few organisms that currently carry only Centers for Disease Control and Prevention (CDC) alpha-numeric designations. The phenotypic characteristics by which these genera are separated are presented in Table 3-1. The genera *Eikenella, Brucella,* and *Francisella,* although possessing the general characteristics of nonfermenters, are grouped in this text with the fastidious, gram-negative bacilli and are discussed in Chapter 6. The currently accepted organism nomenclature and a listing of previous designations are presented in Table 3-2.

METABOLISM OF THE NONFERMENTERS

Bacteria that derive their energy from organic compounds are known as *chemoorganotrophs.* Most of the bacteria encountered in clinical medicine derive energy from the utilization of carbohydrates by one of several metabolic pathways. Detection and measurement of various metabolic products are necessary to identify bacterial species that may be the cause of infectious disease. Some bacteria, such as members of the genus *Moraxella,* do not utilize carbohydrates but derive energy from the degradation of other organic compounds, such as amino acids, alcohols, and organic acids. Space in this text permits only a brief summary of the metabolic pathways used by the nonfermenters, enough to gain a working understanding of terms such as *aerobic, anaerobic, fermentation,* and *oxidation.*

FERMENTATIVE AND OXIDATIVE METABOLISM

The bacterial degradation of carbohydrates proceeds by several metabolic pathways in which hydrogen ions (electrons) are successively transferred to compounds of higher redox potential, with the ultimate release of energy in the form of adenosine triphosphate. All six-, five-, and four-carbon carbohydrates are initially degraded to pyruvic acid, an initial intermediate. Glucose is the main carbohydrate source of carbon for bacteria, and degradation proceeds by three major pathways: the Embden-Meyerhof-Parnas, the Entner-Doudoroff, and the Warburg-Dickens (hexose monophosphate) pathways. As shown in Figure 3-1, glucose is converted to pyruvic acid in each of these three pathways by a different set of degradation steps. Bacteria utilize one or more of these pathways for glucose metabolism, depending on their enzymatic composition and the presence or lack of oxygen.

Embden-Meyerhof-Parnas Pathway

Because glucose is degraded without oxygen, the Embden-Meyerhof-Parnas (EMP) pathway has also been called the *glycolytic* or *anaerobic* pathway; it is used primarily by anaerobic bacteria and, to some degree, by facultatively anaerobic bacteria as well. The intermediate steps in the EMP pathway include the initial phosphorylation of glucose, conversion to fructose-phosphate, and cleavage to form two molecules of glyceraldehyde phosphate, which, through a series of intermediate steps (not shown in Fig. 3-1), forms pyruvic acid. Pyruvic acid acts as an intermediate hydrogen acceptor but is then oxidized by giving up its hydrogen ions to sodium lactate to form lactic acid, or to other or-

(text continues on page 82)

Table 3-1
Identifying Characteristics of Several Genera of Nonfermentative Bacilli

GENUS	METABOLISM	MOTILITY	OXIDASE	GROWTH ON MacCONKEY AGAR	ADDITIONAL CHARACTERISTICS
Acinetobacter	Oxidative or nonsaccharolytic	Nonmotile	Negative	Good growth except for some strains of *A. lwoffii*	Special growth factors are not required. Acid production from glucose is weak (*A. baumannii*) or lacking (*A. lwoffii*). Cells appear coccoid in Gram-stained preparations. Most stains are penicillin resistant.
Alcaligenes	Oxidative	Motile by peritrichous flagella	Positive	Good growth	Obligative aerobe. Glucose may be oxidized slowly (5 days); xylose is oxidized rapidly (24 hours)
	Nonsaccharolytic	Motile by peritrichous flagella	Positive	Good growth	Strict aerobe, although some strains utilize nitrate instead of oxygen as the final electron acceptor.
Bordetella	Oxidative	Variable, one species motile by peritrichous flagella (*B. bronchiseptica*)	Variable, one species negative (*B. parapertussis*)	Growth (*B. parapertussis* and *B. bronchiseptica*). No growth (*B. pertussis*)	Nicotinic acid, cysteine, and methionine required by some strains for growth. Potato glycerol blood agar (Bordet-Gengou) needed for growth of *B. pertussis*, *B. bronchiseptica* rapidly splits urea.
Flavobacterium	Oxidative (some strains are slow fermenters)	Nonmotile	Positive	Poor or negative	Supplemental nitrogen and B-complex vitamins required for growth of many strains. Yellow pigment often produced. No

(continued)

Table 3-1 (continued)

GENUS	METABOLISM	MOTILITY	OXIDASE	GROWTH ON MacCONKEY AGAR	ADDITIONAL CHARACTERISTICS
Flavobacterium (continued)					denitrification of nitrates. Growth optimal at 30°C. All species are resistant to polymyxin B. Most species are weak indole-positive (*F. odoratum* is indole-negative).
Moraxella	Oxidative or nonsaccharolytic	Nonmotile	Positive	Scant or negative	Most strains are fastidious in growth requirements, some requiring serum supplement. Strict aerobes. May appear as coccobacilli on Gram stain. Highly susceptible to penicillin.
Pseudomonas	Oxidative	Motile by means of polar flagella	Positive	Good growth	Monotrichous and multitrichous polar flagella. Special growth factors are not required. Fluorescein pigments are produced by some species. Pyocyanin pigment is produced by one species (*P. aeruginosa*).
Stenotrophomonas (*Xanthomonas*)	Oxidative	Motile by single polar flagellum	Negative or weak	Good growth	Colonies may be yellowish or yellow green. Methionine or cystine is required for growth. Under aerobic conditions acid is readily produced from maltose but not glucose for one species (*S. maltophilia*).

Table 3-2
Nomenclature for Gram-Negative Nonfermentative Bacilli

CURRENT USAGE	PREVIOUS DESIGNATIONS*	COMMENTS
Achromobacter group	*Achromobacter xylosoxidans* *Achromobacter* species CDC Vd-1, Vd-2	Currently no recognized species in genus *Achromobacter*. Type species moved to genus *Alcaligenes;* Vd-1 and Vd-2 moved to genus *Ochrobactrum*.
Acinetobacter baumannii	*Acinetobacter calcoaceticus* var. *anitratus* *Achromobacter anitratus* *Bacterium anitratum* *Herellea vaginicola* Morax-Axenfeld bacillus *Moraxella glucidolytica* var. *nonliquefaciens* *Pseudomonas calcoacetica*	Species name given to *Acinetobacter* genospecies 1. Produces acid from glucose. Can be separated from *Acinetobacter calcoaceticus* (genospecies 1) by growth at 41° and 44°C, production of β-xylosidase, and utilization of malate (*A. baumannii*–positive and *A. calcoaceticus*–negative). Laboratories that do not perform these tests may choose to report these organisms as *A. calcoaceticus*–*A. baumannii* complex. Most *Acinetobacter* strains isolated from human patients belong to this species.
Acinetobacter lwoffii	*Acinetobacter calcoaceticus* var. *lwoffi* *Achromobacter lwoffi* *Mima polymorpha* *Moraxella lwoffi*	Species name given to *Acinetobacter* genospecies 8. Non–glucose-oxidizing strain found in human clinical specimens.
Agrobacterium tumefaciens	CDC Vd-3 *Agrobacterium radiobacter*	
Alcaligenes faecalis	CDC VI *Alcaligenes odorans*	*Alcaligenes odorans* was proposed at a later date for an organism that is a strain of the earlier named *Alcaligenes faecalis*.
Alcaligenes piechaudii		New species. Isolated primarily from human clinical specimens, but some strains are isolated from the environment. Clinical significance is not known. There is one report of otitis media caused by this organism.
Alcaligenes xylosoxidans subsp. *xylosoxidans*	*Achromobacter xylosoxidans* *Alcaligenes denitrificans* subsp. *xylosoxidans* CDC IIIa and IIIb	
Alcaligenes xylosoxidans subsp. *denitrificans*	*Alcaligenes denitrificans* *Alcaligenes denitrificans* subsp. *denitrificans* CDC Vc	
Bordetella bronchiseptica	*Alcaligenes bronchicanis* *Alcaligenes bronchiseptica* *Bordetella bronchicanis* *Brucella bronchiseptica* *Haemophilus bronchiseptica*	Rapid urea–positive

(continued)

Table 3-2 (continued)

CURRENT USAGE	PREVIOUS DESIGNATIONS	COMMENTS
Burkholderia cepacia	*Pseudomonas cepacia* *Pseudomonas multivorans* *Pseudomonas kingae* CDC EO-1	Yellow pigment. Recovered from numerous water sources and wet surfaces. Respiratory pathogen in cystic fibrosis patients.
Burkholderia gladioli	*Pseudomonas gladioli* *Pseudomonas marginata*	Primarily plant pathogen. Has been reported from sputum of patients with cystic fibrosis.
Burkholderia pickettii	*Pseudomonas pickettii* CDC Va-1, Va-2 *Pseudomonas thomasii* (Va-3)	Slow growing, pinpoint colonies after 24 hours on BAP. Rarely associated with infection.
Burkholderia pseudomallei	*Pseudomonas pseudomallei*	Cause of melioidosis in humans
Chryseomonas luteola	CDC Ve-1 *Pseudomonas luteola* *Chryseomonas polytricha*	Yellow pigmented, oxidase-negative, esculin-positive
Comamonas acidovorans	*Pseudomonas acidovorans* *Pseudomonas desmolytica* *Pseudomonas indoloxidans* *Achromobacter cystino-vorum*	Orange indole reaction caused by production of an-phinilic acid from tryptone
Comamonas terrigena	Various species of *Vibrio* *Aquaspriillum aquaticum* E. Falsen Group 10	
Comamonas testosteroni	*Pseudomonas testosteroni* *Pseudomonas desmolytica* *Pseudomonas dacunhae* *Pseudomonas cruciviae*	
Flavimonas oryzihabitans	CDC Ve-2 *Pseudomonas oryzihabitans* *Pseudomonas lacunogenes*	Clinical isolates associated with septicemia and prosthe-tic valve endocarditis. Yellow pigment, oxidase-negative, esculin-negative
Flavobacterium indo-logenes	CDC IIb	
Flavobacterium men-ingosepticum	CDC IIa	Highly pathogenic for premature infants
Flavobacterium odoratum	CDC M-4F	

(continued)

Table 3-2 (continued)

CURRENT USAGE	PREVIOUS DESIGNATIONS	COMMENTS
Moraxella atlantae	CDC M-3	
Moraxella lacunata	*Moraxella liquefaciens*	
Moraxella nonliquefaciens	*Bacillus duplex nonlique-faciens*	
Moraxella osloensis	*Mima polymorpha* var. *oxidans*	
Moraxella phenylpyruvica	CDC M-2	Phenylalanine deaminase–positive
Moraxella species CDC M-5	CDC M-5	Clinical isolates associated with dog bites
Neisseria elongata subsp. *nitroreducens*	*Moraxella* species CDC M-6	Similar to *Moraxella* species except catalase-negative; clinical isolates are associated with endocarditis.
Ochrobactrum anthropi	CDC Vd-1, Vd-2 *Achromobacter* spp. bio. 1 and 2	
Oligella ureolytica	CDC IVe	Rapid urea–positive and phenylalanine deaminase–positive
Oligella urethralis	CDC M-4	Clinical isolates have been from ear and urinary tract infections
Pseudomonas aeruginosa	*Pseudomonas pyocyanea* *Bacterium aeruginosa*	
Pseudomonas diminuta	CDC Ia	
Pseudomonas fluorescens		
Pseudomonas mendocina	CDC Vb-2	
Pseudomonas putida		Belongs to fluorescent group
Pseudomonas stutzeri	CDC Vb-1	Wrinkled colonies. Ubiquitous in soil and water. Rarely associated with infection.
Pseudomonas vesicularis	*Corynebacterium vesiculare*	

(continued)

Table 3-2 (continued)

CURRENT USAGE	PREVIOUS DESIGNATIONS	COMMENTS
Shewanella putrefaciens	*Pseudomonas putrefaciens* *Alteromonas putrefaciens* *Achromobacter putrefaciens* CDC Ib-1, Ib-2	Hydrogen sulfide–positive
Sphingobacterium multi-vorum	CDC IIk-2 *Flavobacterium multivorum*	Yellow pigment, oxidase-positive, esculin-positive
Sphingobacterium spiri-tivorum	CDC IIk-3 *Flavobacterium spiritivorum* *Sphingobacterium versatilis*	Yellow pigment, oxidase-positive, esculin-positive
Sphingomonas pau-cimobilis	*Pseudomonas paucimobilis* CDC IIk-1	
Stenotrophomonas mal-tophilia	*Xanthomonas maltophilia* *Pseudomonas maltophilia* CDC I	Oxidase-negative
Weeksella virosa	CDC IIf *Flavobacterium genitale*	Mucoid and sticky. Difficult to remove from agar. Clinical isolates have been associated with urinary and vaginal infections
Weeksella zoohelcum	CDC IIj	Rapid urea–positive. Associated with dog and cat bites

All CDC alphanumeric designations are Roman numerals and lowercase letters.

ganic salts to form one of several so-called mixed acids. These acids are the end products of glucose metabolism by the EMP pathway, accounting for the drop in *p*H in fermentation tests used for identifying bacteria. Bacteria that possess the appropriate enzyme systems can further degrade these mixed acids into alcohols, CO_2, or other organic compounds.

Entner-Doudoroff Pathway

The Entner-Doudoroff (ED) pathway is also termed the *aerobic pathway* because oxygen is required for glycolysis to occur. Note in the center column of Figure 3-1 that glucose is not converted into two triose carbon molecules as in the EMP pathway; rather, it is oxidized to 6-phosphogluconate and 2-keto-3-deoxy-6-phosphogluconate before form-

ing pyruvic acid. "Oxidation" refers more to the manner in which pyruvic acid transfers its hydrogen ions than to the pathway by which it is formed. Lacking the dehydrogenase enzymes necessary to oxidize pyruvic acid to lactic acid or other "mixed acids," oxidative bacteria transfer the available hydrogen ions from pyruvic acid into the Krebs cycle, where the ions ultimately link with elemental oxygen to form water. Thus, the oxidative metabolism of carbohydrates is presently defined as the energy-yielding reactions that require molecular oxygen (or other nonorganic elements) as the terminal hydrogen (electron) acceptor.

This difference in metabolism necessitates alternate, practical approaches to the identification of oxidative and fermentative bacteria. The acids that are formed in the ED pathway (glucuronic acid and their derivatives) and those produced in the Krebs cycle (citric acid and its derivatives) are extremely

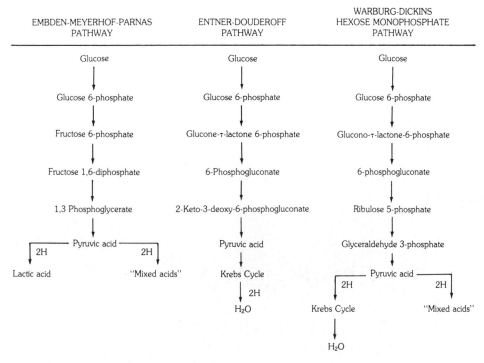

Figure 3-1. Metabolic pathways for the bacterial degradation of glucose.

weak compared with the mixed acids resulting from fermentation. Because the end product of oxidative metabolism is water, gas is not formed from carbohydrates by oxidative organisms. Therefore, test systems with more sensitive detectors of acid production must be used when studying oxidative bacteria, which are discussed in detail later in this chapter. Test systems designed to detect acid production from fermentative bacteria often cannot be applied to oxidative organisms that produce insufficient acids to convert the *p*H indicator.

Warburg-Dickens Hexose Monophosphate Pathway

Facultatively anaerobic bacteria have the capacity to grow on the surface of an agar plate in the presence of oxygen or in an anaerobic environment. Just because a microorganism can grow in an aerobic environment does not necessarily mean that oxygen is metabolically utilized. That is, not all aerobes are oxidative. The term *aerotolerant* is more appropriate for nonoxidative bacteria that are capable of growing in the presence of oxygen but that grow better in an anaerobic environment.

Many of the facultative anaerobes can use either the EMP or the ED pathway, depending on the environmental conditions in which they are growing. The hexose monophosphate pathway (HMP), as shown in the right-hand column of Figure 3-1, is actually a hybrid of the EMP and ED pathways. Note that the initial steps in the degradation of glucose in the HMP pathway parallel those of the ED pathway; later in the HMP scheme, glyceraldehyde-3-phosphate is formed as the precursor of pyruvic acid, similar to the EMP pathway. These organisms appear fermentative in test systems, even though the EMP pathway is not strictly used.

INITIAL CLUES THAT AN UNKNOWN ISOLATE IS A NONFERMENTER

Several characteristics used to make preliminary identification of the nonfermenters are presented in Table 3-1 and Color Plate 3-1. The microbiologist may suspect that an unknown gram-negative bacillus is a member of the nonfermenter group by observing one or more of the following characteristics:

▸ Lack of evidence for glucose fermentation (see Color Plate 3-1A)
▸ Positive cytochrome oxidase reaction (see Color Plate 3-1B)
▸ Failure to grow on MacConkey agar (see Color Plate 3-1C)

Lack of Evidence for Glucose Fermentation

Acids produced by nonfermenters are considerably weaker than the mixed acids derived from fermentative bacteria, thus the pH in fermentation test media, in which a nonfermenter is growing, may not drop sufficiently to convert the pH indicator. The initial clue that an unknown organism is a nonfermenter is usually the lack of acid production in either KIA or TSI media, manifest in each instance as an alkaline (red) slant and an alkaline deep (see Color Plate 3-1A). Before setting up differential systems, it is recommended that the oxidative/fermentative (OF) characteristic of all unknown isolates of gram-negative bacilli be assessed by inoculating a KIA or TSI slant.

Positive Cytochrome Oxidase Reaction

Any colony of a gram-negative bacillus growing on blood agar or other primary isolation media that is cytochrome oxidase–positive can be suspected of belonging to the nonfermentative group (see Color Plate 3-1B). Not all oxidase-positive, gram-negative bacilli are nonfermenters; therefore, the mode of glucose utilization must still be measured (again demonstrating the importance of setting up a KIA or TSI tube). The tests for cytochrome oxidase activity are discussed in Chapter 2. To test the oxidase activity of nonfermenters, the CDC recommends using a 0.5% aqueous solution of tetra-methyl-p-phenylenediamine hydrochloride. This solution is good for 1 week if stored in a dark bottle in the refrigerator at 4° to 10°C. A few drops of reagent can be used to flood the surface of agar medium on which bacterial colonies are growing. The development of a blue color within a few seconds indicates a positive test. Negative reactions can be confirmed using the more sensitive Kovac's method, in which a loopful of organisms is mixed with a few drops of reagent on a piece of filter paper (see Color Plate 3-1B). The development of a dark blue color within 10 seconds indicates a positive test result.

Failure to Grow on MacConkey Agar

A gram-negative bacillus that grows on blood agar but grows poorly or not at all on MacConkey agar should be suspected of belonging to the nonfermentative group. This guideline is far from absolute because many of the fastidious gram-negative bacilli also do not grow on MacConkey agar. The ability of bacteria to grow on MacConkey agar is determined by inspecting with reflected light the surface of plates that have been inoculated and then incubated for 24 to 48 hours. Interpretation of the growth patterns on MacConkey agar is usually not difficult. Organisms that grow well produce colonies that are 3 mm or more in diameter and easy to see. Poorly growing strains produce either widely scattered, tiny pinpoint colonies or absolutely no growth (see Color Plate 3-1C).

TESTS USED IN THE IDENTIFICATION OF NONFERMENTERS

Utilization of Glucose

Most conventional culture media designed to detect acid production from fermentative bacteria, such as the Enterobacteriaceae, are not suitable for the study of nonfermentative bacilli. They do not support the growth of many strains, and the acids produced are often too weak to convert the pH indicator. Hugh and Leifson[13] were the first to design an OF medium that accommodated the metabolic properties of the nonfermentative bacilli. The Hugh-Leifson OF medium contains 0.2% peptone and 1% carbohydrate, so that the ratio of peptone to carbohydrate is 1:5, in contrast to the 2:1 ratio found in media used for carbohydrate fermentation. The decrease in peptone minimizes the formation of oxidative products from amino acids, which tend to raise the pH of the medium and may neutralize the weak acids produced by the nonfermentative bacilli. On the other hand, the increase in carbohydrate concentration enhances acid production by the microorganism. The semisolid consistency of the agar, the use of bromthymol blue as the *p*H indicator, and the inclusion of a small quantity of diphosphate buffer are all designed to enhance the detection of acid.

Two tubes of each carbohydrate medium are required for the test. The medium in one tube is exposed to air; the other is overlaid with sterile mineral oil or melted paraffin (Fig. 3-2). Oxidative microorganisms produce acid only in the open tube exposed to atmospheric oxygen; fermenting organisms produce acid in both tubes; and nonsaccharolytic bacteria are inert in this medium, which remains at an alkaline *p*H after incubation. Color Plate 3-1*D* shows the OF reaction of an oxidative nonfermenter, with only the open tube showing the yellow color of acid production.

Motility

A semisolid agar medium for detecting motility of fermentative organisms may not be suitable for nonfermenting species that grow only on the surface of the agar. If a semisolid agar medium is used for nonfermentative bacilli, one should stab-inoculate only the upper 4 mm of the medium and make

an initial reading within 4 to 6 hours. Many motile strains of nonfermentative bacilli show only an early, faint haziness near the surface of the agar, which tends to disappear with prolonged incubation (see Color Plate 3-1*E*). Readings should again be made at 24 and 48 hours to detect the motility of slowly growing strains. Incubation at 25°C enhances the motility of some strains.

The hanging drop preparation may be more accurate in detecting motility of many species of nonfermentative bacilli. In this technique, a loopful of a 6- to 24-hour, actively growing broth culture that has been incubated at 25°C is placed in the center of a No. 1 coverslip that is inverted and suspended over the concavity of a depression slide. True motility must be differentiated from brownian movement or the flow of fluid beneath the coverslip. Motile bacteria show directional movement and change in position with respect to each other; when brownian movement is the cause of the motion, they maintain the same relative positions.

Pigment Production

A number of pigments are produced by nonfermenters, some of which are helpful in making a

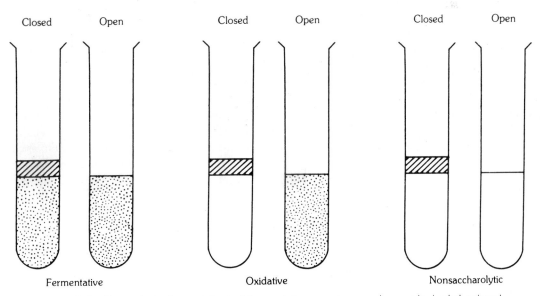

Figure 3-2. The oxidative-fermentative test. Fermentative organisms produce acid in both the closed and open tubes (stippled effect); oxidative organisms provide acid only in the open tube. Asaccharolytic organisms that do not utilize carbohydrates produce no change in either tube.

species identification (see Color Plate 3-1*F*). Water-insoluble pigments include carotenoids (yellow-orange), violacein (violet or purple), and phenazines (red, maroon, yellow) that impart distinctive colors to the colonies; water-soluble and diffusible pigments include fluorescein (pyoverdin), pyocyanin, pyorubin, melanin, and miscellaneous other pigmented byproducts that discolor the culture medium. "Tech" and "Flo" media[14] were developed to enhance formation of the water-soluble pigments pyocyanin and pyoverdin (see Color Plate 3-1*G*). Pigment production can also be enhanced by growing organisms in gelatin-, potato-, or milk-containing media and by incubating them at 25° to 30°C. Pyoverdin may be demonstrated by using a Wood's lamp or, on Flo agar, by the appearance of a yellow pigment in the media (see Color Plate 3-1*G* and *H*).

Hydrolysis of Urea

The test for urea hydrolysis is discussed in Chapter 2.

Nitrate Reduction and Denitrification of Nitrates and Nitrites

The basic principles and procedures for performing the nitrate reduction test are presented in Chapter 2. Denitrification refers to microorganisms that have the capability of reducing nitrate or nitrite (or both) to gaseous nitrogen. Nitrate or nitrite broth with an inverted Durham tube or an agar slant can be used. Because the media contain no carbohydrates, any gas that forms is derived from the nitrate or nitrite, indicating a positive denitrification test. The broth medium containing the inverted Durham tube is easier to interpret since any collection of gas within the inverted tube can be easily visualized.

Indole Production

The basic principles and procedure for determination of indole production are presented in Chapter 2. Minor modifications may be required when detecting indole production by certain weak-reacting nonfermenters. An enriched tryptophan-containing medium, usually heart infusion broth, may be required. Because only small quantities of indole are formed by some nonfermenters, extraction of the culture media by layering a small quantity of xylene or chloroform on the surface may be helpful. Care should be taken to add only a small quantity of extractant, since even minimal dilution may lower the concentration of indole below the sensitivity of detection by either Ehrlich's or Kovac's reagent. The appearance of a fuchsia red color at the interface of the surface of the medium (or the extractant) with the reagent indicates indole formation and constitutes a positive test result.

Decarboxylation

The Moeller method for detecting decarboxylation of an amino acid (described in Chapter 2) is based on a change in *p*H. The development of an alkaline purple color in the test medium, after inoculation with the test organism and incubation at 35°C for 24 to 48 hours, constitutes a positive test result. Many nonfermenters display only weak decarboxylase activity and may produce insufficient amines to convert the *p*H indicator system. The sensitivity of detection can be increased by using only small quantities of substrates (1 to 2 mL) and a heavy inoculum of pregrown organisms in which a high concentration of enzymes has already accumulated and by overlaying the culture medium with 4 mm of petrolatum. It is essential that uninoculated, amino acid–free substrate controls be used to compare the color reactions. The initial conversion of the medium to a yellow color as acids accumulate from the small amount of glucose in the medium is not seen with nonfermenters; rather, the end point reactions are read comparing the strong alkaline purple color reactions with the lighter blue-green hue of the controls. Tubes should be incubated at 35°C for up to 5 days before interpreting the reaction as negative.

Esculin Hydrolysis

Esculin hydrolysis is used primarily as a differential characteristic to distinguish certain *Pseudomonas* species and the Ve group of nonfermenters. Organisms to be tested are inoculated onto the surface of esculin agar slants and observed under ultraviolet light using a Wood's lamp after 24 to 48 hours of incubation. Esculin in the medium fluoresces when observed with Wood's lamp. When esculin is hydrolyzed, the medium turns reddish black and fluorescence is lost, indicating a positive test result.

MEDICALLY IMPORTANT GENERA OF NONFERMENTERS

In the space available here, it is possible to provide only a brief summary of the medically important nonfermenters. Several references can be consulted for an in-depth discussion of the identifying features and clinical syndromes caused by this group of organisms.[7,8,10,11,15,19,24]

CLASSIFICATION OF NONFERMENTERS

Unlike the Enterobacteriaceae the nonfermenting gram-negative bacilli do not fit conveniently into a single family of well-characterized genera. For this reason the study of nonfermenters is often confusing for the beginning microbiologist. The major genera of nonfermenting gram-negative bacilli have been classified into five families (Alcaligenaceae, Cytophagaceae, Methylococcaceae, Pseudomonadaceae, Rhizobiaceae). The remaining genera of clinically important nonfermenters are as yet not assigned to a family and are grouped under the heading Organisms Whose Taxonomic Position Is Uncertain.

Family Alcaligenaceae

This family consists of the genera *Alcaligenes* and *Bordetella*.[6] The biochemical features that differentiate the members of this family, as well as certain other nonfermenters with similar biochemical characteristics, are given in Table 3-3.

Genus *Alcaligenes*

Members of the genus *Alcaligenes* are gram-negative rods that are oxidase-positive, grow on MacConkey agar, and are motile by means of peri-

trichous flagella. Additional differentiating characteristics are given in Table 3-3.

A. faecalis is the most frequently isolated member of the Alcaligenaceae in the clinical laboratory. Members of this species produce strong alkaline reactions in all carbohydrate media. Most strains form characteristic colonies with a thin spreading irregular edge. Some strains (previously named *A. odorans*) produce a characteristic fruity odor (sometimes described as the odor of green apples) and cause a greenish discoloration of blood agar medium. A key biochemical feature of this species is its ability to reduce nitrite but not nitrate. *A. faecalis* exists in the soil and water and has been isolated from many types of clinical specimens. Most infections are opportunistic and acquired from moist items such as nebulizers, respirators, and lavage fluids. Blood, sputum, and urine are common sites of recovery.

A. xylosoxidans and *A. piechaudii* are less commonly recovered species. *A. xylosoxidans* subspecies *xylosoxidans* has been reported as a cause of nosocomial pneumonia, bacteremia, and meningitis. *A. piechaudii* has been isolated mainly from human clinical material, but there is only one report of a possible pathogenic role for this species.[23]

Genus *Bordetella*

The three species *B. pertussis*, *B. parapertussis*, and *B. bronchiseptica* cannot be differentiated genotypically through DNA homology studies, but phenotypically they behave differently. *B. bronchiseptica* is motile by means of peritrichous flagella and grows readily on ordinary media. *B. pertussis* and *B. parapertussis* are nonmotile and require special media for growth. Accordingly, these latter two species will not be discussed in detail here but are covered in Chapter 6. Colonies of *B. bronchiseptica* grow well on blood and MacConkey agar and in 24 hours appear as smooth translucent, colorless colonies about 1.5 mm in diameter. On Gram stain, the organisms appear small and coccobacillary. They have the distinguishing biochemical feature of rapidly converting Christensen's urea agar. Other distinguishing features are given in Table 3-3. *B. bronchiseptica* is found in the respiratory tract of domestic and wild mammalian animals. It is an infrequent isolate in the clinical laboratory, and only a few cases of human infections have been reported.

Table 3-3
Key Characteristics of Alcaligenes, Bordetella, and Related Species

TEST	Alcaligenes				Bordetella Bronchiseptica	IVc-2	Oligella Ureolytica (IVe)	Oligella Urethralis (M-4)
	A. faecalis (odorans)	A. xylosoxidans subsp. xylosoxidans	A. xylosoxidans subsp. denitrificans	A. piechaudii				
Oxidase	+	+	+	+	+	+	+	+
Growth on MacConkey	+	+	+	+	+	+	V (79)	V (83)
Motility	+	+	+	+	+	+	V (84)	−
OF glucose	ALK	A	ALK	ALK	ALK	ALK	AlK	ALK
OF xylose	ALK	A	ALK	ALK	ALK	ALK	AlK	ALK
NO_3 to NO_2	−	V (69)	+	+	+	−	+	−
NO_3 to N_2	−	−	+	−	−	−	V (58)	−
NO_2 to N_2	+	−	+	−	−	−	V (63)	V (33)
Urea	−	−	V (31)	−	++	++	++	−
PAD	−	−	−	−	V (25)	−	+	+
Acetamide	+	V (66)	V (45)	NA	−	−	−	−
6.5% NaCl	+	−	−	+	−	−	−	−
Flagella	Pert.	Pert.	Pert.	Pert.	Pert.	Pert.	P, L	−

+, 90% or more of strains positive; −, 90% or more of strains negative; V, 11%–89% of strains positive; ++, strong positive reaction; A, acid reaction; ALK, alkaline reaction; NA, results not available; numbers in parentheses are percentage strains giving positive reaction; Pert., peritrichous; P, polar; L, lateral.

(Data from Gilardi GL. Identification of glucose-nonfermenting gram-negative rods. New York, North General Hospital, 1990; and Kiredjian M, Holmes B, Kersters K, et al. Alcaligenes piechaudii, a new species from human clinical specimens and the environment. Int J Syst Bacteriol 1986;36:282–287)

Family Cytophagaceae

The members of the Cytophagaceae include the genera *Flavobacterium*, *Sphingobacterium*, and *Weeksella*. The key differentiating features of the clinically significant members of the family are given in Table 3-4. Most species produce yellow-pigmented colonies on blood agar medium, and all are oxidase-positive. All species are nonmotile and negative for nitrate reduction, and most species fail to grow on MacConkey agar. Most species (except *W. virosa*) are polymyxin resistant, a property they share with the pseudomallei group discussed elsewhere in this chapter.

Genus *Flavobacterium*

The flavobacteria occur naturally in soil, water, plants, and foodstuffs. In the hospital environment these bacteria exist in water systems and wet surfaces. *Flavobacterium* species (except *F. odoratum*) are readily distinguished from other nonfermenters by their ability to produce indole in tryptophan broth. The indole reaction is often weak and difficult to demonstrate; therefore, the more sensitive Ehrlich method should be used. *F. indologenes* is the most frequently isolated species from human clinical specimens and is easily recognized by the production of dark yellow colonies. *F. meningosepticum*, in contrast, produces colonies with a very pale yellow pigment that may not be evident on initial examination of colonies at 24 hours. Pigment production may be augmented by incubating the culture for an additional 24 hours at room temperature. *F. odoratum* is distinctive in that it typically forms effuse, spreading colonies that may be confused with the colony morphology of a *Bacillus* species. A telltale feature of *F. odoratum* is a characteristic fruity odor (similar to the odor of *A. faecalis*). Although strains of *F. odoratum* grow on MacConkey agar, the other *Flavobacterium* species generally grow poorly or not at all on this medium. Additional characteristics of *Flavobacterium* species can be found in Table 3-4. *F. meningosepticum* (formerly CDC group IIa) is the species most often associated with significant disease in humans. It is highly pathogenic for premature infants and has been associated with neonatal meningitis; it may also cause pneumonia in adults, usually in immunosuppressed patients.

Weeksella and *Sphingobacterium*

The genus *Weeksella* contains two species, *W. virosa* (formerly CDC group IIf) and *W. zoohelcum* (formerly CDC group IIj). Like the flavobacteria, both species are indole-positive but have the unusual feature of being susceptible to penicillin. *W. virosa* forms mucoid, sticky colonies that are difficult to remove from agar and has been primarily recovered from the urogenital tract of women. *W. zoohelcum* is part of the normal oral and nasal flora of dogs, and, as might be expected, the majority of human isolates have been from dog or cat bites.

The sphingobacteria are differentiated from flavobacteria and weeksellae by their failure to produce indole from tryptophan. Additional differentiating features of these bacteria are given in Table 3-4.

Family Methylococcaceae

Genus *Methylobacterium*

Methylobacterium species are gram-negative, pink-pigmented bacteria. *M. mesophilicum* is the species most often isolated from human clinical specimens. Isolates are reported to be oxidase-positive and motile, but the oxidase reaction may be weak and motility may be difficult to demonstrate. Other key reactions include positive tests for catalase, urease, and amylase. Isolates are slow growing on ordinary media, with best growth occurring on Sabouraud agar, buffered charcoal-yeast extract agar, or Middlebrook 7H11 agar. Optimal growth occurs from 25° to 30°C.

Family Pseudomonadaceae

The genus *Pseudomonas* and some closely related genera, many of which were formerly placed in the genus *Pseudomonas*, make up what is now the Pseudomonadaceae.[21]

Gilardi,[11] after several years of exhaustively observing various phenotypic characteristics, divided the pseudomonads into seven major groups: fluorescent, stutzeri, alcaligenes, pseudomallei, acidovorans, facilis-delafieldii, and diminuta. Parallel to his work has been that of Palleroni[21] and others, who have proposed a taxonomy based on rRNA/DNA homology studies. The Palleroni classifica-

Table 3-4
Key Characteristics of the Family Cytophagaceae*

TEST	FLAVOBACTERIUM			WEEKSELLA		SPHINGOBACTERIUM	
	F. meningosepticum IIa	F. indologenes IIb	F. odoratum M-4F	W. virosa IIf	W. zoohelcum IIj	S. multivorum IIk2	S. spiritivorum IIk3
Oxidase	+	+	+	+	+	+	+
Growth on MacConkey agar	V (26)	-	V (78)	-	-	V (17)	-
Motility	-	-	-	-	-	-	-
OF glucose	A†	A†	-	-	-	A	A
OF mannitol	A†	-	-	-	-	-	A
Indole	+	+	-	+	+	-	-
Starch hydrolysis	-	+	-	-	-	V (79)	-
Esculin	+	+	-	-	-	+	+
ONPG	+	V (41)	-	-	-	+	+
DNase	+	-	+	-	-	-	+
Urea	-	-	+	-	++	+	+
Penicillin	R	R	V	S	S	R	R
Polymyxin	R	R	R	S	R	R	R
Pigment (yellow)	Pale	Bright	Yellow-green	Pale	-	Pale	Pale

+, 90% or more of strains positive; −, 90% or more of strains negative; V, 11%–89% of strains positive; + +, strong positive reaction; A, acid reaction; ALK, alkaline reaction; NA, results not available; R, resistant; S, susceptible; numbers in parentheses are percentage of strains giving positive reaction.

†Delayed reaction.

*(Data from Gilardi GL. Identification of glucose-nonfermenting gram-negative rods. New York, North General Hospital, 1990)

tion places the pseudomonads into one of five rRNA homology groups, which, in turn, include several smaller DNA homology groups. A classification that combines the genotypic grouping of Palleroni and the phenotypic grouping of Gilardi follows:

rRNA Group I
Fluorescent group
> *Pseudomonas aeruginosa*
> *Pseudomonas fluorescens*
> *Pseudomonas putida*

Stutzeri group
> *Pseudomonas stutzeri*
> *Pseudomonas mendocina*
> CDC group Vb-3

Alcaligenes group
> *Pseudomonas alcaligenes*
> *Pseudomonas pseudoalcaligenes*
> *Pseudomonas* species group 1

rRNA Group II
Pseudomallei group
> *Burkholderia mallei*
> *Burkholderia pseudomallei*
> *Burkholderia cepacia*
> *Burkholderia gladioli*
> *Burkholderia pickettii*

rRNA Group III
Acidovorans group
> *Comamonas acidovorans*
> *Comamonas terrigena*
> *Comamonas testosteroni*

Facilis-delafieldii Group
> *Acidovorax delafieldii*
> *Acidovorax facilis*
> *Acidovorax temperans*

rRNA Group IV
Diminuta group
> *Pseudomonas diminuta*
> *Pseudomonas vesicularis*

rRNA Group V
> *Stenotrophomonas maltophilia*

Unknown Nucleic Acid Homology
> *Chryseomonas luteola*
> *Flavimonas oryzihabitans*
> *Shewanella putrefaciens*
> *Sphingomonas paucimobilis*
> *Pseudomonas*-like group 2

Members of this family have the characteristics of being straight or slightly curved, gram-negative bacilli that are strict aerobes; most strains are motile by means of one of more polar flagella; they utilize glucose and other carbohydrates oxidatively and are usually cytochrome oxidase–positive. The key differentiating features of the bacteria making up the Pseudomonadaceae are given in Table 3-5.

The following are the key phenotypic and clinical features of the organisms included in the Pseudomonadaceae.

rRNA Group I

FLUORESCENT GROUP. The species within this group are all characterized by the production of a water-soluble pyoverdin pigment that fluoresces white to blue-green under long-wavelength (400 nm) ultraviolet light. Although all three members of this group produce pyoverdin, only one species, *P. aeruginosa*, produces the distinctive blue, water-soluble pigment pyocyanin (see Color Plate 3-1*G*). The key biochemical features that separate the members of the fluorescent group are given in Table 3-5.

P. aeruginosa is the pseudomonad most frequently recovered from clinical specimens. *P. aeruginosa* infection is especially prevalent among patients with burn wounds, cystic fibrosis, acute leukemia, organ transplants, and intravenous drug addiction. Infections commonly occur at any site where moisture tends to accumulate—tracheostomies, indwelling catheters, burns, the external ear ("swimmer's ear"), and weeping cutaneous wounds. *P. fluorescens* and *P. putida* occur in water and soil and may exist in water sources in the hospital environment. Both are normal flora of the oral cavity and are rare opportunistic pathogens in humans.

STUTZERI GROUP. The organisms in the Stutzeri group are all soil denitrifiers and can grow anaerobically in nitrate- containing media with production of nitrogen gas. Strains are motile by means of polar monotrichous flagella. Characteristics that differentiate members of the Stutzeri group are given in Table 3-5.

P. stutzeri (formerly CDC group Vb-1) is ubiquitous in soil and water and has been recovered from humus, manure, straw, sewage, stagnant wa-

(*text continues on page 94*)

Table 3-5
Key Characteristics of the Family Pseudomonadaceae

	OXIDASE	MOTILITY	PYOVERDIN	GLUCOSE	MALTOSE	LACTOSE	MANNITOL	ARGININE	LYSINE	NO3-NO2	NO3-N2	UREA HYD	ONPG	DNAse	ACETAMIDE	ESCULIN	POLYMYXIN
RNA Group I																	
Genus: *Pseudomonas*																	
Fluorescent Group																	
P. aeruginosa	+	+	+	+	v	–	v	+	–	+	v	v	–	–	+	–	S
P. fluorescens	+	+	+	+	v	–	+	+	–	v	–	v	–	–	–	–	S
P. putida	+	+	+	+	v	–	v	+	–	–	–	v	–	–	–	–	S
Stutzeri Group																	
P. stutzeri	+	+	–	+	+	–	v	–	–	+	+	v	–	–	–	–	S
P. mendocina	+	+	–	+	–	–	–	+	–	+	+	v	–	–	–	–	S
CDC group Vb-3	+	+	–	+	+	–	+	+	–	+	+	v	–	–	–	–	S
Alcaligenes Group																	
P. alcaligenes	+	+	–	–	–	–	–	–	–	v	–	v	–	–	–	NA	S
P. pseudoalcaligenes	+	+	–	–	–	–	–	v	–	+	–	–	–	–	–	–	S
Pseudomonas species group 1	+	+	–	–	–	–	–	v	–	+	+	–	–	–	–	NA	S
RNA Group II																	
Genus: *Burkholderia*																	
Pseudomallei Group																	
B. pseudomallei	+	+	–	+	+	+	+	+	–	+	+	v	–	–	–	v	R
B. cepacia	w	+	–	+	+	+	+	–	+	v	–	v	v	–	v	v	R
B. gladioli	–	+	–	+	–	–	+	–	–	v	–	+	+	–	–	–	R
B. pickettii	+	+	–	+	v	v	v	–	–	v	v	+	–	–	–	–	R

92

RNA Group III

Genus: Comamonas

Acidovorans Group

RNA Group IV

Genus: Pseudomonas

Diminuta Group

RNA Group V

Unknown Nucleic Acid Homology

	OXIDASE	MOTILITY	PYOVERDIN	GLUCOSE	MALTOSE	LACTOSE	MANNITOL	ARGININE	LYSINE	$NO_3^- - NO_2$	$NO_3^- - N_2$	UREA HYD	ONPG	DNAse	ACETAMIDE	ESCULIN	POLYMYXIN
C. acidovorans	+	+	−	−	−	−	+	−	−	+	+	−	−	−	+	−	V
C. terrigena	+	+	−	−	−	−	−	−	−	+	−	−	−	−	−	NA	S
C. testosteroni	+	+	−	−	−	−	−	−	−	+	−	−	−	−	−	NA	S
P. diminuta	+	+	−	V	−	−	−	−	−	−	−	−	−	V	−	−	V
P. vesicularis	+	+	−	V	V	−	−	−	−	−	−	−	V	−	−	+	S
Genus: Stenotrophomonas																	
S. maltophilia	−	+	−	+	++	+	−	−	+	V	−	−	+	+	−	+	S
Genus: Chryseomonas																	
C. luteola	−	+	−	+	+	−	+	V	−	V	−	V	+	−	−	+	S
Genus: Flavimonas																	
F. oryzihabitans	−	+	−	+	+	−	+	−	−	−	−	V	−	−	−	−	S
Genus: Shewanella																	
S. putrefaciens*	+	+	−	+	V	−	−	−	−	+	−	−	−	+	−	−	S
Genus: Sphingomonas																	
S. paucimobilis	+	+	−	+	+	+	−	−	−	−	−	−	+	−	−	+	S

+, 90% or more strains positive; −, 90% or more strains negative; V, 11%–89% of strains positive; ++, strong positive reaction; NA, results not available; R, resistant; S, susceptible; shaded areas indicate key reactions.

*Other key reactions are production of hydrogen sulfide in KIA and ornithine decarboxylase.

(Data from Gilardi GI. Identification of glucose-nonfermenting gram-negative rods. New York, North General Hospital, 1990; and Gilardi GI. Pseudomonas and related genera. In: Balows A, ed. Manual of clinical microbiology. 5th ed. Washington, DC, American Society for Microbiology, 1991;429–441) ter, baby formula, hospital equipment, eye cosmetics, and various clinical specimens.[11] Freshly isolated colonies are adherent and have a characteristic wrinkled appearance, which may be lost after repeated laboratory subculture. *P. mendocina* (formerly CDC group Vb-2) and the unnamed species CDC group Vb-3 are rarely isolated from clinical specimens.

ALCALIGENES GROUP. Organisms in the Alcaligenes group are characterized by being asaccharolytic or only weakly saccharolytic in OF glucose medium. Additional characteristics are given in Table 3-5. Although members of this group are recovered from clinical specimens, their ability to act as human pathogens has only rarely been documented.

rRNA Group II

PSEUDOMALLEI GROUP. All species in rRNA homology group II have been transferred to the new genus *Burkholderia*.[30] The pseudomallei group is easily separated from other groups of pseudomonads by the property of exhibiting resistance to the polymyxin group of antibiotics (polymyxin B and colistin). The biochemical characteristics used to distinguish the members of this group are given in Table 3-5. *B. mallei* is the cause of glanders in horses and is not a human pathogen. The remaining members of this group, however, have all been associated with human disease.

B. pseudomallei causes melioidosis, a glanders-like disease in animals and humans. This organism grows well on standard laboratory media and often produces wrinkled colonies and thus may resemble *P. stutzeri* morphologically. Laboratory workers are advised to use biologic safety hoods when working with this organism because laboratory-acquired infection with *P. pseudomallei* has been reported.[26] Further information on the clinical and laboratory features of melioidosis can be found in the reviews by Dance[4,5] and Leelarasamee and Bovornkitti.[16]

B. cepacia is a phytopathogen that causes onion bulb rot in plants and foot rot (jungle rot) in humans. It has been isolated from numerous water sources and wet surfaces, including detergent solutions and intravenous fluids. Clinical infections include pneumonia and pneumonitis in patients receiving contaminated anesthetics, urinary tract infection in patients receiving contaminated irriga-

tion fluids after catheterization or cystoscopy, septicemia after heart surgery, endocarditis due to contaminated heart valves, conjunctivitis, septic arthritis, and neonatal meningitis.[20] Since the early 1980s, *B. cepacia* has evolved as an opportunistic pathogen in patients with cystic fibrosis.

B. gladioli (formerly named *P. marginata*) is another rare isolate that has been reported in the sputum of patients with cystic fibrosis.[3]

B. pickettii is slow growing and produces only pinpoint colonies on blood agar plates after 24 hours. It is rarely associated with human infections but has been reported to cause nosocomial infections, including bacteremia and urinary tract infections.

rRNA Group III

Willems and colleagues[28] have proposed that the organisms belonging to rRNA group III be recognized as a new bacterial family, the Comamonadaceae.

ACIDOVORANS GROUP. This group consists of the organisms formerly named *Pseudomonas acidovorans*, *Pseudomonas testosteroni*, and *Comamonas terrigena*. All three are now considered to be species of *Comamonas*.[27] A key feature of *Comamonas* species is their inability to utilize glucose, and therefore all species produce an alkaline reaction in OF glucose medium (see Table 3-5). *C. acidovorans* is the most common of this group to be isolated from clinical specimens. It has the unique feature of producing an orange indole reaction owing to the production of anthranilic acid from tryptone. *C. acidovorans* has been isolated from a variety of clinical specimens and is usually considered to be nonpathogenic. *C. testosteroni* is an uncommon isolate in the clinical laboratory despite its wide environmental distribution. *C. terrigena* has not been isolated from human clinical specimens.

FACILIS-DELAFIELDII GROUP. Willems and colleagues have proposed a new genus, *Acidovorax*, that contains the following three species: *Acidovorax facilis* (formerly *Pseudomonas facilis*), *Acidovorax delafieldii* (formerly *Pseudomonas delafieldii*), and *Acidovorax temperans* (for several former *Pseudomonas* and *Alcaligenes* strains).[29] Two of the species, *A. delafieldii* and *A. temperans*, have been isolated from clinical specimens; no information regarding the clinical significance of these organisms is available.[11,29] *Acidovorax* species are oxidase-positive, are motile, and utilize carbohydrates oxidatively.

rRNA Group IV

DIMINUTA GROUP.   This group is represented by two species, *P. diminuta* and *P. vesicularis*. This group is characterized by the presence of a single, tightly coiled, polar flagella. *P. vesicularis* is slow growing and usually requires 48 hours of incubation for colonies to be observed and produce a dark yellow to orange pigment. It is easily separated from all other species of alkaline pseudomonads by virtue of a strong esculin hydrolysis reaction. We have isolated *P. vesicularis* from peritoneal dialysate fluid, a renal dialysis machine, an oral abscess, and a scalp wound. *P. diminuta* has been isolated in pure culture from the blood of three patients at the University of Illinois hospital.

rRNA Group V

STENOTROPHOMONAS MALTOPHILIA.   *Stenotrophomonas* is the new genus name for the organism formerly known as *Xanthomonas maltophilia* and *Pseudomonas maltophilia*.[22] It can be easily distinguished from other pseudomonads by virtue of being lysine and DNAse-positive and oxidase-negative (see Table 3-5). It vigorously attacks OF maltose but is usually negative or only weakly positive in OF glucose in 24 hours. Colonies may appear pale yellow or lavender green on blood agar medium. *S. maltophilia* is ubiquitous and can be recovered from almost any clinical site. It occasionally causes opportunistic infections and is emerging as an important hospital-acquired pathogen. Most strains are resistant to multiple antibiotics.

Unknown Nucleic Acid Homology

GENUS *CHRYSEOMONAS*.   The genus *Chryseomonas* consists of only one species, *C. luteola* (formerly CDC group Ve-1). The organism is motile by means of multitrichous polar flagella, is oxidase-negative, and grows on both MacConkey and blood agar media, producing yellow-pigmented colonies. Additional biochemical features are given in Table 3-5. It is a rare clinical isolate and has been recovered from a variety of clinical specimens, including wound, cervix, urine, and throat specimens.

GENUS *FLAVIMONAS*.   The genus *Flavimonas* is represented by a single species, *F. oryzihabitans* (formerly CDC group Ve-2). *F. oryzihabitans*, like *Chryseomonas luteola*, is motile, is oxidase-negative, and forms yellow-pigmented colonies on blood agar medium. This organism can be differentiated from *C. luteola* by negative reactions for esculin hydrolysis and *ortho*-nitrophenyl-β-D-galactopyranoside (ONPG) and the feature of having a single polar flagellum. Additional differential characteristics are given in Table 3-5. *F. oryzihabitans* has also been recovered from a variety of clinical sites, including wounds, sputum, ear, eye, inhalation therapy equipment, and blood.

GENUS *SHEWANELLA*.   The newly named genus *Shewanella* is composed of three species: *S. putrefaciens* (formerly *Pseudomonas putrefaciens*), *S. hanedai*, and *S. benthica*.[17] All three are generally associated with aquatic and marine habitats, however, the type species, *S. putrefaciens*, has been recovered from human clinical specimens. Strains of *S. putrefaciens* are oxidase-positive and motile by means of polar flagella. They are easily distinguished by virtue of the fact that they are the only nonfermenters that produce hydrogen sulfide in KIA and TSI media (see Table 3-5). Colonies produce an orange-tan pigment on blood agar medium. Although it is an infrequent clinical isolate, *S. putrefaciens* has been isolated from skin ulcers, ear discharge, intra-abdominal abscess, human bile, and blood.[18]

GENUS *SPHINGOMONAS*.   *Sphingomonas paucimobilis* was formerly known as *Pseudomonas paucimobilis* and as CDC group IIk-1. It is a gram-negative, motile rod with a polar flagellum. Few cells are actively motile in broth culture, thus making motility a difficult characteristic to demonstrate. Motility occurs at 18° to 22°C but not at 37°C. The oxidase reaction is positive, although Gilardi[9] has reported that only 90% of the strains are oxidase-positive. Colonies grown on blood agar medium are yellow pigmented; this species is slow growing, and only small colonies may be observed after 24 hours of incubation. Growth occurs at 37°C but not at 42°C, with optimum growth occurring at 30°C.[21] Additional biochemical features are given in Table 3-5. *S. paucimobilis* has been isolated from a variety of clinical specimens, including blood, cerebrospinal fluid, urine, wounds, vagina, and cervix, and from the hospital environment.[12]

Organisms Whose Taxonomic Position Is Uncertain

Genus *Acinetobacter*

Acinetobacter species are nonmotile, oxidase-negative coccobacilli. Studies have revealed that the genus consists of at least 12 DNA hybridization groups referred to as genospecies.[1] Genospecies 2 is the most common genospecies found in human clinical specimens and has been named *A. baumannii*. It includes those isolates previously referred to as *A. calcoaceticus* var. *anitratus*. Further discussion of the taxonomic placement of the genus *Acinetobacter* and the related genus *Moraxella* is found in Chapter 7.

One initial clue that a nonfermenter isolate may belong to the genus *Acinetobacter* is the Gram stain morphology: gram-negative coccobacillary cells often appear as diplococci. After 24 hours of growth on blood agar, the colonies are between 0.5 and 2 mm in diameter, translucent to opaque (never pigmented), convex, and entire. Most strains grow well on MacConkey agar and produce a faint blue tint. Presumptive identification of *Acinetobacter* species can be made on the basis of the lack of cytochrome oxidase activity, lack of motility, and resistance to penicillin.

A. baumannii (formerly *A. calcoaceticus* var. *anitratus*) is the species most prevalent in clinical specimens and most often responsible for hospital-acquired infections. *A. baumannii* is saccharolytic and acidifies most OF carbohydrates; in particular, definitive identification is made by demonstrating the rapid production of acid from lactose (1% and 10% concentrations). In contrast, *A. lwoffii* (genospecies 8) is asaccharolytic. Additional differentiating features of the 12 genospecies can be found in the paper of Bouvet and Grimont.[1]

A variety of human infections have been reported to be caused by *Acinetobacter* species, including pneumonia (most often related to endotracheal tubes or tracheostomies), endocarditis, meningitis, skin and wound infections, peritonitis (in patients receiving peritoneal dialysis), and urinary tract infections.

Genus *Moraxella*

The correct taxonomic placement of the genus *Moraxella* remains a controversy. It has been proposed that the genus *Branhamella* be transferred to the genus *Moraxella* in the Neisseriaceae, a proposal that is included in the most recent edition of *Bergey's Manual of Systematic Bacteriology*.[2] More recently, two new proposals have been made, one assigning *Moraxella* to the new family Moraxellaceae and another assigning *Moraxella* to the new family Branhamaceae. A more detailed review of the taxonomic placement of the genus *Moraxella* is given in Chapter 7.

Several key features make one suspect that an unknown nonfermenter may belong to the genus *Moraxella*. After 24 hours on blood agar, the colonies tend to be small and pinpoint (usually less than 0.5 mm in diameter) with poor or no growth on MacConkey agar. The bacterial cells appear as tiny, gram-negative diplococci or diplobacilli in Gram-stained preparations. Both the cytochrome oxidase and catalase reactions are positive (the former rules out *Acinetobacter* species; the latter rules out *Kingella* species). The inability of *Moraxella* species to form acid from carbohydrates also eliminates most *Neisseria* species from consideration. *Branhamella* (*Moraxella*) *catarrhalis* is also asaccharolytic and may be difficult to distinguish. Most *Moraxella* species are extremely sensitive to low concentrations of penicillin. Examination of Gram-stained smears prepared from the outer zone of inhibition around the penicillin susceptibility disk can be used to distinguish *Neisseria* and *Branhamella* species (which retain their coccoid morphology) from *Moraxella* species (which produce elongated, pleomorphic forms. All *Moraxella* species are nonmotile.

The *Moraxella* species of medical importance are *M. lacunata*, *M. nonliquefaciens*, *M. osloensis*, *M. phenylpyruvica* (CDC group M-2), and *M. atlantae* (CDC group M-3). Species identifications are not made in most laboratories because many strains are fastidious and biochemical reactions are often equivocal. *Moraxella* species are normal flora on mucosal surfaces. They occur most frequently in the respiratory tract and less commonly in the genital tract and occasionally may cause systemic infection.

Other Species of Nonfermenters

There are several other species of nonfermenters of uncertain classification that are infrequently recovered in clinical laboratories. Omitted from discussion here are organisms such as *Ochrobactrum anthropi* and *Agrobacterium tumefaciens*, the names given to the urease-positive "*Achromobacter*" species, formerly designated CDC groups Vd-1,

Vd-2, and Vd-3 and unnamed CDC groups EO-2 and EO-3. Differentiating characteristics for these organisms are given in Table 3-6. Also omitted from discussion are the genus *Oligella* consisting of two species, *O. urethralis* (formerly *Moraxella urethralis* and CDC group (M-4) and *O. ureolytica* (formerly CDC group IVe); and unnamed CDC groups IVc-2. Characteristics that differentiate these species are given in Table 3-3.

APPROACH TO RECOVERY AND IDENTIFICATION OF NONFERMENTERS

Levels of Service in Identification of Nonfermenters

The level to which species identification of nonfermenters is performed depends on the size and purpose of the individual laboratory. Reference laboratories, or universities and clinics, where students and residents are being trained, may be required to identify all recovered nonfermenters to the species level. Laboratories that provide services primarily for the medical community may be prepared to identify only the more frequently encountered species, sending the rare isolates to a reference laboratory. In most clinical laboratories, a single species, namely *P. aeruginosa*, accounts for about two thirds or more of all nonfermentative bacilli isolates, followed in order by *A. anitratus* (now *A. baumannii*), about 7%; *S. maltophilia* and *Flavobacterium* species, about 4% each; and all other nonfermenter species comprising the remaining 20% in about equal proportions.

Identification of Most Common Species

The identification of the two most commonly recovered clinical species, *P. aeruginosa* and *A. baumannii*, is addressed first. Most strains can be iden-

Table 3-6
Characteristics of *Ochrobactrum*, *Agrobacterium*, Saccharolytic *Alcaligens*, and CDC EO Groups

TEST	Ochrobactrum Anthropi VD-1, Vd-2	Agrobacterium Tumefaciens Vd-3	Alcaligenes Xylosoxidans SUBSP. Xylosoxidans	CDC GROUP EO-2	CDC GROUP EO-3
Oxidase	+	+	+	+	+
OF glucose	A	A	A	A	A
OF xylose	A	A	A	A	A
OF lactose	−	A	−	A	A
OF mannitol	V (50)	A	−	V (50)	wk +
NO₃ to NO₂	+	V (84)	+	V (42)	−
NO₃ to N₂	+	−	V (69)	−	−
Urea	+	+	−	+ (75)	+
Phenylalanine deaminase	+	+	−	−	NA
Esculin hydrolysis	V (40)	+	−	−	−
Motility	+	+	+	−	−
Flagella	Pert.	Pert.	Pert.	−	−
Yellow pigment	−	−	−	−	+

+, 90% or more of strains positive; −, 90% or more of strains negative; V, 11%–89% of strains positive; A, acid reaction; ALK, alkaline reaction; NA, results not available; Pert., peritrichous; numbers in parentheses are percentage of strains giving positive reaction.
(Data from Gilardi GL. Identification of glucose-nonfermenting gram-negative rods. New York, North General Hospital, 1990; Moss CW, Wallace PL, Hollis DG, et al. Cultural and chemical characterization of CDC groups EO-2, M-5, and M-6, Moraxella [Moraxella] species, Oligella urethralis, Acinetobacter species, and Psychrobacter immobilis. J Clin Microbiol 1988;26:484–492; and Pickett MJ, Hollis DG, Bottone EJ. Miscellaneous gram-negative bacteria. In: Balows A, ed. Manual of clinical microbiology. 5th ed. Washington, DC, American Society for Microbiology, 1991;410–428)

tified easily on the basis of only a few observations and chemical tests. Not only does the rapid identification of these common isolates provide the physician with immediate information, but it also relieves the laboratory of performing a battery of time-consuming and expensive secondary tests.

Identification of *Pseudomonas aeruginosa*

More than 95% of *P. aeruginosa* strains recovered from clinical specimens can be identified by observing the presence of the following primary characteristics:

▸ Forms large colonies that have a grapelike odor
▸ Produces pyocyanin
▸ Is oxidase-positive (within 10 seconds)

Most strains produce pyocyanin, a water-soluble green phenazine pigment that imparts a greenish color to the culture medium. In fact, it is probable that observing the presence of pyocyanin may be the only characteristic required to identify *P. aeruginosa* because no other nonfermenter synthesizes this pigment. Reyes and coworkers[25] have shown that 98% of the *P. aeruginosa* strains isolated in their laboratory produced pyocyanin on Tech agar within 48 hours and suggest that the use of Tech agar is a satisfactory alternative to the use of extensive identification schemes when *P. aeruginosa* is suspected. Detecting the grapelike odor is also a helpful clue when examining the growth on agar plates. The colonies are large, may be mucoid or dry, and often spread. A few strains of *P. aeruginosa* may produce pigments with other colors — pyorubin (red), pyomelanin (brown to black), and pyoverdin (yellow).

Fluorescein pigment can be visualized by observing the growth on certain media using a long-wavelength ultraviolet light source (*eg*, Wood's lamp); see Color Plate 3-1*H*. Media containing proteose peptone 3 (Difco Laboratories, Detroit, MI) and cations, such as magnesium or manganese, enhance fluorescein synthesis. King's medium B, Sellers' medium, and Mueller-Hinton agar are also suitable for demonstrating fluorescence. The following additional characteristics are helpful in identifying non–pigment-producing strains of *P. aeruginosa*:

▸ Grows at 42°C
▸ Alkalinizes acetamide
▸ Denitrifies nitrates and nitrites
▸ Is motile by way of polar, monotrichous flagellum

In summary, most strains of *P. aeruginosa* can be identified easily by observing the typical large colonies with a blue-green discoloration on primary isolation media and further confirmed by detecting a typical grapelike odor. Demonstration of fluorescein pigment and cytochrome oxidase activity helps to confirm the final identification, and additional tests are usually not required. The typical characteristics by which *P. aeruginosa* is identified are shown in Table 3-5.

Identification of *Acinetobacter baumannii*

Acinetobacter baumannii (formerly *A. calcoaceticus* var. *anitratus*) is the second most frequent nonfermenter encountered in clinical laboratories, but with only about one tenth the frequency of *Pseudomonas aeruginosa*. The following are the characteristics by which a presumptive identification can be made:

▸ Appears as cocci or coccobacilli on Gram stain
▸ Grows well on MacConkey agar (colonies may have a slightly bluish tint, a helpful characteristic when present)
▸ Does not produce cytochrome oxidase
▸ Exhibits rapid utilization of glucose with production of acid
▸ Exhibits rapid utilization of 10% lactose with production of acid
▸ Is nonmotile
▸ Is penicillin resistant

The initial clue is the observation of tiny (1 by 0.7 μm) diplococci on Gram stains prepared directly from clinical materials. When Gram stains are prepared from agar or broth cultures, the cells may appear larger and more like coccobacilli. *Acinetobacter* species are not pigmented when grown on blood agar, a helpful characteristic in differentiating them from certain other nonfermenters, such as occasional oxidase-negative, nonmotile strains of *Pseudomonas cepacia*. Colonies growing on MacConkey agar may produce a faint blue tint or a deeper cornflower blue when observed on eosin methylene blue agar. Resistance to penicillin helps distinguish *A. baumannii* from the highly penicillin-sensitive *Moraxella* species, which also usually appear as coccobacilli in Gram stain. Most strains of *Moraxella* species are also cytochrome oxidase-positive. *A. lwoffii* is nonsaccharolytic and can be differentiated from *A. baumannii* because it produces no acid when grown in media that contain carbohydrates.

Identification of *Stenotrophomonas maltophilia*

Stenotrophomonas maltophilia (formerly *Xanthomonas maltophilia*) is the third most frequent nonfermenter encountered in clinical laboratories. The following are the characteristics by which a presumptive identification can be made:

- Grows well on blood and MacConkey agars
- Does not produce cytochrome oxidase
- Produces acid in OF maltose but may be negative in OF glucose
- Is lysine decarboxylase–positive
- Some strains have yellow pigment

The antibiotic susceptibility pattern can also be a clue to the identification of *S. maltophilia*, which is typically resistant to most antibiotics including the aminoglycosides but is susceptible to trimethoprim-sulfamethoxazole.

PRACTICAL APPROACH TO IDENTIFICATION OF NONFERMENTERS

If an unknown nonfermentative gram-negative bacillus is not *P. aeruginosa*, *A. baumannii*, or *S. maltophilia*, additional characteristics must be determined to make a species identification. Several schemes are currently being used in clinical laboratories. In many laboratories, hybrids of the test procedures used in published schemes are used. Which approach to select is largely one of personal preference, past experience, and the local availability of the culture media required to perform the various tests.

One approach is to divide the various clinically important nonfermentative bacilli into four functional groups based on an immediate assessment of their motility and ability to produce cytochrome oxidase. Based on these two reactions, the clinically important nonfermentative bacilli can be divided into the following four groups:

Oxidase-Negative, Nonmotile
Acinetobacter baumannii
Acinetobacter lwoffii
Bordetella parapertussis

Oxidase-Negative, Motile
Stenotrophomonas maltophilia
Burkholderia cepacia (93% are weak oxidase-positive)
Burkholderia gladioli
Chryseomonas luteola (Ve-1)
Flavomonas oryzihabitans (Ve-2)
Sphingomonas paucimobilis (IIk-1, 94% are oxidase-positive)

Oxidase-Positive, Nonmotile
Flavobacterium species
Oligella urethralis (M-4)
Moraxella species
Sphingobacterium multivorum (IIk-2)
Sphingobacterium spiritivorum (IIk-3)
Weeksella virosa (IIf)
Weeksella zoohelcum (IIj)

Oxidase-Positive, Motile
Oligella ureolytica (IVe)
Ochrobactrum anthropi (Vd-1, Vd-2)
Agrobacterium tumefaciens (Vd-3)
Group IVc-2
Pseudomonas aeruginosa and most other *Pseudomonas* species
Alcaligenes species
Bordetella bronchiseptica
Comamonas species

Definitive identifications of nonfermenters can be made by referring to specific tables that list specific biochemical tests for further differentiation of the species within the grouping. Those interested in pursuing this subject should see the various tables included in Chapter 4 of the *Color Atlas and Textbook of Diagnostic Microbiology*.[15]

COMMERCIAL KIT SYSTEMS

Packaged kit systems have been designed for, or adapted to, the identification of the nonfermentative bacilli. These kits share many of the attributes of packaged systems in general; that is, they are convenient to use, have a long shelf life, and preclude the need for fresh supplies of media and reagents. The packaged systems also provide standardized techniques that are accurate and give reproducible results equal to or better than conventional procedures, with certain exceptions.

Inherent problems in the use of many of the currently available packaged kits for identifying nonfermenters include the (1) tendency for organisms that exhibit weak or delayed biochemical activity to produce false-negative reactions, (2) less than optimal design of many systems for cultivation of certain nonfermenters, and (3) inclusion of some differential tests that may not be applicable to the identification of nonfermenters. Whereas members of the Enterobacteriaceae usually grow rapidly and exhibit active enzymatic activity on a variety of substrates that can readily be detected with kit systems, most nonfermenter species are slow growing and relatively inactive enzymatically. The microbiologist needs considerable experience to interpret some incomplete or weak reactions that may be encountered in the use of these systems.

The following five kit systems have been used with some success in identification of nonfermenting bacilli:

- Oxi/Ferm Tube (Becton Dickinson Microbiology Systems, Cockeysville, MD)
- API 20E (bioMérieux Vitek, Inc, Hazelwood, MO)
- Rapid NFT (bioMérieux Vitek, Inc, Hazelwood, MO)
- UNI-N/F System (Remel Laboratories, Lenexa, KS)
- Minitek System (Becton Dickinson Microbiology Systems, Cockeysville, MD)

Selection of a System

Clinical microbiologists must evaluate parameters such as accuracy, cost effectiveness, and effects on work flow when deciding whether to use a packaged system in identifying nonfermenters. The packaged systems perform with levels of accuracy equal to or better than conventional methods in identifying *P. aeruginosa*, *Acinetobacter* species, and *S. maltophilia*; these metabolically active organisms can also be identified easily by the methods described in this text. Because relatively few nonfermenters, particularly strains of species other than the three just mentioned, are encountered in most

medium-sized or small laboratories, the services of a reference laboratory should be seriously considered. Identifying nonfermenters is not difficult if the microbiologist is willing to devote the time and dedication necessary to achieve an acceptable level of accuracy. Packaged systems can be recommended, provided one understands their shortcomings and is willing to set up supplemental tests to identify weakly reactive or fastidious strains.

REFERENCES

1. Bouvet PJM, Grimont PAD. Taxonomy of the genus *Acinetobacter* with the recognition of *Acinetobacter baumannii* sp. nov., *Acinetobacter haemolyticus* sp. nov., *Acinetobacter johnsonii* sp. nov., and *Acinetobacter junii* sp. nov. and emended descriptions of *Acinetobacter calcoaceticus* and *Acinetobacter lwoffii*. Int J Syst Bacteriol 1986;36:228–240.

2. Bovre K. Family VIII. Neisseriaceae Prevot 1933, 119AL. In: Krieg NR, Holt JG, eds. Bergey's manual of systematic bacteriology. Baltimore, Williams & Wilkins, 1984;1:288–309.

3. Christenson JC, Welch DF, Mukwaya G, et al. Recovery of *Pseudomonas gladioli* from respiratory tract specimens of patients with cystic fibrosis. J Clin Microbiol 1989;27:270–273.

4. Dance DAB. Melioidosis. Rev Med Microbiol 1990;1:143–150.

5. Dance DAB. Melioidosis: the tip of the iceberg. Clin Microbiol Rev 1991;4:52–60.

6. De Ley J, Segers P, Kersters K, et al. Intra- and intergeneric similarities of the *Bordetella* ribosomal ribonucleic acid cistrons: proposal for a new family, *Alcaligenaceae*. Int J Syst Bacteriol 1986;36:405–414.

7. Gilardi GL, ed. Glucose nonfermenting gram-negative bacteria in clinical microbiology. West Palm Beach, FL, CRC Press, 1978.

8. Gilardi GL. Nonfermentative gram-negative rods: laboratory identification and clinical aspects. New York, Marcel Dekker, 1985.

9. Gilardi GL. Cultural and biochemical aspects for identification of glucose-nonfermenting gram-negative rods. In: Gilardi GL, ed. Nonfermentative gram-negative rods: laboratory identification and clinical aspects. New York, Marcel Dekker, 1985:17–84.

10. Gilardi GL. Identification of glucose-nonfermenting gram-negative rods. New York, North General Hospital, 1990

11. Gilardi GL. *Pseudomonas* and related genera. In: Balows A, ed. Manual of clinical microbiology. 5th

ed. Washington, DC, American Society for Microbiology, 1991:429–441.

12. Holmes B, Owen RJ, Evans A, et al. *Pseudomonas paucimobilis*, a new species isolated from human clinical specimens, the hospital environment, and other sources. Int J Syst Bacteriol 1977;27:133–146.

13. Hugh R, Leifson E. The taxonomic significance of fermentative versus oxidative metabolism of carbohydrates by various gram-negative bacteria. J Bacteriol 1953;66:24–26.

14. King EO, Ward MK, Raney DE. Two simple media for the demonstration of pyocyanin and fluorescein. J Lab Clin Med 1954;44:301–307.

15. Koneman EW, Allen SD, Janda WM, Schreckenberger PC, Winn WC Jr. Color atlas and textbook of diagnostic microbiology. 4th ed. Philadelphia, JB Lippincott, 1992.

16. Leelarasamee A, Bovornkitti S. Melioidosis: review and update. Rev Infect Dis 1989;11:413–425.

17. MacDonell MT, Colwell RR. Phylogeny of the Vibrionaceae, and recommendation for two new genera, *Listonella* and *Shewanella*. Syst Appl Microbiol 1985;6:171–182.

18. Marne C, Pallares R, Sitges-Serra A. Isolation of *Pseudomonas putrefaciens* in intraabdominal sepsis. J Clin Microbiol 1983;17:1173–1174.

19. Oberhofer TR. Manual of nonfermenting gram-negative bacteria. New York, John Wiley & Sons, 1985

20. Pallent LJ, Hugo WB, Grant DJW, et al. *Pseudomonas cepacia* as contaminant and infective agent. J Hosp Infect 1983;4:9–13.

21. Palleroni NJ. Family I. Pseudomonadaceae. In: Krieg NR, Holt JG, eds. Bergey's manual of systematic bacteriology. Baltimore, Williams & Wilkins, 1984;1:141–219.

22. Palleroni NJ, Bradbury JF. *Stenotrophomonas*, a new bacterial genus for *Xanthomonas maltophila* (Hugh 1980) Swings et al. 1983. Int J Syst Bacteriol 1993; 43:606–609.

23. Peel MM, Hibberd AJ, King BM, et al. *Alcaligenes piechaudii* from chronic ear discharge. J Clin Microbiol 1988;26:1580–1581.

24. Pickett MJ, Hollis DG, Bottone EJ. Miscellaneous gram-negative bacteria. In: Balows A, ed. Manual of clinical microbiology. 5th ed. Washington, DC, American Society for Microbiology, 1991: 410–428.

25. Reyes EAP, Bale MJ, Cannon WH, et al. Identification of *Pseudomonas aeruginosa* by pyocyanin production in Tech agar. J Clin Microbiol 1981; 13:456–458.

26. Schlech WF, Turchik JB, Westlake RE, et al. Laboratory-acquired infection with *Pseudomonas pseudomallei* (melioidosis). N Engl J Med 1981;305: 1133–1135.

27. Tamaoka J, Ha D-M, Komagata K. Reclassification of *Pseudomonas acidovorans* den Dooren de Jong 1926 and *Pseudomonas testosteroni* Marcus and Talalay 1956 as *Comamonas acidovorans* comb. nov. and *Comamonas testosteroni* comb. nov., with an emended description of the genus *Comamonas*. Int J Syst Bacteriol 1987;37:52–59.

28. Willems A, De Ley J, Gillis M, Kersters K. Comamonadaceae, a new family encompassing the Acidovorans rRNA complex, including *Variovorax paradoxus* gen. nov., comb. nov., for *Alcaligenes paradoxus* (Davis 1969). Int J Syst Bacteriol 1991; 41:445–450.

29. Willems A, Falsen E, Pot B, et al. *Acidovorax*, a new genus for *Pseudomonas facilis*, *Pseudomonas delafieldii*, E. Falsen (EF) group 13, EF group 16, and several clinical isolates, with the species *Acidovorax facilis* comb. nov., *Acidovorax delafieldii* comb. nov., and *Acidovorax temperans* sp. nov. Int J Syst Bacteriol 1990;40:384–398.

30. Yabuuchi E, Kosako Y, Oyaizu H, et al. Proposal of *Burholderia* gen. nov. and transfer of seven species of the genus *Pseudomonas* homology group II to the new genus, with the type species *Burkholderia cepacia* (Palleroni and Holmes 1981) comb. nov. Microbiol Immunol 1992;36:1251–1275.

4

Curved Gram-Negative Bacilli and Oxidase-Positive Fermenters: Campylobacters and Vibrionaceae

The genera of gram-negative bacilli to be discussed in this chapter are divided into two groups as follows:

Curved Gram-Negative Bacilli

Campylobacter species
Helicobacter species
Wolinella succinogenes
Arcobacter species
"*Flexispira rappini*"

Oxidase-Positive Fermenters

Family: Vibrionaceae
Vibrio species
Aeromonas species
Plesiomonas species
Listonella species
Shewanella species
Genus: *Chromobacterium*

CURVED RODS: *CAMPYLOBACTER, HELICOBACTER, WOLINELLA,* AND *ARCOBACTER*

Classification of *Campylobacter* and Related Taxa

All of the named *Campylobacter* species and related taxa belong to the same phylogenetic group, which is referred to as rRNA superfamily VI. Five genera, including *Campylobacter, Arcobacter, Helicobacter, Wolinella,* and "*Flexispira*" are included in rRNA superfamily VI. Characteristics that differentiate between these related genera are listed in Table 4-1.

Further studies have shown that bacterial species included in rRNA superfamily VI can be separated into three distinct rRNA clusters:

rRNA group I: Contains the true *Campylobacter* species—*C. fetus* (type species), *C. coli, C. jejuni, C. lari, C. hyointestinalis, C. concisus, C. mucosalis, C. sputorum, C. upsaliensis, C. curvus, C. rectus,* and two generically misnamed species, *Bacteroides gracilis* and *Bacteroides ureolyticus*

rRNA group II: Contains the *Arcobacter* species—*A. butzleri, A. cryaerophilus,* and *A. nitrofigilis*

rRNA group III: Contains the *Helicobacter* species—*H. pylori, H. mustelae, H. felis, H. nemestrinae, H. cinaedi* (CLO-1), *H. fennelliae* (CLO-2); the unnamed species CLO-3, "*Flexispira rappini*"; and *Wolinella succinogenes*

rRNA Group I: True *Campylobacter* Species

Campylobacter species are microaerophilic (require decreased O_2) and capnophilic (require increased CO_2), curved spiral bacteria that are motile by means of a single unsheathed polar flagellum. These organisms are nonfermentative and nonoxidative in their metabolism, deriving energy from the use of amino acids and four- and six-carbon Krebs cycle intermediates. These organisms used to be classified with *Vibrio* species, until DNA homology studies showed that they were unrelated to the vibrios. Even among the recognized *Campylobacter* species, much genotypic and phenotypic diversity exists. The organisms inhabit a wide variety of ecologic niches and environments. Most species are found in animals (cattle, swine) and cause infertility and abortion.

The *Campylobacter* species that are most frequently isolated in the clinical laboratory are those that cause gastroenteritis, the most common of which is *C. jejuni* subspecies *jejuni*.

CAMPYLOBACTER JEJUNI SUBSPECIES *JEJUNI*
Clinical Significance. *C. jejuni* subspecies *jejuni* is the most important human pathogen among the campylobacters. It has worldwide distribution, being recovered from 4% to 35% of fecal specimens of patients with acute diarrheal disease. In many practice settings, the rate of recovery of *Campylobacter* species exceeds the combined recovery of the time-honored enteric pathogens *Salmonella* species and *Shigella* species. It is also ubiquitous in domestic animals—house pets may carry the organism, and the vast majority of chickens, turkeys, and waterfowl are colonized. Ingestion of raw milk, partially cooked poultry, or contaminated water are the common sources for human infections. Enteritis with this organism is characterized by crampy abdominal pain, bloody diarrhea, chills, and fever. For most persons, the infection is self-limited and resolves in 3 to 7 days. The organism may continue to be excreted by convalescing patients for 2 weeks to 1 month. In cases of severe disease, the patient may be treated with oral erythromycin.

Although enteritis and diarrheal syndromes remain the most common manifestations of *Campylobacter* infections, other diseases have emerged during the past few years. Cases of septic arthritis, meningitis, and proctocolitis secondary to *C. jejuni*

Table 4-1
Characteristics for Differentiating *Arcobacter, Campylobacter, Wolinella, Helicobacter,* and *"Flexispira"*

GENUS	NITRATE REDUCTION	GROWTH ON 0.5% GLYCINE	HYDROLYSIS OF UREA	GROWTH AT 15°C	30°C	42°C	CELL MORPHOLOGY	FLAGELLAR SHEATHS
Arcobacter	+	NA	V	+	+	−	Curved and spiral rods	Absent
Campylobacter	+	V	−	−	+	V	Curved and spiral rods	Absent
Wolinella	+	−	−	−	−	W	Spiral	Absent
Helicobacter	V	+	V	−	V	V	Curved and spiral rods	Present
"Flexispira"	−	+	+	−	−	+	Straight fusiform rods	Present

+, 90% or more of strains positive; −, 90% or more of strains negative; V, 11%–89% of strains positive; W, weak reaction; NA, results not available.
(Modified from Vandamme P, Falsen E, Rossau R, et al. Revision of Campylobacter, Helicobacter, and Wolinella *taxonomy: emendation of generic descriptions and proposal of* Arcobacter gen. nov. Int J Syst Bacteriol 1991;41:88–103)

have been reported.[33] In addition, several new *Campylobacter* and *Campylobacter*-like species, to be discussed later in this chapter, have been discovered, many associated with new clinical syndromes.

Presumptive Identification From Stool. It may be possible to make a presumptive diagnosis of *Campylobacter* enteritis by observing characteristic gram-negative, curved, S-shaped, gull-winged, or long spiral forms in Gram-stained preparations of diarrheal stools (Fig. 4-1). In some laboratories it is common practice to initially examine wet mounts or stained smears of all diarrheal stool specimens for polymorphonuclear leukocytes and the presence of bacterial forms suggestive of *Campylobacter* species. Stool specimens for *Campylobacter* species are not further processed in some laboratories unless polymorphonuclear leukocytes are present. The rationale for this practice is that it is unlikely that *Campylobacter* species will be recovered in clinically significant numbers in stool specimens devoid of leukocytes. The expenditure of time and use of special culture media for specimens in which there is little chance to recover significant microbes is not considered cost effective.

Methods for Laboratory Isolation. Successful isolation of *C. jejuni* from stool depends on the use of selective media (eg, Campy-Thio, Campy-BAP), incubation at an elevated temperature

(42°C), and the proper incubation atmosphere (5% O_2, 10% CO_2, 85% N_2). A membrane filtration technique that is used with nonselective blood agar plates has been reported to be as effective as the use of antibiotic media for the isolation of *C. jejuni*.[35] This method has the advantage of allowing the isolation of antibiotic-sensitive campylobacters.

Various procedures can be used to provide a suitable gaseous atmosphere for cultivating microaerophilic campylobacters. These include evacuation-replacement procedures, disposable gas generators, and the use of the Fortner principle. The use of a

Figure 4-1. Gram stain of *Campylobacter jejuni* illustrating pleomorphic gram-negative bacilli, with short, curved, and spiral forms. Some cells connect to form gull-winged and S shapes.

CO_2 incubator is not recommended for cultivating campylobacters because only strains that are very aerotolerant grow in the atmosphere provided. Likewise, various investigators have emphasized that a candle extinction jar is also not recommended because the O_2 level (12% to 17%) is too high for optimal growth of campylobacters.[23,37]

Several selective media have been developed to allow for the isolation of *C. jejuni* from fecal samples. Merino and colleagues[27] evaluated the efficacy of seven selective *Campylobacter* isolation media. The names of these media, their composition, and a summary of the evaluation of each are included in Table 4-2. Butzler selective medium, Blaser medium (Campy-BAP), and Skirrow blood agar have been used in most clinical laboratories. Merino and colleagues[27] found that Preston *Campylobacter* blood-free medium with cefoperazone yielded the greatest number of *C. jejuni* isolations. Karmali and colleagues[17] found that a blood-free, charcoal-based selective medium (CSM), consisting of Columbia agar base, activated charcoal, hematin, sodium pyruvate, cefoperazone, vancomycin, and cycloheximide, is more selective than Skirrow's medium, and has a higher isolation rate of *C. jejuni* from mixed cultures. Charcoal, hematin, ferrous sulfate, and sodium pyruvate serve as substitutes for blood in growth media for campylobacters. Casein is added to help grow certain strains of nalidixic acid–resistant thermophilic campylobacters that are environmental organisms.

Endtz and colleagues[9] compared a semisolid blood-free selective motility medium with two blood-free CSM, two blood-based media (Skirrow medium and Blaser's Campy-BAP), and the membrane filter technique. They found that CSM was the single best medium; the highest isolation rates were observed when CSM was used in combination with any other media or the filter technique. Endtz and colleagues[9] also reported that extending the incubation time from 48 to 72 hours led to an increase in the isolation rate regardless of the medium used.

Rectal swabs or swab samples of the stool specimen can be inoculated directly to a small area on the surface of one of the recommended selective agar media. Formed stool specimens may also be processed by emulsifying a small portion (peanut sized) in phosphate-buffered saline or broth before inoculating one or two drops to the surface of the agar with a Pasteur pipette; similarly, one or two drops of liquid stool specimens can be inoculated directly.

An outline of a procedure that will allow isolation of enteric campylobacters from fecal samples is included below. This technique is consistent with information from the literature about requirements for cultivation of these bacteria and should be suitable for use in most clinical laboratories:

Procedure for Isolating *C. jejuni* and Other Enteric Campylobacter Species From Fecal Specimens

1. Using a fecal sample or a swab sample in Cary-Blair medium, prepare a turbid suspension of the feces in 10 mL of brain–heart infusion broth. Immediately inoculate one or two plates (two plates are preferable) of a *Campylobacter*-selective medium (best results are obtained with CSM); streak to obtain isolated colonies; and hold in a N_2-holding jar (see Chapter 11) until the remaining media are inoculated.

2. Lightly centrifuge the specimen (at approximately 1000 *g*) for 5 minutes.

3. Remove about 5 mL of the supernatant with a syringe and filter through a sterile 0.65-μL Millipore filter, as described by Butzler.[3] Discard the first 3 mL of fluid and use one or two drops of the remainder to inoculate two plates of chocolate agar without selective agents or a blood agar medium such as the Centers for Disease Control (CDC) anaerobe blood agar that will support the growth of *Campylobacter*. Streak for isolation.

4. Incubate one set of Campy-selective agar and chocolate agar plates at 42°C in an atmosphere of 5% O_2, 10% CO_2, and 85% N_2 and the remaining plates at 35° to 37°C in the same gaseous atmosphere.

5. Inspect the plates after 24, 48, and 72 hours of incubation for colonies characteristic of *Campylobacter* species and identify the isolates with the techniques described in the text. Plates not showing growth after 24 or 48 hours of incubation should be returned for an additional 24 to 48 hours in the same incubator and gaseous atmospheric conditions as described previously.

An alternative membrane filter technique, as described by Steele and McDermott,[35] may be used in combination with a Campy-selective medium with equivalent results:

Table 4-2
Formulas for Selective Media for Isolation of *Campylobacter jejuni*

MEDIUM	BASE	ADDITIVES
Butzler's selective medium	Fluid thioglycollate medium (Difco Laboratories, Detroit, MI)	Agar (3%) Sheep blood (10%) Bacitracin (25,000 IU/L) Novobiocin (5 mg/L) Colistin (10,000 IU/L) Cephalothin (15 mg/L) Actidione (50 mg/L)
Skirrow's blood agar	Blood agar base no. 2 (Oxoid)	Lysed horse blood (7%) Vancomycin (10 mg/L) Polymyxin B (2500 IU/L) Trimethoprim (5 mg/L)
Blaser's medium (Campy-BAP)	*Brucella* agar base (Becton Dickinson Microbiology Systems, Cockeysville, MD)	Sheep blood (10%) Vancomycin (10 mg/L) Trimethoprim (5 mg/L) Polymyxin B (2500 IU/L) Cephalothin (15 mg/L) Amphotericin B (2 mg/L)
Preston *Campylobacter* selective medium	Nutrient broth no. 2 (Oxoid CM67) 1.2% New Zealand agar	5% Saponin-lysed horse blood Trimethoprim (10 μg/mL) Polymyxin B (5 IU/mL) Rifampin (10 μg/mL) Cycloheximide (100 μg/mL)
Preston *Campylobacter* blood-free medium	Nutrient broth no. 2 (Oxoid CM67) 1.2% New Zealand agar	Bacteriologic charcoal Sodium deoxycholate Ferrous sulfate Sodium pyruvate Casein hydrolysate Cefoperazone (32 mg/L)
Butzler virion medium	Columbia agar base (Oxoid CM331)	Defibrinated sheep blood Cefoperazone (15 mg/L) Rifampin (10 μg/L) Colistin (10,000 IU/L) Amphotericin B (2 mg/L)
Modified Preston medium	Nutrient broth no. 2 (Oxoid)	7% defibrinated horse blood Cefoperazone (32 mg/L) Amphotericin B (2 mg/L) Campylobacter growth supplement (Oxoid)

(continued)

Table 4-2 (continued)

MEDIUM	BASE	ADDITIVES
Charcoal-based blood-free selective medium	Columbia agar base (GIBCO)	Activated charcoal (Oxoid) Hematin (0.032 g/L) Sodium pyruvate (0.1 g/L) Vancomycin (20 mg/L) Cefoperazone (32 mg/L) Cycloheximide (100 mg/L)

(Data from Karmali MA, Simer AE, Roscoe M, et al. Evaluation of a blood-free, charcoal-based, selective medium for the isolation of Campylobacter organisms from feces. J Clin Microbiol 1986;23:456–459; and Merino FJ, Agulla A, Villasante PA, et al. Comparative efficacy of seven selective media for isolating Campylobacter jejuni. J Clin Microbiol 1986;24:451–452)

1. Mix 1 g stool in 10 mL of sterile saline containing glass beads. Vortex for 30 seconds.
2. Place a 47-mm, 0.45 Gelman cellulose triacetate membrane filter (Gelman No. 63069) centrally onto the surface of a nonselective *Brucella* agar plate containing 5% sheep blood.
3. Place 8 to 10 drops of fecal suspension on the surface of the filter with a Pasteur pipette. Take care to ensure that the drops do not extend to the edge of the filter.
4. Remove filter and discard 30 minutes after the suspension is applied.
5. Incubate plate in Campy environment as described earlier.

Routine use of enrichment selective "Campy broth" is generally not recommended. Kaplan and coworkers,[16] however, have reported that the use of Blaser Campy-Thio gave a 10% increased yield of *C. jejuni* from stool specimens. This increase may represent low concentrations of organisms that are of questionable clinical significance. Enrichment broths may be beneficial if stool specimens are delayed in transit or left at room temperature too long.

Since campylobacters are microaerophilic, they tend to grow best near the top of the tube. If a *Campylobacter* broth is used, the following procedure for subculture should be followed:

1. Use a Falcon brand polyethylene plastic pipette that can be inverted.
2. Place the tip of the pipette 1 inch below the surface of the medium and continuously withdraw sample while removing the pipette.

3. Invert the pipette to facilitate mixing of the sample.
4. Place three drops on a Campy-BAP plate and streak for isolation.
5. Incubate plate in Campy environment as described earlier.

Identification From Culture. The appearance of colonies on one of the selective *Campylobacter* agars that has been incubated at 42°C in the gaseous environment described previously is already presumptive evidence that the organism is one of the thermophilic *Campylobacter* species (most commonly *C. jejuni*). The morphology of *Campylobacter* species on selective agar varies from flat, gray, irregular-shaped colonies that may be either dry or moist to colonies that are round and convex and glistening with entire edges. There is a tendency for colonies to form confluent growth along the streak lines on the agar surface. Hemolytic reactions are not observed on blood agar. The identification can be further confirmed by performing rapid catalase and cytochrome oxidase tests (*C. jejuni*, *C. coli*, and *C. lari* are positive for both). On occasion, thermophilic bacterial species other than *Campylobacter* species, notably *Pseudomonas aeruginosa*, may break through and grow on the selective media. *P. aeruginosa* also produces cytochrome oxidase and catalase and might be confused with *Campylobacter* species; however, most strains can be differentiated by their production of pyocyanin pigment and the characteristic grape-like odor. Examination of a wet mount of one of the suspected colonies under phase-contrast or darkfield optics may be helpful to visualize the organisms; *Campylobacter* species have a characteristic darting motility.

Gram-stained preparations from colonies of *C. jejuni* after 24 to 48 hours of incubation on blood agar show characteristic gram-negative, curved, S-shaped, gull-winged, or long spiral forms (see Fig. 4-1). Coccoid forms are more commonly seen in older cultures of *C. jejuni*, particularly after colonies have been exposed to ambient air. Since *Campylobacter* species are typically faint staining, we have adopted the practice of extending the staining time of the safranin counterstain to at least 10 minutes to allow for greater staining intensity. Also, the addition of 0.5 g of basic fuchsin per liter of safranin improves the intensity of the counterstain without overstaining the cellular elements.

Once isolated, both subspecies of *C. jejuni* can be easily identified since they are the only campylobacters that hydrolyze hippurate (Table 4-3). In addition, this species is resistant to cephalothin and susceptible to nalidixic acid.

OTHER *CAMPYLOBACTER* SPECIES OF CLINICAL IMPORTANCE. Only the species considered to be of clinical importance are covered in this text. For more information concerning all species of *Campylobacter*, the reader is referred elsewhere.[22]

Campylobacter coli. *C. coli*, closely related to *C. jejuni* and also a cause of diarrhea in humans, shares several cultural characteristics with *C. jejuni*, including susceptibility to nalidixic acid and resistance to cephalothin. *C. coli* can be differentiated from *C. jejuni* by the hippurate hydrolysis test (*C. jejuni* hydrolyzes hippurate; *C. coli* does not). The report when this organism is recovered in laboratories in which the hippurate test is not performed should read "*C. jejuni/coli.*"

***Campylobacter fetus* Subspecies *fetus*.** *C. fetus* subspecies *fetus* is associated primarily with infective abortion in cattle and sheep and is an infrequent cause of human infections. Infections usually result in systemic illness and usually affect debilitated persons with chronic hepatic, renal, or neoplastic disease or with compromised immune function.

***Campylobacter jejuni* Subspecies *doylei*.** A new subspecies of *C. jejuni* has been isolated from human clinical specimens including gastric epithelium biopsies and feces from children with diarrhea. The pathogenicity of the organism remains unknown. *C. jejuni* subspecies *doylei* can be distinguished readily from other campylobacters because it does not reduce nitrates and hydrolyzes hippurate. It is susceptible to cephalothin and therefore will not be recovered on media containing cephalosporin-type antibiotics.

Campylobacter lari. Formerly named *C. laridis*, the organism now known as *C. lari* is thermophilic, halotolerant, and nalidixic acid resistant; otherwise, it shares several features with *C. jejuni* and *C. coli*. Anaerobic growth in the presence of 0.1% trimethylamine oxide (TMAO) and failure to hydrolyze indoxyl acetate help to identify this species (reagents available from Sigma Chemical Co, St Louis, MO). Many laboratories rely on resistance to nalidixic acid to separate *C. lari* from *C. jejuni* and *C. coli*; we have noted a case of *C. jejuni* infection isolated from a patient on ciprofloxacin therapy (a quinolone similar to nalidixic acid) in which resistance to nalidixic acid was developed by the *C. jejuni* isolate. *C. lari* is endemic in sea gulls but causes enteritis simulating *C. jejuni* infections in humans.

Campylobacter upsaliensis. *C. upsaliensis* is catalase-negative or only weakly positive, and thus it has been referred to as the CNW strain of *Campylobacter*. Because weak catalase reactions may also occur for *C. jejuni* subspecies *doylei*, however, the CNW designation no longer holds. Except for the lack of or weak production of catalase, this organism shares several characteristics with pathogenic campylobacters. It is thermophilic (grows at 42°C) and is highly susceptible to drugs that are present in selective isolation media, making them unsuitable for the isolation of *C. upsaliensis*. Goossens and coworkers[12] reported the isolation of 99 strains of *C. upsaliensis* by the filter method, with only 4 strains recovered simultaneously from selective media.

Domestic pets may serve as the reservoir of this species, which was first isolated from healthy dogs, dogs with diarrhea, and, most recently, asymptomatic cats. Data from some reports suggest that this organism may be an opportunistic agent of infections in children.

DEFINITIVE IDENTIFICATION OF CAMPYLOBACTERS. The colonial morphology and Gram stain characteristics of *C. jejuni* as described earlier also pertain to most other *Campylobacter* species.

Table 4-3
Differential Characteristics of Campylobacters and Related Taxa

ORGANISM	CATALASE	NITRATE	HYDROGEN SULFIDE TRIPLE SUGAR IRON	UREASE	INDOXYL ACETATE	HIPPURATE	GROWTH							SUSCEPTIBILITY*	
							25°C	37°C	42°C	MacConkey	0.1% TMAO	1.5% NaCl	1% Glycine	Nalidixic Acid	Cephalothin
RNA Group I															
Campylobacter coli	+	+	−	−	+	−	−	+	+	+	−	−	+	S	R
C. concisus	−	+	+	−	NA	−	−	+	C	+	−	+	C	R	R
C. fetus subsp. fetus	+	+	−	−	−	−	+	+	−	+	−	V	+	R	S
C. fetus subsp. venerealis	+	+	−	−	−	−	+	+	−	+	−	V	−	R	S
C. hyointestinalis	+	+	+	−	−	−	V	+	+	+	+	−	+	R	S
C. jejuni subsp. jejuni	+	+	−	−	+	+	−	+	+	+	−	−	+	S	R
C. jejuni subsp. doylei	V	−	−	−	+	+	−	+	W	NA	−	−	+	S	S
C. lari	+	+	−	−	−	−	−	+	+	+	+	+	+	R	R
C. mucosalis	−	+	+	−	−	−	+	+	C	+	C	C	C	R	S
C. sputorum biovar bubulus	−	+	+	−	−	−	−	+	C	−	+	+	+	R	S
C. sputorum biovar fecalis	+	+	+	−	−	−	−	+	+	+	C	+	+	V	S
C. sputorum biovar sputorum	−	+	+	−	−	−	−	+	+	−	C	+	+	S	S
C. upsaliensis	−(W)	+	−	−	+	−	−	+	+	−	−	−	C	S	S

ORGANISM	CATALASE	NITRATE	HYDRO-GEN SULFIDE TRIPLE SUGAR IRON	UREASE	INDOXYL ACETATE	HIP-PURATE	GROWTH 25°C	37°C	42°C	Mac-Conkey	0.1% TMAO	1.5% NaCl	1% Glycine	SUSCEPTIBILITY* Nal-idixic Acid	Cepha-lothin
RNA Group II															
Arcobacter butzleri	-(W)	+	-	-	+	-	+	+	V	+	NA	V	+	V	R
A. cryaerophilus	+	+	-	-	+	-	+	+	-	-	-	+	-	V	R
A. nitrofigilis	+	+	+	V	-	-	+	+	-	NA	NA	+	-	S	S
RNA Group III															
Helicobacter cinaedi (CLO-1)	+	+	-	-	C	-	-	+	-	-	-	-	+	S	S
H. fennelliae (CLO-2)	+	-	-	-	+	-	-	+	-	-	-	-	+	S	S
CLO-3	+	-	-	++	+	-	-	+	+	NA	NA	NA	+	S	R
H. felis	+	+	-	++	NA	-	-	+	+	NA	NA	-	-	R	S
H. mustelae	+	+	-	++	+	-	-	+	+	NA	NA	-	V	S	R
H. nemestrinae	+	-	-	++	NA	NA	-	+	+	NA	NA	-	NA	R	S
H. pylori	+	-	-	++	-	-	-	+	C	-	-	NA	V	R	S
"Flexispira rappini"	C	-	-	++	NA	-	-	+	+	NA	NA	NA	-(w)	R	R
Wolinella succinogenes	-	+	W	-	-	-	-	+	W	NA	NA	NA	-	R	R

*Susceptibility to antibiotics determined with 30-μg disks.
+, 90% or more of strains positive; –, 90% or more of strains negative; V, 11%–89% of strains positive; + +, strong positive reaction; W, weak reaction; NA, results not available; C, contradictory reports in literature; R, resistant; S, susceptible; TMAO, trimethylamine oxide; shaded areas indicate key reactions.

Table 4-4
Identification of the Most Commonly Encountered Campylobacters

	NALIDIXIC ACID	CEPHALOTHIN	TRIPHENYLTETRAZOLIUM CHLORIDE	HIPPURATE HYDROLYSIS	INDOXYL ACETATE HYDROLYSIS
C. *jejuni* subsp. *jejuni*	S	R	R	+	+
C. *coli*	S	R	R	−	+
C. *fetus* subsp. *fetus*	R	S	S	−	−
C. *lari*	R	R	S	−	−

Definitive species identification depends on the determination of the phenotypic characteristics presented in Table 4-3.

The differential susceptibility to nalidixic acid and cephalothin can be used to differentiate the more commonly encountered *Campylobacter* species (Table 4-4).

LATEX AGGLUTINATION TESTS.   Latex agglutination tests are now available for the identification of *Campylobacter* species and related organisms. Meritec-Campy (jcl) (Meridian Diagnostics, Cincinnati, OH) is a latex agglutination assay that is used for culture isolate identification of *C. jejuni, C. coli,* and *C. lari.* Campyslide (Becton Dickinson Microbiology Systems, Cockeysville, MD) is a latex agglutination assay that can be used for genus-level culture confirmation of four major *Campylobacter* pathogens: *C. jejuni, C. coli, C. lari,* and *C. fetus* subspecies *fetus.* Published evaluations of both of these assays have shown them to be reliable for use in the clinical laboratory.[13,28]

NUCLEIC ACID PROBES.   Nucleic acid probes are also coming on the market for use in the identification of *Campylobacter* species. AccuProbe *Campylobacter* Culture Identification Test (Gen-Probe, Inc, San Diego, CA) is a DNA probe-based test that provides for rapid identification of *C. jejuni, C. coli,* and *C. lari* directly from bacterial colonies. The probe is nonradiometric and is labeled with a chemiluminescent acridinium ester. Reactions are read in a luminometer.

rRNA Group II: *Arcobacter Group*

The *Arcobacter* group consists of those species referred to as the aerotolerant campylobacters because they grow in the presence of atmospheric levels of O_2. Other characteristics useful in distinguishing aerotolerant "*Campylobacter*" species from other campylobacters include hydrolysis of indoxyl acetate; growth at 15°, 25°, and 36°C but not 42°C; and the inability to hydrolyze hippurate (see Table 4-3). The genus includes three species: *A. butzleri, A. cryaerophilus,* and *A. nitrofigilis.*

Most human isolates belong to a single species, *A. butzleri,* that can be separated from the biochemically similar species *A. cryaerophilus* by demonstrating aerotolerance at both 30° and 36°C (*A. cryaerophilus* is aerotolerant at 30° but not at 36°C). In addition, *A. butzleri* grows on MacConkey agar and in glycine- and nitrate-containing media (reducing nitrate to nitrite) and in 1.5% and 3.5% NaCl. Most isolates from humans have been from stools of patients with diarrheal illness; three isolates were from abdominal contents or peritoneal fluids and three isolates were obtained from blood cultures.[21]

rRNA Group III: *Helicobacter, Wolinella, "Flexispira," and Campylobacter-Like Organisms*

This homology group contains three genera and one unnamed *Campylobacter*-like species. The *Helicobacter* species are strict microaerophiles with a spiral or helical morphology. Many species exhibit strong urease activity. "*Flexispira rappini*" is the name proposed for an organism that is closely related to *Helicobacter* but is straight and fusiform rather than curved. The genus *Wolinella* consists of a single species, *W. succinogenes,* that is an obligate anaerobe and requires formate and fumarate for growth. Species included in the genera *Helicobacter* and "*Flexispira*" possess sheathed flagella. No other

Campylobacter or *Wolinella* species possess sheathed flagella (see Table 4-1).

HELICOBACTER PYLORI. This species was initially called *Campylobacter pyloridis* and then *Campylobacter pylori* but has subsequently been transferred to the new genus *Helicobacter.*[11] *H. pylori* is found only on the mucus-secreting epithelial cells of the stomach. Evidence suggests that *H. pylori* is the causative agent of active chronic antral gastritis[25] and may also be a major factor in the pathogenesis of peptic ulcer disease.[32] *H. pylori* gastritis is widespread in many countries in the world and may be one of the most common chronic human infections. The case for *H. pylori* as a causative agent of duodenal ulcer remains controversial.

H. pylori strains are microaerophilic (10% CO_2, 5% O_2, 85% N_2) and will also grow in air with increased (10%) CO_2 content. The optimum temperature for isolation is 35° to 37°C, although some strains will grow at 42°C. High humidity has also been found to favor growth. Most strains take 3 to 5 days to grow, with occasional isolates requiring 7 days of incubation before growth is evident. They can be cultured on nonselective blood-containing media, producing small, translucent, gray colonies. The characteristic Gram stain (small, curved, slightly plump bacilli) and positive reactions for catalase, oxidase, and urease provide an identification.

Specimens for Recovery of *Helicobacter pylori.* For the diagnosis of *H. pylori*–associated gastritis, histologic staining and culturing of biopsy specimens has been considered the gold standard. Suitable specimens include gastric and duodenal biopsy tissue. Specimens should be fresh and not delayed in transport for more than 3 hours. Specimens may be kept for up to 5 hours if stored at 4°C. Tissue should be kept moist by the addition of 2 mL or less of sterile isotonic saline.

Culture and Isolation of *Helicobacter pylori.* Grinding of specimens in a ground-glass grinder yields heavier growth than mincing or rubbing the specimen onto an agar surface. Material should be inoculated onto a nonselective blood agar medium. Poor growth is observed on commercially prepared chocolate agar plates; therefore, use of chocolate agar is not recommended. Because these bacteria are susceptible to cephalothin, *H. pylori* will not grow on Blaser's Campy-BAP or any selective medium containing cephalosporins. Many laborato-

ries have had good results using modified Thayer-Martin agar as a selective medium for isolation of *H. pylori* in mixed cultures. Plates are incubated at 37°C in a humid, microaerophilic environment. We recommend the use of a Campy GasPak jar. Growth is usually observed in 3 to 5 days.

Identification of *Helicobacter pylori.* Colonies of *H. pylori* are small, gray, translucent, and weakly β-hemolytic. Gram stain reveals pale-staining, curved, gram-negative bacteria with characteristic gull-wing and U shapes. Presumptive identification can be made with positive reactions for oxidase and catalase and an extremely rapid (within minutes) urease reaction. Additional identifying characteristics are listed in Table 4-3.

Biopsy Urease Test. A more rapid but somewhat less sensitive and specific technique than the previously mentioned tests is the biopsy urease test. In this test, a medium containing urea and a *p*H-sensitive dye is inoculated with the mucosal biopsy specimen. If urease is present in the specimen, urea is split and ammonia causes a rise in *p*H and subsequent change in the color of the indicator. This test may produce false-negative results if only a small number of organisms are present or false-positive results if other urea-splitting organisms are present.[26]

VIBRIONACEAE AND "AEROMONADACEAE"

Classification of the Vibrionaceae

The name Vibrionaceae was originally proposed by Vernon in 1965 with the intent of grouping a number of genera of organisms that were oxidase-positive and motile by means of polar flagella. This grouping was intended as a convenience for the purpose of differentiating these organisms from the Enterobacteriaceae and did not necessarily imply a taxonomic relationship among the included species. The Vibrionaceae, as presently defined in *Bergey's Manual of Systematic Bacteriology,*[1] includes the following genera: *Vibrio* (27 species), *Aeromonas* (4 species), *Photobacterium* (3 species), and *Plesiomonas* (1 species). In the past decade a variety of methods for nucleic acid analysis have revolutionized microbial taxonomy and have resulted in the restructuring of this family along phylogenetic lines and the establishment of two new genera, *Listonella* and *Shewanella*, and a new family, Aeromonadaceae.[7,24] The correct phylogenic placement of the genus *Plesiomonas* remains unresolved at this time.

Genus *Vibrio*

Vibrio species have both historical and contemporary interest. *V. cholerae* is the etiologic agent of Asiatic cholera in humans, a potentially severe diarrheal disease that has been the scourge of humanity for centuries. The organism was first described and named by Pacini in 1854; 32 years later Koch isolated the organism, which he called "Kommabacillus" because of the characteristic curved or comma-shaped appearance of the individual bacterial cells.

TAXONOMY. The strains of *Vibrio cholerae* that have been recovered from classic cases of pandemic cholera agglutinate in what has been designated 01 antiserum. Strains not agglutinating in this antiserum are called either non-01 *V. cholerae* (if this species is determined biochemically) or a variety of other *Vibrio* species names, such as *V. parahemolyticus*, *V. mimicus*, and so on. Since the non-01 species usually do not cause diarrheal syndromes as severe or potentially life threatening as 01 species, or more commonly may be associated with extraintestinal infections, early differentiation between the two groups can be of considerable clinical importance. Although 35 or more distinct *Vibrio* species have been identified, all but 11 are environmental organisms, called "marine vibrio species," and have not been associated with human infections.[15]

DESCRIPTION AND ASSOCIATED CLINICAL SYNDROMES OF *VIBRIO* SPECIES OF HUMAN IMPORTANCE. The species that are recovered from humans and potentially cause disease can be divided into two groups: *Vibrio cholerae* and the non-cholera vibrios.

VIBRIO CHOLERAE. V. cholerae is the etiologic agent of epidemic and pandemic cholera in humans. Since the first pandemic in 1816 to 1817, six others have followed at about 10- to 15-year intervals through 1889; the latest occurred in 1961, involving the El Tor strain, to be discussed in more detail later. In 1989, there were 48,403 cases of cholera reported to the World Health Organization from 35 countries, reflecting the widespread

nature of the current pandemic.[4] There are at least 60 known somatic (O) serovars, which are all indistinguishable phenotypically and genetically. All of the pandemic strains are agglutinated with a single antiserum that has been designated 01. The 01 type *V. cholerae* strains can be further separated into one of three serogroups: Inaba, Ogawa, and Hikojima.

Epidemic strains of serovar 01 may be further divided into the classic and El Tor biovars. El Tor is an actively β-hemolytic biotype of *V. cholerae* that was isolated at the El Tor Quarantine Station in Egypt. The El Tor strain has been found to be hardier and better capable of surviving in the environment; furthermore, chronic carriers of the El Tor strain have been reported in the literature.[18] The El Tor vibrio is now recognized as a biotype of *V. cholerae* and is responsible for most current epidemic outbreaks of classic cholera. The present pandemic of cholera that began in 1961 is caused by the El Tor biovar, as are the outbreaks identified in the Gulf Coast region of the United States[20] and in South America.[5,6] The classic biovar has almost disappeared except for rare isolations in India.

Cholera in the United States. In 1973, the first case of cholera in the United States since 1911 was reported from Texas. This was followed in 1978 by the report of 11 cases in Louisiana and in 1981 with two additional outbreaks in Texas involving 18 cases. Crabs harvested from nearby estuaries were found to be the vehicle of infection in the Louisiana cases, while the largest of the two Texas outbreaks was traced to contamination of cooked rice after accidental rinsing with water from the environment containing the outbreak strain. It is now known that 44 toxigenic *V. cholerae* 01 infections were acquired in the United States between 1973 and 1987. All resulted from exposures in Louisiana and Texas near the Gulf Coast. In 1991, 26 cases of cholera were reported in the United States; 18 were associated with travel to Latin America. Of these, 11 were related to crabs brought back in suitcases. Between January 1 and August 26, 1992, 96 cases of cholera were reported in the United States, more than in any year since cholera surveillance was begun.[6]

V. cholerae non-01 serotypes 02 to 100 have been associated with isolated cases of diarrheal disease in the United States, although the majority of non-01 strains do not produce cholera toxin but appear to produce an enterotoxin different from cholera toxin. Strains have also been isolated from wounds and systemic infections. Most known cases have occurred in immunocompromised patients, particularly those with hematologic malignancy or cirrhosis.

Pathophysiology of *Vibrio cholerae*–Induced Gastroenteritis. *V. cholerae* is the prototype of diarrheal syndromes in which disease is caused not by tissue invasion of microorganisms but through the production of toxins that interrupt normal intraintestinal exchanges of water and electrolytes. In particular, 01 strains produce a toxin that binds to a receptor on the epithelial cell membrane and activates adenylate cyclase, causing increased levels of cyclic adenosine monophosphate and hypersecretion of salt and water, resulting in the characteristic "rice water" diarrhea of cholera. The result is varying degrees of dehydration and electrolyte imbalance that can lead to metabolic acidosis, hypokalemia, shock, and death in extreme cases.

Treatment of *Vibrio cholerae* Infections. *V. cholerae* is rapidly killed by tetracycline; fluid secretion may, however, persist for several hours after treatment from the effect of toxin already bound to the mucosal cells. Correction of fluid and electrolyte losses is essential with as much as 1 L or more of fluid per hour required. Antibiotic therapy with trimethoprim-sulfamethoxazole or tetracycline will help shorten the duration of the diarrhea.

NON-CHOLERA VIBRIOS. Most cases of *Vibrio* infections in the United States have been caused by nonepidemic species other than *V. cholerae*. The term *non-cholera* is probably a misnomer because many strains can cause severe diarrheal disease in addition to extraintestinal infections that can result in fatal septicemia. In most infections, symptoms are less severe and shorter in duration than is experienced in classic epidemic cholera.

VIBRIO PARAHAEMOLYTICUS. *V. parahaemolyticus* is the most common non-cholera *Vibrio* and causes gastroenteritis in humans after ingestion of contaminated seafood, the mechanism of which has not been elucidated. Symptoms include watery and sometimes bloody diarrhea, abdominal cramps, nausea, vomiting, headache, low-grade fever, and chills. The illness is usually mild to moderate and self-limiting with a duration of 2 or 3 days. Extraintestinal infections by *V. parahaemolyticus* have also been reported, mostly from wounds.

A urea-positive biotype has appeared and has been the cause of several outbreaks, often associated with ingestion of contaminated raw oysters.[30,31]

METHODS FOR LABORATORY ISOLATION OF VIBRIOS. In discussing the laboratory approach to the isolation of *Vibrio* species from clinical specimens, Farmer and colleagues[10] suggest one of the following:

1. Use normal procedures and make no specific effort to search for *Vibrio* species.
2. Use normal procedures and plating media and look for oxidase-positive colonies.
3. Incorporate thiosulfate citrate bile sucrose (TCBS) agar as an extra plate for stool cultures and also for other likely specimens such as those from wounds, blood, eye, and ear.
4. Use other special procedures to enhance the isolation of *V. cholerae*, *V. parahaemolyticus*, and other *Vibrio* species.

For laboratories in the American midwest, where positive cultures for *Vibrio* species may be few, Farmer and colleagues[10] suggest that the first or second approaches may be most appropriate. In laboratories near oceans, particularly those located in endemic areas, the third or fourth approach is indicated. These researchers mention several disadvantages to the routine use of TCBS agar, inluding the increased cost for a relatively low return and the fact that some *Vibrio* species or strains may not grow well on TCBS agar. It is helpful for laboratory personnel to be informed when clinical cases of cholera or extraintestinal *Vibrio* infections are suspected. In these cases, the use of a selective medium or alkaline broth enrichment, to be discussed in a later section, may still be in order.

SPECIMEN COLLECTION, PROCESSING, AND MEDIA SELECTION. Laboratory personnel should be notified if the physician suspects a cholera syndrome or extraintestinal infections with *Vibrio* species. Specimens should be collected as early in the disease as possible. In the acute diarrheal stages of disease, specimens may be collected from the rectum with a soft rubber catheter or a rectal swab or from a small portion of the passed liquid stool. Culturing of vomitus also may be productive of organisms, particularly in the early stages of disease.

Specimens should be transported in closed containers to preserve moisture and transferred to culture media as soon as possible. *Vibrio* species are generally sensitive to drying, exposure to sunlight, and the development of an acid *p*H. They are also easily inhibited by the normal intestinal flora or contaminating organisms. If cultures cannot be set up immediately, *Vibrio* species will remain viable in Cary-Blair semisolid transport medium for an extended time. The use of buffered glycerol saline transport medium should be avoided. If a transport medium is not available, a 2 by ¹/₂ inch strip of thick blotting paper can be soaked in the fecal specimen, placed in a sealed plastic bag, and then mailed to the nearest reference laboratory.[19] Specimens suspicious for harboring *Vibrio* species should be inoculated to 5% sheep blood and MacConkey agar. Whether to also inoculate a plate of TCBS agar or a tube of alkaline peptone water enrichment must be determined by each laboratory supervisor depending on the prevalence of *Vibrio*-related diseases in any given locale. If TCBS agar is not used, β-hemolytic colonies that appear on sheep blood agar after overnight incubation should be tested for cytochrome oxidase activity. Either representative colonies can be individually touched and spot tested for the oxidase reaction using Kovac's reagent or one or two drops of Kovac's reagent can be dropped in an area on the surface of the plate where suspicious colonies are present. The rapid development of a blue color is indicative of a positive test. Oxidase-positive colonies can be transferred to TCBS agar for further species identification using biochemical and other characteristics.

Alkaline peptone water (APW) enrichment broths should be subcultured to TCBS agar for further evaluation of colonies that grow after an additional 24 to 48 hours of incubation. APW, which contains 1% peptone and 1% NaCl at *p*H 8.6, is a simple-to-use enrichment broth that can be recommended in situations where low concentrations of organisms in the specimen are anticipated (eg, in convalescent stages of disease). The high *p*H of the medium serves to suppress the growth of many commensal intestinal bacteria while allowing uninhibited multiplication of *V. cholerae*. Subcultures to TCBS or gelatin agar should be made within 12 to 18 hours since other organisms can begin to overgrow the broth after prolonged incubation. APW is also an excellent transport medium if specimens cannot be immediately delivered to the laboratory for processing. It is recommended that about 1 mL of liquid or 1 g of formed stool be placed into 10 mL of APW in a screw-capped tube; alternatively, rectal swabs can be placed into a tube containing 1 to 2 mL of APW.[19]

PRESUMPTIVE IDENTIFICATION OF *VIBRIO* SPECIES BASED ON COLONIAL AND MICROSCOPIC MORPHOLOGY. Vibrios grow readily on most isolation media; growth of all species is enhanced by adding 1% NaCl to the medium. Colonies are typically smooth, convex, creamy, and gray-white and have entire margins (see Color Plate 4-1*A* through *C*). Rough colonies are occasionally encountered that adhere to the agar. Certain marine vibrios are able to swarm on the surface of agar media, associated with the formation of long cells with lateral flagella. This phenomenon is not seen with most human isolates.

Microscopically, straight or curved gram-negative bacilli are observed (see Color Plate 4-1*D*). The curved character of the cells may be best seen in the early stationary phase in broth cultures; in logarithmic phase, straight and rounded coccoid forms are intermixed. Although a presumptive diagnosis of cholera can be made by observing large numbers of curved bacilli in direct Gram-stained stool specimens, recovery of the organism in culture is needed to make a definitive identification.

The differential reactions on TCBS agar are helpful in making a presumptive identification of *V. cholerae*, *V. alginolyticus*, *V. parahaemolyticus*, and *V. vulnificus*. After 18 to 24 hours of incubation on TCBS agar, *V. cholerae* organisms grow as smooth, yellow colonies, 2 to 4 mm in diameter, with an opaque center and transparent periphery (see Color Plate 4-1*A*). The colonies of *V. alginolyticus*, which also ferment sucrose, will also produce yellow colonies on TCBS agar; *V. parahaemolyticus* and *V. vulnificus*, which do not utilize sucrose, produce blue-green colonies (see Color Plate 4-1*B*). On gelatin agar, *V. cholerae* grow as transparent colonies surrounded by an opaque halo indicating liquefaction of gelatin (see Color Plate 4-1*C*).

BIOCHEMICAL CHARACTERIZATION AND LABORATORY IDENTIFICATION OF *VIBRIO* SPECIES. Members of the genus *Vibrio* are facultative anaerobes capable of both respiratory and fermentative metabolism. Because they grow and react in carbohydrate test media designed for fermentative metabolism, they are classified with the fermenters. The natural habitat for *Vibrio* species is aquatic, in both fresh and salt water. The growth and biochemical reactivity of most species are enhanced in differential test media supplemented with 1% to 2% sodium chloride.

Most *Vibrio* species produce cytochrome oxidase, a characteristic that separates them from the Enterobacteriaceae. Therefore, *Vibrio* species are included in the group of oxidase-positive fermenters—*Aeromonas* species, *Plesiomonas* species, and *Chromobacterium* species—from which they must be differentiated (Table 4-5). Since *V. cholerae* ferments glucose, an acid-deep/alkaline-slant reaction is seen on Kligler iron agar. Since sucrose is also fermented, an acid-deep/acid-slant reaction is seen on triple sugar iron agar. *V. cholerae* produces both lysine and ornithine decarboxylases; *A. hydrophila* and *C. violaceum* are negative for these reactions.

Those laboratory workers who use lysine iron agar to screen stool isolates will note that *V. cholerae* produces a purple-slant/purple-deep reaction because of the decarboxylation of lysine. *A. hydrophila* produces a positive arginine dihydrolase reaction; *V. cholerae* is negative. Most strains of *A. hydrophila* hydrolyze esculin, differentiating it from the other organisms included in Table 4-5. Differences in the utilization of lactose, sucrose, mannitol, and inositol also serve to differentiate these genera.

V. cholerae, including the El Tor biotype, can be distinguished from other *Vibrio* species by the ability to produce a positive string test (see Color Plate 4-1E). To perform this test, bacterial colonies are mixed with a few drops of 0.5% sodium deoxycholate on a glass slide. An inoculating loop is immersed into the mixture and pulled away from the drop. *V. cholerae* produces a long string that becomes more tenacious after 60 seconds or more (other vibrios may give an initial string reaction that diminishes or disappears 45 to 60 seconds later). A positive slide agglutination with polyvalent O antiserum is also helpful in differentiating *V. cholerae* from other closely related strains (see Color Plate 4-1F). The El Tor biotype can be distinguished from classic strains of *V. cholerae* by several characteristics (Table 4-6). El Tor strains are actively β-hemolytic on blood agar (see Color Plate 4-1G) and are capable of agglutinating chicken erythrocytes (see Color Plate 4-1H). The chicken erythrocyte test is performed by mixing a loopful of washed chicken erythrocytes (2.5% suspension in saline) with bacterial cells from a pure culture to be tested. Visible clumping of the erythrocytes indicates the El Tor biotype, in contrast to classic 01 strains of *V. cholerae* that do not

have this property. Classic strains of *V. cholerae* are susceptible to 50 IU of polymyxin B in the disk diffusion test; El Tor strains are resistant. El Tor strains are also Voges-Proskauer–positive, whereas classic strains of *V. cholerae* are Voges-Proskauer–negative. For laboratories capable of performing phage IV susceptibility tests, El Tor strains are resistant to this phage.

Genera *Listonella* and *Shewanella*

The members of the genus *Listonella* are curved, gram-negative bacilli, are motile by monotrichous or peritrichous flagella, and are oxidase-positive. The genus includes three species, *L. anguillara*, *L. damsela*, and *L. pelagia*, all of which were formerly included in the genus *Vibrio*.

Members of the genus *Shewanella* (most notably *S. putrefaciens*) are straight or curved, gram-negative bacilli that are motile by means of a single polar flagellum. Characteristic colonies are dome shaped, circular, slightly viscous or mucoid, and usually red-brown or salmon-pink. They possess cytochrome oxidase activity and produce abundant hydrogen sulfide in Kligler iron agar. Nitrates are reduced to nitrites, and gelatinase, ornithine decarboxylase, and DNase tests are positive. Both *Listonella* and *Shewanella* species are associated with marine environments and are pathogenic for fish. *S. putrefaciens* has been recovered from human clinical specimens and is discussed in Chapter 3.

Classification of *Aeromonas* and *Plesiomonas*

In *Bergey's Manual of Systematic Bacteriology*, *Aeromonas* species are included along with *Vibrio* species and *Plesiomonas shigelloides* in the Vibrionaceae.[1] Based on molecular genetic evidence, MacDonell and Colwell[7,24] have proposed the removal of *Aeromonas* species and placement in a separate family, Aeromonadaceae, and the removal of *Plesiomonas* to the genus *Proteus*. Phenotypic differences between *Vibrio*, *Aeromonas*, and *Plesiomonas* species are listed in Table 4-5.

Genus *Aeromonas*

As the species name *hydrophila* ("water loving") indicates, the natural habitat of *Aeromonas* species is fresh or sea water, where they commonly cause

Table 4-5
Oxidase-Positive, Fermentative, Gram-Negative Bacilli: Differential Characteristics
of *Aeromonas hydrophila, Plesiomonas shigelloides, Chromobacterium violaceum,*
and *Vibrio cholerae*

CHARACTERISTIC	AEROMONAS HYDROPHILA	PLESIOMONAS SHIGELLOIDES	CHROMO-BACTERIUM VIOLACEUM	VIBRIO CHOLERAE
Kligler iron agar (slant/deep/ hydrogen sulfide)	K/A/ −	K − A/A/ −	K/A/ −	K/A/ −
Catalase	+	+	+	+
Esculin	(+)	−	−	−
Motility	+	(+)	+	+
ONPG	+	+	−	+
Indole	(+)	+	−	+
Voges-Proskauer	(−)	−	−	(−)
Lysine decarboxylase	−	+	−	+
Ornithine decarboxylase	−	+	−	+
Carbohydrates				
Lactose	−	(+)	−	−
Sucrose	(+)	−	(−)	+
Mannitol	+	−	−	+
Inositol	−	+	−	−
Growth in peptone, 1% with 0% NaCL	+	+	+	+
7% NaCL	−	−	−	−
11% NaCL	−	−	−	−

+, 90% or more of strains positive; (+), 51%–89% of strains positive; (−), 10%–50% of strains positive; −, less than 10% of strains positive; V, variable; K/A, alkaline/acid; K−A/A, alkaline to acid/acid; ONPG, ortho-nitrophenyl-β-D-galactopyranoside.

Table 4-6
Differentiation Between *Vibrio cholerae* Biotypes

TEST	CLASSIC	EL TOR
String test	+	+
β-Hemolytic on sheep blood agar	−	+
Voges-Proskauer test	−	+
Chicken red blood cell agglutination	−	+
Susceptibility to 50 IU polymyxin B	S	R
Phage IV susceptibility	S	R

+, positive test; −, negative test; S, susceptible; R, resistant.

Table 4-7
Phenotypic Grouping of Currently Recognized Species and Known DNA Hybridization Groups in the Genus *Aeromonas*

DNA HYBRIDIZATION GROUP (GENOSPECIES)	PHENOTYPIC GROUP (PHENONS)	NAMED SPECIES
1	} *A. hydrophila*	*A. hydrophila*
2		Unnamed
3		*A. salmonicida*
4	} *A. caviae*	*A. caviae* (*A. punctata*)*
5A		*A. media*
5B		*A. Media*
6		*A. eucrenophila*
7	} *A. sobria*	*A. sobria*
8		*A. veronii*
9		*A. jandaei*
10/8		*A. venonii*†
11		*A. veronii*-like
12		*A. schubertii*

*A. punctata *has been shown to be identical to* A. caviae.
†DNA groups 8 and 10 have been shown to be identical.
(Modified from Altwegg M, Steigerwalt AG, Altwegg-Bissig R, et al. Biochemical identification of Aeromonas genospecies isolated from humans. J Clin Microbiol 1990;28:258–264)

infectious diseases in cold-blooded aquatic animals. These bacteria also reside in sink traps and drainpipes and can be recovered from tap water faucets and distilled water supplies, which are potential sources of organisms involved in nosocomial infections.

TAXONOMY. There are 12 DNA hybridization groups (also called genospecies) recognized within the genus *Aeromonas*. Because there is a lack of phenotypic characteristics that correlate with each specific genospecies, some of the DNA hybridization groups cannot be phenotypically separated and, therefore, some of the groups have not yet been named. The recognized species and the various DNA hybridization groups are summarized in Table 4-7. The genus *Aeromonas* consists of 10 named species, which can be grouped into two subdivisions as follows:

Psychrophilic group: *Aeromonas salmonicida*. The only species in this group, *A. salmonicida*, is a fish pathogen. It is nonmotile, does not grow at 37°C, and therefore is not important in clinical microbiology.
Mesophilic group: *Aeromonas hydrophila* group. Members of this group grow at 37°C and are motile. This group comprises 11 DNA hybridization groups and includes several named species. It can be divided into three principal phenotypic groups (called phenons) which are equivalent to the species *A. hydrophila*, *A. caviae*, and *A. sobria*, as shown in Table 4-7.

CLINICAL SIGNIFICANCE. The mesophilic group of motile species are considered to be potential human pathogens; *A. salmonicida*, the only member of the psychrophilic group, has not been recovered from humans. The role of *Aeromonas* species as potential agents of human gastrointestinal disease has still not been resolved. Published reports differ on the significance of finding *Aeromonas* species in the stool of patients with diarrhea. The differences in findings may be related to geographic location, season of collection, or the culture media used for isolation. In spite of this uncertainty, four types of infection caused by *Aeromonas* have been outlined[36]:

Cellulitis and wound infections: Infections after exposure to contaminated water, soil, or food, with highest incidence in warm seasons.
Acute diarrheal disease of short duration: The diarrhea is most commonly watery in consistency with a disease syndrome that closely mimics cholera.
Septicemia: Patients with hepatobiliary disease are particularly susceptible to *A. hydrophila* septicemia.
Miscellaneous infections: Urinary tract, wound, hepatobiliary, meningeal, and ear infections and en-

docarditis and septicemia secondary to *Aeromonas hydrophila* have been reported.

LABORATORY RECOVERY OF *AEROMONAS* SPECIES FROM CLINICAL SPECIMENS. Differential or selective agars should be utilized when *Aeromonas* is suspected as the etiologic agent of gastroenteritis or when fecal specimens are submitted for work-up on patients whose peak of diarrheal symptoms has subsided. Most strains grow on selective enteric media as lactose fermenters and, therefore, may be overlooked as unimportant or commensal enteric organisms.

Blood agar (with or without ampicillin): Blood agar can be made selective by incorporation of 10 μg/mL ampicillin. Janda and associates[14] recommend the use of a selective sheep blood agar containing ampicillin (SB-A agar) to improve the recovery of *Aeromonas* species from stool specimens.

Alkaline peptone water: Initially developed for isolation of *Vibrio* species, alkaline peptone water (APW; pH 8.6) can be used to recover aeromonads present in low numbers (10 colony-forming units per milliliter) in stools. After overnight enrichment, APW is subcultured to the agar medium of choice.

Cefsulodin irgasan novobiocin (CIN) agar: Originally developed for the isolation of *Yersinia enterocolitica*, CIN agar is also suitable for recovery of *Aeromonas* from feces.

Enteric agars: Deoxycholate, MacConkey, and xylose lysine deoxycholate were found to give the highest overall plating efficiencies of eight routine enteric agars tested for recovery of *Aeromonas* species from feces.[8]

LABORATORY IDENTIFICATION OF *AEROMONAS* SPECIES. *Aeromonas* species are cytochrome oxidase–positive and can be quickly excluded from the Enterobacteriaceae by performing an oxidase test. A drop or two of tetramethyl-*p*-phenylenediamine-dihydrochloride (oxidase reagent) can be placed on surface colonies and observed for the evolution of a black discoloration characteristic of the colonies of *Aeromonas* species. Mesophilic *Aeromonas* species are motile with polar rather than peritrichous flagella similar to *Pseudomonas* species. *Aeromonas* species can be differentiated from *Pseudomonas* because they utilize glucose fermentatively rather than oxidatively and most *Aeromonas* species

are indole-positive (*Pseudomonas* species are negative). The biochemical differentiation of the clinically important *Aeromonas* species is shown in (Table 4-8).

Namdari and Bottone[29] also describe the suicide phenomenon for the rapid differentiation of *Aeromonas* species. This phenomenon is expressed when unknown strains are grown in broth media containing 0.5% glucose. The supplied glucose suppresses the tricarboxylic acid cycle, resulting in accumulation of acetic acid and cell death. *A. hydrophila* is nonsuicidal, aerogenic, and esculin-positive; *A. sobria* is suicide-variable, aerogenic, and esculin-negative; and *A. caviae* is suicidal, anaerogenic, and esculin-positive.

Genus *Plesiomonas*

The term *plesiomonas* is derived from the Greek word meaning "neighbor," indicating a close association with *Aeromonas*. As mentioned previously, *Aeromonas* species are being reclassified within their own family and *Plesiomonas* is believed to be more closely related to *Proteus* than *Aeromonas*.[24] Presently, *Plesiomonas* remains in the Vibrionaceae and *P. shigelloides* is the only species in the genus.

P. shigelloides is ubiquitous in surface waters and in soil and commonly infects various cold-blooded animals (frogs, snakes, turtles, lizards). Humans become infected primarily by ingesting contaminated or unwashed food. Although less frequently recovered from human feces than *Aeromonas* species, *Plesiomonas*-induced gastroenteritis has been reported in both children and adults.

Plesiomonas-related gastroenteritis in humans usually manifests as a mild watery diarrhea in which the stools are free of blood and mucin. Severe colitis or a cholera-like illness may be seen in patients who are immunosuppressed or who have gastrointestinal malignancies. The infection is more prevalent in the subtropical and tropical regions of the world and during the warm summer months. A few isolated cases of extraintestinal infections including septicemia, neonatal meningitis, cellulitis, septic arthritis, and acute cholecystitis have also been reported.

LABORATORY ISOLATION AND IDENTIFICATION. *P. shigelloides* is a straight, rounded, short, motile gram-negative bacillus with polar, generally lophotrichous flagella (*Vibrio* species and *Aeromo-*

Table 4-8
Differentiation of *Plesiomonas shigelloides* and Clinically Important *Aeromonas* Species

ORGANISM	β-HEMOLYSIS Sheep Blood	OXIDASE	MOTILITY	DNase	INDOLE	VOGES-PROSKAUER	DECARBOXYLASES Lysine	DECARBOXYLASES Ornithine	DECARBOXYLASES Arginine	ESCULIN	GAS FROM GLUCOSE	L-Arabinose	FERMENTATION Sucrose	FERMENTATION Mannitol	FERMENTATION Inositol
A. hydrophila group															
A. hydrophila	+	+	+	+	+	+	+	–	+	+	+	+	+	+	–
A. caviae group															
A. caviae	–	+	+	+	+	–	–	–	+	+	–	+	+	+	–
A. media	NA	+	–	+	V	–	–	–	+	+	–	+	–	NA	NA
A. sobria group															
A. sobria	+	+	+	+	+	+	+	+	+	–	+	V	+	+	–
A. veronii	+	+	+	NA	+	+	+	–	–	+	+	–	+	+	–
A. jandaei	+	+	+	+	+	V	+	–	+	–	+	–	–	+	–
A. schubertii	V	+	+	NA	–	–	+	–	+	–	–	–	–	–	–
A. trota	+	+	+	+	+	–	+	+	+	–	+	–	–	+	–
P. shigelloides	–	+	+	–	+	–	+	+		–	–	–	–	–	+

+, 90% or more of strains positive; –, 90% or more of strains negative; V, 11%–89% of strains positive; NA, results not available; shaded areas indicate key reactions.

nas species are monotrichous). The organism grows well on sheep blood agar and on most enteric media. Isolates are nonhemolytic on sheep blood agar and in 24 hours at 30° to 35°C (growth is optimum at 30°C); colonies average 1.5 mm in diameter and are gray, shiny, smooth, and opaque and may be slightly raised in the center. *P. shigelloides* is readily isolated on enteric agars such as MacConkey, deoxycholate, Hektoen, and xylose lysine deoxycholate. Ampicillin-containing selective media that are frequently used for the isolation of *Aeromonas* species are not suitable for the isolation of *P. shigelloides*.

Glucose is fermented; therefore, the butt portion of Kligler iron agar or triple sugar iron agar tubes appears yellow. *P. shigelloides* appears as a non–lactose fermenter on MacConkey agar and may be confused with *Shigella* species. The cytochrome oxidase reaction is positive, and indole is produced. *P. shigelloides* decarboxylates arginine, lysine, and ornithine. It does not produce DNAse or extracellular proteases, and it ferments inositol but not mannitol. These are key characteristics by which it is separated from *Aeromonas* species. Additional key identifying characteristics are listed in Table 4-8.

P. shigelloides can be resistant to penicillin, ampicillin, carbenicillin, and other β-lactamase sensitive penicillins. Most strains are susceptible to the aminoglycosides, chloramphenicol, tetracycline, trimethoprim-sulfamethoxazole, and the quinolones ciprofloxacin and norfloxacin.[2,34]

Genus *Chromobacterium*

Brief mention of the genus *Chromobacterium* is made here because some strains are oxidase-positive fermenters and can be confused with *Aeromonas* species and *Vibrio* species. *Chromobacterium violaceum* is the species most commonly encountered in clinical laboratories, although it is seldom associated with human disease. *C. violaceum* grows well on blood agar, and most strains produce abundant violet pigment that makes recognition easy. Select biochemical characteristics are shown in Table 4-6. In addition, the ability of the organism to utilize citrate, reduce nitrates, and strongly hydrolyze casein is also helpful in making a final definitive identification.

REFERENCES

1. Baumann P, Schubert RHW. Family II. *Vibrionaceae* Vernon 1965, 5245[AL]. In: Krieg NR, Holt JG, eds. Bergey's manual of systematic bacteriology. Vol 1. Baltimore, Williams & Wilkins, 1984;1:516–550.

2. Brenden RA, Miller MA, Janda JM. Clinical disease spectrum and pathogenic factors associated with *Plesiomonas shigelloides* infections in humans. Rev Infect Dis 1988;10:303–316.

3. Butzler JP. Infections with *Campylobacter*. In: Williams JD, Heremann W, eds. Modern topics in infectious diseases. London, Medical Books Ltd, 1978:214–239.

4. Centers for Disease Control. Cholera—worldwide, 1989. MMWR 1990;39:365–367.

5. Centers for Disease Control. Cholera—Peru, 1991. MMWR 1991;40:108–110.

6. Centers for Disease Control. Update: cholera—western hemisphere, 1992. MMWR 1992;41:667–668.

7. Colwell RR, MacDonell MT, De Ley J. Proposal to recognize the family Aeromonadaceae fam. nov. Int J Syst Bacteriol 1986;36:473–477.

8. Desmond E, Janda JM. Growth of *Aeromonas* species on enteric agars. J Clin Microbiol 1986;23:1065–1067.

9. Endtz HP, Ruijs GJHM, Zwinderman AH, et al. Comparison of six media, including a semisolid agar, for the isolation of various *Campylobacter* species from stool specimens. J Clin Microbiol 1991;29:1007–1010.

10. Farmer JJ III, Hickman-Brenner FW, Kelly MT. *Vibrio*. In: Lennette EH, ed. Manual of clinical microbiology. 4th ed. Washington, DC, American Society for Microbiology, 1985:282–301.

11. Goodwin CS, Armstrong JA, Chilvers T, et al. Transfer of *Campylobacter pylori* and *Campylobacter mustelae* to *Helicobacter* gen. nov. as *Helicobacter pylori* comb. nov. and *Helicobacter mustelae* comb. nov., respectively. Int J Syst Bacteriol 1989;39:397–405.

12. Goossens H, Pot B, Vlaes L, et al. Characterization and description of "*Campylobacter upsaliensis*" isolated from human feces. J Clin Microbiol 1990;28:1039–1046.

13. Hodinka RL, Gilligan PH. Evaluation of the Campyslide agglutination test for confirmatory identification of selected *Campylobacter* species. J Clin Microbiol 1988;26:47–49.

14. Janda JM, Dixon A, Raucher B, et al. Value of blood agar for primary plating and clinical implications of simultaneous isolation of *Aeromonas hydro-*

phila and *Aeromonas caviae* from a patient with gastroenteritis. J Clin Microbiol 1984;20:1221–1222.

15. Janda JM, Powers C, Bryant RG, et al. Current perspectives on the epidemiology and pathogenesis of clinically significant *Vibrio* spp. Clin Microbiol Rev 1988;1:245–267.

16. Kaplan RL, Barrett JE, Landau W, et al. The value of Campy thio in the recovery of *Campylobacter*: an analysis of three years experience. Presented before the annual meeting of the American Society for Microbiology, abstract C-77, 1984:249.

17. Karmali MA, Simor AE, Roscoe M, et al. Evaluation of a blood-free, charcoal-based, selective medium for the isolation of *Campylobacter* organisms from feces. J Clin Microbiol 1986;23:456–459.

18. Kelly MT. Cholera: a worldwide perspective. Pediatr Infect Dis 1986;5:S101–S105.

19. Kelly MT, Hickman-Brenner FW, Farmer JJ III. *Vibrio*. In: Balows A, ed. Manual of clinical microbiology. 5th ed. Washington, DC, American Society for Microbiology, 1991:384–395.

20. Kelly MT, Peterson JW, Sarles HE Jr, et al. Cholera on the Texas gulf coast. JAMA 1982;247:1598–1599.

21. Kiehlbauch JA, Brenner DJ, Nicholson MA, et al. *Campylobacter butzleri* sp. nov. isolated from humans and animals with diarrheal illness. J Clin Microbiol 1991;29:376–385.

22. Koneman EW, Allen SD, Janda WM, Schreckenberger PC, Winn WC Jr, eds. Color atlas and textbook of diagnostic microbiology. 4th ed. Philadelphia, JB Lippincott, 1992:243–277.

23. Luechtefeld NW, Reller LB, Blaser MJ, et al. Comparison of atmospheres of incubation for primary isolation of *Campylobacter fetus* subsp. *jejuni* from animal specimens: 5% oxygen versus candle jar. J Clin Microbiol 1982;15:53–57.

24. MacDonell MT, Colwell RR. Phylogeny of the Vibrionaceae and recommendation for two new genera, *Listonella* and *Shewanella*. Syst Appl Microbiol 1985;6:171–182.

25. Marshall BJ. *Campylobacter pyloridis* and gastritis. J Infect Dis 1986;153:650–657.

26. McNulty CAM, Dent JC, Uff JS, et al. Detection of *Campylobacter pylori* by the biopsy urease test: an assessment in 1445 patients. Gut 1989;30:1058–1062.

27. Merino FJ, Agulla A, Villasante PA, et al. Comparative efficacy of seven selective media for isolating *Campylobacter jejuni*. J Clin Microbiol 1986;24:451–452.

28. Nachamkin I, Barbagallo S. Culture confirmation of *Campylobacter* spp. by latex agglutination. J Clin Microbiol 1990;28:817–818.

29. Namdari H, Bottone EJ. Suicide phenomenon in mesophilic aeromonads as a basis for species identification. J Clin Microbiol 1989;27:788–789.

30. Nolan CM, Ballard J, Kaysner CA, et al. *Vibrio parahaemolyticus* gastroenteritis: an outbreak associated with raw oysters in the Pacific northwest. Diagn Microbiol Infect Dis 1984;2:119–128.

31. Oberhofer TR, Podgore JK. Urea-hydrolyzing *Vibrio parahaemolyticus* associated with acute gastroenteritis. J Clin Microbiol 1982;16:581–583.

32. Peterson WL. *Helicobacter pylori* and peptic ulcer disease. N Engl J Med 1991;324:1043–1048.

33. Quinn TC, Goodell SE, Fennell C, et al. Infections with *Campylobacter jejuni* and *Campylobacter*-like organisms in homosexual men. Ann Intern Med 1984;101:187–192.

34. Reinhardt JF, George WL. *Plesiomonas shigelloides*-associated diarrhea. JAMA 1985;253:3294–3295.

35. Steele TW, McDermott SN. Technical note: the use of membrane filters applied directly to the surface of agar plates for the isolation of *Campylobacter jejuni* from feces. Pathology 1984;16:263–265.

36. Von Graevenitz A, Altwegg A. *Aeromonas* and *Plesiomonas*. In: Balows A, ed. Manual of clinical microbiology. 5th ed. Washington, DC, American Society for Microbiology, 1991:396–401.

37. Wang W-LL, Luechtefeld NW. Effect of incubation atmosphere and temperature on isolation of *Campylobacter jejuni* from human stools. Can J Microbiol 1983;29:468–470.

5

Haemophilus

Members of the genus *Haemophilus* are small, non-motile, gram-negative bacilli that require growth factors present in blood; the genus name is derived from the Greek words meaning "blood loving." Some *Haemophilus* species require X factor, which is probably not a single substance but rather a group of heat-stable tetrapyrrole compounds that are provided by several iron-containing pigments (eg, hemin and hematin). These compounds are used in the synthesis of catalases, peroxidases, and cytochromes of the electron transport system. Most *Haemophilus* species also require V factor, which is nicotinamide adenine dinucleotide (NAD, coenzyme I) or nicotinamide adenine dinucleotide phosphate (NADP, coenzyme II).

Both X and V factors are found within blood cells, including the sheep erythrocytes found in blood agar formulations routinely used in clinical laboratories. Sheep blood also contains enzymes that slowly hydrolyze V factor. Consequently, V factor–dependent haemophili do not generally grow on sheep blood agar in which the erythrocytes are intact. Gentle heating during the addition of blood to the molten agar base results in lysis of erythrocytes, liberation of both X and V factors, and inactivation of enzymes that hydrolyze V factor. Most laboratories rely on chocolate agar for the recovery of *Haemophilus* species from clinical specimens. *Haemophilus* species are also able to grow on blood agar containing intact 5% horse blood or rabbit blood. On these media, some *Haemophilus* species are β-hemolytic, which is a useful property for identification.

Even though most *Haemophilus* species are unable to grow on sheep blood agar, tiny colonies of the organisms may occasionally be observed on this medium as pinpoint growth around colonies of other organisms in mixed cultures. These colonies also appear as "satellite" colonies within the hemolytic zone of a "staph streak" on sheep blood agar. The lysed erythrocytes in the agar surrounding the *Staphylococcus aureus* streak provide X factor, and the staphylococcal cells themselves secrete V factor during logarithmic growth. The staph streak technique can be used to recover *Haemophilus* species from clinical specimens and is also a useful presumptive identification test (called the satellite test) for members of this genus.

TAXONOMY AND CLINICAL SIGNIFICANCE OF *HAEMOPHILUS* SPECIES

The genus *Haemophilus* is classified in the family Pasteurellaceae, which also includes members of the genera *Pasteurella* and *Actinobacillus*.[50] There are 10 human species and several animal species in the genus (Table 5-1). Although the genus *Haemophilus* has traditionally been defined by the requirement of its members for X and V factors, nucleic acid hybridization and cell wall studies over the past several years have demonstrated that growth factor requirements may not be an exclusive feature of *Haemophilus*. For example, certain V factor–dependent avian haemophili (eg, *H. avium*) were shown to be genetically more closely related to the type species of the genus *Pasteurella* (*P. multocida*; see Chapter 6) than to the type species of the

Table 5-1

Human and Animal Species in the Genus *Haemophilus*

HUMAN SPECIES	ANIMAL SPECIES
H. influenzae	H. equigenitalis (mares)
H. parainfluenzae	H. somnus (cattle)
H. haemolyticus	H. parasuis (swine)
H. parahaemolyticus	H. paragallinarum (poultry)
H. aphrophilus	H. paracuniculus (rabbits)
H. paraphrophilus	H. agni (sheep)
H. paraphrophaemolyticus	H. haemoglobinophilus (dogs)
H. aegyptius	Actinobacillus (Haemophilus) pleuropneumoniae (swine)
H. segnis	Actinobacillus (Haemophilus) avium (poultry)
H. duccreyi	

genus *Haemophilus* (*H. influenzae*). Human species are, for the most part, associated with the upper respiratory tract, except for *H. ducreyi*, which is a primary pathogen of the genital tract. Infections in humans caused by *Haemophilus* species, the appropriate specimens for culture, and the clinical manifestations of these infections are summarized in Table 5-2.

A full discussion of the clinical syndromes associated with *Haemophilus* species infections is beyond the scope of this chapter. In brief, meningitis is one of the more common manifestations, affecting 8000 to 10,000 persons in the United States annually, occurring primarily in children between 1 month and 2 years of age. Prior nasopharyngeal colonization in a susceptible host leads to invasion of the bloodstream and subsequent seeding of the meninges. Onset of meningeal signs and symptoms may be abrupt or insidious, with the latter being the most common pattern. The infection is contagious, and family members 4 years of age or younger are at increased risk of acquiring infection.

Other infections include epiglottitis and obstructive laryngitis, otitis media, sinusitis, chronic bronchitis, pneumonia, and bacteremia. Epiglottitis is often associated with laryngeal edema and upper airway obstruction, representing an acute medical emergency. Acute otitis media presents as ear pain with or without drainage, fever, and other

Table 5-2
Infectious Diseases Associated with *Haemophilus* Species

DISEASE	SPECIES	SPECIMENS FOR CULTURE	CLINICAL MANIFESTATIONS
Meningitis	*H. influenzae* type b (rarely other capsular types)	Cerebrospinal fluid; blood	Meningeal signs (headache, stiff neck), generally insidious onset; fever; seizures; usually seen in children 1 month to 2 years old
Acute pharyngitis and laryngeotracheo-bronchitis	*H. influenzae* type b	Posterior pharyngeal swab; laryngeal secretions	Inflamed mucous membranes, with swelling and yellow exudate; sore throat with stridor and cough; similar to croup if the laryngeal mucosa is involved
Epiglottitis	*H. influenzae* type b (rarely other capsular types)	Blood; laryngeal secretions	Rapid onset and progression of sore throat; dysphagia and upper airway obstruction; red and swollen epiglottis; may require tracheostomy to establish airway
Bronchitis	*H. influenzae* (often nontypeable strains)	Sputum; transtracheal aspirates; bronchial washings	Persistent, nonproductive cough; wheezing and dyspnea; disease is usually chronic with periodic purulent exacerbations
Acute sinusitis	*H. influenzae* (usually nontypeable strains); rarely *H. parainfluenzae*	Sinus aspirates; surgical specimens	Frontal headaches; facial pain, swelling and redness of suborbital and periorbital tissues; sinus empyema
Otitis media	*H. influenzae* (usually nontypeable strains)	Swab of pus in the ear canal; needle aspiration or myringotomy; suspected systemic disease may require collection of cerebrospinal fluid or blood cultures	Pain and fullness in the ears, usually bilateral; bulging, opaque tympanic membranes; fever, irritability, and vomiting may be noted in children; concomitant systemic disease should be suspected
Pneumonia	*H. influenzae* type b; nontypeable strains recovered from elderly patients	Sputum; transtracheal aspirates; bronchial washings	Cough, sputum production, and pleuritic pain, distribution tends to be lobar or segmental, simulating pneumococcal pneumonia; bacteremic pneumonia caused by nontypeable strains seen in elderly persons
Endocarditis	*H. aphrophilus;* *H. paraphrophilus;* *H. parainfluenzae;* *H. influenzae* (rare)	Blood	Chills, spiking fevers, leukocytosis, and secondary complications such as anemia, weight loss, malaise, and anorexia; mitral and aortic valves are most commonly involved; high incidence of arterial embolization
Genital tract infection; postpartum bacteremia; neonatal sepsis with meningitis	*H. influenzae* (nontypeable); *H. parainfluenzae*	Urethral and endocervical specimens; blood; fetal tissues; cerebrospinal fluid	Urethritis characterized by a thin, mucoid discharge; organisms may be recovered from cervical and blood cultures of women with postpartum fever; may also be cultured from multiple genital sites (eg, Bartholin's glands, endometrium), placenta, amniotic fluid, and neonatal body fluids (blood, cerebrospinal fluid)

(continued)

Table 5-2 (continued)

DISEASE	SPECIES	SPECIMENS FOR CULTURE	CLINICAL MANIFESTATIONS
Conjunctivitis	*H. aegyptius*	Conjunctival swab specimens	Characterized by mucopurulent conjunctival discharge; hyperemic conjunctivae, and diffusely injected sclera; spread to others by infectious secretions on towels, hands, and other fomites
Brazilian purpuric fever	*H. aegyptius* (BPF clone)	Blood; conjunctivae; skin lesions; oropharynx	Fever, abdominal pain with vomiting; petechial and hemorrhagic skin lesions; symptoms mimic meningococcal meningitis, but meningitis is not present; previous or concurrent conjunctival infection with *H. aegyptius* BPF clone usually found
Chancroid	*H. ducreyi*	Swabs obtained from genital ulcers; aspirates of swollen lymph nodes (buboes); endocervical specimens	Sexually transmitted disease characterized by painful, ulcerative genital lesions and enlarged, suppurative inguinal lymph nodes; may progress to abscess formation and fistula formation if left untreated

secondary systemic signs and symptoms of infection. The role of *H. influenzae* as a cause of sinusitis is questionable; evidence exists that these bacterial agents may represent secondary invaders after viral sinus infection. Similarly, the role of *H. influenzae* in chronic bronchitis is not clear, although several observations and experimental data suggest its role in chronic bronchitis, particularly as the cause of acute exacerbations. Cases have been reported in which *H. influenzae* bronchitis may extend to pneumonia in elderly patients with underlying respiratory diseases (chronic obstructive pulmonary disease, bronchiectasis) or systemic conditions such as immunodeficiency, diabetes, alcoholism, and neoplasms. The pneumonia is characteristically lobar, segmental, and purulent, closely simulating pneumococcal pneumonia. Bacteremia is a frequent and early manifestation of acute *H. influenzae* type b infection. Septic arthritis and osteomyelitis may also complicate *H. influenzae* bacteremia.

In addition to causing various disease syndromes, encapsulated *H. influenzae* (capsular serotypes a, b, c, d, e, and f) may also be found as a part of the normal upper respiratory tract flora of both children and adults. Colonization by capsular serotype b strains is found in 2% to 6% of children but may be as high as 60% among children in day care centers.[7,39] Therefore, recovery of *H. influenzae* from sputum specimens may reflect merely the presence of these organisms as a part of the normal nasopharyngeal flora and not the etiology of a disease process per se. In those persons with preexisting or chronic respiratory ailments, such as bronchitis, chronic obstructive pulmonary disease, bronchiectasis, bronchogenic carcinoma, and sinusitis, however, both encapsulated (typeable) and nonencapsulated (nontypeable) *H. influenzae* may cause severe respiratory tract infections.[7,40] Most infections are caused by *H. influenzae* strains belonging to capsular serotype b.[39] The reasons for the virulence of type b organisms and their ability to cause rapidly progressive and even life-threatening infections remain unclear, although their resistance to phagocytosis and intracellular killing by neutrophils afforded by the PRP capsule is an important factor.[49]

In the United States, *H. influenzae* type b is associated with about 16,000 cases of invasive disease in children 5 years of age and younger each year.[4] Most *Haemophilus* infections occur in children between the ages of 2 months and 5 years; most systemic type b infections affect children aged 2 years and younger.[50] It is recognized that inadequate levels of protective, anti-PRP bactericidal antibodies at this age play a major role in the development of disease. Immunity in the neonate is probably acquired by transplacental antibodies that are lost within the first few months of life. These antibodies generally reappear later, after exposure to the type b organisms or to other microbial antigens that engender cross-reactive antibodies. Most persons who develop systemic *H. influenzae* type b disease have low or undetectable levels of anti-PRP capsular antibodies. The antigenic capabilities of native, purified PRP and the protection afforded by anti-PRP antibodies were exploited in the first *H. influenzae* type b vaccine preparations.[3] It was found that the purified PRP failed to elicit protective levels of antibody in infants and young children, the groups most at risk for serious illness. Immune responses were consistently seen only in children older than 2 years of age.[19,47] Furthermore, the vaccine did not predictably elicit a "booster" response on subsequent antigenic challenge.

Because of the poor immunogenicity of the purified capsular polysaccharide and the demonstrated lack of efficacy in children younger than 18 months of age, clinical trials were subsequently undertaken with several polysaccharide/protein conjugate vaccines.[8,57] With this approach, it was hoped that the immunogenicity of the PRP material would be enhanced, with the protein "carrier" acting as an adjuvant. With the use of the conjugate vaccines, clinical trials have indeed demonstrated protective responses in much younger children.[1,15] Three conjugate vaccines for *H. influenzae* type b have now been approved by the Food and Drug Administration. After clinical trials, two of the vaccines were licensed for use in infants as young as 2 months of age, and the third was licensed for children as young as 15 months of age.[8,15]

LABORATORY APPROACH TO THE DIAGNOSIS OF *HAEMOPHILUS* INFECTIONS

Direct Examination of Clinical Material

Gram and Methylene Blue Stains

A rapid presumptive diagnosis of *H. influenzae* infection can be made by direct examination of appropriate clinical material using Gram stain. If

sufficient amounts (ie, more than 1 to 2 mL) of cerebrospinal fluid are received, the specimen should be centrifuged to obtain a pellet of material for examination and culture. Otherwise, the uncentrifuged specimen should be examined directly. On Gram-stained preparations, *Haemophilus* organisms appear as small, pale-staining, gram-negative coccobacilli (Color Plate 5-1*A*). Occasionally, slender filamentous cells may be observed. Because of the small size, cellular pleomorphism, and the poor staining of some strains with safranin, a simultaneously prepared smear may be stained with methylene blue to aid in the detection of these small bacterial cells. In the latter preparation, the organisms appear as blue-black coccobacilli against a light blue-gray background. Although *H. influenzae* may be the likely pathogen on the basis of the Gram-stained appearance and the patient's clinical presentation, the organisms cannot be identified on the basis of the Gram-stained smear alone. Furthermore, negative results on Gram stain do not rule out the possibility of *Haemophilus* infection because very few organisms may be present in the specimen.

Detection of Type b Capsular Antigen

For rapid diagnosis of *H. influenzae* type b infections, immunologic techniques are available for the detection of the type b PRP capsular antigen in cerebrospinal fluid, serum, and urine. The methods that are used in most laboratories are latex particle agglutination (LA) and staphylococcal protein A coagglutination (COA). Antibodies prepared against the *H. influenzae* type b PRP capsular antigen (or against capsular material of the other agents of bacterial meningitis) are bound to latex beads (LA) or to staphylococcal cells (COA) "carriers." Mixture of the appropriate body fluid containing the antigen with the sensitized LA or COA reagent results in visible agglutination or clumping of the reagent within seconds to minutes. Commercial LA kits include the Directigen Meningitis Test (Becton-Dickinson Microbiology Systems, Cockeysville, MD), the Bactigen *H. influenzae* type b (Wampole Laboratories, Cranbury, NJ), and the Wellcogen *H. influenzae* type b (Murex, Norcross, GA). The commercial COA test is the Phadebact *H. influenzae* type b (Karo Bio Diagnostics AB, Huddinge, Sweden). Several studies indicate that LA is probably the most sensitive method for the detection of capsular antigens in body fluids.[11,24,33]

Recovery of *Haemophilus* Species in Culture

Optimal recovery of *Haemophilus* species from clinical specimens depends on proper collection and transport of specimens and the use of appropriate culture media and incubation environments. Because these organisms are fastidious, specimens containing them should not be exposed to drying or to extremes in temperature. Crucial specimens such as cerebrospinal fluid should be hand-carried to the clinical laboratory as soon after collection as possible. Conventional sheep blood agar is not suitable for recovery of *Haemophilus* species that require V factor for growth owing to the presence of V factor–inactivating enzymes in native sheep blood. Rabbit or horse blood does not contain these enzymes, and agar media containing either of these blood products will support the growth of most *Haemophilus* species. Media that contain rabbit blood or horse blood are not routinely used in most clinical laboratories, so other techniques or media must be used if *Haemophilus* organisms are to be isolated. Regardless of the media employed, isolation of *Haemophilus* requires incubation in a moist environment with increased CO_2 (3% to 5%). This is provided by modern CO_2 incubators or by candle extinction jars.

Primary isolation of *Haemophilus* species from clinical specimens is accomplished by using chocolate agar, *Haemophilus* isolation agar, or the *Staphylococcus* streak technique.

Chocolate Agar

Chocolate agar is prepared by adding sheep blood to an enriched agar base medium that is at a high enough temperature (ie, about 80°C) to lyse the red blood cells and release X and V factors. Prolonged heating must be avoided to prevent inactivation of heat-labile V factor. For quality control and other technical purposes, most clinical laboratories purchase chocolate agar and other bacteriologic media from commercial vendors. Commercially prepared chocolate agar usually contains a synthetic mixture of hemin (X factor) and a "cocktail" of chemically defined growth factors added to gonococcal (GC) agar base medium.

The disadvantage of using chocolate agar for primary isolation of *Haemophilus* species is that the medium does not allow the determination of hemolytic properties, which help to differentiate *H. haemolyticus* and *H. parahaemolyticus* from *H. influenzae*. It is, however, an excellent medium for the recovery of other fastidious organisms, such as *Neisseria meningitidis* and *Neisseria gonorrhoeae*, from specimens that are not commonly contaminated with other organisms, such as cerebrospinal fluid or joint fluid. Because *Haemophilus* species are common inhabitants of the upper respiratory tract (including both hemolytic and nonhemolytic species), many laboratories have adopted *Haemophilus* isolation agar for recovery of these organisms from respiratory tract specimens. Selective chocolate agar–based media containing various antibiotics (eg, vancomycin, bacitracin, and clindamycin) have been described but are not widely used.[10] The gray mucoid colonies of *H. influenzae* type b growing on chocolate agar are shown in Color Plate 5-1*B*.

Haemophilus Isolation Agar

Many commercial media companies market antibiotic-containing media for the selective isolation of *Haemophilus* species from respiratory tract specimens. These media contain beef heart infusion, peptones, yeast extract, and defibrinated horse blood (5%), which contains both X and V factors. In addition, bacitracin (300 mg/L) is added to inhibit the other normal respiratory tract flora, including staphylococci, micrococci, neisseriae, and streptococci. Besides the selective recovery of *Haemophilus* species from heavily mixed cultures, the hemolytic properties of certain haemophili can be determined directly on primary isolation.

Staphylococcus Streak Technique

Many bacteria and yeasts synthesize and secrete V factor during growth on bacteriologic media. In mixed cultures, *Haemophilus* species that require V factor may grow as pinpoint colonies around the colonies of these other microorganisms. This phenomenon is called *satellitism*. This property provides a technique for detecting these organisms in mixed cultures as well as a presumptive test for genus-level identification. A colony of a possible *Haemophilus* species can be subcultured to a sheep blood agar plate and streaked as a lawn. With the use of an inoculating wire, a single streak of a V factor–producing organism, such as *Staphylococcus aureus*, is made through the inoculum of the possible *Haemophilus*. After overnight growth in a CO_2-enriched environment, tiny moist colonies of the haemophili may be observed within the hemolytic area adjacent to the staphylococcal growth (see Color Plate 5-1C). X factor–dependent haemophili will also grow as satellite colonies because hemin and hematin are released from the lysed red blood cells by the action of staphylococcal hemolysins. This method may be used for presumptive identification of *Haemophilus* species when species-level identification is not required or essential (eg, upper respiratory tract specimens).

Identification of *Haemophilus* Species

Identification Procedures

In the clinical laboratory, commonly encountered *Haemophilus* species are identified on the basis of their hemolytic reactions on horse blood agar and their growth requirements for X and V factors. The method using filter paper disks or strips impregnated with X factor, V factor, or both is routinely used to determine these growth requirements. The organism to be identified is streaked as a lawn on media deficient in growth factors. Trypticase-soy agar is recommended as the medium of choice for performance of the growth factor determination procedure.[13] It is important when selecting colonies from primary culture plates for this test that none of the chocolate agar or other blood-containing media are transferred to the factor determination plate. Suspending the organism in factor-deficient broth before plate inoculation is one way to reduce carryover of growth factors and consequent false-positive results.

The X and V factor disks or strips are placed on the agar surface about 1 to 2 cm apart. If a disk or strip containing both factors is also used, the disks may be more widely spaced on the agar surface. The plates are incubated in 3% to 5% CO_2 at 35°C for 18 to 24 hours, and the patterns of growth around the disks or strips are observed. Differentiation of *Haemophilus* species is then made on the basis of the growth patterns shown Color Plate 5-1D.

The δ-aminolevulinic acid (ALA)-porphyrin test, originally described by Kilian,[29] is another method for determining X factor requirements. The reaction utilized in this test is a direct assessment of the ability of a *Haemophilus* strain to synthesize protoporphyrin intermediates in the biosynthetic pathway to hemin from the precursor compound δ-aminolevulinic acid. Strains that require exogenous X factor for growth (ie, *H. influenzae* and *H. haemolyticus*) are incapable of synthesizing protoporphyrins from ALA and, consequently, are negative with this test. Strains that do not require exogenous X factor for growth (ie, *H. parainfluenzae* and *H. parahaemolyticus*) possess the enzymes that synthesize protoporphyrin compounds from the ALA substrate and are, consequently, ALA-porphyrin test–positive.

Commercially available ALA-impregnated filter paper disks (Difco Laboratories, Detroit, MI; Remel Laboratories, Lenexa, KS) or growth media containing the ALA reagent (Remel Laboratories) may also be used to perform the ALA-porphyrin test.[16,32] With the disk method, the impregnated disk is moistened with water and inoculated with organisms from growth media. After 4 hours, the disk is observed under ultraviolet light (Wood's light). Brick-red fluorescence in the area of organism deposition indicates a positive test result; bluish fluorescence constitutes a negative test result. With the ALA agar medium, the organism is inoculated onto the medium and incubated overnight. The next day the growth is examined under a Wood's light for brick-red fluorescence. The ALA-porphyrin test is shown in Color Plate 5-1E.

Serotyping of *Haemophilus influenzae*

Although most *H. influenzae* strains recovered from systemic infections belong to serotype b, the other serotypes (ie, types a, c, d, e, and f) have also been recovered from infectious processes in both children and adults.[12,18,53] The easiest technique for serotyping isolates is slide agglutination.[22] A dense suspension of the organism is prepared in saline. Single drops of the suspension are placed in each of a series of circles on a glass slide corresponding to the number of sera to be tested, plus a saline control. Type-specific antisera are added to each of the test circles, and the slide is rotated. Rapid (less than 1 minute) agglutination of organisms by a specific antiserum and the absence of agglutination in the saline control identifies the isolate as a specific serotype. Polyvalent and type-specific antisera for *H. influenzae* are commercially available from Murex (Norcross, GA) and Difco Laboratories (Detroit, MI).

A coagglutination culture confirmation test (Phadebact Haemophilus Test, Karo Bio Diagnostics AB, Huddinge, Sweden) is also available for simultaneous identification and serotyping of H. influenzae type b from primary culture media. This kit contains a vial of staphylococcal cells sensitized with type b antisera (test reagent) and a second vial of staphylococci sensitized with antisera to type a, c, d, e, and f (control reagent). Colonies from the growth media are mixed with each of the two reagents on a cardboard slide. After mixing, the slide is rocked for 30 to 60 seconds. Visible agglutination of the mixture with the test reagent but not the control reagent identifies the isolate as H. influenzae type b. This test has been shown to be highly sensitive and specific for identifying type b H. influenzae.[52]

Biotyping of Haemophilus influenzae and Haemophilus parainfluenzae

In his taxonomic study of the genus Haemophilus, Kilian[29] introduced the use of biochemical tests for identifying and characterizing haemophili. Based on the results of three tests—indole production, urease activity, and ornithine decarboxylase activity—Kilian divided H. influenzae strains into four biotypes, which were designated I through V.[31] These biotypes were independent of the serotype of the organism; that is, organisms of different serotypes or nontypeable strains could have the same pattern of biotyping reactions. With the use of these same tests, four additional H. influenzae biotypes (V, VI, VII, and VIII) have also been described.[20,54]

Similarly, seven biotypes of H. parainfluenzae (designated I through IV and VI through VIII) have been delineated with the same three tests. The biochemical tests for an H. influenzae biotype I strain are shown in Color Plate 5-1F.

Biochemical characterization of Haemophilus species has yielded valuable epidemiologic information, and specific biotypes have been associated with different types of infections, sources of isolation, antigenic properties, and antimicrobial resistance patterns.[18,31,36] In a survey of 130 H. influenzae strains from cases of meningitis, 93.1% were biotype I, while 4.6% and 2.3% were biotypes II and IV, respectively.[31] All but one strain in this series were type b. Other studies have also noted the association between H. influenzae biotypes II and III and conjunctival infections.[2] As mentioned previously, biotype IV H. influenzae strains have been documented as pathogens in obstetric, gynecologic, perinatal, and neonatal infections[34,48,56] and have been isolated from men with nongonococcal urethritis.[55] Initial studies suggested that resistance to ampicillin was associated primarily with biotype I and II strains of H. influenzae, but it now appears that this characteristic is more generally distributed among the various biotypes of both H. influenzae and H. parainfluenzae.

Biochemical Methods and Kit Systems for Haemophilus Identification

The RIM (Rapid Identification Method)-H system (Austin Biological Laboratories, Austin, TX) is a commercially available method that uses buffered carbohydrates (glucose, lactose, and sucrose) along with a substrate blank and a rapid ALA-porphyrin test to identify Haemophilus species. In an evaluation of this identification method,[46] 100% of 76 H. influenzae strains and 92% of 23 H. parainfluenzae strains were correctly identified. Hemolysis on horse blood agar was required to differentiate H. haemolyticus from H. influenzae and H. parahaemolyticus from H. parainfluenzae.

Biochemical identification methods have been exploited in the development of other commercial kit systems and reagents that use modified conventional tests along with novel chromogenic enzyme substrates for both identifying and biotyping of Haemophilus isolates. The RapID NH panel (Innovative Diagnostics Systems, Inc, Atlanta, GA), the Neisseria-Haemophilus Identification (NHI) card (bioMérinex Vitek, Hazelwood, MO; see Color Plate 5-1G), and the Haemophilus-Neisseria Identification (HNID) panel (American MicroScan, Sacramento, CA; see Color Plate 5-1H), identify these organisms within 4 hours of inoculation with a pure culture.[13,25,26] All three systems will identify the species and generate a biotype based on the urease, ornithine decarboxylase, and indole tests.

Several commercially available systems designed for identifying enteric bacteria (eg, the API 20E, the Micro ID, and the Minitek System) have also been used to biotype Haemophilus strains.[6,28] Reagent-impregnated disks (Remel Laboratories,

Lenexa, KS) for performing urease and ornithine decarboxylase tests can also be used along with the spot indole test for rapid (1 hour) biotyping of individual isolates. In fact, the spot indole test alone can provide a presumptive identification of *H. influenzae* in respiratory tract specimens because indole-positive biotype II strains represent 40% to 70% of the *H. influenzae* strains found in these specimens.[58]

Laboratory Diagnosis of *Haemophilus ducreyi* Infection

Gram-stained smears of the suppurative exudate from the genital lesions of chancroid and from suppurating lymph nodes may reveal the organism. On properly collected and prepared smears, *H. ducreyi* appear as pale-staining gram-negative coccobacilli, often arranged in groups having a "school-of-fish" appearance. They may be found inside and outside polymorphonuclear cells.

It has been historically reported that *H. ducreyi* is extremely difficult to culture and identify. As a result of improvements in media quality, however, several studies have reported that isolation of the organism is relatively easy.[21,44] Aspirates from the lesion or an adjacent swollen lymph node or a swab specimen from the base of a thoroughly cleansed lesion should be promptly inoculated onto growth media. Several media have been described for isolation of *H. ducreyi*. GC agar base containing 1% to 2% hemoglobin, 5% fetal calf serum, 1% Iso-Vitalex enrichment, and vancomycin (3 g/mL) has been used successfully, as has Mueller-Hinton agar with 5% chocolatized horse blood, 1% IsoVitalex enrichment, and vancomycin (3 g/mL).[38] Vancomycin is added to inhibit gram-positive organisms (eg, staphylococci and streptococci) that may be present as contaminants or superinfecting bacteria in the chancroid lesion.

Commercial chocolate agar media generally support the growth of *H. ducreyi*; vancomycin disks may be placed in various quadrants of a chocolate plate to help detect the organisms in mixed cultures. It is recommended that more than one medium (eg, one with and one without vancomycin) be used and that multiple appropriate specimens be collected. Media are incubated at 33° to 35°C in 3% to 5% CO_2 with high humidity and are inspected daily for 10 days. Most isolates cultured

directly from clinical specimens produce visible growth in 2 to 4 days.

Colonies of *H. ducreyi* are small, nonmucoid, and gray, yellow, or tan. The colonies can characteristically be "nudged" along the agar surface with a bacteriologic loop, are difficult to pick up, and produce a nonhomogeneous, "clumpy" suspension in saline. On Gram stain the organisms appear as gram-negative coccobacilli. *H. ducreyi* is catalase-negative and oxidase-positive; the oxidase reaction is usually delayed and develops only after 15 to 20 seconds with the tetramethyl-*p*-phenylenediamine dihydrochloride reagent.[38] Because of the fastidious nature of *H. ducreyi*, growth factor requirements cannot be demonstrated with factor-impregnated disk or strip techniques. The ALA-porphyrin test is negative, indicating that exogenous hemin is required for growth. The organism is biochemically inert, except for positive nitrate reduction and alkaline phosphatase tests.[21] Shawar and coworkers[51] examined 25 *H. ducreyi* strains and found that all isolates gave unique and consistent enzymatic reactions on the RapID ANA system (Analytab Products, Inc, Plainview, NY), which is used for the identification of clinically significant anaerobic bacteria (see Chapter 11).

ANTIMICROBIAL SUSCEPTIBILITY OF *HAEMOPHILUS* SPECIES

Resistance to Ampicillin and Chloramphenicol in *Haemophilus influenzae*

By 1974, it was found that certain strains of *H. influenzae* were indeed ampicillin resistant on the basis of their ability to produce β-lactamase enzymes capable of hydrolyzing and inactivating ampicillin. A national collaborative susceptibility study found that 20% of *H. influenzae* strains obtained from medical centers throughout the country produced β-lactamase.[14] Because of this, chloramphenicol was frequently administered along with or substituted for ampicillin in empiric therapy for serious *H. influenzae* infections. Strains of *H. influenzae* have, however, been isolated that are resistant to chloramphenicol or to both ampicillin and chloramphenicol.[5,17,45] In recent years, β-lactamase-mediated ampicillin resistance has been found in encapsulated *H. influenzae* non–type b isolates, nontypeable *H. influenzae* strains, and *H. parainfluenzae* organisms.[43]

In addition to β-lactamase production, some *H. influenzae* strains have been isolated that are resistant to ampicillin but do not produce β-lactamase enzymes.[37,45] Resistance to ampicillin in these strains is due to alterations in both the penicillin-binding proteins in the cell wall and to altered permeability of the cell membrane to the antimicrobial agents.[37] Susceptibility of *Haemophilus* species to ampicillin and other antimicrobial agents can be determined by disk diffusion and either broth or agar dilution procedures.[27,41,42] These methods are described in Chapter 12.

Resistance to chloramphenicol, the other antimicrobial agent traditionally used in the treatment of serious *H. influenzae* disease, has also appeared in these microorganisms.[5,9] Although the prevalence of these strains is not high, the microbiologist should be aware of the methods required for their detection in the clinical laboratory. Most chloramphenicol-resistant *H. influenzae* strains elaborate an enzyme called chloramphenicol acetyltransferase (CAT),[35] which prevents the antimicrobial from its normal function of inhibiting bacterial protein synthesis.

Ampicillin remains the drug of choice for the treatment of *H. influenzae* meningitis caused by ampicillin-susceptible strains.[50] Acceptable alternative agents include cefotaxime, ceftriaxone, and chloramphenicol. For ampicillin-resistant strains, ceftriaxone is the drug of choice. With the availability of more defined standards for *H. influenzae* susceptibility testing,[41,42] surveillance of resistance patterns among *Haemophilus* isolates can now be performed more readily and reliably.

REFERENCES

1. Ahonkhai VI, Lukacs LJ, Jonas LC, et al. *Haemophilus influenzae* type b conjugate vaccine (meningococcal protein conjugate) (Pedvax HIB): clinical evaluation. Pediatrics 1990;85:676–681.
2. Albritton WL, Brunton JL, Meier M, et al. *Haemophilus influenzae*: Comparison of respiratory tract isolates with genitourinary tract isolates. J Clin Microbiol 1982;16:826–831.
3. Ambrosino DM, Landesman SH, Gorham CC, et al. Passive immunization against disease due to *Haemophilus influenzae* type b: Concentrations of antibody to capsular polysaccharide in high-risk children. J Infect Dis 1986;153:1–7.
4. American Academy of Pediatrics, Committee on Infectious Diseases. *Haemophilus influenzae* type b conjugate vaccines: immunization of children at 15 months of age. Pediatrics 1990;86:794–796.
5. Azemun P, Stull T, Roberts M. Rapid detection of chloramphenicol resistance in *Haemophilus influenzae*. Antimicrob Agents Chemother 1981;20:168–170.
6. Back AE, Oberhofer TR. Use of the Minitek system for biotyping *Haemophilus* species. J Clin Microbiol 1978;7:312–313.
7. Berk SL, Holtzclaw SA, Weiner SL, et al. Nontypeable *Haemophilus influenzae* in the elderly. Arch Intern Med 1982;142:537–539.
8. Black SB, Shinefield RA, Hiatt B, et al. Efficacy of HbOC conjugate *Haemophilus influenzae* type b vaccine in a study population of 48,000 infants. In: Program and Abstracts of the 30th Interscience Conference on Antimicrobial Agents and Chemotherapy. Atlanta, 1990.
9. Burns JL, Mendelman PM, Levy J, et al. A permeability barrier as a mechanism of chloramphenicol resistance in *Haemophilus influenzae*. Antimicrob Agents Chemother 1985;27:46–54.
10. Chapin KC, Doern GV. Selective recovery of *Haemophilus influenzae* from specimens contaminated with upper respiratory tract flora. J Clin Microbiol 1983;17:1163–1165.
11. Collins JK, Kelly MT. Comparison of Phadebact coagglutination, Bactigen latex agglutination, and counterimmunoelectrophoresis for detection of *Haemophilus influenzae* type b antigens in spinal fluid. J Clin Microbiol 1983;17:1005–1008.
12. Controni G, Rodriguez WJ, Chang MJ. Meningitis caused by *Haemophilus influenzae* type e, biotype IV. South Med J 1982;75:78.
13. Doern GV, Chapin KC. Laboratory identification of *Haemophilus influenzae*: effects of basal media on the results of the satellitism test and evaluation of the RapID NH system. J Clin Microbiol 1984;20:599–601.
14. Doern GV, Jorgensen JH, Thornsberry C, et al. National collaborative study of the prevalence of antimicrobial resistance among clinical isolates of *Haemophilus influenzae*. Antimicrob Agents Chemother 1988;32:180–185.
15. Eskola J, Peltola H, Takala AK, et al. Efficacy of *Haemophilus influenzae* type b polysaccharide-diphtheria toxoid conjugate vaccine in infancy. N Engl J Med 1987;317:717–722.
16. Gadbury JL, Amos MA. Comparison of a new commercially prepared porphyrin test and the conventional satellite test for the identification of

Haemophilus species that require X factor. J Clin Microbiol 1986;23:637–639.

17. Givner LB, Abramson JS, Wasilauskas B. Meningitis due to *Haemophilus influenzae* type b resistant to ampicillin and chloramphenicol. Rev Infect Dis 1989;11:329–334.

18. Granato PA, Jurek EA, Weiner LB. Biotypes of *Haemophilus influenzae*: Relationship to clinical source of isolation, serotype, and antibiotic susceptibility. Am J Clin Pathol 1983;79:73–77.

19. Granoff DM, Munson RS. Prospects for prevention of *Haemophilus influenzae* type b disease by immunization. J Infect Dis 1986;153:448–461.

20. Gratten M. *Haemophilus influenzae* biotype VII. J Clin Microbiol 1983;13:1015–1016.

21. Hannah P, Greenwood JR. Isolation and rapid identification of *Haemophilus ducreyi*. J Clin Microbiol 1982;7:39–43.

22. Himmelreich CA, Barenkamp SJ, Storch GA. Comparison of methods for serotyping *Haemophilus influenzae*. J Clin Microbiol 1986;21:159–160.

23. Holmes RL, DeFranco LM, Otto M. Novel method of biotyping *Haemophilus influenzae* that uses API 20E. J Clin Microbiol 1982;15:1150–1152.

24. Ingram DL, Pearson AW, Occhiuti AR. Detection of bacterial antigens in body fluids with the Wellcogen *Haemophilus influenzae* b, *Streptococcus pneumoniae*, and *Neisseria meningitidis* (ACYW135) latex agglutination tests. J Clin Microbiol 1983;18:1119–1121.

25. Janda WM, Bradna JJ, Ruther P. Identification of *Neisseria* spp., *Haemophilus* spp, and other fastidious gram-negative bacteria with the MicroScan *Haemophilus Neisseria* identification panel. J Clin Microbiol 1989;27:869–873.

26. Janda WM, Malloy PJ, Schreckenberger PC. Clinical evaluation of the Vitek *Neisseria-Haemophilus* identification card. J Clin Microbiol 1987;25:37–41.

27. Jorgensen JH, Howell AW, Maher LA. Antimicrobial susceptibility testing of less commonly isolated *Haemophilus* species using *Haemophilus* test medium. J Clin Microbiol 1990;28:985–988.

28. Kilian M. A rapid method for the differentiation of *Haemophilus* stains: the porphyrin test. Acta Pathol Microbiol Scand [B] 1974;82:935–942.

29. Kilian M. A taxonomic study of the genus *Haemophilus* with the proposal of a new species. J Gen Microbiol 1976;93:9–62.

30. Kilian M, Biberstein EL. Genus II. *Haemophilus*. In: Krieg NR, Holt JG, eds. Bergey's manual of systematic bacteriology. Baltimore, Williams & Wilkins, 1984;1:558–559.

31. Kilian M, Sorensen I, Frederiksen W. Biochemical characteristics of 130 recent clinical isolates from *Haemophilus influenzae* meningitis. J Clin Microbiol 1979;9:409–412.

32. Lund ME. Filter paper porphyrin production test for identification of *Haemophilus*. Clin Microbiol Newsletter 1981;3:27–29.

33. Marcon MJ, Hamoudi AC, Cannon HJ. Comparative laboratory evaluation of three antigen detection method for diagnosis of *Haemophilus influenzae* type b disease. J Clin Microbiol 19:1984;333–337.

34. Martel AY, St. Laurent G, Dansereau LA, et al. Isolation and biochemical characterization of *Haemophilus* species isolated simultaneously from the oropharyngeal and anogenital areas. J Clin Microbiol 1989;27:1486–1489.

35. Matthews HW, Baker CN, Thornsberry C. Relationship between in vitro susceptibility test results for chloramphenicol and production of chloramphenicol acetyltransferase by *Haemophilus influenzae*, *Streptococcus pneumoniae* and *Aerococcus* species. J Clin Microbiol 1988;26:2387–2390.

36. Matthews JS, Reynolds JA, Weesner DE, et al. Rapid species identification and biotyping of respiratory isolates of *Haemophilus*. J Clin Microbiol 1983;18:472–475.

37. Mendelman PM, Chaffin DO, Stull TL, et al. Characterization of non–beta-lactamase–mediated ampicillin resistance in *Haemophilus influenzae*. Antimicrob Agents Chemother 1984;26:235–244.

38. Morse SA. Chancroid and *Haemophilus ducreyi*. Clin Microbiol Rev 1989;2:137–157.

39. Moxon ER. *Haemophilus influenzae*. In: Mandell GL, Douglas RG Jr, Bennett JE, eds. Principles and practice of infectious diseases. New York, Churchill Livingstone, 1990:1722–1729.

40. Murphy TF, Apicella MA. Nontypeable *Haemophilus influenzae*: a review of clinical aspects, surface antigens and human immune response to infection. Rev Infect Dis 1987;147:838–846.

41. National Committee for Clinical Laboratory Standards. Performance standards for antimicrobial disk susceptibility tests (approved standard, NCCLS document M2-A4). 4th ed. Villanova, PA, National Committee for Clinical Laboratory Standards, 1988.

42. National Committee for Clinical Laboratory Standards. Methods for dilution antimicrobial susceptibility tests for bacteria that grow aerobically (approved standard, NCCLS document M7-A2). 2nd ed. Villanova, PA, National Committee for Clinical Laboratory Standards, 1990.

43. Needham C. *Haemophilus influenzae*: antibiotic susceptibility. Clin Microbiol Rev 1988;1:218–227.

44. Oberhofer TR, Back AE. Isolation and cultivation of *Haemophilus ducreyi*. J Clin Microbiol 1982; 15:625–629.

45. Offit PA, Campos JM, Plotkin SA. Ampicillin-resistant, beta-lactamase–negative *Haemophilus influenzae* type b. Pediatrics 1982;69:230–231.

46. Palladino S, Leahy BJ, Newall TL. Comparison of the RIM-H rapid identification kit with conventional tests for the identification of *Haemophilus* species. J Clin Microbiol 1990;28:1862–1863.

47. Pincus DJ, Morrison D, Andrews C, et al. Age-related response to two *Haemophilus influenzae* type b vaccines. J Pediatr 1982;100:197–201.

48. Quentin R, Musser JM, Mellouett M, et al. Typing of urogenital, maternal, and neonatal isolates of *Haemophilus influenzae* and *Haemophilus parainfluenzae* in correlation with clinical course of isolation and evidence for a genital specificity of *Haemophilus influenzae* biotype IV. J Clin Microbiol 1989;27:2286–2294.

49. Robbins JB, Schneerson R. Polysaccharide–protein conjugates: a new generation of vaccines. J Infect Dis 1990;161:821–832.

50. Saez-Llorens X, McCracken GH. Bacterial meningitis in neonates and children. Infect Dis Clin North Am 1990;4:623–644.

51. Shawar R, Sepulveda J, Clarridge JE. Use of the RapID-ANA system and sodium polyanethol sulfonate disk susceptibility testing in identifying *Haemophilus ducreyi*. J Clin Microbiol 1990;28: 108–111.

52. Shively RG, Shigei JT, Peterson EM, et al. Typing of *Haemophilus influenzae* by coagglutination and conventional slide agglutination. J Clin Microbiol 1981;14:706–708.

53. Slater LN, Guarnaccia J, Makintubee S, et al. Bacteremic disease due to *Haemophilus influenzae* capsular type f in adults: report of five cases and review. Rev Infect Dis 1990;12:628–635.

54. Sottnek FO, Albritton WL. *Haemophilus influenzae* biotype VIII. J Clin Microbiol 1984;20:815–816.

55. Sturm AW. *Haemophilus influenzae* and *Haemophilus parainfluenzae* in nongonococcal urethritis. J Infect Dis 1986;153:165–167.

56. Wallace RJ, Baker CJ, Quinones F, et al. Nontypeable *Haemophilus influenzae* (biotype IV) as a neonatal, maternal, and genital pathogen. Rev Infect Dis 1983;5:123–136.

57. Ward J, Brenneman G, Letson GW, et al. Limited efficacy of a *Haemophilus influenzae* type b conjugate vaccine in Alaska Native infants. N Engl J Med 1990;323:1393–1401.

58. Welch DF, Ahlin PA, Matsen JM. Differentiation of *Haemophilus* spp. in respiratory cultures by a spot indole test. J Clin Microbiol 1982;15: 216–219.

6

Miscellaneous Fastidious Gram-Negative Bacilli

INTRODUCTION TO THE FASTIDIOUS GRAM-NEGATIVE BACILLI

The fastidious gram-negative bacteria considered in this chapter are isolated infrequently but, nonetheless, may cause serious infections in humans. In many cases, these organisms occur in specific clini-
cal settings, so an understanding of the disease process and the condition of the patient may help tremendously in the laboratory's efforts to recover these organisms from clinical specimens. For example, a history of indolent, insidious symptoms with the presence of vegetations on the heart valves as determined by echocardiogram is the clinical setting for endocarditis due to the HACEK group

of organisms. A history of recurring febrile episodes in a patient who works in the meat-packing industry may lead one to suspect *Brucella* infection. Cultures from dog bite wounds will frequently grow *Pasteurella multocida* or the fastidious organism formerly called CDC group DF-2 (*Capnocytophaga canimorsus*).[22] Obviously, the physician caring for the patient and the microbiologist handling the specimens must be engaged in close communication for the successful diagnosis and treatment of these unusual infections.

THE HACEK ORGANISMS

The organisms constituting the HACEK group include fastidious gram-negative bacteria that are all part of the normal human oropharyngeal or urogenital flora. Under certain circumstances they can cause serious disease. These organisms are found mainly in association with endocarditis, bacteremia, and mixed-flora wound infections. *HACEK*, the mnemonic used to group these organisms together, stands for *Haemophilus aphrophilus/paraphrophilus* (H), *Actinobacillus actinomycetemcomitans* (A), *Cardiobacterium hominis* (C), *Eikenella corrodens* (E), and *Kingella* species (K). All of these bacteria are slow growing, requiring 48 to 72 hours of incubation before adequate growth is apparent. When grown in blood cultures, detection of these organisms may take from a few days to 2 weeks or longer in some cases. All of them require or are stimulated by the presence of CO_2, necessitating incubation in a candle jar or a CO_2 incubator. Optimal growth is achieved only on enriched media, such as chocolate or blood agar, and no growth is seen on selective enteric media such as MacConkey or eosin methylene blue (EMB) agar. Although not an absolute requirement, hemin in the medium generally enhances initial recovery of the organisms. Once these organisms are recovered in pure culture, identification is fairly easy if appropriate media and techniques are employed.

Haemophilus aphrophilus and Haemophilus paraphrophilus

Haemophilus aphrophilus and *H. paraphrophilus* have been implicated in a wide variety of human infectious processes.[13,15,107] These infections include sinusitis, otitis media, pneumonia, empyema, septicemia, endocarditis, septic arthritis, osteomyelitis, soft tissue abscesses, wound infections, necrotizing fasciitis, meningitis, brain abscess, and laryngoepiglottitis. Trauma, neutropenia, malignancy, and cancer chemotherapy are apparently predisposing factors for infections with these organisms.[43] Of the *Haemophilus* species presented in Chapter 5, *H. aphrophilus* and *H. paraphrophilus* are the most common ones recovered from patients with endocarditis. The incidence of endocarditis caused by these organisms is highest in young to middle-aged adults and may or may not be associated with preexisting valvular disease.[13,15,61] *H. aphrophilus* and *H. paraphrophilus* grow slowly on agar medium. Colonies are small after 24 hours; 48 to 72 hours incubation is required before colony morphology can be ascertained and sufficient growth is available for preliminary identification tests. Microcolonies growing in broth tend to adhere to the sides of the tube, a characteristic these organisms share with *A. actinomycetemcomitans*. On chocolate agar colonies measure less than 0.5 to 1 mm after 48 hours, are convex and granular, and have a yellowish pigment (Color Plate 6-1*A*). A distinct odor like grade-school paste may be noted. The organisms do not grow on MacConkey agar or other selective/differential enteric media. On primary isolation, *H. aphrophilus* may require X factor (hemin); this requirement is lost on subculture. Because of the lack of factor requirements for growth, *H. aphrophilus* will grow on sheep blood agar and brain–heart infusion agar without supplementation. Short, pale-staining gram-negative coccobacilli are seen in Gram-stained preparations (see Color Plate 6-1*B*).

H. paraphrophilus is biochemically similar to *H. aphrophilus*, except that V factor (nicotinamide adenine dinucleotide [NAD]) is required for growth (Table 6-1). Consequently, this species does not grow on sheep blood agar and will not grow on brain-heart infusion or trypticase-soy agar without NAD supplementation (eg, a V factor disk or strip). *H. aphrophilus* and *H. paraphrophilus* are positive in the δ-aminolevulinic acid (ALA)-porphyrin test (they do not require exogenous hemin for growth), are negative for the three reactions used for biotyping of *Haemophilus* species (urease, indole and ornithine carboxylase), and readily hydrolyze *ortho*-nitrophenol-β-D-galactopyranoside (ONPG). Catalase is not produced, and acid is produced from both glucose and lactose. These characteristics differentiate *H. aphrophilus* and *H.*

Table 6-1

Biochemical Characteristics for Identification of *Haemophilus aphrophilus*, *Haemophilus paraphrophilus*, and *Actinobacillus actinomycetemcomitans*

CHARACTERISTIC	*H. aphrophilus*	*H. paraphrophilus*	*A. actinomycetemcomitans*
Hemolysis on sheep blood agar	−	−	−
Oxidase	−*	−*	−*
Catalase	−	−	+
Reduction of NO_3 to NO_2	+	+	+
Requirement for X factor	−	−	−
Requirement for V Factor	−	+	−
Indole	−	−	−
Urease	−	−	−
Ornithine decarboxylase	−	−	−
Hydrolysis of esculin	−	−	−
Hydrolysis of ortho-nitrophenyl-β-D-galactopyranoside	+	+	−
Gas from glucose	+	+	V
Production of acid from:			
Glucose	+	+	+
Maltose	+	+	+†
Fructose	+	+	+
Sucrose	+	+	−
Lactose	+	+	−
Xylose	−	−	V
Mannitol	−	−	V‡
Mannose	+	+	+
Galactose	+	−	V
Melibiose	−	+	−
Trehalose	+	+	−
Melezitose	−	+	NA
Raffinose	+	−	−

+, positive reaction; −, negative reaction; V, variable reaction; NA, not available.
*Few strains may produce weak or delayed positive reactions.
†Rare strains may be maltose-negative.
‡Most strains are mannitol-positive.

paraphrophilus from *A. actinomycetemcomitans*, which is catalase-positive and does not ferment lactose. Most strains are oxidase-negative, although a delayed, weak, or equivocal oxidase reaction may be observed with some isolates. *H. paraphrophilus* can be differentiated from *H. aphrophilus* by its requirement for V factor and by utilization patterns for galactose, melibiose, melezitose, and raffinose. The biochemical features of *H. aphrophilus* and *H. paraphrophilus* are shown in Table 6-1 along with those of *A. actinomycetemcomitans*.

    H. aphrophilus and *H. paraphrophilus* are generally susceptible to tetracycline, chloramphenicol, streptomycin, and the other aminoglycosides. Although most strains are also susceptible to penicillin and ampicillin, isolates resistant to these antimicrobials have been reported; some of these resistant isolates produced β-lactamase enzymes.[81]

Actinobacillus actinomycetemcomitans

The genus *Actinobacillus* contains many species,[111,121] only one of which will be discussed here. *A. actinomycetemcomitans* is a small gram-negative coccobacillus that is associated with endocarditis, bacteremia, wound infection, and dental infections. Although the organism has frequently been coisolated with *Actinomyces israelii* from actinomycotic abscesses, it has also been isolated from similar lesions in the absence of the anaerobic actinomycetes. The most common infection associated with *A. actinomycetemcomitans* is subacute bacterial endocarditis. Several cases of endocarditis caused by this organism have been reported in the literature; most of these were in persons with valvular damage due to congenital heart diseases.[2,33,62,82,86] Prosthetic mitral valve and aortic valve endocarditis have also been reported in persons with both tissue (eg, porcine) or mechanical valve replacements.[147] A principal predisposing factor in the development of native or prosthetic valve endocarditis with this organism is poor dentition or recent dental manipulations.[6] Complications of this infection include the formation of emboli, congestive heart failure, glomerulonephritis, need for placement of prosthetic valves due to native valvular damage, prosthetic heart valve replacement, hematogenous dissemination of the organisms to distant sites, and death.[62,82] Research in the area of dental microbiology has also established an important role for *A. actinomycetemcomitans* in periodontal disease.

A. actinomycetemcomitans grows slowly on chocolate and blood agars, with visible colonies appearing after 48 to 72 hours. Colonies of *A. actinomycetemcomitans* are nonhemolytic, small, smooth, and translucent and have slightly irregular edges (see Color Plate 6-1*C*). Fresh clinical isolates are adherent to the agar and are difficult to emulsify. On prolonged incubation (5 to 7 days), colonies may develop a central density that takes on the appearance of a four- or six-pointed star. On repeated subculture the surface structure of the colonies become less marked and become less adherent. As with *H. aphrophilus*, growth in broth is scant and adherent to the sides of the tube. On Gram stain the organisms appear as pale staining, gram-negative coccobacilli. On repeated subculture longer cells may be noted on stained smears (see Color Plate 6-1*D*).

Characteristics for the identification of *A. actinomycetemcomitans* include lack of growth on Mac-Conkey and other enteric agars and positive reactions for catalase production and nitrate reduction. The organism is oxidase-negative (occasional strains may be weakly positive), is urease-negative,

does not produce indole, and does not require X or V factors.[127] Lysine and ornithine decarboxylase and arginine dihydrolase reactions are negative. Most strains strongly ferment glucose, fructose, and mannose. Acid production from maltose, mannitol, and xylose may vary. *A. actinomycetemcomitans* can be differentiated from *H. aphrophilus* in that the former is catalase-positive and ONPG-negative and acid is not produced from lactose, sucrose, or trehalose (see Table 6-1).

A. actinomycetemcomitans is generally susceptible to tetracyclines, streptomycin, and chloramphenicol.[152] Ceftriaxone and rifampin have also been shown effective both in vitro and in vivo. Variable susceptibility to penicillin, ampicillin, erythromycin, and the aminoglycosides has been reported. In vitro studies indicate that combinations of various therapeutic agents for the treatment of *A. actinomycetemcomitans* endocarditis may be synergistic, additive, or antagonistic.[152] Hence, the efficacy of combination therapy cannot be predicted and these properties must be determined for individual strains.

Cardiobacterium hominis

Cardiobacterium hominis has the unique characteristic of being associated exclusively with endocarditis.[60,125,151] It may be isolated from the human upper respiratory tract as a part of the normal flora, but, because of its slow growth rate, it is rarely noted in these specimens. As with the other organisms described, this organism enters the bloodstream and usually infects previously diseased heart valves.[151] *C. hominis* endocarditis has also been reported in persons with no evidence of previous heart disease. Prosthetic valve endocarditis associated with this organism may also occur.[151] The infection follows a very subacute course, with an insidious onset and vague symptoms. Consequently, the physician must have a high index of suspicion that he or she is dealing with this organism and should inform the laboratory so that extra efforts to recover the organism may be taken. Patients frequently have a history of having had dental work performed before the onset of symptoms of endocarditis.

Since *C. hominis* is associated with endocarditis, it will be isolated from blood cultures. The organism grows slowly and may be recovered in essentially all commercially available blood culture media. No visible change in the blood culture medium (eg, hemolysis, pellicle formation, turbidity) will be noted, so frequent blind subcultures of macroscopically negative blood culture bottles to chocolate and blood agars should be performed. In our experience, the BACTEC radiometric blood culture system (Becton Dickinson Microbiology Systems, Cockeysville, MD) has been able to detect growth of the organism after 3 to 5 days. Characteristically, the growth indices on the BACTEC system will increase in small increments over time when bottles become positive with this organism.

Gram stains of positive blood bottles may not reveal the organism; a low-speed centrifugation to remove red blood cells and a high-speed centrifugation to pellet small numbers of organisms may aid in their visualization. On Gram staining, the organisms may appear gram-variable, with a tendency for the cells to retain the crystal violet dye at the poles. Individual cells may appear swollen at one or both ends, resulting in teardrop-, dumbbell-, and lollipop-shaped organisms.[125] The morphology of the individual cells is dependent on the type of culture medium used. In media containing yeast extract, cells may appear as uniform, gram-negative bacilli. Often, the cells will assume rosette-shaped clusters or picket-fence arrangements (see Color Plate 6-1E).

On blood and chocolate agars *C. hominis* grows as very small, glistening, opaque colonies, generally after 48 to 72 hours at 35°C in 5% to 7% CO_2 (see Color Plate 6-1F). Some strains may also pit the agar on further incubation. No growth is observed on MacConkey agar or other enteric selective or differential agars. The organism is oxidase-positive, catalase-negative, nitrate-negative, and urease-negative. The positive oxidase and negative nitrate reduction reactions help to differentiate this organism from *H. aphrophilus* and *A. actinomycetemcomitans* but is similar to reactions seen for *Eikenella*, *Kingella*, and *Suttonella* (Table 6-2).

The most helpful feature for identifying this organism is the production of indole. A tryptone broth should be heavily inoculated (with a swab) and incubated for 48 hours. Extraction with xylene or chloroform and use of Ehrlich's reagent rather than Kovac's reagent allows the detection of the small amounts of indole produced. The spot indole reagent (*p*-amino cinnamaldehyde) may or may not detect indole production by *C. hominis*. Hydrogen

sulfide production can be detected using lead acetate strips. *C. hominis* produces acid from glucose, fructose, sucrose, mannose, and sorbitol; acid production from maltose and mannitol is variable (most strains are positive). Lactose, xylose, galactose, trehalose, and raffinose are not fermented (see Color Plate 6-1G).

C. hominis strains are generally susceptible to most antimicrobial agents, including penicillin, ampicillin, cephalothin, aminoglycosides, chloramphenicol, and tetracycline. Patients with *C. hominis* endocarditis are generally treated with penicillin alone or penicillin combined with an aminoglycoside. The organism is resistant to vancomycin and erythromycin.

Eikenella corrodens

Eikenella corrodens is a part of the normal flora of the mouth and upper respiratory tract.[24] In this location the organism is most frequently associated with dental and periodontal infections, head and neck infections, otitis media, mastoiditis, and respiratory tract infections.[132] By extension from periodontal, middle ear, or sinus infections, the organism may enter the central nervous system, leading to meningitis and brain or paraspinal abscesses. Bacteremia and endocarditis caused by *E. corrodens* may also occur; most of these infections have been in immunocompromised hosts, intravenous drug abusers, or persons with previous valvular damage who had recently had extensive dental work.[89,93] Prosthetic valve endocarditis and infections of indwelling vascular prostheses associated with *E. corrodens* have also been reported.[34] *E. corrodens* bacteremia with or without endocarditis may also occur in persons with underlying disease (eg, rheumatoid arthritis, cancer).[47]

In recent years, *E. corrodens* has been isolated from cutaneous and subcutaneous abscesses and cellulitis associated with the injection of drugs ("skin popping"), in which needles are lubricated with saliva before introduction of the needle into the skin or where the drug is dissolved in saliva before injection.[93] *E. corrodens* may also be isolated from infections of the hand after clenched-fist injuries resulting from fist fights.[66] Traumatic implantation of the organism into the subcutaneous tissue by this or other mechanisms (eg, puncture wounds) may result in extension of the organism into the

Table 6-2
Biochemical Characteristics for Identification of *Cardiobacterium hominis*, *Eikenella corrodens*, *Kingella* species, and *Suttonella indologenes*

CHARACTERISTIC	C. hominis	E. corrodens	K. kingae	K. denitrificans	S. indologenes
Hemolysis on sheep blood agar	−	−	+*	−	−
Oxidase	+	+	+	+	+
Catalase	−	−†	−	−	−
Reduction of NO_3 to NO_2	−	+	−	+	−
Reduction of NO_2 to gas	+	−	+	+	+
Indole	+	−	−	−	+
Urease	−	−	−	−	−
Ornithine decarboxylase	−	+	−	−	−
Hydrolysis of esculin	−	−	−	−	−
Hydrolysis of ortho-nitrophenyl-β-D-galactopyranoside	−	−	−		
Gas from glucose	−	−	−		
Production of acid from:					
Glucose	+	−	+	+	+
Maltose	+‡	−	+	−	+
Fructose	+	−	−	−	+
Sucrose	+	−	−	−	+
Lactose	−	−	−	−	−
Xylose	−	−	−	−	−
Mannitol	+‡	−	−	−	−
Mannose	+	−	−	−	+
Galactose	−	−	−	−	−
Trehalose	−	−	−	−	−
Raffinose	−	−	−	−	−
Sorbitol	+	−	−	−	−

+, positive reaction; −, negative reaction.
*Most strains produce a "soft" β-hemolysis on sheep blood agar.
†Rare strains may be weakly catalase-positive.
‡Rare strains may be maltose- or mannitol-negative.

bone, resulting in osteomyelitis and septic arthritis.[28,114] In these settings the organism is usually recovered in mixed culture with other facultative organisms (α- and β-hemolytic streptococci, *Staphylococcus aureus*, coagulase-negative staphylococci, enteric gram-negative bacilli) and obligate anaerobes (*Peptostreptococcus* species, oral *Bacteroides/Porphoromonas* species). *E. corrodens* may also be recovered from the gastrointestinal tract and, in this milieu, may be present in mixed culture with facultative and anaerobic gut flora in the settings of abdominal and biliary abscesses and peritonitis.[24]

E. corrodens can be recovered on blood and chocolate agar and does not grow on MacConkey agar. Colonies are small (0.5 to 1 mm) after 48 hours.

About 50% of isolates may "pit" the agar as they grow, and both pitting and nonpitting variants may be observed in the same culture (see Color Plate 6-1*H*). A pale yellow pigment (observed best on a white swab swept through growth on a chocolate agar plate) is usually produced, and most strains have an odor suggestive of sodium hypochlorite (ie, Chlorox bleach) when grown on commercial chocolate and blood agars. On Gram stain the organisms appear as regular, slender gram-negative bacilli or coccobacilli with rounded ends.

Biochemical characteristics of both pitting and nonpitting *E. corrodens* strains are uniform. The organisms are oxidase-positive and catalase-negative, although rare strains may be weakly catalase-positive. The organism reduces nitrate to nitrite and does not require X or V factors, although hemin is necessary for aerobic growth. Indole and urease are not produced, but most strains are lysine- and ornithine decarboxylase–positive. Unlike the other organisms in the HACEK group, *E. corrodens* does not produce acid from carbohydrates. Consequently, in some texts the organism is grouped with the nonfermentative bacteria, although its cultural characteristics correspond more to those of the fastidious gram-negative bacteria. The phenotypic characteristics of *E. corrodens* are presented in Table 6-2, along with the other oxidase-positive, catalase-negative fastidious HACEK bacteria.

Most *E. corrodens* strains are susceptible to ampicillin, ticarcillin, carbenicillin, tetracycline, and chloramphenicol and are resistant to the penicillinase-resistant penicillins (eg, methicillin, dicloxacillin, nafcillin, and oxacillin), clindamycin, lincomycin, vancomycin, and the aminoglycosides. Penicillin susceptibility may vary from strain to strain. Most isolates are variably susceptible to the first-generation cephalosporins. Although they are rare, β-lactamase–positive strains of *E. corrodens* have been reported.[67]

Kingella Species and *Suttonella indologenes*

Although they are part of the normal upper respiratory and genitourinary tract flora of humans, *Kingella* species, and *K. kingae* in particular, may be occasionally isolated from significant infections. *K. kingae* appears to have a specific tissue tropism for cardiac, valvular, joint space, and skeletal tissue; therefore, it has been associated primarily with endocarditis and bone and joint infections.[99,141] The portal of entry for the organism into the bloodstream is probably through a breach in the oropharyngeal mucosa. Many patients are noted to have poor oral hygiene, pharyngitis, or mucosal ulcerations from treatment for other conditions (eg, radiation therapy). *K. kingae* endocarditis, as with the other fastidious bacteria discussed thus far, primarily occurs in those persons with underlying heart disease (congenital malformation, rheumatic heart disease, mitral valve prolapse) or cardiac prostheses, although cases in persons with no previous heart disease have been reported.[106,155]

Among bone and joint infections, septic arthritis with osteomyelitis is the most common clinical presentation.[35] These localized infections result from hematogenous spread of the organism. Interestingly, *K. kingae* arthritis and osteomyelitis are most often seen in infants and young children usually 5 years of age and younger.[19,31] Many of these children also have significant underlying conditions such as acute lymphocytic leukemia or congenital heart disease. Septicemia with *K. kingae* may also mimic systemic neisserial infections in its clinical presentation.[140]

K. denitrificans and *S. indologenes* (formerly *K. indologenes*) have rarely been isolated from clinically significant infections.[36] *K. denitrificans* has been cultured from the throat and the genitourinary tract; a single report has appeared citing it as a cause of endocarditis.[65] *S. indologenes* has been isolated from human eye infections and was first reported in association with a case of prosthetic valve endocarditis in 1987.[79,135]

Kingella species are plump gram-negative bacilli or coccobacilli that sometimes occur in pairs or short chains. They are oxidase-positive and, unlike *Neisseria* and *Moraxella* species, catalase-negative. All species grow on chocolate and blood agars and do not grow on MacConkey agar or other enteric media. Multiple colony types may be produced in a single culture. *K. kingae* is β-hemolytic on sheep blood agar and may "pit" or corrode the agar surface, particularly on primary isolation. The hemolytic reaction is "soft," resembling group B streptococci, and may only be noted in areas of confluent growth or after the removal of the colony from the agar surface. *S. indologenes* is distinguished by its ability to produce indole. Like *C. hominis*, this characteristic should be determined in tryptone broth with xylene extraction and addition of Ehrlich's indole reagent. *K. denitrificans* was originally called "TM-1" and was first recognized by its ability to grow on Thayer-Martin medium.[76] *K. denitrificans* will also produce acid from glucose in supplemented media, rapid carbohydrate degradation tests, and various kit systems; because of this it may be misidentified as *N. gonorrhoeae* particularly in specimens from the genitourinary tract.[74,77,78] This organism, unlike the other species in the genus, reduces nitrate to nitrite, and most strains will also reduce nitrite to nitrogen gas on prolonged incubation. *S. indologenes* may be differentiated from *C. hominis*, which it closely resembles, by appearance on Gram stain, positive alkaline phosphatase activity, and failure to produce acid from mannitol and sorbitol.[26,36] *E. corrodens* may be differentiated from both *C. hominis* and *Kingella* species by its Gram stain morphology, its failure to ferment carbohydrates, and its positive ornithine decarboxylase reaction. Biochemical reactions for identification of *Kingella* species and *S. indologenes* are presented in Table 6-2.

Kingella/Suttenella species are usually susceptible to peniicillin, ampicillin, oxacillin, cephalosporins of all generations, chloramphenicol, the aminoglycosides, trimethoprim-sulfamethoxazole, and ciprofloxacin. Some strains may be relatively resistant to erythromycin, and most strains are resistant to clindamycin and lincomycin.

OTHER MISCELLANEOUS FASTIDIOUS GRAM-NEGATIVE BACTERIA

Capnocytophaga Species

Capnocytophaga species are gliding, gram-negative bacteria that are a part of the normal oropharyngeal flora. They are implicated to play a role (along with *A. actinomycetemcomitans*) in the pathogenesis of periodontal disease in humans. In recent years, *Capnocytophaga* species have also been reported as a cause of sepsis in patients with malignancy, granulocytopenia, and other severe underlying illnesses (eg, myeloblastic leukemia, acute lymphocytic leukemia, adenocarcinoma, multiple myeloma, Hodgkin's disease, endometrial carcinoma).[7,52,64] In virtually all cases, bacteremic episodes with this organism coincided with periods of profound granulocytopenia due to the underlying disease or the administration of cytotoxic chemotherapeutic agents. Oral ulcerations and bleeding gums have been characteristically found in these patients, thus establishing the route of entry for the organism into the bloodstream. The organism is most frequently isolated form respiratory sources (gingival crevices, the oropharynx, periodontal pockets, saliva) and is occasionally isolated from blood and cerebrospinal fluid. Rarely, the organism may be recovered from the vagina, the cervix, pleural fluid, amniotic fluid, and conjunctivae. Cases of endocarditis and cervical lymphadenitis in nonimmunocompromised hosts caused by *Capnocytophaga* species have also been reported.[95,108]

Capnocytophaga species are slow growing, with colonies becoming visible generally after 48 hours of incubation and developing a characteristic morphology after this time. All species require a CO_2-enriched environment for growth; this may be provided in a CO_2 incubator or a candle jar. The colonies of the organism are yellow, tan, or slightly pinkish and have marginal finger-like projections (gliding motility) appearing as a film surrounding the central area of the colony. The central part of the colonies also have a moist, mottled, or sweaty appearance. The organism grows on blood and chocolate agar but not on MacConkey agar. Good growth may also be observed on modified Thayer-Martin agar because of its resistance to vancomycin, colistin, and trimethoprim. The organisms are gram-negative, are fusiform, and may appear straight or slightly curved (see Color Plate 6-1*I*). Pleomorphism and variations in the size of the cells is characteristic, with swollen or large coccoid cells being seen in older cultures. All species are catalase- and oxidase-negative and produce acid from glucose, maltose, sucrose, and mannose, but not from ribose, xylose, mannitol, or sorbitol (see Color Plate 6-1*J*).[129] Indole and urease are not produced, and all decarboxylase reactions are negative.

Most strains are susceptible to penicillin, ampicillin, cefaclor, clindamycin, chloramphenicol, carbenicillin, cefaperazone, and tetracycline.[134] Many strains also demonstrate susceptibility to metronidazole, erythromycin, and cefamandole. Variable susceptibility may be seen for the various types of first-generation cephalosporins (cephalothin, cefazolin, cephalexin and cephradine). The organisms are generally resistant to aminoglycosides (kanamycin, gentamicin, tobramycin, amikacin, netilmicin, and neomycin), colistin, and vancomycin.

DF-2 and DF-2–Like Bacteria: *Capnocytophaga canimorsus* and *Capnocytophaga cynodegmi*

CDC group DF-2 was originally isolated in 1976 from blood and cerebrospinal fluid cultures of a patient who became symptomatic after suffering a dog bite. Subsequently, several case reports describing similar organisms were published and, through 1987, over 150 isolates of the organism were sent to the Special Bacteriology Branch of the CDC.[50,73] Based on genetic relatedness and phenotypic characteristics, DF-2 and a group of "DF-2–like" organisms have been classified as new

Capnocytophaga species. CDC group DF-2 is now called *Capnocytophaga canimorsus* (Latin for "dog bite") and the DF-2–like strains are now called *Capnocytophaga cynodegmi* (Greek for "dog bite").[22] Although these organisms are genotypically and phenotypically different from the previously described *Capnocytophaga* species, they are similar to them with respect to Gram stain morphology, cellular fatty acids, gliding-type motility, and cultural conditions for growth.

DF-2 infections are generally associated with dog bites or close contact with dogs.[50] Susceptible hosts generally have underlying diseases or conditions that predispose them to severe infection with the organism. These conditions include hepatic disease secondary to alcoholism, previous splenectomy related to other medical circumstances, Hodgkin's disease, pulmonary fibrosis, malabsorption syndrome, renal disease, chronic obstructive pulmonary disease, peptic ulcer disease, and the use of systemic or topical corticosteroids.[57,73] The frequently noted association of systemic DF-2 infection with asplenia strongly suggests that the reticuloendothelial system plays an important role in containing the infection. Major clinical features of these infections have included wound infection with cellulitis, meningitis, fulminant bacteremia with septic shock, hypotension, renal failure, disseminated intravascular coagulation, hemorrhagic skin lesions reminiscent of meningococcal disease, and bacterial endocarditis.[5,57,73] DF-2 has also been isolated from the oropharynx and saliva of dogs. A case of corneal ulcer with perforation caused by DF-2 has also been reported.[84] In this case, the patient had sustained a scratch on the cornea from his dog that was treated with, among other things, topical prednisone. DF-2 infections have also been reported occasionally in immunocompetent hosts and in persons with no known contact with dogs or other animals. Interestingly, a few cases of DF-2 infection, including keratitis and systemic infection, have occurred in persons who sustained bites or scratches from domestic cats.[27] DF-2 is usually recovered from blood cultures, although other specimens (wound cultures, aspirates from cellulitis) may also be submitted.

The organism has been recovered in several types of blood culture media, and growth is generally slow. The lysis-centrifugation method (Isolator, Wampole Laboratories, Cranbury, NJ) has also been used successfully for isolation.[138] In most reports cultures become positive 3 to 7 days after collection. The organism grows on both blood and chocolate agar that is incubated at 35°C and in a CO_2 incubator or a candle jar. Poor growth on routine sheep blood agar has been attributed to the use of a trypicase-soy base; better growth is seen when a heart infusion base is employed. Commercial supplemented chocolate agars containing Iso-Vitalex or other similar enrichments are satisfactory. Pinpoint colonies appear after 3 or 4 days of incubation. After a few more days the colonies appear circular, smooth, and convex. On Gram stain the bacteria appear as thin, fusiform bacilli that are 2 to 4 μm long. Some cells may appear slightly curved. Like the other fastidious bacteria discussed thus far, no growth is observed on Mac-Conkey agar. DF-2 (*C. canimorsus*) and DF-2–like (*C. cynodegmi*) bacteria are catalase- and oxidase-positive. These two reactions differentiate them from the other *Capnocytophaga* species, which are both oxidase- and catalase-negative. Both species are also arginine dihydrolase– and ONPG-positive. Lysine and ornithine decarboxylase tests are negative. *C. canimorsus* and *C. cynodegmi* are differentiated by carbohydrate utilization tests, with the latter organism producing acid from a wider variety of sugars.

In 1988, Verghese and associates reported on a broth dilution technique using Schaedler broth as the growth medium.[142] All eight DF-2 strains tested were susceptible to all antibiotics except aztreonam. These antimicrobial agents included penicillin, erythromycin, ticarcillin, piperacillin, cefazolin, cefaperazone, cefotaxime, ceftazidime, gentamicin, amikacin, chloramphenicol, trimethoprim-sulfamethoxazole, and ciprofloxacin. Antibiotics that are generally more active against grampositive organisms, such as vancomycin, clindamycin, erythromycin, and rifampin were also active against DF-2. These data support the clinical efficacy observed with penicillin (mean penicillin minimal inhibitory concentration = 0.04 μg/mL $\pm$ 0.01 μg/mL for all strains tested).

CDC Group DF-3

CDC group DF-3 is an uncommon isolate, although a few cases have been reported in the recent medical literature. The first case, reported in 1988, involved multiple isolations of the organism in pure culture from the stool of an elderly woman with common variable hypogammaglobulinemia of long standing.[144] The second case, also reported in

1988, occurred in a 24-year-old man with a relapse of acute lymphocytic leukemia.[10] During intensive chemotherapy and irradiation, the patient became profoundly granulocytopenic, and during this period multiple blood cultures were drawn to determine the etiology of low-grade fevers. The organism was isolated from blood cultures collected during this time.

Blum and coworkers reported the recovery of DF-3 from the stool of eight patients presenting with diarrhea of varying degrees of severity. All patients were immunocompromised or had severe underlying conditions. Treatment can eliminate the organism from the stool, and a carrier state can occur.

DF-3 does not grow well on standard enteric isolation media such as MacConkey, *Salmonella Shigella* (SS), or xylose-lysine-deoxycholate (XLD)

agar or most selective Campy media incubated at 42°C (an exception is CVA-Campy medium, which does not contain cephalothin or trimethoprim). Thus, the organism will not be recovered from routine stool cultures in most laboratories unless a specific search is made. Cefoperazone-vancomycin-amphotericin blood agar incubated at 35°C is selective for the recovery of DF-3 from stool cultures. Pinpoint colonies become visible after 24 hours incubation at 35°C in CO_2. After 48 to 72 hours the colonies are gray-white, smooth, and nonhemolytic. On Gram stain the organisms appear as gram-negative coccobacilli. Both clinical reports also mention that a sweet odor is produced by the organism on agar media.[10,144] Both oxidase and catalase reactions are negative, and nitrate is not reduced. Biochemical characteristics are shown in Table 6-3.

Table 6-3
Biochemical Characteristics for Identification of CDC Groups DF-3, EF-4a, EF-4b, HB-5, M-5, and M-6
(*Neisseria elongata* subspecies *nitroreducens*)

CHARACTERISTIC	DF-3	EF-4a	EF-4b	HB-5	M-5	M-6
Hemolysis on sheep blood agar	−	−*	−*	−	−	−
Oxidase	−	+	+	V†	+	+
Catalase	−	+	+	−	V	−
Growth on MacConkey agar	−	V	V	V	V	V
Reduction of NO_3 to NO_2	−	+	+	+	−	+
Reduction of NO_2 to gas	NA	V	−	−	V	+
Indole	V‡	−	−	+	−	−
Urease	−	−	−	−	−	−
Arginine dihydrolase	NA	V	V	−	−	−
Lysine decarboxylase	−	−	−	−	−	−
Ornithine decarboxylase	−	−	−	−	−	−
Esculin hydrolysis	+	−	−	−	−	−
Gas from glucose	−	−	−	+	−	−
Production of acid from:						
Glucose	+	+§	+‖	+	−	−/W+
Maltose	+	−	−	−	−	−
Fructose	NA	−	−	+	−	−
Sucrose	+	−	−	−	−	−
Lactose	+	−	−	−	−	−
Xylose	−	−	−	−	−	−
Mannitol	−	−	−	−	−	−
Mannose	−	−	−	+	−	−

+, positive; −, negative; V, variable; −/W+, negative or weakly positive; NA, not available.
*Some strains may show weak α-hemolysis.
†Weak or delayed positive reactions may be noted with some strains.
‡In one report, the organism was indole-positive; in the second report, the organism was indole-negative.
§Acid is produced from glucose by fermentation.
‖Acid is produced from glucose by oxidation.

Antimicrobial susceptibility of these DF-3 isolates was determined by disk diffusion and broth dilution methods.[10,144] DF-3 strains are resistant to several agents, including penicillin, ampicillin, aminoglycosides, cephalosporins (first, second, and third generation), erythromycin, and vancomycin. Isolates are susceptible to trimethoprim-sulfamethoxazole and chloramphenicol, and variably susceptible (possibly method dependent) to clindamycin, tetracycline, and imipenem.

CDC Group EF-4a and EF-4b

Formerly a group of uncertain taxonomic affiliation, these bacteria have recently been classified as unnamed members of the family Neisseriaceae.[122] CDC group EF-4 (eugonic fermenter 4) is a rare human isolate that is a part of the normal oral flora of cats and dogs.[12] Consequently, it has been isolated from human wounds resulting from scratches and bites from these animals. Some strains have a distinct popcorn odor and develop a yellow pigment. Biochemical characteristics for identification of group EF-4 strains are shown in Table 6-3.

CDC Group HB-5

CDC group HB-5 isolates have been recovered primarily from the genitourinary tract and related specimens (ie, vagina, cervix, urethra, Bartholin's glands and amniotic fluid). They have also been identified in cases of male urethritis, pelvic inflammatory disease, and Bartholin's gland abscesses, with the suggestion that this organism may be a sexually transmitted pathogen.[11] This organism has also been isolated on occasion from blood, wounds, perianal lesions, and abscesses.

HB-5 strains are gram-negative coccobacilli and bacilli that grow on both blood agar and chocolate agar; ability to grow on MacConkey agar is variable. After 24 hours of incubation in a CO_2 environment, colonies are pinpoint, nonhemolytic, smooth, and white. The distinguishing characteristic of HB-5 is that it produces indole in tryptone broth. As with *C. hominis* the amount of indole formed is small, so xylene extraction of the broth and use of Ehrlich's indole reagent are required for its detection. Biochemical tests for identification of CDC group HB-5 are shown in Table 6-3.

CDC Group M-5

CDC group M-5 organisms used to be classified with the *Moraxella* and "*Moraxella*-like" bacteria but have recently been incorporated into the emended family Neisseriaceae along with the CDC group EF-4 organisms.[122] Like EF-4, these bacteria are associated with infected dog bites. They are generally susceptible to antimicrobial agents. Characteristics for identification are shown in Table 6-3.

CDC Group M-6 (*Neisseria elongata* Subspecies *nitroreducens*)

Along with Group M-5, these organisms were previously included among the moraxellae. Using DNA relatedness techniques, Grant and associates have shown that M-6 strains are actually *Neisseria* species that are similar to *N. elongata*, the only rod-shaped member of the genus.[69] CDC group M-6 organisms are now incorporated as a subspecies of *N. elongata* called *N. elongata* subspecies *nitroreducens*. These organisms have been isolated from blood cultures of patients with endocarditis.[110] Biochemical characteristics are shown in Table 6-3.

Streptobacillus moniliformis

Streptobacillus moniliformis is a fastidious gram-negative bacillus that is normally found in the oropharynx of rodents—including wild rats, laboratory rats and mice, and domesticated rodents (eg, gerbils)—and can be transmitted to humans by bites from these animals.[4] *S. moniliformis* is a fastidious, pleomorphic gram-negative bacillus that tends to form long, thin (about 1 μm), filamentous single cells that may be over 100 μm long and may fold into loops and coils. On prolonged incubation, bulbous or sausage-shaped swelling may appear along the filament, causing the organism to resemble a string of beads. On enriched, serum-containing media, the organisms appear as regular, thin, fusiform bacteria with rounded or pointed ends. The organism may also lose its cell wall and exist as an "L-form." *S. moniliformis* is microaerophilic and growth in liquid medium usually requires serum (10% to 20%) supplementation.

In humans, the organism causes a disease called rat-bite or Haverhill fever when it is acquired by ingestion of the organism. The latter name comes from Haverhill, Massachusetts, where this organism was recovered from blood cultures of several patients during a local outbreak of the disease.[112] After an incubation period of 7 to 10 days after the bite of a rat or the ingestion of food or water contaminated with rat excrement, there is an abrupt onset of high fever, chills, headache, muscle aches, vomiting, and other constitutional symptoms. A few days after disease onset, a rash appears on the extremities (including the palms and soles), and some patients may develop severe joint pain or frank arthritis.[90] The disease may resolve spontaneously with no residual symptoms or may develop into a chronic, periodically febrile condition.

Diagnosis of rat bite or Haverhill fever is made by recovery of the organism from blood cultures.[41] Because the organism is inhibited by the anticoagulant sodium polyanetholsulfonate (SPS), blood (10 mL) must be anticoagulated with citrate (10 mL sodium citrate, 2.5%) before processing. The citrated blood cells are sedimented by centrifugation, and the packed cells are inoculated onto agar medium (heart infusion agar) containing 10% sterile decomplemented horse serum and 0.5% yeast extract. The inoculum is gently spread over the agar surface. A broth medium of similar ingredients (heart infusion broth with serum and yeast extract) is also inoculated with the packed cells. The medium is incubated at 35°C in a candle jar or a CO_2 incubator. Other specimens (eg, citrated joint fluid, aspirates, abscess material) may be cultured in the same manner. In broth medium the organism grows as small "puff balls" near the bottom of the tube or bottle and overlying the red blood cells and stroma.

On serum-enriched agar medium, growth may appear within 2 to 3 days or may require a week or more. Colonies are small, white, smooth, and buttery in consistency. The L-phase variants form spontaneously under or around the existing colonies and have the typical "fried egg" morphology that is seen with *Mycoplasma* species (see Chapter 17). Identification of *S. moniliformis* is accomplished by observing the typical gram-negative, filamentous morphology on Gram staining and by performing biochemical identification tests in serum-supplemented medium.[126] These tests must be incubated for 3 weeks before final interpretations are made. Rapid identification of the organism may also be accomplished by fatty acid profile

Table 6-4
Biochemical Characteristics for Identification of *Streptobacillus moniliformis*

CHARACTERISTIC	REACTION
Oxidase	−
Catalase	−
Nitrate reduction	−
Indole	−
Urease	−
Esculin hydrolysis	+
Production of hydrogen sulfide (lead acetate)	+
Alkaline phosphatase	+
Gas production from glucose	−
Acid production from:	
Glucose	+
Maltose	+
Fructose	+
Sucrose	V
Lactose	V
Xylose	−
Mannitol	−
Mannose	+

+, positive; −, negative; V, variable.

analyses using gas–liquid chromatography.[123] The reactions of *S. moniliformis* in various biochemical identification tests are shown in Table 6-4.

In vitro antimicrobial susceptibility data indicate that *S. moniliformis* is susceptible to penicillin and ampicillin, with erythromycin and gentamicin having less activity.[41] The drug of choice for treatment is penicillin, although cephalothin, tetracycline, and streptomycin have also shown clinical efficacy.

PASTEURELLA SPECIES

Members of the genus *Pasteurella* are gram-negative bacilli that are found primarily in animals. These bacteria have certain phenotypic characteristics in common.[16,29,91] They are all nonmotile, gram-negative, facultatively anaerobic bacilli. Most species are oxidase-, catalase-, and alkaline phosphatase–positive and reduce nitrate to nitrite. Most species produce acid from glucose, fructose, mannose, and sucrose, and none of them hydrolyze starch or salicin. They are all generally susceptible to penicillins and cephalosporins.

Members of the genus *Pasteurella* and those species of *Actinobacillus* of significance for humans are difficult to distinguish from one another on the basis of phenotypic characteristics. Members of both genera are characteristically oxidase- and catalase-positive gram-negative coccobacilli that reduce nitrate to nitrite, and several members of both genera also produce urease.[44] Genetic studies using type strains of the two genera have supported the transfers of three *Pasteurella* species (*P. ureae*, *P. haemolytica*, and *P. pneumotropica*) to the genus *Actinobacillus*.[91,101,102]

The habitats and clinical significance of *Pasteurella* species and the *Pasteurella* (*Actinobacillus*)

species are described briefly in Table 6-5. The present discussion will be restricted to the agents in the genus *Pasteurella* and *Pasteurella* (*Actinobacillus*) group that have been associated with human disease.

Pasteurella *multocida*

Pasteurella multocida is the species that is most frequently recovered from human specimens and is also recovered from a wide variety of animals. The organism can commonly be cultured from the oral cavities of healthy domesticated cats (70% to 90%) and dogs (40% to 66%),[12] but it is also found in a wide variety of other animals, including cattle, horses, swine, sheep, fowl, rodents, rabbits, mon-

Table 6-5
Current *Pasteurella* Species and *Pasteurella* (*Acticobacillus*) Species

SPECIES/SUBSPECIES	HABITAT AND CLINICAL SIGNIFICANCE IN HUMANS (IF ANY)
P. multocida subsp. *multocida*	Respiratory tract of nonhuman mammals, birds; clinical isolate from infections in humans
P. multocida subsp. *septica*	Same as above
P. multocida subsp. *gallicida*	Same as above; also associated with fowl cholera
P. ureae (*A. ureae*)	Uncommon respiratory tract commensal of humans; rare human infections reported
P. pneumotropica (*A. pneumotropica*)	Respiratory tract of guinea pigs, rats, hamsters, cats, and dogs; rarely isolated from humans
P. haemolytica (*A. haemolytica*)	Pneumonic infections in cattle; mastitis in ewes; septicemia in goats and sheep; rare human isolates reported
P. aerogenes	Normal flora in intestinal tract of swine; human infection following a swine bite
Pasteurella species new species 1 (also called *Pasteurella* "gas")	Upper respiratory tract flora of dogs and cats; associated with dog and cat bite wounds; human endocarditis also reported
P. dagmatis	Respiratory tract of dogs and cats; animal bite wounds and systemic infections in humans
P. gallinarum	Respiratory tract of chickens and hens
P. canis	Respiratory tract of dogs; dog bite wound in humans; respiratory tract of calves
P. stomatis	Respiratory tracts of dogs and cats
P. anatis	Intestinal tract flora of ducks
P. langaa	Respiratory tract flora of chickens and other fowl
P. avium	Respiratory tract flora of healthy fowl
P. volantium	Respiratory tract flora of healthy fowl
P. bettii	Human Bartholin's gland and human finger abscesses
P. lymphangitidis	Bovine lymphangitis
P. mairi	Abortion in sows and sepsis in piglets
P. testudinis	Parasitic in certain species of desert tortoises
P. trehalosii	Septicemia in adolescent lambs
Pasteurella species A	Unnamed species; respiratory tract flora of chickens
Pasteurella species B	Unnamed species; respiratory tract flora of chickens

keys, lions, panthers, lynx, birds, reindeer, and buffalo. In some animals this organism causes serious infections.

In humans, *P. multocida* causes several types of infections; most of these follow some sort of contact with domesticated animals. Local wound infections in humans are associated with cat bites, cat scratches, or dog bites.[9] These local wound infections are characterized by rapid development of pain, erythema, swelling, cellulitis, and purulent or serosanguineous drainage at the site of the wound. Local complications include osteomyelitis of the bones near the bite wound site due to traumatic implantation of the organisms or extension of the cellulitis and septic arthritis. Since the wound is generally on the hand, bone and joint complications are usually seen at this site. Serious localized complications most frequently follow cat bites in which the wound may be deep, forceful, and traumatic to underlying tissues.[145]

P. multocida may also be isolated from the respiratory tract, where it may exist as a commensal or as a cause of pneumonia, empyema, bronchitis, sinusitis, tonsillitis, and otitis media.[130] These patients will also usually have some history of animal exposure.

P. multocida has also been the etiologic agent of other life-threatening systemic infections.[145] Bacteremia may occur by spread of the organism from a localized bite wound or may result from hematogenous spread from a localized infected site elsewhere. Bacteremia with this organism occurs in the settings of preexisting liver disease or other underlying conditions. Central nervous system infections caused by *P. multocida* have included meningitis, subdural empyema, and brain abscess. Other complicated infections in which this organism has been isolated are intraabdominal wound infections, spontaneous bacterial peritonitis, intraabdominal and hepatic abscess, chorioamnionitis with neonatal sepsis, diffuse female genital tract infections, Bartholin's gland abscess, and upper and lower urinary tract infections.[145]

P. multocida is generally not difficult to isolate and identify, although knowledge of the specimen type and a history of exposure to animals (eg, "cat bite wound" on the requisition) increases the index of suspicion that this organism may be present. The organism grows well on chocolate and sheep blood agar where it forms smooth, gray colonies that are 0.5 to 2 mm after 24 hours of incubation in CO_2. The organism is nonhemolytic and does not grow on MacConkey agar, EMB agar, or other types of selective or differential enteric media. Isolates from respiratory tract specimens may be mucoid. A characteristic odor (like *Escherichia coli* but more pungent) is frequently noted, perhaps as a result of the formation of large amounts of indole by the organism. *P. multocida* is oxidase-, catalase-, ornithine decarboxylase–, and indole-positive, and urease-negative. The spot indole test using the *p*-aminocinnamaldehyde reagent is generally strongly positive. *P. multocida* produces acid, but no gas, from glucose, sucrose, and mannitol but not from maltose or lactose.

Antimicrobial susceptibility testing and clinical response of infected patients indicate that *P. multocida isolates* are generally susceptible to a wide variety of antimicrobial agents.[131] The organism is susceptible to penicillin, ampicillin, broad-spectrum penicillins (eg, carbenicillin, ticarcillin, piperacillin, mezlocillin), second-generation cephalosporins (cefotaxime, cefoperazone), third-generation cephalosporins (cefuroxime, ceftazidime, ceftizoxime), tetracycline, and chloramphenicol. Less activity has been noted for the first-generation cephalosporins, such as cephalothin and cefazolin, and the semisynthetic penicillins such as methicillin and oxacillin.

Other *Pasteurella* Species

Pasteurella (Actinobacillus) ureae, *P. (A.) pneumotropica*, *P. (A.) haemolytica*, and *P. aerogenes* are rarely associated with human infections and will not be further discussed here but are more fully discussed elsewhere.[20,70,94,103,105]

BORDETELLA SPECIES

The genus *Bordetella* contains four species: *B. pertussis*, *B. parapertussis*, *B. bronchiseptica*, and *B. avium*.[83,113] Genetic studies have shown that these organisms are very closely related to each other. Members of the genus *Bordetella* are small and gram-negative coccobacilli on primary isolation. On subculture, they tend to become more pleomorphic. They are obligately aerobic and are not very metabolically active. They are nonmotile except for *B. bronchiseptica*, which possesses peritrichous flagella. Unlike *Haemophilus* species, these organisms do not require X and V factors. Primary isolation of *B. pertussis*, in particular, requires the addition of charcoal, ion exchange resins, or 15% to 20% blood to neutralize the growth-inhibiting effects of such substances as unsaturated fatty acids, sulfides, and peroxides. Isolation of this organism requires enriched media, while the other species can be grown on simpler media.

B. pertussis causes the syndrome called pertussis or "whooping cough."[41] The organism is acquired through droplet infection and is highly contagious, with an attack rate of greater than 90% in nonimmunized persons. The clinical illness can be divided into three stages. The *prodromal* or *catarrhal stage* begins 5 to 10 days after acquisition of the organism and is characterized by nonspecific cold or flu symptoms. The disease is highly communicable at this stage since large numbers of organisms are present in the upper respiratory tract. Cultures collected at this time have the greatest likelihood of being positive. A cough appears late in this stage and increases in persistence, severity, and frequency. This evolves into the *paroxysmal stage* after 7 to 14 days. This stage is characterized by the staccato cough with the inspiratory "whoop" heard at the end of the coughing spell. Inspiratory efforts are futile during the coughing paroxysm, and the whoop is caused by the inspiration of air through the swollen and narrowed glottis. The coughing spell is frequently followed by vomiting. This stage may be so severe as to sometimes require intermittent ventilatory assistance. The *convalescent stage* generally begins within 4 weeks of onset and, during this time, there is a decrease in the frequency and severity of the coughing spells. Complications that may occur during the course of the disease include secondary bacterial infections and otitis media, central nervous system symptoms, such as convulsions and high fever, particularly with the presence of intervening secondary infections, and inguinal hernia or rectal prolapse associated with the severe coughing.

Despite the availability of an effective vaccine, pertussis continues to be a problem of worldwide importance.[56] Before the availability of the vaccine, the disease was primarily seen in children 1 to 5 years of age; infants were spared because of the presence of transplacental antibody from previous exposure or disease in the adult. With the institution of widespread vaccination in the 1960s, the

yearly incidence of disease dwindled. Since most adults do not receive booster vaccinations, many children are now born without passively transferred antibody. In the period from 1982 to 1985, more than half of the reported cases of pertussis occurred in children younger than 1 year old. Added to this are the large number of susceptible adults whose vaccine-induced immunity has waned. Atypical respiratory infections in adults may actually represent pertussis disease that is ameliorated by the presence of low levels of antibody.[119] *B. pertussis* may also be an opportunistic agent in adults; the organism has been isolated from the respiratory tracts of patients with acquired immunodeficiency syndrome.[104]

B. parapertussis is associated with a pertussis-like illness in humans as well, but it is generally milder in clinical presentation. Outbreaks of *B. parapertussis* have, however, been reported in which the illness has been severe and resulted in death, particularly in very young children.[88] *B. bronchiseptica* causes respiratory tract infections (eg, bronchitis, pneumonia, otitis media, atrophic rhinitis) in dogs and cats and may be isolated as a commensal from the human upper respiratory tract.[42] It may also cause infections primarily in immunocompromised hosts.[63] Cases of sepsis, meningitis, and pneumonia caused by *B. bronchiseptica* have been reported in patients with underlying liver disease, alcoholism, asplenia, Hodgkin's disease, chronic renal failure, systemic lupus erythematosus, and severe hypertension.[32,133] Since *B. pertussis* preferentially attaches to the ciliated epithelium in the upper respiratory tract, the specimen of choice is a nasopharyngeal swab.[56,92] For the recovery of *Bordetella* species, two specimens are usually collected by passing a small nasopharyngeal swab posteriorly through each nostril until the tip reaches the posterior nasopharynx. The swabs are left in place for 30 to 60 seconds to allow organisms to adsorb onto the swab. Fine-tipped, alginate (Ultrafine Calgiswab, Inolex Corp.) or Dacron swabs (Spectrum Laboratories, Inc, Los Angeles, CA) on the end of a fine, flexible metal wire are the optimal specimen collection devices.[56,121] Cotton-tipped swabs should not be used, because cotton material is actually inhibitory to the organism.

Special media are required for the isolation of *B. pertussis*. The classic medium used for this organism is Bordet-Gengou (BG) agar. This medium is prepared from potatoes to impart a high starch content. The starch neutralizes toxic materials that may be present in the agar or in the specimen itself.

In 1977, Regan and Lowe described a medium containing charcoal and horse blood that has demonstrated superiority to BG agar in several studies.[56,117] Although originally described as a transport/enrichment medium, Regan-Lowe agar formulations are available both as a semisolid transport/enrichment medium and as a solid medium for organism isolation. The formula for Regan-Lowe (RL) medium is shown below (per liter distilled water):

- Charcoal agar (Oxoid CM 119), 51 g
- Horse blood, defibrinated, 100 mL
- Cephalexin, 0.04 g
- Amphotericin B (optional), 0.05 g
- Final pH, 7.4

The semisolid transport/enrichment medium is identical in formula to the isolation medium shown above, except that the charcoal agar is present in half strength (ie, 25.5 g/L) and is dispensed into sterile screw-capped tubes rather than into 100-mm Petri dishes. It is also recommended that some of the medium be prepared without cephalexin so that both selective and nonselective media are available for recovery of the organisms.

Optimally, media should be directly inoculated at the time of specimen collection onto both selective (methicillin- or cephalexin-containing) and nonselective media. If a transport system is used, the Regan-Lowe (RL) semisolid medium is optimal, since Stuart and Amies transport medium formulations are not suitable for maintaining the viability of pertussis organisms. Specimens transported in semisolid RL medium can be subcultured on receipt to RL isolation medium or BG medium with and without cephalexin (or methicillin). The transport medium is then incubated along with the primary plate and subcultured to RL agar after 48 hours enrichment at 35°C in 5% to 7% CO_2. All plates should be held for at least 7 days.

In addition to culture, direct fluorescent antibody (DFA) tests are also used to detect *B. pertussis* directly on smears prepared from nasopharyngeal specimens. Although DFA tests do provide rapid results, it is well accepted that culture on appropriate media is more sensitive than DFA.[72] On DFA, the organisms appear as small, coccobacilli with bright, apple-green peripheral fluorescence. They

may appear singly, in pairs, or in clusters. In smears prepared from highly tenacious specimens, the organisms may appear adherent to the mucous strands.

On culture, colonies of *B. pertussis* may be observed after 2 to 4 days. Growth is usually apparent sooner on antibiotic-free medium, but this is not always the case. Plates should be examined under a dissecting microscope (10 ×) with oblique incident light to determine colony characteristics. Fresh clinical isolates of *B. pertussis* on BG agar appear as smooth, shiny colonies with a high, domed profile. Classically, they are described as resembling small droplets of mercury. Colonies on BG may be slightly β-hemolytic, particularly in the more confluent areas of growth or after prolonged incubation. On RL agar medium, colonies are small, domed, and shiny, with a white mother-of-pearl opalescence. *B. parapertussis* colonies grow more rapidly, are more β-hemolytic, and are gray or slightly brown. *B. bronchiseptica* colonies are apparent within 24 hours, are large and more flat, and have a dull rather than a shiny appearance. The latter species resembles a nonfermentative gram-negative rod (like an *Alcaligenes* species) in the appearance of its colonies and the production of a distinct "nonfermenter" odor. Gram stain morphology of these organisms also differs. *B. pertussis* appears as small, pale-staining coccobacilli, while *B. parapertussis* and *B. bronchiseptica* are more definitely rod shaped. Because of the pale staining of the organisms, the safranin counterstain should be left on the slide for at least 2 minutes.

Once isolated, *B. pertussis* is generally identified by the fluorescent antibody test, since the organism is so inert in biochemical identification tests (Table 6-6). Serologic methods may be used to identify *B. parapertussis* as well, but biochemical methods may provide a presumptive identification.

Pertussis is generally treated with erythromycin for at least 2 weeks to prevent relapse. Administration of this antibiotic even during the paroxysmal stage shortens the severity and the duration of illness. In vitro, *B. pertussis* is susceptible to a wide variety of antimicrobial agents, including ampicillin-amoxicillin, trimethoprim-sulfamethoxazole, rifampin, and ciprofloxacin.[87] These other drugs have been used and will eliminate the organism from the respiratory tract, but clinical experience indicates that erythromycin is superior. In addition, most strains are resistant to tetracycline.

Table 6-6
Biochemical Characteristics for Identification of *Bordetella pertussis, Bordetella parapertussis, Bordetella bronchiseptica,* and *Bordetella avium*

CHARACTERISTIC	B. Pertussis	B. Parapertussis	B. Bronchiseptica	B. Avium
Respiratory tract Growth on:	+	+	+	+
Bordet-Gengou agar	3–6 days	1–3 days	1–2 days	2 days
Chocolate agar	–	1–3 days	1–2 days	2 days
MacConkey agar	–	–	+	+
Urease	–	+ (24 hours)	+ (4 hours)	–
Motility	–	–	+	+*
Nitrate reduction	–	–	+	–†
Growth on citrate	–	+	+	+
Growth, carbon source:				
Glucose	NA	–	–	–
Acetate	NA	–	+	V
Succinate	NA	–	+	+
Pyruvate	NA	+	+	+
Brown pigment in heart infusion agar with L-tyrosine (1 g/L)	–	+	–	–

+, positive reaction; –, negative reaction; V, variable; NA, not available.
*Motility is more pronounced at 25°C.
†In serum-supplemented medium, nitrate is reduced.

The other *Bordetella* species are more resistant to antimicrobial agents than *B. pertussis*.

BRUCELLA SPECIES

Brucellosis (infection with *Brucella* species) is worldwide in distribution and has been known historically as undulant fever, Bang's disease, Gibralter fever, Mediterranean fever, and Malta fever. The organism was first isolated in 1887 by Sir David Bruce, who recovered a suspect organism from the spleens of British soldiers dying of Malta fever. It was later found that goat's milk and products produced from it (eg, goat cheese) were the source of the infection in these soldiers. Subsequently, several other similar organisms were recovered from cattle and sows and from humans exposed to these animals and their products. The disease, therefore, is a zoonosis and is of great economic importance to the livestock industry in certain parts of the world. In developed countries, human infections are most commonly associated with meat-packing and dairy-related occupations.[153] In the United States, most reported cases have come from California, Iowa, Virginia, and Texas, reflecting the animal husbandry, cattle, and dairy industries central to the economy of those states.

The incidence of human brucellosis in the United States has declined steadily as a result of control measures implemented in the livestock industry. These measures include vaccination of young animals, and slaughter of older animals with serologic evidence of infection.[153] Human brucellosis is, however, underdiagnosed and underreported, with estimates that at least 25 cases go unrecognized for every case that is diagnosed.[153] With the increasing popularity of international travel, cases of brucellosis are being seen in the United States that are imported from areas of the world where the disease is still endemic.[8] *B. melitensis*, the organism most commonly implicated, is found in the Mediterranean, Latin America, and Asia. *B. abortus* is found worldwide, and *B. suis* is endemic in the southern United States, Southeast Asia, and Latin America. *B. canis* infections are seen in Latin America, Central Europe, and Japan. During the past 5 to 10 years, increasing numbers of *Brucella* infections have been diagnosed in Texas and California among persons who have ingested Mexican cheese prepared from unpasteurized goat's milk.[136] Similar cases are being seen among travelers to Italy, France, Greece, Spain, and Mexico on their return to this country.[8] Occasionally, brucellosis has been acquired as a result of laboratory accidents, such as spills or aerosolization while working with the organisms.

Brucella species are facultative intracellular organisms and the disease spectrum is partially explained by the ability of the organism to evade host defense mechanisms by its intracellular existence. Brucellae are transmitted to humans by three principal routes: (1) direct contact with infected animal tissues, (2) ingestion of contaminated meats or dairy products, and (3) inhalation of aerosolized organisms.[153] Once in the host, the organisms are phagocytized but are able to survive within these cells, presumably by inactivating the intracellular myeloperoxidase-peroxide defense mechanisms. The organisms are carried into the lymph nodes and the bloodstream and become sequestered in various parts of the reticuloendothelial system (ie, the liver sinusoids, spleen, and bone marrow).

Brucella infections may be difficult to diagnose because of the wide spectrum of clinical manifestations associated with them. After an incubation period of about 3 weeks (with a range of from 1 week to 2 or 3 months), the onset of symptoms may be abrupt or may develop over a period of several days. Fever, night sweats, chills, and malaise, often accompanied by severe headache, myalgias, and arthralgias, are the nonspecific symptoms seen in most cases of brucellosis. Lymphadenopathy, splenomegaly, and hepatomegaly may also be present. The name *undulant fever* has been attached to brucellosis because of the periodic nocturnal fever that may occur over weeks, months, or even years.[153] Symptoms of infection may wax and wane over prolonged periods as a result of the containment of the organisms in granulomas in the tissues and the subsequent release of organisms (or organism components such as lipopolysaccharides) back into the circulation. Therefore, the disease presents nonspecifically and assumes the characteristics of a debilitating, chronic illness. These patients are frequently pancultured to determine an etiology for a fever of unknown origin.

Because *Brucella* species infect the reticuloendothelial system, the specimens of choice in suspected cases of brucellosis primarily include blood and bone marrow specimens.[68] Because of the documented risk of laboratory-acquired infections due to *Brucella* species, all work with specimens suspected of harboring *Brucella* and all manipulations of *Brucella* cultures should be performed in a biologic safety cabinet with recommended precautions for Biosafety Level 3 organisms (eg, mycobacteria, *Francisella tularensis*).[30] Procedures that are known to generate aerosols (eg, aspiration of liquid with syringes, mixing on a "vortex" mixer, vigorous bulb pipetting) should be kept to a minimum. Obviously, to comply with these guidelines, close communication among the laboratory director, the technologists, and the physicians caring for patients with "possible" brucellosis is necessary.

Because of the slow growth of the organism, blood cultures and supplemental broth cultures should be incubated at 35°C for 4 to 6 weeks with frequent blind subcultures to chocolate and blood agar.[156] Radiometric detection by the BACTEC system may or may not detect the organism, and, if so, it may require at least 10 days of incubation before a positive growth index value is obtained. In our laboratory, we have recovered *Brucella* species from BACTEC blood cultures after 5 to 7 days of incubation.

Brucella species are identified on the basis of carbon dioxide requirements for growth, biochemical tests (hydrogen sulfide production, urease), growth in the presence of thionine and basic fuchsin dyes, and agglutination in antisera. A presumptive identification of a "possible *Brucella* species" can be made when a slow-growing, faintly staining, minute coccobacillus is recovered from blood or bone marrow cultures of a "compatible" patient; that is, one with a history of possible occupational exposure, "exotic" travel, or ingestion of uncooked meats or unpasteurized dairy products. *Brucella* species grow slowly on blood and chocolate agars, but not on MacConkey, EMB, or other "enteric" media. Good growth will also be obtained on buffered charcoal yeast extract (BCYE) agar used for isolation of *Legionella* species.[92] Both the oxidase and catalase tests are positive for all *Brucella* species. *B. melitensis*, *B. suis*, and *B. abortus* all produce urease; with a heavy inoculum, *B. suis* strains usually will be urease-positive on Christensen's urea medium within 5 minutes. Methods using monoclonal antibodies for culture confirmation of *Brucella* species have also been described.[120]

Isolates suspected of being a *Brucella* species should be sent to a reference laboratory for identification.

The treatment of human brucellosis is a controversial area because of the spectrum of disease, the possibility of chronic infection, and the development of complications. Because the organism is an intracellular parasite, prolonged therapy is also necessary. Doxycycline (a tetracycline derivative) and rifampin for at least 6 weeks is a currently recommended treatment regimen; both drugs can be given orally. Streptomycin and tetracycline may also be used, but the former drug must be given daily by injection.[115] Brucellosis has also been successfully treated with other drugs, including the quinolones.[14]

FRANCISELLA TULARENSIS

Tularemia, the disease caused by the fastidious gram-negative coccobacillus *Francisella tularensis*, is also a disease of animals that humans acquire by contact with them.[45,51] Reservoirs of the bacterium in nature include rabbits, rodents, squirrels, deer, and raccoons; domestic animals such as cats and dogs may also become infected. The organism is transmitted among animals by ticks and biting flies such as deerflies. Transovarial transmission of *F. tularensis* occurs in the tick, thus providing a constant source of the organism in the environment. Infections in humans are most commonly acquired by bites from infected ticks or deerflies or by direct contact with blood or internal organs of infected animals (eg, as would occur when skinning game). Eating contaminated animal meat, ingestion of contaminated water, or inhalation of the organism in aerosols may also lead to infection. The organism is highly contagious—as few as 10 organisms administered subcutaneously or 25 organisms given by the aerosol route are enough to cause infection, and the bacterium can easily penetrate minute breaks in the skin. Cases of tularemia have resulted from laboratory accidents that have occurred during processing of infected specimens, isolation of the organism, or working with large numbers of the organisms in research. Although the disease has been reported throughout the United States, most cases now occur in the southern and south-central states, including Missouri, Kansas, Arkansas, Oklahoma, and Texas.

F. tularensis strains can be subdivided into *F. tularensis* biogroup *tularensis* and *F. tularensis* biogroup *palearctica* on the basis of acid production from glycerol. *F. novicida* and *F. philomiragia* are two other species recently discovered[75] but will not be further discussed here.

Clinical tularemia can be divided into six major syndromes that are delineated by the mode of organism acquisition.[45,51,53] *Ulceroglandular tularemia* is the most common form (70% to 85% of cases). The patient presents with an ulcerated skin lesion, usually at the site of a tick bite, along with painful regional lymphadenopathy. Other features (eg, headache, fever, chills, sweating, coughing) also are present. *Glandular tularemia* (2% to 12% of cases) is characterized by lymphadenopathy and fever, but no skin lesion may be readily apparent. *Typhoidal tularemia* (7% to 14% of cases) presents as an acute onset of fever and systemic illness with no initial skin lesion or lymphadenopathy. In this form, blood and sputum cultures may be positive and the mortality rate is usually high. *Oculoglandular tularemia* (1% to 2% of cases) results from inoculation of the organism into the conjunctivae, with severe conjunctivitis and regional lymphadenopathy. *Oropharyngeal tularemia* (2% to 4% of cases) describes those cases in which the primary lesion is in the oropharynx, and the patient presents with an exudative pharyngitis suggestive of severe streptococcal pharyngitis, diphtheria, or Vincent's disease. *Pneumonic tularemia* (8% to 13% of cases) may occur as a complication of all of the other forms as a result of seeding of the pulmonary tract during bacteremia or as a clinical entity resulting from inhalation of the organisms in an aerosol. Radiographic examinations may show involvement of one or more lobes, with pleural effusions, pneumonic infiltrates, abscess formation, and hilar lymphadenopathy.

Because this organism can penetrate through small breaks in the skin, it is considered potentially dangerous to handle specimens or cultures of the organism. As with *Brucella* infections, the disease may not be suspected, and considerable time may be spent handling specimens and cultures before this diagnosis is entertained. If the clinical history suggests the possibility of tularemia, all specimens and cultures should be processed in a biological safety cabinet, gloves should be worn during all procedures, and any procedures that may generate aerosols should be avoided.[30]

F. tularensis is a small, pale-staining, gram-negative coccobacillus. The organism has a growth requirement for the amino acids cysteine and cystine, and the classically described medium for isolation was called cysteine-blood agar. *F. tularensis* will grow on commercially available chocolate agar, however, since this hemin-containing medium is supplemented with a growth enrichment (eg, Iso-Vitelex, Becton Dickinson Microbiology Systems, Cockeysville, MD) that contains cysteine and other nutrients required by fastidious bacteria. Like the brucellae, this organism is also able to grow on BCYE agar, the medium used for isolation of *Legionella* species.[116] *F. tularensis* is obligately aerobic; growth is stimulated by increased CO_2 and may require take 3 to 5 days before colonies are visible on agar medium. All suspicious specimens should be sent to a public health reference laboratory for identification.

The drug of choice for treatment of tularemia is the aminoglycoside streptomycin, with gentamicin being an acceptable alternative. Other agents, such as tetracycline and chloramphenicol, have been used but are associated with a higher rate of relapse. Intravenous therapy with erythromycin has also been used successfully.

LEGIONELLA SPECIES

During the summer of 1976, an explosive outbreak of pneumonia of unknown etiology occurred among persons who attended an American Legion convention in Philadelphia.[55] Persons who developed the multisystemic illness that included pneumonia were said to have legionnaires' disease.[25] At autopsy, patients typically showed severe confluent lobar pneumonia with or without abscesses.[17,150] A major medical mystery was solved when the etiologic agent, a fastidious bacterium later named *Legionella pneumophila*, was isolated by Dr. Joseph McDade, who was then working at the Center for Disease Control in Atlanta.[98]

Legionella species are non–spore-forming, narrow, gram-negative bacilli, 0.3 to 0.9 μm in width that vary from short forms 1.5 to 2 μm in length to longer filamentous forms.[21,23] They are usually short and thin or coccobacillary when seen in direct smears of clinical specimens but more variable in length after growth in culture media (Color Plate 6-2*A*), with forms greater than 20 μm long not unusual. Legionellae stain much more readily

with the Diff-Quick, Giemsa, or Gram-Weigert stains than they do with Gram stain in touch preparations of fresh tissue imprints, smears of bronchial alveolar lavage fluid, or sputum.

The Legionellaceae are aerobic and nutritionally fastidious. They require L-cysteine and iron salts for growth, which are provided in BCYE agar but do not grow on the usual blood agar and differential agar media commonly used for respiratory specimens in clinical microbiology laboratories. Growth on BCYE agar with no growth on blood agar is one of the most useful presumptive clues that an isolate could be a species of *Legionella*. Colonies of *Legionella* typically appear on BCYE agar after 2 to 3 days of incubation in areas that have been heavily inoculated. If only a few organisms are present, however, and if the plates have been lightly inoculated, isolated colonies may take several more days to develop.

Clinical Spectrum of Legionellosis

Legionnaires' disease occurs both sporadically in the form of community-acquired pneumonia[25,37,99,149] and in epidemics.[11] In addition to classic legionnaires' disease, a mild form of illness, Pontiac fever, occurs. Legionellosis has most commonly been recognized as a form of pneumonia (see Color Plate 6-2*A* and *B*).[153] The earliest symptoms typically include a rundown feeling, muscle aches, and a slight headache. During the first day, patients commonly experience a rapid onset of dry cough and elevated temperature (102° to 104°F or higher) with chills. Abdominal pain and gastrointestinal symptoms (nausea, vomiting, and diarrhea) occur in many patients. A summary of clinical manifestations is given in Table 6-7.

In recent years, the clinical spectrum of legionellosis has expanded. The illness may involve essentially any organ system in the body, with or without pneumonia. Examples of selected manifestations of extrapulmonary involvement follow. Nearly half the patients with legionnaires' disease show central nervous system manifestations such as headache, lethargy, confusion, stupor, ataxia, and seizures.[80] Other patients have focal signs and symptoms suggesting brain abscess or encephalitis mimicking herpes encephalitis.[3,115] *L. pneumophila* serogroup 1 has been demonstrated in lymph nodes, spleen, kidney, and bone marrow and has

Table 6-7
Clinical Manifestations in Two Kinds of Legionellosis

	LEGIONNAIRES' DISEASE	PONTIAC FEVER
Mortality	15%–30%	0%
Incubation period	2–10 days	1–2 days
Symptoms	Fever, chills, cough, myalgia, headache, chest pain, sputum, and diarrhea (and confusion or other mental states in some)	Similar to influenza: fevers, chills, and myalgia (and cough, chest pain, and confusion in some)
Lung	Pneumonia and pleural effusion (lung abscess in some)	Pleuritic pain; no pneumonia, no lung abscess
Kidney	Renal failure (proteinuria, azotemia, and hematuria in some)	No renal manifestations
Liver	Modest liver function abnormalities	No liver function abnormalities
Gastrointestinal tract	Watery diarrhea, abdominal pain, and nausea and vomiting	No abnormalities
Central nervous system	Somnolence, delirium, disorientation, confusion, and obtundation (seizure rarely documented)	No central nervous system manifestations

(Data from references 55, 148, 154, and 157)

been documented in acute myocarditis,[146,149] prosthetic valve endocarditis,[97] pericarditis,[96] and hemodialysis fistula infections.[149] Reports of extrapulmonary manifestations have been more commonly associated with *L. pneumophila* than with other species. For a review of manifestations of illness produced by *Legionella* species other than *L. pneumophila*, see the article by Fang and colleagues.[49]

Predisposing Factors

Legionnaires' disease usually occurs in middle-aged or older persons. It must be included in the differential diagnosis of immunosuppressed patients who develop fever and pulmonary infiltrates;[71,124] of patients who develop pneumonia not responsive to penicillins, cephalosporins, or aminoglycosides; and

of patients with severe pneumonia, especially when there is no readily apparent alternative diagnosis. In hemodialysis, renal transplant and cardiac transplant patients, for example, legionnaires' disease has been a major cause of morbidity and mortality.[85,137,154]

The usual source of *Legionella* in hospitalized patients is water (mainly the hot water system), especially from showers and baths,[46] and from cooling towers that are part of the building's air conditioning system.[1,59] Other documented sources have included humidifiers, respiratory therapy equipment (masks and handheld nebulizers, washed with contaminated tap water), and whirlpools.[48] Early diagnosis of legionellosis and epidemiologic surveillance of cases within the hospital are needed not only for prompt and effective therapy of those infected but also to aid in instituting control measures to prevent subsequent cases.

Laboratory Diagnosis

Selection, Collection, and Transport of Specimens

The broad clinical spectrum and severe morbidity and mortality of legionnaires' disease emphasize the need for rapid and accurate laboratory diagnosis. When legionellosis is suspected clinically, lower respiratory tract specimens should be collected for both culture and DFA testing. Appropriate specimens for culture and DFA examinations include expectorated sputum, materials collected using bronchoscopy (bronchial brush, biopsy, lavage, or washings), transtracheal aspirates, closed- and open-lung biopsy material, fine needle aspirates of lung, and pleural fluid. Although culture using current media and methods, as described below, is more sensitive than the DFA procedure for demonstrating *Legionella*, it is recommended that both be done.[40,148]

Primary recovery of *Legionella* species on solid media has been successful from closed- and open-lung biopsy material, pleural fluid and transtracheal aspirates, bronchial alveolar lavage samples, and sputum. *L. pneumophila*, on a few occasions, has been recovered from blood cultures using conventional media supplemented with L-cysteine and ferric pyrophosphate, or using BACTEC radiometric aerobic and anaerobic media without any special supplements.[39,118] As mentioned earlier, legionellae may also be encountered (rarely) in extrapulmonary sites. The practical value of seeking *Legionella* in blood cultures or extrapulmonary sites has not been established.

Isolation of *Legionella* Species From Clinical Specimens

Bacteriologic culture of *Legionella* is the preferred method to diagnose legionellosis.[40,157] The recommended nonselective solid medium for isolation of legionellae is BCYE agar, which contains L-cysteine, ferric pyrophosphate, ACES (N-[2-acetamido]-2-aminoethanesulfonic acid) buffer, α-ketoglutaric acid, and activated charcoal.[29] The medium is available commercially from several manufacturers. In addition to BCYE agar, it is recommended that one or more selective media be used to avoid overgrowth by normal flora and the possibility that other organisms may inhibit the growth of *Legionella* species. Antibiotics have been added to the BCYE agar base, resulting in reasonably effective selective media. One useful example is BCYE agar base supplemented with cefamandole, polymyxin B, and anisomycin (BMAP agar); a second medium contains glycine, vancomycin, polymyxin B, and anisomycin ("modified Wadowsky-Yee" or MWY medium).

Identification of *Legionella* Species

The colonies that appear on BCYE agar after 2 to 3 days of incubation typically are variable in size (punctate or up to 4 mm). They are glistening, convex, circular, and slightly irregular and have an entire margin (see Color Plate 6-2*E*). When examined under a dissecting microscope (7× to 15× magnification), *Legionella* colonies appear to have crystalline internal structures within the colonies or a speckled, opalescent appearance similar to that of *Fusobacterium nucleatum* (see Color Plate 6-2*F*). *L. bozemanii*, *L. dumoffii*, and *L. gormanii* show a blue-white fluorescence under long-wavelength (366 nm) ultraviolet light.

Colonies suspected of being *Legionella* should be subcultured onto an ordinary unsupplemented 5% sheep blood agar plate of L-cysteine–deficient BCYE agar. Organisms that grow on 5% sheep blood, L-cysteine-deficient BCYE agar, or other routine media (such as MacConkey agar) are probably not *Legionella*. Pure culture isolates of gram-negative bacilli with typical colony characteristics of *Legionella* as described earlier should be confirmed using the DFA test. The organisms appear as apple-green staining bacilli (see Color Plate 6-2*D*). The services of a reference laboratory may be advisable if local resources do not permit accurate species identifications.

DIRECT FLUORESCENT ANTIBODY PROCEDURE. In performing the DFA test, specific antibody in the form of fluorescein isothiocyanate (FITC)-labeled polyvalent antiserum (conjugate) directed against the antigen to be detected is usually purchased commercially. Commercial suppliers of FITC, as well as control sera and other reagents for *Legionella* DFA testing, include MarDx Diagnostics, Inc (Scotch Plains, NJ), Meridian Diagnostics, Inc (Cincinnati, OH), Organon Teknika Corporation (Durham, NC), and Genetic Systems (Seattle, WA). Genetic Systems markets a monoclonal antibody conjugate that has the advantage of decreasing the number of false-positive reactions while retaining the ability to react with many serotypes of *L. pneumophila*.[49] This reagent cannot, however, be recommended for DFA studies of potable water or other samples from manmade water systems, and its performance in natural habitat water studies is uncertain.[143]

When performing the test, the directions of the manufacturer of the DFA kit should be followed exactly. When the test is properly performed, bacteria can be seen (using a fluorescence microscope) as brilliantly fluorescing, yellow-green rods (see Color Plate 6-2*D*).

NUCLEIC ACID PROBES FOR DETECTION OF *LEGIONELLA* SPECIES. A DNA probe test kit for detection of Legionella is now commercially available from Gen-Probe, Inc (San Diego, CA). The kit, which contains a genus-specific iodine 125–labeled cDNA probe, was developed for in-solution hybridization of *Legionella* ribosomal ribonucleic acid in clinical specimens. The sensitivity of the DNA probe was reported to be 70% to 75%, and the specificity was 99% to 100%.[38,109] The probe was found to identify all *Legionella* species correctly to the genus level when colonies were taken from plate cultures and did not cross react with any bacteria other than legionellae in culture.[38] Drawbacks of the probe test is the cost (use a relatively expensive radioactive probe with a short half-life and the need for a gamma counter) and the fact that the test is not sufficiently sensitive to replace culture for *Legionella* species.

Antimicrobial Susceptibility and Treatment

Erythromycin has been effective in reducing the case mortality rate and remains the drug of choice in the treatment of legionellosis.[54,149,154] Rifampin is known to be active in vitro[139] and could be given in addition to erythromycin to certain patients who are seriously ill or who fail to respond to erythromycin alone. Rifampin should not be given alone. In vitro antimicrobial susceptibility testing of *Legionella* isolates has not been standardized and does not correlate with the clinical response to antibiotic therapy; therefore, it should not be attempted in hospital diagnostic laboratories.[149]

IDENTIFICATION OF FASTIDIOUS GRAM-NEGATIVE BACILLI USING PACKAGED KIT SYSTEMS

Commercial kit systems are also available for assistance in identifying many of the fastidious gram-negative species. The RapID NH system (Innovative Diagnostics Systems, Inc, Atlanta, GA) includes *H. aphrophilus* and *H. paraphrophilus*, *A. actinomycetemcomitans*, *C. hominis*, *E. corrodens*, *Kingella* species, and *P. multocida* in its data base. The newly reformatted panel has, however, not been extensively evaluated. The Vitek Neisseria-Haemophilus Identification (NHI) Card (bioMérieux Vitek, Inc, Hazelwood, MO) includes all the HACEK group organisms in its data base. In the single published evaluation, the NHI card provided definitive identifications for these organisms or indicated the correct identification among a choice of two or three possible identifications.[78] The performance of selected modified conventional tests is suggested by the data base of the computer-assisted identification system. The MicroScan Haemophilus-Neisseria Identification (HNID) panel (American MicroScan, Sacramento, CA) currently lists only *H. aphrophilus* and *H. paraphrophilus* in its data base. Janda and colleagues, however, tested several strains of fastidious gram-negative species (including *A. actinomycetemcomitans*, *C. hominis*, *E. corrodens*, and *Kingella* species) and found that unique biochemical profiles were produced.[60] Agreement was noted between the modified conventional tests on the panel (carbohydrate fermentations, indole, urease, ornithine decarboxylase) and conventional identification procedures.

REFERENCES

1. Addis DG, Davis JP, LaVenture M, et al. Community-acquired legionnaires' disease associated with a cooling tower: evidence for longer-distance transport of *Legionella pneumophila*. Am J Epidemiol 1989;130:557–568.
2. Ah Fat LNC, Patel BR, Pickens S. *Actinobacillus actinomycetemcomitans* endocarditis in hypertrophic obstructive cardiomyopathy. J Infect 1983;6:81–84.

3. Anderson BB, Sogaard I. Legionnaires' disease and brain abscess. Neurology 1987;37:333–334.

4. Anderson LC, Leary SL, Manning PJ. Rat-bite fever in animal research laboratory personnel. Lab Anim Sci 1983;33:292–294.

5. Andrews JH, Waters MJ. Dysgonic fermenter 2 septicemia. Rev Infect Dis 1988;10:1063.

6. Anolik R, Berkowitz RJ, Campos JM, et al. *Actinobacillus* endocarditis associated with periodontal disease. Clin Pediatr 1981;20:653–655.

7. Appelbaum PC, Ballard JO, Eyster ME. Septicemia due to *Capnocytophaga* (*Bacteroides ochraceus*) in Hodgkin's disease. Ann Intern Med 1979;90:716–717.

8. Arnow PM, Smaron M, Ormiste V. Brucellosis in a group of travelers to Spain. JAMA 1984;251:505–507.

9. Arons MS, Fernando L, Polayes IM. *Pasteurella multocida*: the major cause of hand infections following domestic animal bites. J Hand Surg 1982;7:47–52.

10. Aronson NE, Zbick CJ. Dysgonic fermenter 3 bacteremia in a neutropenic patient with acute lymphocytic leukemia. J Clin Microbiol 1988;26:2213–2215.

11. Baddour LM, Gelfand MS, Weaver RE, et al. CDC group HB-5 as a cause of genitourinary tract infection in adults. J Clin Microbiol 1989;27:801–805.

12. Bailie WE, Stowe EC, Schmitt AM. Aerobic flora of oral and nasal fluids of canines with reference to bacteria associated with bites. J Clin Microbiol 1978;7:223–231.

13. Bauer CL, Walker WJ. *Haemophilus aphrophilus* endocarditis: successfully treated with ampicillin and streptomycin. Calif Med 1966;104:475–479.

14. Baykal M, Akalin HE, Firat M, et al. In vitro activity and clinical efficacy of ofloxacin in infections due to *Brucella melitensis*. Rev Infect Dis 1989;11(Suppl 3):S993–S994.

15. Bieger RC, Brewer NS, Washington JA. *Haemophilus aphrophilus*: a microbiologic and clinical review and report of 42 cases. Medicine (Balt) 1978;57:345–355.

16. Bisgaard M, Falsen E. Reinvestigation and re-classifiecation of a collection of 56 human isolates of Pasteurellaceae. Acta Pathol Microbiol Immunol [B] 1986;94:215–222.

17. Blackmon JA, Chandler FW, Cherry WB, et al. Legionellosis. Am J Pathol 1981;103:429–465.

18. Boenning DA, Fleisher GR, Campos JM. Dog bites in children: Epidemiology, microbiology, and penicillin prophylactic therapy. Am J Emerg Med 1983;1:17–21.

19. Blum R, Koneman EW, Berry C, Phillips M, Hamilos D. Clinical significance of dysgonic fermenter 3 (DF-3) isolated from stool. J Clin Microbiol 1992;30:396–400.

20. Brass EP, Wray LM, McDuff T. *Pasteurella ureae* meningitis associated with endocarditis. Eur Neurol 1983;22:138–141.

21. Brenner DJ, Feeley JC, Weaver RE. Family VII. Legionellaceae Brenner, Steigerwalt and McDade 1979. 658. In: Kreig NR, Holt JG, eds. Bergey's manual of systematic bacteriology. Baltimore, Williams & Wilkins, 1984.

22. Brenner DJ, Hollis DG, Famming R, et al. *Capnocytophaga canimorsus* sp. nov. (formerly CDC group DF-2) and *C. cynodegmi* sp. nov., a cause of localized wound infection following dog bite. J Clin Microbiol 1989;27:231–235.

23. Brenner DJ, Steigerwalt AG, McDade JE. Classification of legionnaires' bacterium: *Legionella pneumophila*, genus novum, species nova, of the family Legionellaceae, family nova. Ann Intern Med 1979;90:656–658.

24. Brooks GF, O'Donoghue JM, Rissing JP, et al. *Eikenella corrodens*, a recently recognized pathogen. Medicine (Balt) 1974;53:325–342.

25. Broome CV, Fraser DW. Epidemiologic aspects of legionellosis. Epidemiol Rev 1979;1:1–16.

26. Bruun B, Ying Y, Kirkegaard E, et al. Phenotypic differentiation of *Cardiobacterium hominis*, *Kingella indologenes*, and CDC group EF-4. Eur J Clin Microbiol 1984;3:230–235.

27. Carpenter PD, Heppner BT, Gnann JW. DF-2 bacteremia following cat bites: report of two cases. Am J Med 1987;82:621–623.

28. Carruthers MM, Sommers HM. *Eikenella corrodens* osteomyelitis. Ann Intern Med 1973;79:900.

29. Carter GR. Genus I. *Pasteurella* Trevisan 1887. 94[AL]. Nom. cons. Opin. 13, Jud. Comm. 1954, 153. In: Kreig NR, Holt JG, eds. Bergey's manual of systematic bacteriology. Baltimore, Williams & Wilkins, 1984;1:552–557.

30. Centers for Disease Control. Biosafety in microbiological and biomedical laboratories. 2nd ed. Atlanta, Centers for Disease Control, 1988.

31. Chanal C, Tiget F, Chapius P, et al. Spondylitis and osteomyelitis caused by *Kingella kingae* in children. J Clin Microbiol 1987;25:2407–2409.

32. Chang KC, Zakheim RM, Cho CT, et al. Post-traumatic purulent meningitis due to *Bordetella bronchiseptica*. J Pediatr 1975;86:639–640.

33. Chowdhury MNH, Al-Nozha M, Husian IS, et al. Endocarditis due to *Actinobacillus actinomycetemcomitans*. J Infect 1985;10:158–162.

34. Decker MD, Graham BS, Hunter EB, et al. Endocarditis and infections of intravascular devices due to *Eikenella corrodens*. Am J Med Sci 1986;292:209–212

35. De Groot R, Glover D, Clausen C, et al. Bone and

joint infections caused by *Kingella kingae*: six cases and review of the literature. Rev Infect Dis 1988; 10:998–1004.

36. Dewhirst FE, Paster BJ, LaFontaine S, et al. Transfer of *Kingella indologenes* (Snell and Lapage 1976) to the genus *Suttonella* gen. nov. as *Suttonella indologenes* comb. nov.; transfer of *Bacteroides nodosus* (Beveridge 1941) to the genus *Dichelobacter* gen. nov. as *Dichelobacter nodosus* comb. nov.; and assignment of the genera *Cardiobacterium*, *Dichelobacter*, and *Suttonella* to Cardiobacteriaceae fam. nov. in the gamma division of Proteobacteria on the basis of 16S rRNA sequence comparisons. Int J Syst Bacteriol 1990;40:426–433.

37. Edelstein PH. Improved semi-selective medium for isolation of *L. pneumophila* from clinical and environmental specimens. J Clin Microbiol 1981; 14:298–303.

38. Edelstein PH, Bryan RN, Enns RK, et al. Retrospective study of Gen-Probe Rapid Diagnostic System for detection of legionellae in frozen clinical respiratory tract samples. J Clin Microbiol 1987;25:1022–1026.

39. Edelstein PH, Meyer RD, Finegold SM. Isolation of *Legionella pneumophila* from blood. Lancet 1979;1:750–751.

40. Edelstein PH, Meyer RD, Finegold SM. Laboratory diagnosis of legionnaires' disease. Am Rev Respir Dis 1988;121:317–327.

41. Edwards R, Finch RG. Characterization and antibiotic susceptibilities of *Streptobacillus moniliformis*. J Med Microbiol 1986;21:39–42.

42. Ehrhardt M, Lynch KM, Tyson GM, et al. *Bordetella bronchiseptica*: pathogen vs. commensal. Clin Microbiol Newsl 1986;8:26–27.

43. Enck RE, Bennett JM. Isolation of *Haemophilus aphrophilus* from an adult with acute leukemia. J Clin Microbiol 1976;4:194–195.

44. Escande F, Grimont F, Grimont PAD, et al. Deoxyribonucleic acid relatedness among strains of *Actinobacillus* spp. and *Pasteurella ureae*. Int J Syst Bacteriol 1984;34:309–315.

45. Evans ME, Gregory DW, Schaffner W, et al. Tularemia: a 30-year experience with 88 cases. Medicine (Balt) 1985;64:251–269.

46. Ezzeddine H, VanOssel C, et al. *Legionella* spp. in a hospital hot water system: effect of control measures. J Hosp Infect 1989;13:121–131.

47. Fainstein V, Luna MA, Bodey GP. Endocarditis due to *Eikenella corrodens* in a patient with acute lymphocytic leukemia. Cancer 1981;48:40–42.

48. Fallon RJ, Rowbotham TJ. Microbiological investigations into an outbreak of Pontiac fever due to *Legionella micdadei* associated with use of a whirlpool. J Clin Pathol 1990;43:479–483.

49. Fang GD, Yu VL, Vickers BS. Disease due to the Legionellaceae (other than *Legionella pneumophila*): historical, microbiological, clinical and epidemiological review. Medicine 1989;68:116–132.

50. Findling JW, Pohlmann GP, Rose HD. Fulminant gram-negative bacillemia (DF-2) following a dog bite in an asplenic woman. Am J Med 1980; 68:154–156.

51. Finley CR, Hamilton BW, Hamilton TR. Tularemia: a review. Mo Med 1986;83:741–743.

52. Forlenza SW, Newman NG, Lipsey AI, et al. *Capnocytophaga* sepsis: a newly recognized entity in granulocytopenic patients. Lancet 1980;1: 567–568.

53. Francis E. Tularemia. JAMA 1925;84:1243–1250.

54. Frazer DW, McDade JE. Legionellosis. Sci Am 1979;241:82–99.

55. Frazer DW, Tsai T, Orenstein W, et al. Legionnaires' disease. I. Description of an epidemic of pneumonia. N Engl J Med 1977;297:1189–1197.

56. Friedman RL. Pertussis: the disease and new diagnostic methods. Clin Microbiol Rev 1988;1: 365–376.

57. Fumarola D. Increasing evidence for the pathogenic role of DF-2 organisms. Rev Infect Dis 1988;10:668.

58. Gadberry JL, Zipper R, Taylor JA, et al. *Pasteurella pneumotropica* isolated from bone and joint infections. J Clin Microbiol 1984;19:926–927.

59. Garbe PL, Davis BJ, Weisfeld JS, et al. Nosocomial legionnaires' disease: epidemiologic demonstration of cooling towers as a source. JAMA 1985;254:521–524.

60. Geraci JE, Greipp PR, Wilkowske CJ, et al. *Cardiobacterium hominis* endocarditis: four cases with clinical and laboratory observations. Mayo Clin Proc 1978;53:49–53.

61. Geraci JE, Wilcowske CJ, Wilson WR, et al. *Haemophilus* endocarditis: report of 14 patients. Mayo Clin Proc 1977;52:209–215.

62. Geraci JE, Wilson WR, Washington JA. Infective endocarditis caused by *Actinobacillus actinomycetemcomitans*: report of four cases. Mayo Clin Proc 1980;55:415–419.

63. Ghosh HK, Tranter J. *Bordetella bronchicanis* (*bronchiseptica*) infections in man: review and a case report. J Clin Pathol 1979;32:546–548.

64. Gilligan PH, McCarthy LR, Bissett BK. *Capnocytophaga ochracea* septicemia. J Clin Microbiol 1981;13:643–645.

65. Goldman IS, Ellner PD, Francke EL, et al. Infective endocarditis due to *Kingella denitrificans*. Ann Intern Med 1980;93:152–153.

66. Goldstein EJC, Miller TA, Citron DM, et al. Infections following clenched fist injury: a new perspective. J Hand Surg 1978;3:455–457.

67. Goldstein EJC, Sutter VL, Finegold SM. Susceptibility of *Eikenella corrodens* to ten cephalosporins. Antimicrob Agents Chemother 1978;14: 639–641.

68. Gotuzzo E, Carrillo C, Guerra J, et al. An evaluation of diagnostic methods for brucellosis: the value of bone marrow culture. J Infect Dis 1986; 153:122–125.

69. Grant PE, Brenner DJ, Steigerwalt AG, et al. *Neisseria elongata* subsp. *nitroreducens* subsp. nov., formerly CDC group M-6, a gram-negative bacterium associated with endocarditis. J Clin Microbiol 1990;28:2591–2596.

70. Grewal P, Fonseca K, Andrews HJ. *Pasteurella ureae* meningitis and septicemia. J Infect 1983; 7:74–76.

71. Gump DW, Frank RO, Winn WC Jr, et al. Legionnaires' disease in patients with associated serious disease. Ann Intern Med 1979;90:638–642.

72. Halperin SA, Bortolussi R, Wort J. Evaluation of culture, immunofluorescence, and serology for the diagnosis of pertussis. J Clin Microbiol 1989; 27:752–757.

73. Hicklin H, Verghese A, Alvarez S. Dysgonic fermenter 2 septicemia. Rev Infect Dis 1987;9: 884–890.

74. Hollis DG, Sottnek FO, Brown WJ, et al. Use of the rapid carbohydrate fermentation test in determining carbohydrate reactions of fastidious bacteria in clinical laboratories. J Clin Microbiol 1980;12:520–623.

75. Hollis DG, Weaver RE, Steigerwalt AG, et al. *Francisella philomiragia* comb. nov. (formerly *Yersinia philomiragia*) and *Francisella tularensis* biogroup Novicida (formerly *Francisella novicida*) associated with human disease. J Clin Microbiol 1989;27:1601–1608.

76. Hollis DG, Wiggins GL, Weaver RE. An unclassified gram-negative rod isolated from the pharynx on Thayer-Martin medium (selective agar). Appl Microbiol 1972;24:772–777.

77. Janda WM, Bradna JJ, Ruther P. Identification of *Neisseria* spp., *Haemophilus* spp., and other fastidious gram-negative bacteria with the MicroScan *Haemophilus-Neisseria* identification panel. J Clin Microbiol 1989;27:869–873.

78. Janda WM, Malloy PJ, Schreckenberger PC. Clinical evaluation of the Vitek *Neisseria-Haemophilus* identification card. J Clin Microbiol 1987;25:37–41.

79. Jenny DB, Letendre PW, Iverson G. Endocarditis caused by *Kingella indologenes*. Rev Infect Dis 1987;9:787–788.

80. Johnson JD, Raff MY, Van Arsdall JA. Neurologic manifestations of legionnaires' disease. Medicine 1984;63:303–310.

81. Jones RN, Slepack J, Bigelow J. Ampicillin-resistant *Haemophilus paraphrophilus* laryngo-epiglottitis. J Clin Microbiol 1976;4:405–407.

82. Kaplan AH, Weber DJ, Oddone EZ, et al. Infection due to *Actinobacillus actinomycetemcomitans*: 15 cases and review. Rev Infect Dis 1989;11:46–63.

83. Kersters K, Hinz K-H, Hertle A, et al. *Bordetella avium* sp. nov., isolated from the respiratory tracts of turkeys and other birds. Int J Syst Bacteriol 1984;34:56–70.

84. Kiel RJ, Crane LR, Aguilar WA, et al. Corneal perforation caused by dysgonic fermenter-2. JAMA 1987;23:3269–3270.

85. Korvick JA, Yu VL. Legionnaires' disease: an emerging surgical problem. Ann Thorac Surg 1987;43:341–347.

86. Kristinsson KG, Thorgeirsson G, Holbrook WP. *Actinobacillus actinomycetemcomitans* and endocarditis. J Infect Dis 1988;157:599.

87. Kurzynski TA, Boehm DM, Rott-Petri JA, et al. Antimicrobial susceptibilities of *Bordetella* species isolated in a multicenter pertussis surveillance project. Antimicrob Agents Chemother 1988;32: 137–140.

88. Linnemann CC, Perry EB. *Bordetella parapertussis*: recent experience and a review of the literature. Am J Dis Child 1977;131:560–563.

89. Maia A, Goldstein FW, Acar JF, et al. Isolation of *Eikenella corrodens* from human infections: report of six cases. J Infect Dis 1988;2:347–353.

90. Mandel DR. Streptobacillary fever, an unusual cause of infectious arthritis. Cleve Clin Q 1985; 51:203–205.

91. Mannhein W. Family III. Pasteurellaceae Pohl 1981a, 382 VP. In: Krieg NR, Holt JG, eds. Bergey's manual of systematic bacteriology. Baltimore, Williams & Wilkins, 1984;1:557–558.

92. Marcon MJ, Hamoudi AC, Cannon HJ, et al. Comparison of throat and nasopharyngeal swab specimens for culture diagnosis of *Bordetella pertussis* infection. J Clin Microbiol 1987;25:1109–1110.

93. Marcus HR, Phelps CM. *Eikenella corrodens* subacute bacterial endocarditis: mixed infection in an amphetamine abuser. NY State J Med 1977;77: 2259–2261

94. Marriott DJ, Brady LM. *Pasteurella ureae* meningitis. Med J Aust 1983;2:455–456.

95. Matlow A, Velland H. *Capnocytophaga*: a pathogen in immunocompetent hosts. J Infect Dis 1985; 152:233–234.

96. Mayrock R, Skale B, Kohler RB. *Legionella pneumophila* pericarditis proved by culture of pericardial fluid. Am J Med 1983;75:534–536.

97. McCabe RE, Baldwin JC, McGregor CA, et al. Prosthetic valve endocarditis caused by *Legionella pneumophila*. Ann Intern Med 1984;100:525–527.

98. McDade JE, Shepard CC, Fraser DW, et al. Le-

gionnaires' disease: isolation of a bacterium and demonstration of its role in other respiratory disease. N Engl J Med 1977;297:1197–1203.

99. Morrison VA, Wagner KF. Clinical manifestations of *Kingella kingae* infections: case report and review. Rev Infect Dis 1989;11:776–782.

100. Moss CW, Wallace PL, Hollis DG, et al. Cultural and chemical characteristics of CDC groups EO-2, M-5 and M-6, *Moraxella* (*Moraxella*) species, *Oligella urethralis*, *Acinetobacter* species, and *Psychrobacter immobilis*. J Clin Microbiol 1988;26:484–492.

101. Mutters R, Ihm P, Pohl S, et al. Reclassification of the genus *Pasteurella* Trevisan 1887 on the basis of deoxyribonucleic acid homology, with proposals for the new species *Pasteurella dagmatis*, *Pasteurella canis*, *Pasteurella stomatis*, *Pasteurella anatis*, and *Pasteurella langaa*. Int J Syst Bacteriol 1985;35:309–322.

102. Mutters R, Peichulla K, Mannheim W. Phenotypic differentiation of *Pasteurella sensu stricto* and *Actinobacillus* group. Eur J Clin Microbiol 1984;3:225–229.

103. Mutters R, Pohl S, Mannheim W. Transfer of *Pasteurella ureae* Jones 1962 to the genus *Actinobacillus* Brumpt 1910: *Actinobacillus ureae* comb. nov. Int J Syst Bacteriol 1986;36:343–344.

104. Ng VL, York M, Hadley WK. Unexpected isolation of *Bordetella pertussis* from patients with acquired immunodeficiency syndrome. J Clin Microbiol 1989;27:337–338.

105. Noble RC, Marek BJ, Overman SB. Spontaneous bacterial peritonitis caused by *Pasteurella ureae*. J Clin Microbiol 1987;25:442–444.

106. Odum L, Jensen KT, Slotsbjerg TD. Endocarditis due to *Kingella kingae*. Eur J Clin Microbiol 1984;3:263–266.

107. Page MI, King EO. Infection due to *Actinobacillus actinomycetemcomitans* and *Haemophilus aphrophilus*. N Engl J Med 1966;275:181–188.

108. Parenti DM, Snydman DR. *Capnocytophaga* species: infections in nonimmunocompromised and immunocompromised hosts. J Infect Dis 1985; 151:140–147.

109. Pasculle AW, Veto GE, Krystofiak S, et al. Laboratory and clinical evaluation of a commercial DNA probe for the detection of *Legionella* spp. J Clin Microbiol 1989;27:2350–2358.

110. Perez RE. Endocarditis with *Moraxella*-like M-6 after cardiac catheterization. J Clin Microbiol 1986;24:501–502.

111. Phillips JE. Genus III. *Actinobacillus* Brumpt 1910, 849[AL]. In: Krieg NR, Holt JG, eds. Bergey's manual of systematic bacteriology. Baltimore, Williams & Wilkins, 1984;1:570–575.

112. Pilsworth R. Haverhill fever. Lancet 1983;2: 236–237.

113. Pittman M. Genus *Bordetella* Moreno-Lopez 1952, 178[AL]. In: Krieg NR, Holt JG, eds. Bergey's manual of systematic bacteriology. Baltimore, Williams & Wilkins, 1984;1:388–393.

114. Polin K, Shulman ST. *Eikenella corrodens* osetomyelitis. Pediatrics 1981;70:462–463.

115. Potasman S, Liberson A, Krimerman S. *Legionella* infection mimicking herpes encephalitis. Crit Care Med 1990;18:453–454.

116. Raad I, Rand K, Gaskins D. Buffered charcoal-yeast extract medium for the isolation of brucellae. J Clin Microbiol 1990;28:1671–1672.

117. Regan J, Lowe F. Enrichment medium for the isolation of *Bordetella pertussis*. J Clin Microbiol 1977;6:303–309.

118. Rihs JD, Yu BL, Zuravleff JJ, et al. Isolation of *Legionella pneumophila* from blood with the BACTEC system: a prospective study yielding positive results. J Clin Microbiol 1985;22: S422–S424.

119. Robertson PW, Goldberg H, Jarvie BH, et al. *Bordetella pertussis* infection: a cause of persistent cough in adults. Med J Aust 1987;147:522–525.

120. Roop RM, Preston-Moore D, Bagchi T, et al. Rapid identification of smooth *Brucella* species with a monoclonal antibody. J Clin Microbiol 1987;25:2090–2093.

121. Ross PW, Cumming CG. Isolation of *Bordetella pertussis* from swabs. Br Med J 1981;282:23–26.

122. Rossau R, Vandenbussche G, Thielemans S, et al. Ribosomal ribonucleic acid cistron similarities and deoxyribonucleic acid homologies of *Neisseria*, *Kingella*, *Eikenella*, *Simonsiella*, *Alysiella*, and Centers for Disease Control Groups EF-4 and M-5 in the emended family Neisseriaceae. Int J Syst Bacteriol 1989;39:185–198.

123. Rowbotham TJ. Rapid identification of *Streptobacillus moniliformis*. Lancet 1983;2:567.

124. Saravolatz LD, Burch KH, Fisher E, et al. The compromised host and legionnaires' disease. Ann Intern Med 1979;90:533–537.

125. Savage DD, Kagan RL, Young NA, et al. *Cardiobacterium hominis* endocarditis: description of two patients and characterization of the organism. J Clin Microbiol 1977;5:75–80.

126. Savage N. Genus *Streptobacillus* Levaditi, Nicolau, and Poincloux 1925, 1188[AL]. In: Krieg NR, Holt JG, eds. Bergey's manual of systematic bacteriology. Baltimore, Williams & Wilkins, 1984;1: 598–600.

127. Slots J. Salient biochemical characteristics of *Actinobacillus actinomycetemcomitans*. Arch Microbiol 1982;131:60–67.

128. Sneath PHA, Stevens M. *Actinobacillus rossii* sp. nov., *Actinobacillus seminis* sp. nov. nom. rev., *Pasteurella bettii* sp. nov., *Pasteurella lymphangitidis* sp nov., *Pasteurella mairi* sp. nov., and *Pasteurella*

trehalosi sp. nov. Int J Syst Bacteriol 1990;40: 148–153.

129. Socransky SS, Holt SC, Tanner ACR, et al. *Capnocytophaga*: a new genus of gram-negative gliding bacteria. III. Physiological characterization. Arch Microbiol 1979;122:29–33.

130. Starkebaum GA, Plorde JJ. *Pasteurella* pneumonia: report of a case and review of the literature. J Clin Microbiol 1977;5:332–335.

131. Stevens DL, Higbee JW, Oberhofer TR, et al. Antibiotic susceptibilities of human isolates of *Pasteurella multocida*. Antimicrob Agents Chemother 1979;16:322–324.

132. Stoloff AL, Gillies ML. Infections with *Eikenella corrodens* in a general hospital: a report of 33 cases. Rev Infect Dis 1986;8:50–53.

133. Stroll DB, Murphey SA, Ballas SK. *Bordetella bronchiseptica* infection in stage IV Hodgkin's disease. Postgrad Med J 1981;57:723–724.

134. Sutter VL, Pyeatt D, Kwok YY. In vitro susceptibility of *Capnocytophaga* strains to 18 antimicrobial agents. Antimicrob Agents Chemother 1981;20:270–271.

135. Sutton RGA, O'Keeffe MF, Bundock MA, et al. Isolation of a new *Moraxella* from a corneal abscess. J Med Microbiol 1972;5:148–150.

136. Taylor JP, Purdue JN. The changing epidemiology of human brucellosis in Texas, 1976–1986. Am J Epidemiol 1989;130:160–165.

137. Thatcher WL, Benson RF, Hawes L, Brenner DJ. Characterization of a *Legionella anisa* strain isolated from a patient with pneumonia. J Clin Microbiol 1990;28:122–123.

138. Tison DL, Latimer JM. Lysis centrifugation-direct plating technique for isolation of group DF-2 from the blood of a dog bite victim. (Letter) J Infect Dis 1986;153:1001–1002.

139. Thornsberry C, Baker CM, Kirvin LA. In vitro activity of antimicrobial agents of legionnaires' disease bacterium. Antimicrob Agents Chemother 1978;13:78–80.

140. Toshniwal R, Draghi TC, Kocka FE, et al. Manifestations of *Kingella kingae* infections in adults: resemblance to neisserial infections. Diagn Microbiol Infect Dis 1986;5:81–85.

141. Verbruggen A-M, Hauglustaine D, Schildermans F, et al. Infections caused by *Kingella kingae*: reports of four cases and review. J Infect 1986;13: 133–142.

142. Verghese A, Hamati F, Berk S, et al. Susceptibility of dysgonic fermenter 2 to antimicrobial agents in vitro. Antimicrob Agents Chemother 1988;32:78–80.

143. Vickers RM, Stout JE, Yu VL. Notes: failure of a diagnostic monoclonal immunofluorescent reagent to detect *Legionella pneumophila* in environmental samples. Appl Envron Microbiol 1990;56: 2912–2914.

144. Wagner DK, Wright JJ, Ansher AF, et al. Dysgonic fermenter 3–associated gastrointestinal disease in a patient with common variable hypogammaglobulinemia. Am J Med 1988;84: 315–318.

145. Weber DJ, Wolfson JS, Swartz MN, et al. *Pasteurella multocida* infections: report of 34 cases and review of the literature. Medicine (Balt) 1984;63:133–154.

146. White HJ, Felton WW, Sun CN. Extrapulmonary histopathologic manifestation of legionnaires' disease: evidence for myocarditis and bacteremia. Arch Pathol Lab Med 1980;104:287–289.

147. Wilson ME. Prosthetic valve endocarditis and paravalvular abscess caused by *Actinobacillus actinomycetemcomitans*. Rev Infect Dis 1989;11: 665–667.

148. Winn WC Jr. Legionellosis. In: Wentworth BB, ed. Diagnostic procedures for bacterial infections. Washington, DC, American Public Health Association, 1987:318–334.

149. Winn WC Jr. Legionnaires' disease: historical perspective. Clin Microbiol Rev 1988;1:60–81.

150. Winn WC Jr, Myerowitz RL. The pathology of the *Legionella* pneumonias: a review of 74 cases and the literature. Hum Pathol 1981;12:401–422.

151. Wormser GP, Bottone EJ. *Cardiobacterium hominis*: review of microbiologic and clinical features. Rev Infect Dis 1983;5:680–691.

152. Yogev R, Shulman D, Shulman ST, et al. In vitro activity of antibiotics alone and in combination against *Actinobacillus actinomycetemcomitans*. Antimicrob Agents Chemother 1986;29:179–181.

153. Young EJ. Human brucellosis. Rev Infect Dis 1983;5:821–842.

154. Yu VL. *Legionella pneumophila* (legionnaires' disease). In: Mandell GL, Douglas RG, Bennett JE, eds. Principles and practice of infectious diseases. 3rd ed. New York, John Wiley & Sons, 1990: 1764–1774.

155. Zeimis RT, Hanley OQ. Endocarditis caused by *Kingella kingae*: case report and review. Lab Med 1985;16:547–550.

156. Zimmerman SJ, Gillikin S, Sofat N, et al. Case report and seeded blood culture study of *Brucella* bacteremia. J Clin Microbiol 1990;28:2139–2141.

157. Zuravleff JJ, Yu VL, Shonnard JW, et al. Diagnosis of legionnaires' disease: an update of laboratory methods with new emphasis on isolation by culture. JAMA 1983;250:1981–1985.

7

Neisseria *Species* *and* Moraxella catarrhalis

INTRODUCTION TO THE FAMILY NEISSERIACEAE

Taxonomy of the Family Neisseriaceae

When the last edition of *Bergey's Manual of Systematic Bacteriology* was published in 1984 the Neisseriaceae included four genera: *Neisseria, Moraxella, Kingella,* and *Acinetobacter.*[85] Since then, several changes in the composition of the Neisseriaceae have been proposed and are likely to be adopted. These changes are based primarily on deoxyribonucleic acid (DNA)–ribosomal ribonucleic acid (rRNA) homology studies.[22,73] Table 7-1 summarizes the old classification and the newly emended classification system for the Neisseriaceae.[72] As can be seen, most of the individual *Neisseria* species are recognized in both schemes.

The familial position of "*M. catarrhalis,*" the other moraxellae, and *Acinetobacter* species is unclear. Two proposals are under consideration, a discussion of which is beyond the scope of this text. Rossau and associates[74] have proposed a new family called the Moraxellaceae based on DNA–ribosomal RNA hybridization. The second proposal of Catlin creates a new family called the Branhamaceae.[15] Interested readers should consult the references cited for more information.

General Characteristics of the Genus *Neisseria* and of *Moraxella catarrhalis*

Members of the genus *Neisseria* are coccoid or rod-shaped gram-negative organisms that frequently occur in pairs or short chains. The coccoid organisms have adjacent sides flattened, giving them a coffee bean shape. All species in the genus *Neisseria* inhabit mucous membrane surfaces of warm-blooded hosts. These organisms are nonmotile and do not form spores. Most species grow optimally at 35° to 37°C. They are capnophilic and grow best in a moist environment. At the present time, *Neisseria* species (except for the three *N. elongata* subspecies) are the only true coccoid members of the Neisseriaceae.[72,85] *N. elongata* subspecies are short rods that sometimes occur in pairs or short chains. All species in the genus are oxidase positive and (except for *N. elongata* subspecies *elongata* and *nitroreducens*) catalase positive.[6,39]

Diplococcal members of the genus that are found in humans include *N. gonorrhoeae, N. meningitidis, N. lactamica, N. sicca, N. subflava* (including biovars *subflava, flava,* and *perflava*), *N. mucosa, N. flavescens, N. cinerea,* and *N. polysaccharea.*[57] In addition, a new organism called *N. gonorrhoeae* subspecies *kochii* has also been described that is both phenotypically and genetically related to *N. gonorrhoeae. N. canis* and *N. denitrificans* are found as normal respiratory tract flora in cats and guinea pigs, respectively.[85] Most species in the genus *Neisseria* are a part of the commensal flora of the human upper respiratory tract. These organisms are, however, being reported more and more frequently as etiologic agents of significant infectious processes. The clinical significance of the major pathogenic *Neisseria* will now be considered.

CLINICAL SIGNIFICANCE OF *NEISSERIA* SPECIES AND *MORAXELLA CATARRHALIS*

Neisseria gonorrhoeae

Neisseria gonorrhoeae is the causative agent of gonorrhea, a bacterial infection of considerable public health significance. More than 3 million persons in the United States are estimated to acquire gonococcal infection each year. In males, *N. gonorrhoeae* causes an acute urethritis with dysuria and urethral discharge.[47] The incubation period between acquisition of the organism and the onset of symptoms ranges from 1 to 10 days, with the average being about 5 days. Most men with gonorrhea have acute symptoms, but asymptomatic infections in men have been reported.[18] If left untreated, the ascending infection may result in gonococcal prostatitis, epididymitis, periurethral abscess, and urethral stricture. Homosexual and bisexual men may also acquire oropharyngeal and rectal gonococcal infections by engaging in unprotected oral or anal intercourse with an infected partner.

In females, the primary infection is present in the endocervix, with concomitant urethral infection occurring in 70% to 90%. Patients may present with cervicovaginal discharge, lower abdominal pain, dysuria, and abnormal or intermenstrual bleeding.[47] Symptoms of uncomplicated endocervical infection often resemble those of other conditions such as cystitis or vaginitis. Infection of Bar-

Table 7-1
Classification of Organisms Within the Family Neisseriaceae

GENUS AND SPECIES IN *BERGEY'S MANUAL* (1984)	GENUS AND SPECIES IN PROPOSED SCHEME 1989[72]	COMMENTS
Neisseria species	*Neisseria* species	
N. gonorrhoeae	N. gonorrhoeae	
	"N. kochii"	Not included in 1989 scheme but accepted in other reports
N. meningitidis	N. meningitidis	
N. lactamica	N. lactamica	
N. sicca	N. sicca	
N. subflava	N. subflava	Biovars *flava, subflava,* and *perflava* recognized only in 1989 scheme
N. mucosa	N. mucosa	
N. flavescens	N. flavescens	
N. cinerea	N. cinerea	
	N. polysaccharea	Species described by Riou, 1987
	N. macacae	Species found in monkeys
N. elongata subsp. *elongata*	N. elongata subsp. *elongata*	
N. elongata subsp. *glycolytica*	N. elongata subsp. *glycolytica*	
	N. elongata subsp. *nitroreducens*	Formerly CDC group M-6
N. canis	N. canis	Respiratory flora, cats
N. denitrificans	N. denitrificans	Respiratory flora, guinea pigs
Kingella species	*Kingella* species	
K. kingae	K. kingae	
K. denitrificans	K. denitrificans	
K. indologenes	Not included	Now classified as *Suttonella indologenes* in the *Cardiobacteriaceae (see Chapter 6)*
Acinetobacter species	Not included	Family affiliation uncertain
Moraxella species	Not included	Family affiliation uncertain; family moraxellaceae and family Branhamellaceae proposed
"Psychrobacter immobilis"	Not included	Added to the Neisseriaceae as described by Bovre in 1986
	Eikenella species	Not formerly included in a designated family (see Chapter 6)
	Simonsiella species	*Simonsiella* species and *Alysiella* species are aerobic, gram-negative gliding bacteria that are found normally in the oral cavities of humans and animals; nonpathogenic
	Alysiella species	
	CDC group EF-4a	These organisms are found as normal flora in the oral cavities of dogs and cats and may be isolated from infected dog and cat bite or scratch wounds (see Chapter 6)
	CDC group EF-4b	
Not included	CDC group M-5	Asaccharolytic, nitrate-negative *Moraxella*-like organisms also associated with infected dog bites (see Chapter 6)

tholin's glands and the periurethral glands of the external female genitalia may be seen in about one third of women with genital tract infection. Women may also acquire pharyngeal or rectal gonococcal infections by engaging in orogenital and anogenital sexual practices; in some cases the anal canal may become secondarily infected by cervical secretions owing to the proximity of the rectum to the vagina. Ascending gonococcal infection in the female may result in acute salpingitis, which can lead to scarring of the fallopian tubes, ectopic pregnancies, and sterility.[47] Symptoms of gonococcal salpingitis include lower abdominal pain, abnormal cervical discharge and bleeding, pain on motion, fever, and peripheral leukocytosis.

In a small percentage (0.5% to 3%) of infected persons, gonococci may invade the bloodstream, resulting in disseminated gonococcal infection.[47] Disseminated gonococcal infection is characterized by fever, hemorrhagic skin lesions (usually located on the hands or feet), and migratory joint pain. Organisms from the bloodstream may localize in one or more joints to cause a purulent and destructive gonococcal arthritis, commonly involving the wrist, fingers, knees, or ankles. This infection occurs more frequently in females than males and is often temporally related to menstruation. Repeated bouts of disseminated gonococcal infection have also been observed in persons with certain complement deficiencies.[71] Systemic dissemination from localized extragenital infections may also occur.

Ocular gonococcal infections are primarily seen in neonates who acquire the organism during passage through an infected birth canal ("ophthalmia neonatorum"). Ocular infections may also be seen in adults who become inoculated with infected genital secretions.[47] Laboratory personnel who work with live and lyophilized cultures of the organism may also become accidentally infected if care is not taken to protect the eyes when working with the organism.

Neisseria meningitidis

Neisseria meningitidis is a primary pathogen that causes a spectrum of infectious processes, ranging from occult sepsis with rapid recovery to fulminant, overwhelming disease resulting in death.[2] Individual patients may manifest only limited aspects of the clinical spectrum; others may progress across this spectrum, sometimes with alarming rapidity. The most serious clinical manifestation of meningococcal disease is meningitis, and *N. meningitidis* is the second leading cause of meningitis in the United States.[41] The classic signs of meningitis, such as confusion, headache, fever, and nuchal rigidity, may be seen only in about one half of the patients.[2] Vomiting may also be a part of the clinical presentation, particularly in children. Blood cultures may or may not be positive. Meningococcemia and widespread dissemination of the organism is heralded by the rapid development of small hemorrhagic skin lesions called petechiae. These lesions are indicators of bleeding complications and coagulopathies that are caused by the organism. Fulminant, rapidly progressive disease may result in coalescence of petechial lesions to form areas of cutaneous hemorrhagic necrosis. Death may supervene as a result of disseminated intravascular coagulation. In these fatal cases, autopsies after reveal terminal myocarditis or the lesions of disseminated intravascular coagulation, with microthrombi and thromboses observed in many organs. The classic findings of acute hemorrhage into the adrenal glands represent the anatomic hallmark of Waterhouse-Friderichsen syndrome.

N. meningitidis may also cause acute and chronic bloodstream infection (meningococcemia) without meningitis.[2] In the acute form, the patient usually presents with a slight fever and symptoms of a respiratory tract infection. Meningococci are recovered from blood cultures, but the patient is usually clinically well by this time, and no treatment or a short course of therapy is administered. With chronic meningococcemia, the patient is generally symptomatic, with fever, rash, and occasionally arthritis. This form of meningococcal disease has been noted to recur in some patients, and it has been shown that such persons frequently have underlying deficiencies in certain complement components (a similar picture to that seen with the gonococcus), particularly the terminal components of the cascade.[63]

The pathogenesis of meningococcal disease is poorly understood. Humans are the only natural host for *N. meningitidis*, and the organism is spread by means of respiratory droplets. The organism may be asymptomatically carried in the oropharynx and nasopharynx of a variable percentage of persons, and the rate of carriage is related to several factors, including age, socioeconomic class, and the presence of actual disease in a community.[11] In some persons the organism leaves the upper respiratory tract and invades the bloodstream to initiate systemic disease. The virulence of individual meningococcal strains is related to the capsular polysaccharide serogroup and protein serotypes within each serogroup. Thirteen meningococcal serogroups (A, B, C, D, H, I, K, L, X, Y, Z, W135, and 29E) are recognized, with most serious infections being associated with organisms belonging to groups A, B, C, and Y.[9,32,41,77]

The diagnosis of meningococcal meningitis constitutes a medical emergency since overwhelming infection may develop rapidly. Bloodstream invasion may seed other body sites, resulting in meningococcal arthritis, osteomyelitis, and pericarditis.[2] Meningococcal pneumonia can also occur, particularly in older persons with preexisting pulmonary diseases. *N. meningitidis* may occasionally be isolated from anogenital sites and may cause infections that are clinically indistinguishable from gonococcal infections, such as acute purulent urethritis, cervicitis, and proctitis.[48]

Other *Neisseria* Species

Neisseria lactamica, N. sicca, N. subflava (biovars *flava, subflava,* and *perflava*), *N. mucosa, N. flavescens, N. cinerea, N. polysaccharea,* and *N. elongata* are all members of the normal flora of the human upper respiratory tract. The traditional "nonpathogenic" or "saprophytic" neisseriae (*N. lactamica, N. sicca, N. subflava* biovars, *N. mucosa,* and *N. flavescens*) are rare causes of significant infections, including osteomyelitis, pleuropulmonary infections, endophthalmitis, ophthalmia neonatorum, Bartholin's gland abscess, pericarditis, cellulitis, empyema, and urethritis.[3,31,35,45] *N. subflava* biovars, *N. mucosa, N. sicca,* and *N. flavescens* have been most frequently reported as agents of endocarditis, particularly in those patients who have prosthetic heart valves or who are intravenous drug abusers.[10,16,34,78] *N. lactamica,* an organism that is of special concern since it is able to grow on selective media for gonococci and meningococci (see later), has been isolated from genital sites and from cerebrospinal fluid and blood.[40,44] The other "nonpathogenic" species have been infrequently isolated from these specimens.[20,45] Rare strains of these organisms may present therapeutic dilemmas, since some may be penicillin resistant because of elaboration of β-lactamase enzymes. In these cases the isolates must be identified and susceptibility tests should be performed. Some of the more recently described species have also been reported as opportunistic pathogens in compromised hosts.

Neisseria cinerea has been recovered as the cause of nosocomial pneumonia in a patient with acquired immunodeficiency syndrome and as an agent of lymphadenitis.[8,17] *N. cinerea* has also been associated with syndromes similar to those caused by gonococci, such as ophthalmia neonatorum and proctitis.[5,27] The "species" *N. gonorrhoeae* subspecies *kochii* (or "*N. kochii*") has been isolated from patients with conjunctivitis in rural Egypt; no isolates have been described from the United States.[67] *N. polysaccharea,* another respiratory commensal organism, has not yet been described as part of a pathologic process. *N. canis* and *N. denitrificans* are animal strains isolated from the upper respiratory tracts of cats and guinea pigs, respectively. *N. denitrificans* has not been associated with human disease, but *N. canis* has been recovered from human wounds resulting from cat bites.[42]

The only rod-shaped member of the genus *Neisseria* is *N. elongata.* Up until 1990 this species contained two subspecies, *elongata* and *glycolytica.* These organisms are normally found in the human upper respiratory tract, and neither of these subspecies has been implicated in human infections. *N. elongata* subspecies *nitroreducens,* a newly reclassified organism, was formerly called CDC group M-6.[39] This "*Moraxella*-like" bacterium has been shown to be related to the *Neisseria* species, in general, and to *N. elongata* isolates, in particular, on the basis of genetic studies, cellular fatty acid composition, and phenotypic properties. *N. elongata* subspecies *nitroreducens* is also found normally in the oropharynx of humans and has been reported as an opportunistic agent of endocarditis and as a cause of osteomyelitis after oral surgery.[33,81] The organism has also been isolated from urine and appendiceal tissue.[39]

Moraxella catarrhalis

During the past 10 years, the organism formerly called *Neisseria catarrhalis, Branhamella catarrhalis, Branhamella (Moraxella) catarrhalis,* and now *Moraxella catarrhalis* has received a great deal of attention as an emerging human pathogen.[14] Before 1990, it was believed that *M. catarrhalis* was a part of the normal human upper respiratory tract flora. Studies by Vaneechouette and colleagues[83] and Knapp and Hook[58] have now shown that the organism is found in the upper respiratory tracts of only 1.5% to 5.4% of healthy adults and is actually more common in the respiratory tracts of healthy children (50.8%) and elderly adults (26.5%). Furthermore, when isolated from adults with respiratory tract disease, the organism is more frequently found in specimens judged to represent lower respiratory tract secretions than in those specimens determined to have large amounts of oropharyngeal contamination. The organism is, thus, not a significant part of the normal upper respiratory tract flora and may be involved in respiratory tract infections more frequently than previously believed.[83] The more frequent recovery of this organism from the respiratory tracts of children and the elderly does support the role of this organism in certain childhood infections (otitis media, acute sinusitis) and lower respiratory tract infections (bronchitis, pneumonia) in older persons.

Infections of the respiratory tract account for the majority of clinical conditions involving *M. catarrhalis* as an etiologic agent. These infections include otitis media, sinusitis, bronchitis, and pneumonia.[43,65,84,88] Although otitis media caused by this organism may occur in all age groups, most studies have centered on this organism's role in pediatric infection. In a study by Van Hare and coworkers,[84] *M. catarrhalis* was the only bacterial pathogen isolated from middle ear fluid of 40 (11%) of 355 children with acute otitis media and was co-isolated with either *Haemophilus influenzae* or *Streptococcus pneumoniae* in 21 (6%) of the patients. The bacteriologic findings with acute otitis media are mirrored in studies of acute sinusitis in the same age groups. With the use of carefully collected maxillary sinus aspirates from children with acute sinusitis, *M. catarrhalis* may be isolated in either pure or mixed cultures from 2% to 16% of patients.[65] Acute sinus infections in adults have also been associated with this organism, but with less frequency than in children.

Lower respiratory tract infections due to *M. catarrhalis* occur predominantly in immunocompromised hosts, particularly those persons with chronic obstructive pulmonary disease.[43,76,88] Immunologic abnormalities due to underlying diseases such as diabetes or alcoholism are also important contributing factors. *M. catarrhalis* is most frequently associated with clinical findings of acute bronchitis, with pneumonia being seen less often. Patients with bronchitis due to this organism usually present with increasing production of purulent sputum and mild respiratory distress without fever. Pneumonic involvement is heralded by the appearance of low-grade fever, dyspnea, and production of increasing amounts of purulent sputum.[76] Progres-

sion to respiratory failure has been observed in some cases. Radiologically, the disease usually appears as patchy infiltrates in both lungs, although lobar involvement has also been documented.[43]

M. catarrhalis also has been isolated from patients with bacteremia, endocarditis, meningitis, conjunctivitis, urogenital tract infections, and wound infections.[14,24] Bacteremia and endocarditis have usually occurred in persons who were immunosuppressed by underlying diseases, treatment of other conditions, or various types of surgical procedures. Such conditions have included leukemias and lymphomas, immunoglobulin deficiency states, and acquired immunodeficiency syndrome.[14] Conjunctival infections caused by *M. catarrhalis* have been documented in both the neonatal period and later in childhood. "Ophthalmia neonatorum" due to this organism is believed to result either from acquisition of the organism at birth from the mother's colonized genital tract or from respiratory tract secretions of the child's caretakers.[14] Recovery of this organism from the genital tract of either men or women is rare, but *M. catarrhalis* has been reported as a cause of a gonorrhea-like urethritis in a few cases.[24] Because of its close resemblance to *Neisseria* species and the frequency of isolation of this organism in the clinical laboratory, methods for identifying *M. catarrhalis* will be discussed after the discussion of those methods used for the *Neisseria* species.

ISOLATION OF THE PATHOGENIC *NEISSERIA* SPECIES

Isolation of *Neisseria gonorrhoeae*

Specimen Collection

As with other pathogenic microorganisms, successful isolation depends on the collection of proper specimens, and this is particularly important for the recovery of *N. gonorrhoeae*. Since this organism can cause infection at a variety of body sites, the collection of appropriate specimens for culture and diagnosis is dependent on the sex and sexual practices of the patient and on the clinical presentation. In all cases, specimens from genital sites (male urethra, female endocervix) should be collected. If the patient has a history of orogenital or anogenital sexual contacts, appropriate oropharyngeal or anal canal specimens are also collected. In suspected cases of disseminated disease, blood cultures and specimens from genital and extragenital sites should be obtained. Appropriate sites for culture are summarized in Table 7-2.

Specimens should be collected with dacron or rayon swabs. Some lots of calcium alginate may be toxic to certain gonococcal strains.[61] Cotton swabs may also be used. Some brands of cotton contain fatty acids that may be inhibitory for gonococci; therefore, calcium alginate and cotton swabs should be used only if the specimen is inoculated directly onto growth media or transported in nonnutritive media containing charcoal to adsorb or neutralize inhibitory materials. Instruments used to aid in the proper collection of specimens (eg, vaginal specula) should be lubricated with warm water or saline since various water- and oil-based lubricants may also be inhibitory. Direct smears for Gram stain should be prepared from urethral and endocervical sites and should be collected with a separate swab. For smear preparation, the swab should be rolled gently over the surface of a glass slide in one direction only. This technique will minimize distortion and breakage of polymorphonuclear leukocyte and will preserve the characteristic appearance of the microorganisms. Smears from normally sterile or minimally contaminated sites (eg, joint fluid, skin lesions) should also be prepared. Table 7-3 describes collection procedures for the recovery of *N. gonorrhoeae* from different anatomic sites.

Specimen Transport

Although maximal recovery of gonococci is obtained when specimens are plated directly onto growth medium after collection, this technique might not always be possible or practical, particularly in busy clinics or hospital emergency departments. For these situations, various types of transport systems are available.

NONNUTRITIVE SWAB TRANSPORT SYSTEMS. Stuart's or Amie's buffered semisolid transport medium can be used for the transport of swab specimens for *N. gonorrhoeae*. These systems are easy to use, are readily available in most clinic and hospital situations, and require no special equipment or storage conditions. Specimens sent to the laboratory in swab transport systems must be processed within 6 hours of collection, however, since there is a decrease in the numbers of viable organisms after this time. With these systems, long delays in transport and exposure to extremes in temperature (eg, refrigeration) may compromise successful recovery of the organism. As mentioned previously, transport medium containing activated charcoal is preferable if cotton swabs are used for the collection of the specimen. Some of the newer semisolid transport formulations (eg, APO-Swab, Apotex, Inc, Windsor, Ontario) are also satisfactory for maintaining viability of *N. gonorrhoeae* for short periods of time.

CULTURE MEDIA TRANSPORT SYSTEMS. Transport of specimens on culture media presents certain advantages and several systems for this purpose are commercially available. These include JEMBEC (*James E. Martin biological environmental chamber*)[66] plates containing various formulations of selective media and the Gono-Pak[21] (Becton Dickinson Microbiology Systems, Cockeysville, MD). With these systems, the medium is inoculated with the specimen and placed in an

Table 7-2
Body Sites to Culture for *Neisseria gonorrhoeae*

PATIENT	PRIMARY SITE(S)	SECONDARY SITE
Female	Endocervix	Rectum, urethra, pharynx
Male, heterosexual	Urethra	Pharynx
Male, homosexual/bisexual	Urethra, rectum, pharynx	
Female, disseminated infection	Blood, endocervix, rectum	Pharynx, skin lesions,* joint fluid†
Male, disseminated infection	Blood, urethra	Pharynx, rectum, skin lesions,* joint fluid†

*If present.
†Culture if arthritis present.

Table 7-3
Specimen Collection Procedures for Diagnosis of Gonococcal Infections

BODY SITE	COLLECTION PROCEDURE
Male urethra	Purulent discharge may be expressed by stripping the penis anteriorly and collecting the material on a swab. Specimens from asymptomatic males are obtained by inserting a calcium alginate naso-pharyngeal swab 2 to 3 cm into the urethra. The swab is gently rotated as it is withdrawn.
Endocervix	After the speculum is in place, remove any cervical mucus with cotton or gauze. Insert the swab and collect the specimen with a gentle side-to-side motion. Allow time for the organisms to adsorb onto the swab surface. Sample any purulent cervical discharge that may be present.
Rectum	Insert the swab 4 to 5 cm into the anal canal and gently move it from side to side to sample the anal crypts. Allow a few seconds for the organisms to adsorb onto the swab and gently rotate the swab during withdrawal. If heavy fecal contamination is observed on the swab, collect another specimen with a fresh swab.
Oropharynx	With the aid of a tongue depressor, firmly swab the tonsillar areas and the posterior pharynx.
Blood	After venipuncture, inoculate suitable blood culture media (trypticase soy broth, Columbia broth) containing sodium polyanethol sulfonate (SPS). If SPS Vacutainer tubes are used for blood collection, transfer the blood specimen from the tube into culture media as soon as possible, since exposure to high concentrations of SPS may be inhibitory to gonococci.
Joint fluid	Material should be aspirated with a needle and syringe and hand-carried to the laboratory.
Skin lesions	Punch biopsy specimens are collected and placed in a sterile container with a small amount of broth or sterile saline and hand-carried to the laboratory.
Conjunctivae	Collect conjunctival discharge from the inner aspect of the lower eyelid with a small nasopharyngeal swab. Prepare smears for Gram stain as described above.

impermeable plastic bag with a bicarbonate–citric acid pellet. Contact of the pellet with moisture (by evaporation of water from the medium during incubation [JEMBEC] or by crushing an ampoule of water adjacent to the pellet [Gono-Pak]) generates a CO_2-enriched environment within the bag. Incubation for at least 18 to 24 hours at 35°C before transport to a reference laboratory allows outgrowth of the organisms and minimizes the loss of viability that may be encountered with swab transport systems.

Selective Culture Media

A variety of enriched selective media for culture of *N. gonorrhoeae* are available and include modified Thayer-Martin (MTM) medium, Martin-Lewis (ML) medium, New York City (NYC) medium, and the new GC-Lect medium (Becton Dickinson Microbiology Systems, Cockeysville, MD). All of these formulations contain antimicrobial agents that inhibit other microorganisms and allow the selective recovery of both *N. gonorrhoeae* and *N. meningitidis*. Table 7-4 shows the concentrations of antimicrobial agents present in MTM, ML, NYC and GC-Lect agar media.

Vancomycin and colistin, antimicrobials present in all four formulations, inhibit gram-positive and gram-negative bacteria (including saprophytic *Neisseria* species), respectively. Lincomycin present in GC-Lect agar provides additional activity against gram-positive contaminant bacteria.[29] Trimethoprim is added to inhibit the swarming of *Proteus* species present in rectal and, occasionally, cervicovaginal specimens.[80] Nystatin, amphotericin B, or anisomycin is added to inhibit yeasts and molds. MTM, ML, and GC-Lect are chocolate agar–based media that are supplemented with growth factors for fastidious microorganisms, while NYC medium is a clear peptone-cornstarch agar–based medium containing yeast dialysate, citrated horse plasma, and lysed horse erythrocytes.[30] All of these media allow selective recovery of *N. gonorrhoeae* from body sites harboring a large endogenous bacterial flora, and all of these media are commercially available in either petri dishes or JEMBEC plates. The formulas for these media are available in general media references. Various modifications of selective media have also been described, such as a hemoglobin-free formulation of NYC agar.[38]

Table 7-4
Antimicrobial Agents in Selective *Neisseria* Media

ANTIMICROBIAL AGENT	MEDIA			
	Modified Thayer-Martin	Martin-Lewis	New York City	GC-Lect
Vancomycin (μg/mL)	3	4	2	2
Lincomycin (μg/mL)	—	—	—	1
Colistin (μg/mL)	7.5	7.5	5.5	7.5
Nystatin (μg/mL)	12.5	—	—	—
Anisomycin (μg/mL)	—	20.0	—	—
Amphotericin B (μg/mL)	—	—	1.2	1.5
Trimethoprim (μg/mL)	5	5	3	5

Inoculation and Incubation of Culture Media

Media for isolation of *Neisseria* should be at room temperature before inoculation and should not be excessively dry or moist. Specimens collected on swabs are firmly rolled in a "Z" pattern on selective media and cross-streaked with a bacteriologic loop. If nonselective media are also inoculated, these plates should be streaked for isolation. The plates are incubated in a CO_2 incubator or a candle extinction jar at 35°C to 37°C. The CO_2 level of the incubator should be 3% to 7% and should not exceed this since some organisms will actually be inhibited at higher CO_2 concentrations. The CO_2 level in a candle extinction jar is about 3%. The atmosphere should be moist, and with candle jars the moisture evaporating from the medium is usually sufficient for organism growth. CO_2 incubators not equipped with humidifiers may be kept moist by placing a pan of water on the lower shelf. If candle jars are used, candles should be made of white wax or beeswax; scented or colored candles release volatile products during burning and extinction that may inhibit the growth of the organisms.

Isolation of *Neisseria meningitidis*

Specimen Collection and Transport

Specimens helpful in the diagnosis of meningococcal disease include cerebrospinal fluid, blood, aspirates and biopsy specimens, and nasopharyngeal and oropharyngeal swabs. Occasionally, meningococci may be sought in sputum and transtracheal aspirates. Genital isolates of *N. meningitidis* may be recovered using the collection and inoculation procedures described for *N. gonorrhoeae*. Specimen collection and processing procedures are summarized in Table 7-5. Incubation conditions for the isolation of *N. meningitidis* are the same as those described for *N. gonorrhoeae*. Meningococci grow well on all selective media for the pathogenic *Neisseria*. Recovery of both gonococci and meningococci from blood cultures may be adversely affected by the anticoagulant sodium polyanetholsulfonate that is present in blood culture media. This effect may be alleviated by addition of sterile gelatin (1% final concentration) to the medium or by processing the blood specimen by lysis-centrifugation.[28,69,79]

IDENTIFICATION OF PATHOGENIC *NEISSERIA* SPECIES

Presumptive Identification of *Neisseria gonorrhoeae*

Colony Morphology

Gonococci produce several colony types in culture. In Kellogg's scheme, these types are termed T1 through T5 and are described in terms of colony size and other colonial characteristics (eg, coloration, topography of the colonies, reflection of

Table 7-5
Specimen Collection Procedures for Isolation of *Neisseria meningitidis*

SPECIMEN	COLLECTION PROCEDURE
Cerebrospinal fluid	In cases of suspected meningococcal meningitis, as much cerebrospinal fluid as possible (at least 1 mL) should be sent for culture, since small numbers of organisms may be present. Cerebrospinal fluid specimens should be hand-carried to the laboratory after collection and must not be refrigerated. The specimen should be centrifuged and the supernatant saved for use in antigen detection procedures. Part of the pellet should be used to prepare a smear for Gram staining, and the rest should be inoculated onto chocolate and blood agar. A supplemented back-up broth (eg, brain-heart infusion broth with 1% IsoVitalex) should also be inoculated with some of the pellet.
Blood	Blood should be cultured as described for gonococci. Direct inoculation of blood culture bottles is preferred over sodium polyanethol sulfonate (SPS) Vacutainer tubes owing to the recognized inhibitory effects of SPS on meningococci. This inhibition may be overcome by the addition of 1% (final volume) sterile gelatin to the blood culture medium. It has also been demonstrated that lysed blood can neutralize the inhibitory and cidal effects of SPS on meningococci and that the processing of blood by lysis-centrifugation overcomes the SPS effects on these organisms.
Petechiae	Specimens from petechial skin lesions may be collected by injection and aspiration of a small amount of sterile saline at the edge of the lesion using a tuberculin syringe. Aspirates are cultured directly on chocolate and blood agars. Since some of the lesions are a result of immunologic phenomena, culture of skin lesions may be noncontributory for diagnosis.
Nasopharyngeal swabs	Nasopharyngeal swabs are particularly important for detecting colonization of persons who are close contacts to cases of meningococcal disease and for carrier surveys. For these specimens, a fine swab on a flexible metal wire (eg, a calcium alginate nasopharyngeal swab) is passed through the oropharynx and behind the uvula, where the nasopharynx is sampled. In most cases, carefully collected throat swabs will provide the same information. These specimens are inoculated onto a selective medium such as modified Thayer-Martin agar.
Biopsy tissue	Biopsy specimens should be hand-carried to the laboratory in sterile containers. Specimens should be moistened with sterile saline or broth and should not be refrigerated. In the laboratory, tissue specimens should be aseptically teased apart and cultured on chocolate and blood agar. A portion of the specimen should also be placed in a suitable supplemented back-up broth medium.
Aspirates	Aspirates from closed spaces are collected with a needle and syringe and are inoculated onto chocolate and blood agars and into a suitable back-up broth.

light).[56] On the individual cellular level, organisms comprising colony types T1 and T2 possess pili on the cell surface, while cells in colony types T3, T4, and T5 lack pili. Isolates obtained on primary cultures are predominantly of the T1 and T2 colony types. These colonies tend to be small, glistening, and raised (see Color Plate 7-1*B*). With subculture of individual T1 and T2 colonies the culture can be maintained in these colony types. Organism suspensions prepared from 18- to 24-hour cultures containing primarily T1 and T2 colony types tend to be smooth and homogeneous. With nonselective subculture (ie, a "sweep" of growth), the other colony types will become more evident, with all colonies eventually becoming the T3, T4, and T5 varieties. These types are larger, are flatter, and do not have the characteristic glistening highlights of the T1 and T2 colony types. Cultures containing these large colony types are difficult to suspend with either a swab or a loop, since the colonies become gummy and rubbery owing to autolysis and release of cellular DNA. The presence of all of these colony types on a subculture from a primary plate may frequently give the appearance of a mixed culture. Careful scrutiny and subculture with the use of a dissecting microscope (10×) enables one to become familiar with these colony types. Variation in colony type is invariably seen with fresh isolates of *N. gonorrhoeae* and occasional isolates of *N. meningitidis*.

Gram Stain and Oxidase Test

Primary plates for isolation of *N. gonorrhoeae* should be examined after 24, 48, and 72 hours incubation using a hand lens or, preferably, a dissecting microscope. Smears prepared from suspicious colonies should be examined with the Gram stain, and an oxidase test should be performed. The Gram stain of the colony should show uniform, characteristic gram-negative diplococci. Some of the organisms may appear as tetrads, particularly on smears prepared from young colonies. Organisms on smears prepared from older cultures may appear swollen and display a wide variation in counterstaining intensity. This step is essential for presumptive identification since other organisms may occasionally grow on selective media, particularly from oropharyngeal specimens.

The best oxidase test results are obtained with the tetramethyl derivative of the oxidase reagent (N', N', N', N'-tetramethyl-*p*-phenylenediamine dihydrochloride, 1% aqueous solution). This solution is placed on a piece of filter paper and a portion of the colony is rubbed onto the reagent with a platinum loop, a cotton swab, or a wooden applicator stick. With fresh cultures a dark purple color will appear within 10 seconds. Excellent results are obtained with the oxidase reagents that are packaged in crushable glass ampules (eg, Difco Oxidase Reagent, Difco Laboratories, Detroit, MI).

Superoxol Test

Superoxol is another helpful test for the rapid presumptive identification of *N. gonorrhoeae*. Superoxol is 30% hydrogen peroxide (not the 3% solution routinely used for the catalase test). *N. gonorrhoeae* strains produce immediate, brisk bubbling when some of the colony material is emulsified with the reagent on a glass slide. *N. meningitidis* and *N. lactamica*, the other species that grow on selective media, produce weak, delayed bubbling. In a study using this test on organisms recovered on selective media, all 201 gonococci tested produced immediate, vigorous bubbling in Superoxol, while 241 of 242 meningococci and 1 of 2 *N. lactamica* strains produced negative or delayed, weak positive reactions.[75]

Differentiation of Other Organisms on Selective Media

Both the presumptive and confirmatory identification of *Neisseria* species is dependent on the ability to differentiate these organisms from others that may also grow on selective media. These organisms include *Kingella denitrificans*, *Moraxella* species (other than *M. catarrhalis*), *Acinetobacter* species, and *Capnocytophaga* species. *K. denitrificans* grows well on MTM medium and produces colony types that resemble those of *N. gonorrhoeae*. A rapid test that is useful in presumptively identifying gonococci and differentiating it from *K. denitrificans* is the catalase test. Gonococci will produce vigorous bubbling when growth from the plate is immersed in 3% hydrogen peroxide. *K. denitrificans* produces a negative catalase reaction. *Moraxella* species are, like gonococci, oxidase positive and catalase positive.

Moraxella species can be differentiated from *Neisseria* by the penicillin disk test.[13] The organism is subcultured to a trypticase-soy blood agar plate and streaked for confluent growth. A 10-unit penicillin disk is then placed on the inoculum. After overnight incubation in CO_2, a Gram stain is prepared from growth at the edge of the zone of inhibition. *Neisseria* species and *M. catarrhalis* will retain their coccal morphology, although the cells may appear swollen. Coccobacillary *Moraxella* species form long filaments or spindle-shaped cells under the influence of subinhibitory concentrations of penicillin. *Acinetobacter* species can be differentiated by their negative oxidase reaction. *Capnocytophaga* species appear as pale-staining, gram-negative, slightly curved, fusiform bacteria and are both oxidase- and catalase-negative. On prolonged incubation (ie, more than 48 hours) these organisms tend to spread, owing to gliding motility, and may impede recovery of gonococci from oropharyngeal specimens.

Criteria for Presumptive Identification of *Neisseria gonorrhoeae*

Oxidase-positive, gram-negative diplococci that are recovered from urogenital sites and that grow on selective media may be presumptively identified as *N. gonorrhoeae*. Confirmatory identification tests are recommended for all isolates and are required for identification of isolates from extragenital sites (ie, throat, rectum, blood, joint fluid, cerebrospinal fluid). Furthermore, suspect gonococci isolated from children should also be confirmed by more than one method since certain social and medicolegal issues are raised on the release of the results.[87]

In sexually transmitted disease clinics the diagnosis of gonococcal urethritis in men is frequently made by the observation of gram-negative intracellular diplococci on a smear prepared from the urethral discharge. When properly performed, the Gram stain is highly sensitive and specific for diagnosis in men. In women, a Gram stain of a carefully collected endocervical specimen may also be very helpful in diagnosis. Gram-stained smears of such specimens have a sensitivity of 50% to 70% depending on the adequacy of the specimen and the patient population. An endocervical smear showing gram-negative intracellular diplococci, particularly from a woman with other signs and symptoms of gonococcal infection, is highly predictive (see Color Plate 7-1*A*).[64] In asymptomatic women, however, the predictive value of the Gram stain is much lower. At any rate, the Gram stain should not be relied on for diagnosis of endocervical or extragenital infections and culture is necessary for making a diagnosis of gonococcal infection at these sites.

Identification Tests for *Neisseria* Species

Confirmatory tests for gonococci, meningococci, and other *Neisseria* species include carbohydrate utilization tests, chromogenic enzyme substrate tests, and serologic tests employing fluorescent antibody or staphylococcal coagglutination for culture confirmation of *N. gonorrhoeae*.

Carbohydrate Utilization Tests

CONVENTIONAL CTA CARBOHYDRATES. The conventional technique for the identification of *Neisseria* species employs cystine tryptic digest semisolid agar base (CTA) medium containing 1% carbohydrates and a phenol red *p*H indicator. The usual test battery includes CTA-glucose, CTA-maltose, CTA-sucrose, and CTA-lactose, plus a carbohydrate-free CTA control (eg, Remel Laboratories, Lenexa, KA). The lactose structural analogue, *ortho*-nitrophenyl-β-D-galactopyranoside (ONPG), may be substituted for the lactose tube, and the addition of fructose to the test battery is helpful for identifying the various *N. subflava* biovars.[57] Some commercial CTA formulations may be supplemented with ascitic fluid to support the growth of more fastidious organisms. CTA media are inoculated with a dense suspension of the organism to be identified from a pure 18- to 24-hour culture on chocolate agar. The inoculum is either prepared in 0.5 mL of saline and divided among the tubes, or each tube is individually inoculated with a loopful of the organism. The inoculum is restricted to the top one-half inch of the agar-deep tubes. The tubes are incubated in a non-CO_2 incubator at 35°C with the caps tightened firmly. With a heavy inoculum, most isolates produce a detectable change in the color of the phenol-red indicator within 24 hours. If the inoculum is heavy enough, many strains will change the indicator within 4 hours. Some fastidious gonococcal strains may require 24 to 72 hours to produce sufficient acid to change the indicator (see Color Plate 7-1*C*).

RAPID CARBOHYDRATE UTILIZATION TEST. This test is a non–growth-dependent method for the detection of acid production from carbohydrates. In this method, small volumes of phosphate buffered saline (PBS, *p*H 7.0) with phenol-red indicator are dispensed in nonsterile tubes to which single drops of 20% filter-sterilized carbohydrates are added. A dense suspension of the organism is prepared in the PBS solution with a bacteriologic loop; this suspension may be mixed on a vortex mixer to disperse clumps. One drop of this suspension is added to each of the carbohydrate-containing tubes. The tubes are incubated for 4 hours at 35°C in a non-CO_2 incubator or a water bath. This method is very economical, the reagents are easy to prepare and inoculate, and the results are clear cut.

Several modifications of the rapid carbohydrate utilization test are commercially available and include the Minitek system (Becton Dickinson Microbiology Systems, Cockeysville, MD), the RIM *Neisseria* test (Austin Biological Laboratories, Austin, TX), and the API QuadFERM + (Analytab Products, Inc, Plainview, NY; see Color Plate 7-1*D*).[23,26,53,55]

Chromogenic Enzyme Substrate Tests

These identification systems use specific biochemical substrates that, on hydrolysis by bacterial enzymes, yield a colored end product that is detected directly (eg, a yellow nitrophenol or nitroaniline product) or after the addition of a diazo-dye coupling reagent (ie, cinnamaldehyde reagent for detection of free β-naphthylamide). The use of these systems is restricted to those species that are

Table 7-6
Enzyme Activities Used for Identification of the Pathogenic *Neisseria* Species
and *Moraxella catarrhalis*

ORGANISM	β-GALACTOSIDASE	γ-GLUTAMYL AMINOPEPTIDASE	HYDROXYPROLYL AMINOPEPTIDASE
N. lactamica	+	−	+
N. meningitidis	−	+	V
N. gonorrhoeae	−	−	+
*M. catarrhalis**	−	−	−

+, positive reaction; −, negative reaction; V, variable reaction.
*Presumptive identification only.

able to grow on selective media (MTM, ML, NYC or GC-Lect media), that is, *N. gonorrhoeae, N. meningitidis,* and *N. lactamica.* Since some strains of *M. catarrhalis* grow on selective media, these systems will also provide a presumptive identification of this organism. The enzymatic activities that are detected in these systems include β-galactosidase, γ-glutamylaminopeptidase, and hydroxyprolylaminopeptidase (Table 7-6 and Color Plate 7-1*E*). β-Galactosidase and γ-glutamylaminopeptidase are specific for *N. lactamica* and *N. meningitidis,* respectively. Absence of these activities and presence of hydroxyprolylaminopeptidase identifies an organism as *N. gonorrhoeae. M. catarrhalis* lacks all three of these activities. The commercial systems that utilize this approach are the Gonochek II (DuPont deNemours Co, Wilmington, DE) and the Identicult-*Neisseria* (Adams Scientific, West Warwick, RI).[23,26,52]

Immunologic Methods for Culture Confirmation of *Neisseria gonorrhoeae*

FLUORESCENT MONOCLONAL ANTIBODY TEST. Identification of *N. gonorrhoeae* by fluorescent antibody (FA) techniques is fast and can identify both living and nonviable organisms. The FA procedure uses monoclonal antibodies that recognize epitopes on Protein I, the principal outer membrane protein of *N. gonorrhoeae.*[62,86] The commercial monoclonal FA test (*Neisseria gonorrhoeae* Culture Confirmation Test, Syva Co, Palo Alto, CA) is performed by preparing a light suspension of the organism in 5 μL of water on an FA slide, allowing the suspension to dry, heat fixing the specimen, overlaying the smear with the FA reagent, and

incubating the smear for 15 minutes. The smear is rinsed, air dried, mounted with a coverslip, and examined with a fluorescence microscope. Gonococci appear as apple-green fluorescent diplococci (see Color Plate 7-1*F*). The advantages of the Syva FA test include its rapidity, the ability to test colonies directly from primary cultures, and the small amount of growth required for test performance. The Syva FA test is not intended for direct detection and identification of organisms on smears from patient specimens.

COAGGLUTINATION TESTS. These tests make use of the ability of Protein A on *Staphylococcus aureus* cells to bind immunoglobulin G molecules by their Fc region. Binding of antigonococcal antibody to killed *S. aureus* cells and subsequent mixture with a suspension of gonococci causes visible agglutination of the suspension. Coagglutination tests for the identification of *N. gonorrhoeae* include the Phadebact GC OMNI (Karo-Bio Diagnostics AB, Huddinge, Sweden), the GonoGen I test (New Horizons Diagnostics, Columbia, MD), and the Meritec GC test (Meridian Diagnostics, Cincinnati, OH; see Color Plate 7-1*G*).[1,12,54]

Multitest Identification Systems

Three kit systems are available that can be used not only for identifying *Neisseria* species but also for identifying other fastidious gram-negative organisms. These systems are the RapID NH (*Neisseria-Haemophilus*) system (Innovative Diagnostic Systems, Norcross, GA), the Vitek NHI (*Neisseria-Haemophilus* Identification) card (bioMérieux Vitek, Inc, Hazelwood, MO), and the *Haemophilus-*

Neisseria identification (HNID) panel (American MicroScan, Sacramento, CA).[49,50] All of these systems use modified conventional tests (eg, acid production from carbohydrates, urease, indole, ornithine decarboxylase) and the chromogenic substrates described previously to provide 4-hour identifications of *Neisseria, Haemophilus,* and other fastidious gram-negative bacteria encountered in clinical specimens.

Neisseria gonorrhoeae Culture Confirmation Probe Test—AccuProbe

Nucleic acid probe technology has also been applied to the culture confirmation of *N. gonorrhoeae.*[54] The Accuprobe *Neisseria gonorrhoeae* Culture Confirmation Test (Gen-Probe, Inc, San Diego, CA) identifies the organism by the detection of specific rRNA sequences that are unique to *N. gonorrhoeae.* In the test, the organism is lysed and mixed with a chemiluminescent-labeled single-stranded DNA probe that is specifically complementary to gonococcal rRNA. After the hydridization occurs, the DNA probe/rRNA double-stranded complex is selected by a chemical process. The presence of the probe in the double-stranded material is detected by addition of reagents that hydrolyze the chemiluminescent tag on the probe, thereby releasing light energy. This energy is detected in a chemiluminometer instrument, and the result is reported as positive or negative.

Direct Detection Nucleic Acid Probe—PACE System

A nucleic acid probe has become available for the direct detection of gonococci in urogenital specimens. The PACE (Probe Assay-Chemiluminescence Enhanced, Gen-Probe, Inc, San Diego, CA) system for *N. gonorrhoeae* is a nonisotopic chemiluminescent DNA probe that hydridizes specifically with gonococcal rRNA. Specimens are collected as for culture and are placed in a transport/lysing solution. The assay requires about 2 hours to perform. In an evaluation of the Gen-Probe PACE system on 209 male urethral and 203 female endocervical specimens, Granato and Franz[37] reported that the test had an overall sensitivity and specificity of 90% and 99.4%, respectively, in comparison with culture on selective medium.

ADDITIONAL CULTURAL CHARACTERISTICS OF *NEISSERIA* SPECIES AND *MORAXELLA CATARRHALIS*

The following sections present helpful features for the laboratory identification and characterization of the gram-negative cocci. Suggestions for the performance of differential and confirmatory tests described in the previous section plus additional test procedures are also described. All of the characteristics for identification of *Neisseria* species and *M. catarrhalis* are shown in Table 7-7.

Neisseria gonorrhoeae and *Neisseria meningitidis*

The culture and identification methods discussed throughout this chapter provide adequate information for the isolation and identification of *N. gonorrhoeae.* Additional tests may be necessary to identify isolates other than *N. gonorrhoeae.* These other tests apply specifically to meningococci, the "saprophytic" *Neisseria,* and *M. catarrhalis.*

On Gram-stained smears prepared from clinical specimens, particularly cerebrospinal fluid, *N. meningitidis* appears as gram-negative diplococci both inside and outside polymorphonuclear cells. Organisms may display considerable size variation and tend to resist decolorization. Heavily encapsulated strains may have a distinct pink halo around the cells. Since the presence of inflammatory cells has prognostic value (eg, with fulminant, rapidly fatal disease, many organisms and few inflammatory cells are present), the Gram stain report to the physician should include quantitation of both organisms and polymorphonuclear leukocytes.

In addition to Gram stain and culture of the cerebrospinal fluid, laboratory personnel may also perform direct antigen detection tests for meningococcal capsular polysaccharides.[60] The available direct antigen tests will detect capsular antigens of groups A, B, C, Y, and W135. These reagents are available from several vendors (latex tests: Hynson, Westcott, and Dunning, Baltimore, MD; Murex Diagnostics, Norcross, GA; coagglutination tests: Pharmacia Diagnostics, Huddinge, Sweden). Although positive test results with these reagents are

Table 7-7
Biochemical Characteristics for Identification of *Neisseria* Species, Other Neisseriaceae, and *Moraxella catarrhalis*

SPECIES	CATALASE*	SUPEROXOL†	GROWTH ON MTM, ML, NYC, OR GC-LECT	ACID PRODUCTION FROM					NO₃	NO₂‡	POLYSACCHARIDE FROM 5% SUCROSE	GROWTH AT 35°C ON NUTRIENT AGAR	DNase PRODUCTION	TRIBUTYRIN HYDROLYSIS
				Glucose	Maltose	Fructose	Sucrose	Lactose						
N. gonorrhoeae	+	+	+	+	-	-	-	-	-	-	-	-	-	-
N. meningitidis	+	-	+	+	+	-	-	-	-	V	-	-	-	-
N. lactamica	+	-	+	+	+	-	-	+	-	V	-	-	-	-
N. cinerea	+	-	-§	-	-	-	-	-	-	+	-	-	-	-
N. flavescens	+	-	V	-	-	-	-	-	-	-	+	+	-	-
N. subflava														
Biovar subflava	+	-	-	+	+	-	-	-	-	+	-	+	-	-
Biovar flava	+	-	-	+	+	+	-	-	-	+	-	+	-	-
Biovar perflava	+	-	V	+	+	+	+	-	-	+	+	+	-	-
N. sicca	+	-	-	+	+	+	+	-	-	+	+	+	-	-
N. mucosa	+	-	-	+	+	+	+	-	+	+	+	+	-	-
N. polysaccharea	+	-	+	+	+	-	-	-	-	V	+	+	-	-
N. elongata														
Subsp. elongata	-	-	-	W⁺	-	-	-	-	-	+	-	+	-	-
Subsp. glycolytica	+	-	-	-/W⁺	-	-	-	-	-	+	-	+	-	-
Subsp. nitro-reducens	-	-	-	-/W⁺	-	-	-	-	+	+	-	+	-	-
"N. kochii"	+	+	-	+	-	-	-	-	-	-	-	+	-	-
M. catarrhalis	+	-	V	-	-	-	-	-	+	+	-	+	+	+
K. denitrificans	-	-	+	+	-	-	-	-	+	+	-	-	-	-

+, positive reaction; −, negative reaction; V, variable reaction; W⁺, weak positive reaction; −/W⁺, negative to weak positive reaction; MTM, modified Thayer-Martin medium; ML, Martin-Lewis medium; NYC, New York City medium; GC-LECT, GC selective medium.

*Catalase test performed with 3% hydrogen peroxide.

†Superoxol test performed with 30% hydrogen peroxide.

‡Results shown indicate use of nitrite broth containing 0.1% nitrite. Some gonococci are able to reduce 0.01% nitrite.

§Some N. cinerea stains have been isolated on selective media but generally do not grow well on subculture because of colistin susceptibility.

helpful for early diagnosis, a negative test does not rule out meningitis caused by any of the organisms that commonly occur. These tests should always be performed in conjunction with Gram stain and culture on both enriched solid media and in a suitable enriched broth (eg, brain–heart infusion broth with IsoVitalex, Becton Dickinson Microbiology Systems, Cockeysville, MD).

Meningococci grow well on both blood and chocolate agars, as well as on the selective media for the pathogenic *Neisseria* (see Color Plate 7-1*H*). Cerebrospinal fluid specimens should be cultured on nonselective media (as described in Table 7-5), while specimens that may harbor other organisms (eg, oropharyngeal and nasopharyngeal swab specimens) should be inoculated onto both selective and nonselective media. Plates are incubated in 5% to 7% CO_2 at 35°C and inspected after 24, 48, and 72 hours. For cerebrospinal fluid specimens in which no growth is evident on the primary plates, the enriched backup broth should be subcultured to solid media before a final report is issued.

Slide agglutination is the most commonly used technique for serogrouping meningococci. Antisera for the major meningococcal serogroups is available from Burroughs-Wellcome Corporation (Research Triangle Park, NC) and from Difco Laboratories (Detroit, MI). Some of these nongroupable strains may actually be *N. polysaccharea* isolates; testing for production of polysaccharide from sucrose will help to identify this species.[4]

Other *Neisseria* Species

Neisseria lactamica

Neisseria lactamica resembles *N. meningitidis* in colony morphology and was initially thought to be a lactose-positive variant of *N. meningitidis*.[46] This species is resident in the throat and is found more frequently in children than in adults.[36] *N. lactamica* grows on selective media; produces acid from glucose, maltose, and lactose; and hydrolyzes ONPG. Some strains may produce false-positive reactions with certain commercial coagglutination tests (eg, the Phadebact GC OMNI test).[53]

Neisseria cinerea

Neisseria cinerea has generated considerable interest since this organism produces colonies that resemble the large colony types of *N. gonorrhoeae* and that may yield results consistent with *N. gonorrhoeae* in some identification tests.[7] Although this organism is part of the commensal flora of the upper respiratory tract, it has been isolated from other sites as well. The initial report regarding this organism described strains that had been isolated from cervical cultures on ML medium.[59] Dossett and associates[27] also reported on the isolation of this organism from a rectal culture of an 8-year-old child with proctitis.

N. cinerea grows on both blood and chocolate agar. On chocolate agar after 24 hours of incubation, colonies are about 1 mm in diameter and are smooth with entire edges. The organism does not produce acid from carbohydrates in either CTA base media or the rapid carbohydrate degradation test. Weak positive reactions with glucose after overnight incubation have been reported with the Minitek system,[7] and its positive hydroxyprolyl aminopeptidase reaction may also produce misidentifications of *N. cinerea* as *N. gonorrhoeae*.[49,52] Most *N. cinerea* isolates, however, do not grow well on selective media; this characteristic precludes the testing of this organism on chromogenic substrate tests such as the Gonochek II and the Identicult-*Neisseria*. *N. cinerea* can be differentiated from the asaccharolytic species *N. flavescens* by its inability to produce polysaccharide from sucrose and the lack of a discernible yellow pigment. This species can also be separated from *M. catarrhalis*, another asaccharolytic species, by its negative nitrate reduction, DNase, and tributyrin hydrolysis reactions (see Table 7-7).

A helpful test for differentiating *N. cinerea* from *N. gonorrhoeae* is the colistin susceptibility test.[57] A suspension of the organism is prepared in broth (corresponding to a 0.5 MacFarland turbidity standard), and is swabbed on a chocolate or blood agar plate as for a Bauer-Kirby disk diffusion susceptibility test. A 10-μg colistin disk is placed and the plate is incubated in CO_2 for 18 to 24 hours. *N. cinerea* is colistin susceptible and will have a zone of greater than or equal to 10 mm around the disk. *N. gonorrhoeae* will generally grow up to the edge of the disk.

Neisseria flavescens

Neisseria flavescens is found in the respiratory tract and is rarely associated with infectious processes.

This organism grows as smooth yellowish colonies on both blood and chocolate agar. In addition to growth on nutrient agar at 35°C, most strains will also grow at room temperature on chocolate or blood agar. This organism is able to synthesize iodine-positive polysaccharides from sucrose and can be differentiated from *M. catarrhalis* by its inability to reduce nitrate and its negative DNAse and tributyrin hydrolysis reactions.

Neisseria subflava Biovars, Neisseria sicca, *and* Neisseria mucosa

Identification of the "nonpathogenic" *Neisseria* species is not generally necessary unless the organism is determined to be clinically significant or if the organism is isolated from a systemic site (eg, blood, cerebrospinal fluid) or in pure culture. Identification is based on colony morphology, growth on simple nutrient medium, inability to grow on selective media, acid production from carbohydrates, reduction of nitrate and nitrite, and synthesis of a starch-like polysaccharide from sucrose.

Neisseria polysaccharea

Neisseria polysaccharea is a newly described species that is found in the human oropharynx. It is an oxidase-positive, catalase-positive, gram-negative diplococcus that forms smooth yellow colonies.[70] At 24 hours the organism forms colonies of about 2 mm in diameter on MTM agar. Acid is produced from glucose and maltose but not from fructose, sucrose, or lactose. Nitrate is not reduced, while nitrite frequently is reduced. Strains of this organism can be differentiated from *N. meningitidis* by the polysaccharide synthesis test; *N. polysaccharea* produces iodine-positive polysaccharide from sucrose, while *N. meningitidis* does not.[4]

Neisseria elongata Subspecies

Neisseria elongata subspecies *elongata*, *glycolytica*, and *nitroreducens* are the only rod-shaped members of the genus *Neisseria*. The first two subspecies were recognized in the last edition of *Bergey's Manual* as *Neisseria* species,[6,85] while the last subspecies, formerly known as CDC group M-6, has been reclassified in the genus.[39] Although subspecies *elongata* and *glycolytica* are members of the human

upper respiratory tract flora and are nonpathogens, subspecies *nitroreducens* has been isolated from infectious processes.[33,81] These subspecies can be differentiated on the basis of catalase reactivity, acid production from glucose, and reduction of nitrate (see Table 7-7).

Moraxella catarrhalis

Moraxella catarrhalis grows well on both blood and chocolate agars, and some strains will also grow well on MTM and other selective media. Colonies are generally gray to white, opaque and smooth. The organism is asaccharolytic in carbohydrate-degradation tests and may actually turn peptone-based identification media alkaline. Most strains reduce nitrate and nitrite and produce DNase. DNase activity is detected by heavily spot-inoculating a plate of DNase test medium containing toluidine blue 0 on an area the size of a dime. After overnight incubation, hydrolysis of the DNA is detected by a change in the color of the medium around and under the inoculum from blue to pink. *S. aureus* and *S. epidermidis* strains are also inoculated onto the plate as positive and negative test controls, respectively. A 2-hour acidometric DNase test is included on the API QuadFERM + strip. In our evaluation of this system, all *M. catarrhalis* strains tested were DNase-positive after 2 hours of incubation.[55]

M. catarrhalis may also be distinguished from *Neisseria* species by its ability to hydrolyze ester-linked butyrate groups (butyrate esterase). This enzyme activity is detected with a substrate called tributyrin. A rapid fluorescent tributyrin hydrolysis test that utilized 4-methylumbelliferyl butyrate as a substrate was reported by Vaneechoutte and associates.[82] In this study all 62 *M. catarrhalis* strains were positive with this test within 5 minutes, while all other *Neisseria* species tested were negative. Janda and Ruther[51] evaluated a rapid tributyrin hydrolysis test called BCAT CONFIRM (Adams Scientific, West Warwick, RI). This test uses a microcupule containing a disk impregnated with tributyrin. Eight drops of a balanced salts–phenol red solution are added to the cupule, and several colonies of the isolate are then emulsified in the capule. A change in the color of the indicator from red to yellow indicates hydrolysis of tributyrin and a positive test (see Color Plate 7-1*I*). In this study, all 68 *M. catarrhalis* strains were positive on the BCAT CONFIRM within 30 minutes, while all *Neisseria* species were negative. A very rapid (2.5 minute) and reliable indoxyl-butyrate hydrolysis spot test has also been described[19] and is commercially available (Remel Laboratories, Lenexa, KS; Carr-Scarborough Microbiologicals, Stone Mountain, GA). The newly reformated RapID NH system (Innovative Diagnostic Systems, Inc, Atlanta, GA) also contains a fatty acid ester hydrolysis test to assist in the identification of *M. catarrhalis.*

Most clinically significant *M. catarrhalis* strains also produce an inducible, cell-associated β-lactamase.[25] Because of its inducible nature, rapid acidometric β-lactamase tests (ie, those that rely on conversion of hydrolysis of penicillin to penicilloic acid) may yield false-negative results. Best results are obtained with the iodometric method or with the chromogenic cephalosporin test[68] (see Color Plate 7-1*J*).

Antimicrobial susceptibility testing of *N. gonorrhoeae*, other *Neisseria* species, and *M. catarrhalis* is discussed in Chapter 12.

REFERENCES

1. Anand CM, Gubash SM, Shaw H. Serologic confirmation of *Neisseria gonorrhoeae* by monoclonal antibody-based coagglutination reagents. J Clin Microbiol 1988;26:2283–2286.

2. Apicella MA. *Neisseria meningitidis.* In: Mandell GL, Douglas RG Jr, Bennett JE, eds. Principles and practice of infectious diseases. 3rd ed. New York, Churchill Livingstone, 1990:1600–1613.

3. Berger SA, Gorea A, Peysser MR, et al. Bartholin's gland abscess caused by *Neisseria sicca.* J Clin Microbiol 1988;26:1589.

4. Bouquete MT, Marcos C, Saez-Nieto JA. Characterization of *Neisseria polysaccharea* sp. nov. (Riou, 1983) in previously identified noncapsulated strains of *Neisseria meningitidis.* J Clin Microbiol 1986;23:973–975.

5. Bourbeau P, Holla V, Peimontese S. Ophthalmia neonatorum caused by *Neisseria cinerea.* J Clin Microbiol 1990;28:1640–1641.

6. Bovre K, Holten E. *Neisseria elongata* sp. nov., a rod-shaped member of the genus *Neisseria:* re-evaluation of cell shape as a criterion for classification. J Gen Microbiol 1970;60:67–75.

7. Boyce JM, Mitchell EB. Difficulties in differentiating *Neisseria cinerea* from *Neisseria gonorrhoeae* in rapid systems used for identifying pathogenic *Neisseria* species. J Clin Microbiol 1985;22:731–734.

8. Boyce JM, Taylor MR, Mitchell EB, et al. Nosocomial pneumonia caused by a glucose-metabolizing strain of *Neisseria cinerea.* J Clin Microbiol 1985;21:1–3.

9. Brandstetter RD, Blaikr RJ, Roberts RB. *Neisseria meningitidis* serogroup W-135 disease in adults. JAMA 1981;246:2060–2061.

10. Brodie E, Adler JL, Daly AK. Bacterial endocarditis due to an unusual species of encapsulated *Neisseria: Neisseria mucosa* endocarditis. Am J Dis Child 1971;122:433–437.

11. Broome CV. The carrier state: *Neisseria meningitidis.* J Antimicrob Chemother 1986;18(Suppl A):25–34.

12. Carlson BL, Calnan MB, Goodman RE, et al. Phadebact monoclonal GC OMNI test for confirmation of *Neisseria gonorrhoeae.* J Clin Microbiol 1987;25:1982–1984.

13. Catlin BW. Cellular elongation under the influence of antibacterial agents: way to differentiate coccobacilli from cocci. J Clin Microbiol 1975;1:102–105.

14. Catlin BW. *Branhamella catarrhalis:* an organism gaining respect as a pathogen. Clin Microbiol Rev 1990;3:293–330.

15. Catlin BW. Branhamaceae fam. nov., a proposed family to accommodate the genera *Branhamella* and *Moraxella.* Int J Syst Bacteriol 1991;41:320–323.

16. Clark H, Patton RD. Post-cardiotomy endocarditis due to *Neisseria perflava* on a prosthetic aortic valve. Ann Intern Med 1968;68:386.

17. Clausen CR, Knapp JS, Totten PA. Lymphadenitis due to *Neisseria cinerea.* Lancet 1984;1:908.

18. Crawford G, Knapp JS, Hale J. Asymptomatic gonorrhea in men: caused by gonococci with unique nutritional requirements. Science 1977;196:1352–1353.

19. Dealler SF, Abbott M, Croughan MJ, et al. Identification of *Branhamella catarrhalis* in 2.5 min with an indoxyl butyrate strip test. J Clin Microbiol 1989;27:1390–1391.

20. Demmler GJ, Couch RS, Taber LH. *Neisseria subflava* bacteremia and meningitis in a child: report of a case and review of the literature. Pediatr Infect Dis 1985;4:286.

21. DeVaux DL, Evans GL, Arndt CW, et al. Comparison of the Gono-Pak system with the candle extinction jar for recovery of *Neisseria gonorrhoeae.* J Clin Microbiol 1987;25:571–572.

22. Dewhirst FE, Paster BJ, Bright PL. *Chromobacterium, Eikenella, Kingella, Neisseria, Simonsiella,* and *Vitreoscilla* species comprise a major branch of the beta group *Protobacteria* by 16s ribosomal nucleic acid sequence comparison: transfer of *Eiken-*

ella and *Simonsiella* to the Family Neisseriaceae (emend.). Int J Syst Bacteriol 1989;39:258–266.

23. Dillon JR, Carballo M, Pauze M. Evaluation of eight methods for identification of pathogenic *Neisseria* species: *Neisseria*-Kwik, RIM-N, Gonobio Test, Minitek, Gonochek II, GonoGen, Phadebact Monoclonal GC OMNI test, and Syva MicroTrak test. J Clin Microbiol 1988;26:493–497.

24. Doern GV, Gantz NM. Isolation of *Branhamella (Neisseria) catarrhalis* from men with urethritis. Sex Transm Dis 1982;9:202–204.

25. Doern GV, Tubert TA. Detection of beta-lactamase activity among clinical isolates of *Branhamella catarrhalis* with six different beta-lactamase assays. J Clin Microbiol 1987;25:1380–1383.

26. Dolter J, Bryant L, Janda JM. Evaluation of five rapid systems for the identification of *Neisseria gonorrhoeae*. Diagn Microbiol Infect Dis 1990;13:265–267.

27. Dossett JH, Applebaum PC, Knapp JS, et al. Proctitis associated with *Neisseria cinerea* misidentified as *Neisseria gonorrhoeae* in a child. J Clin Microbiol 1985;21:575–577.

28. Eng J, Holten E. Gelatin neutralization of the inhibitory effect of sodium polyanethol sulfonate on *Neisseria meningitidis* in blood culture media. J Clin Microbiol 1977;6:1–3.

29. Evans GL, Kopyta DL, Crouse K. New selective medium for the isolation of *Neisseria gonorrhoeae*. J Clin Microbiol 1989;27:2471–2474.

30. Faur YC, Weisburd MH, Wilson ME, et al. A new medium for the isolation of pathogenic *Neisseria* (NYC medium). Health Lab Sci 1973;10:44–54.

31. Feder HM, Garibaldi RA. The significance of nongonococcal, nonmeningococcal *Neisseria* isolates from blood cultures. Rev Infect Dis 1984;6:181–188.

32. Galaid EI, Cherubin CE, Marr JS. Meningococcal disease in New York City, 1973–1978: recognition of groups Y and W135 as frequent pathogens. JAMA 1980;224:2167–2171.

33. Garner J, Briant RH. Osteomyelitis caused by a bacterium known as M-6. J Infect (England) 1986;13:298–300.

34. Gay RM, Sevier RE. *Neisseria sicca* endocarditis: report of a case and review of the literature. J Clin Microbiol 1978;8:729–732.

35. Gini GA. Ocular infection in a newborn caused by *Neisseria mucosa*. J Clin Microbiol 1987;25:1574–1575.

36. Gold R, Goldschneider I, Lepow ML, et al. Carriage of *Neisseria meningitidis* and *Neisseria lactamica* in infants and children. J Infect Dis 1978;137:112–121.

37. Granato PA, Franz MR. Use of the Gen-Probe PACE system for the detection of *Neisseria gonor-*

rhoeae in urogenital samples. Diagn Microbiol Infect Dis 1990;13:217–221.

38. Granato PA, Schneible-Smith C, Weiner LB. Primary isolation of *Neisseria gonorrhoeae* on hemoglobin-free New York City medium. J Clin Microbiol 1981;14:206–209.

39. Grant PE, Brenner DJ, Steigerwalt AG, et al. *Neisseria elongata* subsp. *nitroreducens* subsp. nov., formerly CDC group M-6, a gram-negative bacterium associated with endocarditis. J Clin Microbiol 1990;28:2591–2596.

40. Greenberg LW, Kleinerman E. *Neisseria lactamica* meningitis. J Pediatr 1978;93:1061–1062.

41. Greenlee JE. Approaches to diagnosis of meningitis: cerebrospinal fluid evaluation. Infect Dis Clin North Am 1990;4:583–598.

42. Guibourdenche M, Lambert T, Riou JY. Isolation of *Neisseria canis* in mixed culture from a patient after a cat bite. J Clin Microbiol 1989;27:1673–1674.

43. Hager H, Verghese A, Alvarez S, et al. *Branhamella catarrhalis* respiratory infections. Rev Infect Dis 1987;9:1140–1149.

44. Hansman D. Meningitis caused by *Neisseria lactamica*. N Engl J Med 1978;299:491.

45. Herbert DA, Ruskin J. Are the "non-pathogenic" neisseriae pathogenic? Am J Clin Pathol 1981;75:739–741.

46. Hollis DG, Wiggins GL, Weaver RE. *Neisseria lactamica* sp. n., a lactose-fermenting species resembling *Neisseria meningitidis*. Appl Microbiol 1969;17:71–77.

47. Hook EW, Handsfield HH. Gonococcal infections in the adult. In: Holmes KK, Mardh P-A, Sparling PF, Weisner PJ, eds. Sexually transmitted diseases. 2nd ed. New York, McGraw-Hill, 1990:149–165.

48. Janda WM, Bohnhoff M, Morello JA, et al. Prevalence and site-pathogen studies of *Neisseria meningitidis* and *N. gonorrhoeae* in homosexual men. JAMA 1980;244:2060–2064.

49. Janda WM, Bradna JJ, Ruther P. Identification of *Neisseria* spp., *Haemophilus* spp., and other fastidious gram-negative bacteria with the MicroScan *Haemophilus-Neisseria* identification panel. J Clin Microbiol 1989;27:869–873.

50. Janda WM, Malloy PJ, Schreckenberger PC. Clinical evaluation of the Vitek *Neisseria-Haemophilus* identification card. J Clin Microbiol 1987;25:37–41.

51. Janda WM, Ruther P. B.CAT CONFIRM: a rapid test for confirmation of *Branhamella catarrhalis*. J Clin Microbiol 1989;27:1130–1131.

52. Janda WM, Sobieski V. Evaluation of a ten-minute chromogenic substrate test for identification of pathogenic *Neisseria* species and *Branhamella catar-*

rhalis. Eur J Clin Microbiol Infect Dis 1987;7: 25–29.

53. Janda WM, Ulanday MG, Bohnhoff M, et al. Evaluation of the RIM-N, Gonochek II, and Phadebact systems for the identification of pathogenic *Neisseria* spp. and *Branhamella catarrhalis*. J Clin Microbiol 1985;21:734–737

54. Janda WM, Wilcoski LM, Senf KL, et al. Comparison of monoclonal antibody-based methods and a nucleic acid probe for culture confirmation of *Neisseria gonorrhoeae*. [Abstr C-40] Presented before the annual meeting of the American Society of Microbiology, 1991:348.

55. Janda WM, Zigler KL, Bradna JJ. API Quad-FERM+ with rapid DNase for identification of *Neisseria* spp. and *Branhamella catarrhalis*. J Clin Microbiol 1987;25:203–206.

56. Kellogg DS, Peacock WL, Deacon WE, et al. *Neisseria gonorrhoeae*: I. Virulence genetically linked to clonal variation. J Bacteriol 1963;94:1274–1279.

57. Knapp JS. Historical perspectives and identification of *Neisseria* and related species. Clin Microbiol Rev 1988;1:415–431.

58. Knapp JS, Hook EW. Prevalence and persistence of *Neisseria cinerea* and other *Neisseria* spp. in adults. J Clin Microbiol 1988;26:896–900.

59. Knapp JS, Totten PA, Mulks MH, et al. Characterization of *Neisseria cinerea*, a non-pathogenic species isolated on Martin-Lewis medium selective for pathogenic *Neisseria* spp. J Clin Microbiol 1984;19:63–67.

60. Kurzynski TA, Kimball JL, Polyak MB. Evaluation of the Phadebact and Bactigen reagents for detection of *Neisseria meningitidis* in cerebrospinal fluid. J Clin Microbiol 1985;21:989–990.

61. Lauer BA, Masters HB. Toxic effect of calcium alginate swabs on *Neisseria gonorrhoeae*. J Clin Microbiol 1988;26:54–56.

62. Laughon BE, Ehret JM, Tanino TT, et al. Fluorescent monoclonal antibody for confirmation of *Neisseria gonorrhoeae* cultures. J Clin Microbiol 1987;25:2388–2390.

63. Lee TJ, Snyderman R, Patterson J. *Neisseria meningitidis* bacteremia in association with deficiency of the sixth component of complement. Infect Immun 1979;24:656–658.

64. Lossick JG, Smeltzer MP, Curran JW. The value of the cervical Gram stain in the diagnosis of gonorrhea in women in a sexually transmitted diseases clinic. Sex Transm Dis 1982;9:124–127.

65. Marchant CD. Spectrum of disease due to *Branhamella catarrhalis* in children with particular reference to acute otitis media. Am J Med 1990;88(Suppl 5A):15S–19S.

66. Martin JE, Jackson RL. A biological environmen-

tal chamber for the culture of *Neisseria gonorrhoeae*. J Am Vener Dis Assoc 1975;2:28–30.

67. Mazloum H, Totten PA, Brooks GF, et al. An unusual *Neisseria* isolated from conjunctival cultures in rural Egypt. J Infect Dis 1986;154:212–224.

68. Montgomery K, Raymundo L, Drew WL. Chromogenic cephalosporin spot test to detect beta-lactamase in clinically significant bacteria. J Clin Microbiol 1979;9:205–207.

69. Pai CH, Sorger S. Enhancement of recovery of *Neisseria meningitidis* by gelatin in blood culture media. J Clin Microbiol 1981;14:20–23.

70. Riou JY, Guibourdenche M. *Neisseria polysaccharea* sp. nov. Int J Syst Bacteriol 1987;37:163–165.

71. Ross SC, Densen P. Complement deficiency states and infection: epidemiology, pathogenesis and consequences of neisserial and other infections in an immune deficiency. Medicine 1984;63:243–273.

72. Rossau R, Vandenbussche G, Thielemans S, et al. Ribosomal ribonucleic acid cistron similarities and deoxyribonucleic acid homologies of *Neisseria*, *Kingella*, *Eikenella*, *Simonsiella*, *Alysiella*, and Centers for Disease Control groups EF-4 and M-5 in the emended family Neisseriaceae. Int J Syst Bacteriol 1989;39:185–198.

73. Rossau R, Van Landschoot A, Mannheim W, et al. Inter- and intrageneric similarities of ribosomal nucleic acid cistrons of the Neisseriaceae. Int J Syst Bacteriol 1986;26:323–332.

74. Rossau R, Van Landschoot A, Gillis M, et al. Taxonomy of Moraxellaceae fam. nov., a new bacterial family to accommodate the genera *Moraxella*, *Acinetobacter*, *Psychrobacter* and related organisms. Int J Syst Bacteriol 1991;41:310–319.

75. Saginur R, Clecner B, Portnoy J, et al. Superoxol (catalase) test for identification of *Neisseria gonorrhoeae*. J Clin Microbiol 1982;15:475–477.

76. Sarubbi FA, Myers JW, Williams JJ, et al. Respiratory infections caused by *Branhamella catarrhalis*. Am J Med 1990;88(Suppl 5A):9S–14S.

77. Schwartz B, Moore PS, Broome CV. Global epidemiology of meningococcal disease. Clin Microbiol Rev 1989;2(Suppl):S118–S124.

78. Scott RM. Bacterial endocarditis due to *Neisseria flava*. J Pediatr 1971;78:673–675.

79. Scribner RK. Neutralization of the inhibitory effect of sodium polyanethol sulfonate on *Neisseria meningitidis* in blood cultures processed with the DuPont Isolator system. J Clin Microbiol 1984;20:40–42.

80. Seth A. Use of trimethoprim to prevent overgrowth by *Proteus* in the cultivation of *Neisseria gonorrhoeae*. Br J Vener Dis 1970;46:201–202.

81. Simor AE, Salit IE. Endocarditis caused by M-6. J Clin Microbiol 1983;17:931–933.

82. Vaneechoutte M, Verschraegen G, Claeys G, et al.

Rapid identification of *Branhamella catarrhalis* with 4-methylumbelliferyl butyrate. J Clin Microbiol 1988:26:1227–1228.

83. Vaneechoutte M, Verschraegen G, Claeys G, et al. Respiratory tract carrier rates of *Moraxella (Branhamella) catarrhalis* in adults and children and interpretation of the isolation of *M. catarrhalis* from sputum. J Clin Microbiol 1990;28:2674–2680.

84. Van Hare GF, Shurin PA, Marchant CD, et al. Acute otitis media caused by *Branhamella catarrhalis*: biology and therapy. Rev Infect Dis 1987;9: 16–27.

85. Vedros NA. Genus I. *Neisseria* Trevisan 1885, 105[AL]. In: Krieg NR, Holt JG, eds. Bergey's manual of systematic bacteriology. Baltimore, Williams & Wilkins,, 1984;1:190–196.

86. Welch WD, Cartwright G. Fluorescent monoclonal antibody compared with carbohydrate utilization for rapid identification of *Neisseria gonorrhoeae*. J Clin Microbiol 1988;26:293–296.

87. Whittington WL, Knapp JS. Trends in resistance of *Neisseria gonorrhoeae* to antimicrobial agents in the United States. Sex Transm Dis 1988;15:202–210.

88. Wright PW, Wallace RJ, Shepherd JR. A descriptive study of 42 cases of *Branhamella catarrhalis* pneumonia. Am J Med 1990;88(Suppl 5A):2S–8S.

8

Staphylococci and Related Organisms

THE FAMILY MICROCOCCACEAE: TAXONOMY AND CLINICAL SIGNIFICANCE

In the latest edition of *Bergey's Manual of Systematic Bacteriology*, the Micrococcaceae includes four genera: *Planococcus, Micrococcus, Stomatococcus,* and *Staphylococcus*.[9,10,39,41,42] The members of this family can be differentiated from members of the Streptococcaceae by the catalase test. Members of the Micrococcaceae are catalase-positive, while members of the Streptococcaceae are catalase-negative. *Planococcus* species are asaccharolytic, motile, gram-positive cocci that are associated with marine environments. They are not implicated in human infections. *Micrococcus* species are found in the environment and as transient members of the microflora on the skin of humans and several other mammals. They are occasionally isolated from human clinical specimens, where they usually represent contaminants from the skin or mucous membrane surfaces or from the environment. *Stomatococcus mucilaginosus*, the single member of the genus *Stomatococcus*, is an encapsulated gram-positive coccus that is a part of the normal human respiratory tract flora.[9,10] This organism has been associated with endocarditis related to cardiac catheterization and intravenous drug use, bacteremia and central venous catheter infection, and peritonitis during chronic ambulatory peritoneal dialysis.[8,14,48,49,51,52]

The genus *Staphylococcus* is composed of 28 accepted or proposed species, 14 of which may be encountered in human clinical specimens (Table 8-1).[35,36,38–40,54–56] Staphylococci are generally found on the skin and mucous membranes of humans and other animals. Some of the pathogenic staphylococci in both humans and animals produce an enzyme called *coagulase*, and detection of this enzyme is used in the laboratory to identify these organisms.[27,63] Among the staphylococci, the coagulase-positive species *S. aureus* and two coagulase-negative species, *S. epidermidis* and *S. saprophyticus*, are seen most frequently in human infections.

Staphylococcus aureus

Staphylococcus aureus is by far the most important human pathogen among the staphylococci. Although this organism is frequently a part of the normal human microflora, it can cause significant opportunistic infections under the appropriate conditions.[12,67] Factors that may predispose a person to serious *S. aureus* infections include the following:

- Defects in leukocyte chemotaxis, either congenital (eg, Wiskott-Aldrich syndrome, Down's syndrome, Job's syndrome) or acquired (eg, diabetes mellitus, rheumatoid arthritis)
- Defects in opsonization by antibodies (eg, hypogammaglobulinemia)
- Defects in intracellular killing of bacteria after phagocytosis (eg, chronic granulomatous disease)
- Skin injuries (eg, burns, surgical incisions, eczema)

- Presence of foreign bodies (eg, sutures, intravenous lines, prosthetic devices)
- Infection with other agents, particularly viruses (eg, influenza)
- Chronic underlying diseases such as malignancy, alcoholism, and heart disease
- Therapeutic or prophylactic antimicrobial administration

Under these circumstances, *S. aureus* may cause a variety of infectious processes ranging from relatively benign skin infections to life-threatening systemic illnesses.[67] Skin infections include simple folliculitis (superficial infection surrounding the hair follicles) and impetigo (a superficial skin infection frequently seen in children), as well as furuncles and carbuncles involving subcutaneous tissues and causing systemic symptoms, such as fever. *S. aureus* is frequently isolated from postsurgical wound infections, which may serve as a nidus for the development of systemic infections. Community-acquired staphylococcal bronchopneumonia is usually seen in elderly persons and is associated with viral pneumonia as a predisposing factor. Nosocomial pneumonia due to *S. aureus* occurs in the clinical settings of obstructive pulmonary disease, intubation, and aspiration. Underlying malignant diseases are recognized as important risk factors for the development of *S. aureus* bacteremia. Bacteremia may also "seed" distant sites throughout the body, leading to endocarditis, osteomyelitis, pyoarthritis, and metastatic abscess formation, particularly in the skin, the subcutaneous tissues, lungs, kidneys, and brain. Staphylococcal toxins are also responsible for toxic epidermal necrolysis (staphylococcal scalded skin syndrome) and toxic shock syndrome.[11,57] *S. aureus* strains may also cause food poisoning owing to the elaboration of exotoxins during growth in contaminated foods.

Coagulase-Negative Staphylococci

In the past, coagulase-negative staphylococci were generally considered to be contaminants having little clinical significance. During the past 2 decades, however, these organisms have become recognized as important agents of human disease.[5,13,19,45,50,60,69] Although several different species of coagulase-negative staphylococci have been described (see Table 8-1), relatively few ofthem cause infections in humans. As more laboratories attempt to iden-

Table 8-1
Human, Animal, and Environmental *Staphylococcus* Species

SPECIES	COMMENTS
Staphylococci Found in Humans and Nonhuman Primates	
S. aureus	See text
S. epidermidis	See text
S. saprophyticus	See text
S. hominis	Found on human skin; infrequently isolated from clinical specimens
S. haemolyticus	Part of the human normal skin flora; also found in nonhuman primates and occasionally recovered from human clinical specimens. Strains of *S. haemolyticus* that are resistant to vancomycin (MICs of ≥8 μg/mL) have been reported in the clinical setting of prolonged vancomycin administration, suggesting selection of resistant clones of previously susceptible organisms.
S. schleiferi	Newly described species recovered from human wounds and blood cultures
S. lugdunensis	Newly described species isolated from human blood cultures, wounds, abscesses, lymph node tissue, and an intrauterine device
S. warneri	Found on human and nonhuman primates; not known to be a pathogen
S. simulans	Rarely associated with human infections; found on healthy skin and in the urethras of healthy women
S. capitis	Part of the normal human flora; found surrounding the sebaceous glands on the scalp and forehead; not implicated in infections
S. auricularis	Found on humans, particularly in the external auditory canal; rarely seen in infections
S. cohnii	Contains two subspecies and has been recovered from human infections in a few cases; found on the skin
S. xylosus	Found in both human and nonhuman primates; reported as a cause of human urinary tract infections and pyelonephritis
S. saccharolyticus	Found on human mucous membranes; first case of endocarditis reported in 1990
Staphylococci Found in Other Animals	
S. hyicus	Found in pigs and cattle and in cow's milk; associated with infections in these animals
S. chromogenes	Formerly a subspecies of *S. hyicus*; causes cutaneous infections in cattle
S. sciuri	Found normally in rodents and other small mammals
S. gallinarum	Found in poultry; nonpathogenic
S. intermedius	Found on mammals, particularly carnivores, and on certain birds; opportunistic pathogen in these animals
S. lentus	Part of the normal skin flora of sheep and goats
S. caprae	Found occasionally on goats
S. equorum	Rare equine species of undetermined pathogenic significance
S. delphini	Newly described coagulase-positive species; causes purulent skin lesions in dolphins
S. felis	Newly described species; causes otitis, cystitis, abscesses, wounds, and other cutaneous infections in cats
S. muscai	Newly described species found on the bodies of flies
S. piscifermentans	Found in fish, in fish food products, and from soy sauce mash
Other Staphylococcal Species (Mostly Environmental)	
S. carnosus	Used as a starter culture in the processing of meats such as salami and sausage
S. caseolyticus	Saprophytic species found in milk and other dairy products
S. kloosii	Newly described species; uncertain clinical significance and taxonomic status
S. arlettae	Newly described species; undetermined clinical significance and uncertain taxonomic status

tify the coagulase-negative staphylococci, however, infections caused by other species are being recognized more frequently.[22,29,32,61,68] The types of infections associated with coagulase-negative staphylococci include the following:

- Nosocomial and community-acquired urinary tract infections
- Infections of indwelling devices (eg, prosthetic heart valves, intravenous catheters, joint prostheses, hemodialysis and cerebrospinal shunts, pacemakers, peritoneal dialysis catheters)
- Bacteremia in compromised hosts (premature infants, patients with cardiovascular or neoplastic diseases, patients with hematologic malignancies, burn patients, trauma patients, transplant recipients, patients with congenital defects)
- Osteomyelitis (postsurgical infections, prosthesis-associated infections, trauma-associated infections)
- Postsurgical endophthalmitis

Staphylococcus epidermidis

When clinical findings are correlated with the isolation of coagulase-negative staphylococci, *S. epidermidis* is by far the most frequently recovered organism, accounting for 50% to over 80% of isolates.[4] Infections caused by *S. epidermidis* include endocarditis of native and prosthetic valves, intravenous catheter infections, cerebrospinal fluid shunt infections, peritoneal dialysis catheter-associated peritonitis, bacteremia, osteomyelitis, vascular graft infections, prosthetic joint infections, and urinary tract infections.[4,5,28,34,50,66]

Staphylococcus saprophyticus

The coagulase-negative species *S. saprophyticus* deserves special mention, since this species is a well-documented pathogen causing primarily acute urinary tract infections in young women.[25,30] In this population, *S. saprophyticus* is the second most common cause of cystitis after *Escherichia coli*. In urine specimens from these patients the organism is frequently present in quantities less than 100,000 colony-forming units per milliliter but will be detected in sequential specimens from infected patients. This organism has also been implicated in pyelonephritis, in urethritis in men and women,

and in catheter-associated urinary tract infections in elderly men.

Other Coagulase-Negative Staphylococci

Other staphylococcal species are found in both humans and animals as part of the normal flora and as infectious agents.[17,31] Other species are environmental and are used in the food industry.[53] Although coagulase-negative species other than *S. epidermidis* and *S. saprophyticus* are not frequently recovered from significant infections, several other species have been reported principally in wounds, urinary tract infections, bacteremia, and endocarditis. Implicated species include *S. haemolyticus, S. hominis, S. warneri, S. simulans, S. schleiferi, S. saccharolyticus, S. lugdunensis,* and *S. schleiferi*.[19,22,23,61,68] *S. haemolyticus* has demanded increased interest owing to the emergence of vancomycin resistance in this species.[58,59,64] The coagulase-negative staphylcocci, their ecologic niches, and clinical significance are summarized in Table 8-1.

DIFFERENTIATION OF THE MEMBERS OF THE FAMILY MICROCOCCACEAE

Direct Gram-Stained Smears

On direct Gram-stained smears from clinical specimens, staphylococci appear as gram-positive or gram-variable cocci ranging from 0.5 μm to over 1 μm in diameter. The organisms may appear singly, in pairs, in short chains, or in clusters, both within and outside polymorphonuclear cells (Color Plate 8-1A). Variations in cell size and reaction to Gram staining are probably due to the action of the inflammatory cells and their hydrolytic enzymes on the bacterial cells. On direct smears, pairs and short chains of organisms cannot be differentiated from streptococci, micrococci, or peptostreptococci, although streptococci frequently appear as chains of diplococci rather than as chains of discrete, individual cells. Reports of direct smears should include quantitation of cell types and microorganisms (eg, "many polymorphonuclear leukocytes, moderate gram-positive cocci"). If the

Gram-stained appearance is more typical, a report of "gram-positive cocci resembling staphylococci" can be issued, with culture confirmation to follow.

Colony Morphology

Micrococcus and *Staphylococcus* species form distinctive colonies on sheep blood agar. Micrococci generally grow more slowly, often requiring 48 hours of incubation before typical colony morphology can be discerned. After this time, micrococcal colonies are 1 to 2 mm in diameter, are dull, and have a high convex profile with entire edges. Some strains produce pigments and will appear yellow, pink, orange, or tan, while others will be off-white or bone white.[41] Colonies of most staphylococcal species grow more rapidly and are 1 to 2 mm in diameter after 24 hours of incubation, although some (eg, *S. warneri, S. simulans*) may form smaller colonies during this time. Colonies are usually smooth, are butyrous, and have a low convex profile with an entire edge. Colonies of some *S. aureus* strains may be pigmented yellow or yellow-orange, while other strains may produce off-white or gray colonies (see Color Plate 8-1*B*). The latter strains may resemble group D streptococci and enterococci (catalase-negative). Pigment production in both *S. aureus* and among the coagulase-negative staphylococci may become apparent or more pronounced after incubation at room temperature. Often, strains of some staphylococcal species will show considerable variation in the size of colonies on the same culture plate, giving the appearance of a mixed culture. Some *S. aureus* and some coagulase-negative species may have a distinct or hazy zone of β-hemolysis around the colonies; this hemolytic property may become apparent only after prolonged incubation.

Colonies of *S. mucilaginosus* are gray to white and may be mucoid. They tend to adhere to the agar and, when removed from the media, are difficult to emulsify.

The Catalase Test

The Micrococcaceae are differentiated from the Streptococcaceae by the *catalase test*. This test detects the presence of cytochrome oxidase enzymes in the Micrococcaceae. The test is performed with 3% hydrogen peroxide (H_2O_2) on a glass slide. Immediate and vigorous bubbling indicates conversion of the hydrogen peroxide to water and oxygen (see Color Plate 8-1*C*). The test is performed by transferring growth from the center of a colony to the surface of a glass slide. A drop of 3% hydrogen peroxide is added and observed for the sustained appearance of bubbles or effervescence. Ideally, the catalase test should be performed from a medium that does not contain blood, since red blood cells may produce a weakly positive catalase reaction. Since most clinical laboratories recover staphylococci on either nonselective or selective blood-containing media (eg, sheep blood agar and CNA agar, respectively), care should be taken to sample only the tops of colonies for the catalase test to avoid carryover of blood and possible false-positive reactions. This can be done most expeditiously with a wooden applicator stick. Rare strains of staphylococci may be catalase-negative,[62] and some enterococci (ie, fecal streptococci; see Chapter 9) produce a "pseudocatalase" and are weakly reactive with hydrogen peroxide. *Stomatococcus mucilaginosus* is usually catalase-negative or weakly positive.[9,10]

Methods for Differentiating Micrococci and Staphylococci

Several methods are available for differentiating *Micrococcus* and *Staphylococcus* species, the two catalase-positive genera most frequently seen in the clinical laboratory. Some require special media and prolonged incubation, while others are commercially available and provide results within 18 to 24 hours or less. Table 8-2 lists the test methods and results for *Micrococcus* and *Staphylococcus* species. In most clinical microbiology laboratories, the furazolidone disk test, the Taxo A bacitracin disk test, and the modified oxidase test are probably the most logical choices, since they are rapid, reliable, inexpensive, and commercially available.

Inhibition by Furazolidone

Inhibition by furazolidone[6,15,65] is performed as a disk susceptibility procedure using commercially available disks (FX disk, 100 µg, Becton Dickinson Microbiology Systems, Cockeysville, MD). The procedure is performed by preparing a suspension

Table 8-2
Methods for the Differentiation of *Micrococcus* and *Staphylococcus* Species

METHOD	REACTION FOR	
	Micrococcus	*Staphylococcus*
Acid production from glucose under anaerobic conditions	−	+
Resistance to lysostaphin	+	−
Production of acid from glucose aerobically in the presence of 0.4 µg/mL erythromycin	−	+
Inhibition by furazolidone (100-µg furazolidone disk)	−	+
Modifed oxidase test	+	−
Inhibition by bacitracin (0.04-IU Taxo A disk)	+	−

of the test organism in distilled water or broth equivalent to a 0.5 MacFarland turbidity standard. A swab is saturated with this organism suspension and spread onto one half of a blood agar plate. A 100-µg furazolidone disk is placed aseptically in the center of the inoculated area. The plate is incubated at 35°C in an ambient air incubator for 18 to 24 hours and observed for a zone of growth inhibition around the disk. Staphylococci are inhibited by furazolidone and show zones of 15 mm or more, while micrococci are resistant and show zones of 6 (no zone) to 9 mm (see Color Plate 8-1*D*).[9] Coagulase-negative staphylococci that are resistant to furazolidone may, however, be seen occasionally.

Resistance to Bacitracin

Resistance to bacitracin[6,20] employs the same bacitracin disk used for the presumptive identification of group A, β-hemolytic streptococci. A lawn of growth is prepared on a Mueller-Hinton agar or a blood agar plate as described earlier for the FX disk test, and a bacitracin differential disk (Taxo A, 0.04 units bacitracin, Becton Dickinson Microbiology Systems, Cockeysville, MD) is placed on the inoculum. After overnight incubation, zone sizes are measured. Staphylococci are resistant and grow to the edge of the disk, while micrococci are susceptible, producing zones of 10 mm or greater.[6]

Modified Oxidase Test

The modified oxidase test[6,21] is also commercially available as Microdase Test Disks from Remel Lab-

oratories (Lenexa, KS). Filter paper disks impregnated with tetramethyl-*p*-phenylenediamine dihydrochloride (oxidase reagent) in dimethyl sulfoxide (DMSO) are used. The DMSO renders the cells permeable to the reagent. A colony from the growth medium is removed with an applicator stick and rubbed onto the disk. The development of a blue-purple color within 30 seconds indicates a positive test. No color development within this time is a negative test. Micrococci are modified oxidase-positive, while staphylococci are modified oxidase-negative.

IDENTIFICATION OF *STAPHYLOCOCCUS AUREUS*

The single most reliable characteristic for identifying *S. aureus* is the coagulase test. The conventional coagulase test may be performed by the following slide or tube methods.

Slide Coagulase Test

Most strains of *S. aureus* have a *bound coagulase* or *"clumping factor"* on the surface of the cell wall. This factor reacts directly with fibrinogen in plasma, causing rapid cell agglutination. The test is performed by placing two drops of sterile water or saline on a glass slide within circular areas drawn with a wax pencil. A portion of a well-isolated colony of the organism to be tested is emulsified in the liquid within each of the circles. A drop of coagulase plasma is added to one of the suspensions and mixed with a wooden applicator stick; similarly, a drop of water or saline is added and mixed in the other suspension as a control. The suspension is then observed for agglutination (see Color Plate 8-1*E*).

The test can be performed with growth from blood agar, colistin–nalidixic acid (CNA) agar, or other nonselective nutrient medium but should not be performed from media having a high salt content (eg, mannitol salts agar) since the high salt causes some strains to autoagglutinate. Any strain that is negative with the slide coagulase test must be confirmed with a tube coagulase test because strains deficient in clumping factor will usually produce free coagulase. The human coagulase-negative species *S. lugdunensis* and *S. schleiferi* also produce clumping factor and will be positive with the slide test.[22,29] These species are tube coagulase-negative.

Tube Coagulase Test

The coagulase detected by this method is secreted extracellularly and reacts with a substance in the plasma called *"coagulase-reacting factor"* to form a complex, which, in turn, reacts with fibrinogen to form fibrin (clot formation; see Color Plate 8-1*F*). The test is performed by emulsifying a small amount of the colony growth of the organism in a tube containing 0.5 mL of coagulase plasma. The tube is incubated tube at 35°C for 4 hours and observed for clot formation by gently tipping. If no clot is observed, the tube is reincubated at room temperature and read again after 18 hours. The 4-hour reading is necessary since some strains will produce fibrinolysin on prolonged incubation at 35°C, causing dissolution of the clot during the incubation period.[43] Weak coagulase producers require prolonged incubation to become positive. Rare *S. aureus* strains may be coagulase-negative, and some animal isolates (*S. intermedius*, *S. hyicus*, and *S. delphini*) may be coagulase-positive.[16,27,63]

The recommended medium for both tests is rabbit plasma with EDTA. Citrated plasma should not be used since organisms that are able to utilize citrate (eg, *Enterococcus* species) will yield positive results if they are inadvertently mistaken for staphylococci. This error can be avoided by always performing a catalase test first. Human plasma (eg, outdated material from blood banks) contains variable amounts of coagulase reacting factor and antistaphylococcal antibodies and should not be used.

Alternative Coagulase Test Procedures

Latex Agglutination

Latex agglutination uses latex beads coated with plasma. Fibrinogen bound to the latex detects clumping factor. In addition, immunoglobulin molecules also present on the beads detect Protein A, the staphylococcal cell wall protein that is able to bind IgG molecules by the Fc region. Mixing of the test reagent with colonial material from an agar plate results in rapid clumping of the latex–organism suspension (see Color Plate 8-1*G*). Several products that use this approach are commercially available and include StaphAUREX (Murex Diagnostics), Sero-STAT Staph (Scott Laboratories, Fiskeville, RI), Staphylatex (Baxter Health Care Products, McGaw Park, IL), Accu-Staph (Carr-Scarborough Microbiologicals, Stone Mountain, GA), Bacto-Staph (Difco Laboratories, Detroit, MI), and Veri-Staph (Zeus Technologies, Raritan, NJ) In addition, *S. lugdunensis* and *S. schleiferi*, two recently described human staphylococcal isolates, both produce clumping factor and may be positive with these rapid procedures.[22]

Passive Hemagglutination

Passive hemagglutination procedures use sheep red blood cells that are sensitized with fibrinogen to detect clumping factor on the surface of *S. aureus* cells. Two commercial kits — Staphyloslide (Becton Dickinson Microbiology Systems, Cockeysville, MD) and Hemastaph (Remel Laboratories, Lenexa, KS) — are available. Some workers prefer these tests to the latex agglutination tests because a nonsensitized red blood cell suspension is included as a negative control for each test.

Several evaluations comparing latex and passive hemagglutination kits with the 4- and 24-hour tube coagulase tests have been published. These kits have sensitivities and specificities of 94% to 100% and 93% to 100%, respectively.[1,7,18,33,46,47,70]

Other Identification Tests

DEOXYRIBONUCLEASE (DNase) TEST. Some *S. aureus* strains may produce weak or equivocal tube coagulase reactions, and rare isolates may indeed be coagulase-negative. In these cases, it may be helpful to perform other tests that correlate highly with coagulase production. S. aureus produces both DNase and a thermostable endonuclease.[26,44] Both of these enzymes hydrolyze nucleic acid (ie, DNA). DNase can be detected by heavily spot-inoculating several colonies of the organism on DNase test medium containing the metachromatic dye toluidine blue O (commercially available from several vendors). After 24 hours of incubation at 35°C, the medium under and around the inoculum turns from azure blue to pink, indicating hydrolysis of the DNA.

THERMOSTABLE ENDONUCLEASE TEST. For this test, the same DNase test medium is used, only 3-mm holes are cut into the agar with a sterile cork borer and the wells are filled with a 24-hour broth culture of the test organism that has been boiled in a water bath for 15 minutes. The plate is incubated overnight at 35°C. S. aureus strains will show a pink zone surrounding the well containing the boiled suspension.

MANNITOL FERMENTATION.   In addition to the above tests, S. aureus, unlike S. epidermidis and several other coagulase-negative species, is able to ferment mannitol. This property is exploited in epidemiologic studies to detect S. aureus in soil and feces and in screening nasal carriers of S. aureus. The medium used is mannitol salt agar. This medium contains mannitol (1%), 7.5% sodium chloride, phenol red, and peptones. The high salt concentration discourages the growth of other organisms (except for enterococci) and selectively recovers staphylococci. S. aureus can be detected by the presence of a yellow zone around isolated colonies, indicating acid production from mannitol (see Color Plate 8-1H). Other infrequently isolated staphylococcal species may also produce acid from mannitol, however, so mannitol-positive organisms recovered on this medium should be checked for coagulase production as well.

IDENTIFICATION OF COAGULASE-NEGATIVE STAPHYLOCOCCI

As described earlier, S. epidermidis and S. saprophyticus are the most frequently isolated and clinically significant coagulase-negative staphylococci

in the clinical laboratory. Because of the recognized clinical significance of S. saprophyticus in urinary tract infections and the emerging role of S. epidermidis as an important human pathogen, many laboratories employ methods for confirmatory identification of these two species. In addition, kit systems are available that enable the laboratory to identify not only S. epidermidis and S. saprophyticus but also several of the other human and animal staphylococci that have been described.

Susceptibility to Novobiocin

Three human staphylococcal species (S. saprophyticus, S. cohnii, and S. xylosus) and six animal species (S. sciuri, S. lentus, S. gallinarum, S. kloosii, S. equorum, and S. arlettae) are resistant to novobiocin, with minimal inhibitory concentrations of greater than or equal to 1.6 µg/mL.[37,40] Since novobiocin-resistant species other than S. saprophyticus are infrequently encountered in human clinical specimens, the novobiocin susceptibility test provides a useful method for S. saprophyticus identification. The novobiocin test is performed as a disk susceptibility test, using a 5-µg disk, after a procedure similar to that described for the furazolidone test. Strains resistant to novobiocin show zones measuring 6 (no zone) to 12 mm; susceptible strains have zones of 16 to 27 mm (see Color Plate 8-1I). This test was originally described using a medium called P agar, which is not available commercially. Studies with the routine media mentioned previously have shown that comparable results are obtained.[24]

Commercial Identification Systems

Several commercial kits are available for the identification of coagulase-negative staphylococci. All of these kits use modified carbohydrate fermentation tests, adaptations of standard bacteriologic identification tests (eg, nitrate reduction, urease, Voges-Proskauer), and novel chromogenic enzyme substrate tests for organism identification. These systems are adapted to the particular format used by the manufacturer (eg, strip with small cupules, microtiter trays, plastic cards). Available kits include Staph-IDENT (Analytab Products, Inc, Plainview, NY), Staph-TRAC (Analytab Products; see Color Plate 8-1J), ID32 STAPH (bioMérieux SA, France), Minitek Gram-Positive (Becton Dickinson Microbiology Systems, Cockeysville, MD),

Vitek Gram-Positive Identification (GPI) Card (Vitek Systems, Inc, Hazelwood, MO), MicroScan Gram-Positive Combo Panel (Baxter Healthcare Corporation, McGaw Park, IL), and the Sceptor Gram-Positive MIC/ID Panel (Becton Dickinson Microbiology Systems).[2,3]

IDENTIFICATION OF *MICROCOCCUS* SPECIES

Micrococci are not generally identified to species level in clinical laboratories since they are rarely clinically significant. By using the tests described earlier and in Table 8-2, laboratories may issue reports of "*Micrococcus* species" without further testing. These organisms are also included in the data bases of some of the commercial kit systems used in laboratories.

IDENTIFICATION OF *STOMATOCOCCUS MUCILAGINOSUS*

As mentioned previously, *S. mucilaginosus* is a resident of the human upper respiratory tract and has been isolated from blood cultures of patients with endocarditis secondary to cardiac catheterization and intravenous drug use.[8,14,48,49,51,52] *S. mucilaginosus* colonies are generally mucoid, clear to white, and adherent to the agar surface. They appear on Gram-stained smears as large gram-positive cocci arranged in pairs or clusters. They are weakly catalase-positive, although some strains are catalase-negative. *S. mucilaginosus* can be differentiated from *Micrococcus* and *Staphylococcus* species by their failure to grow on nutrient agar medium containing 5% sodium chloride and by the presence of a capsule.[9,10] These organisms are also included in the data base of the Staph-TRAC, Staph-IDENT, and ID32 STAPH systems. Biochemical characteristics for identification are presented in Table 8-3.

LABORATORY APPROACH TO IDENTIFICATION OF STAPHYLOCOCCI

Because staphylococci are among the most frequently isolated organisms in the clinical laboratory, decisions must be made on how far to go in identifying them. This is especially true regarding the coagulase-negative organisms. Many laboratories have adopted rapid coagulase procedures (ie, latex or hemagglutination tests), so these tests may quickly be performed on colonies that look like staphylococci and are catalase-positive. If the colonies are coagulase-positive, the organism is identified as *S. aureus*. For isolates that are coagulase-negative, a furazolidone or bacitracin disk test, or the modified oxidase test, may be performed to differentiate coagulase-negative staphylococci from *Micrococcus* species. Significant staphylococcal isolates from urine cultures should also be tested for susceptibility to novobiocin to identify *S. saprophyticus*.

Complete species identification using a kit method or the reference procedure should be reserved for clinically significant isolates. These may include isolates that have been recovered from multiple sets of blood cultures, from infected intravenous catheters (when the patient may have the same isolate in multiple blood cultures), or from other normally sterile sites where what appears to be the same coagulase-negative *Staphylococcus* organism has been repeatedly isolated. Decisions involving further identification of these organisms should be made on a case-by-case basis with input

Table 8-3
Biochemical Characteristics of *Stomatococcus mucilaginosus*

CHARACTERISTIC	REACTION
Acetoin production (VP test)	+
Hydrolysis of gelatin	+
Growth under anaerobic conditions	+
Catalase	V
Growth on nutrient agar with 5% NaCl	−
Coagulase	−
Alkaline phosphatase	−
Acid production from:	
Glucose	+
Sucrose	+
Fructose	+
Salicin	+
Mannose	V
Trehalose	V
Mannitol	−
Sorbitol	−

+, *positive reaction;* −, *negative reaction; V, variable reaction.*

from both the laboratory and the physicians caring for the patient.

REFERENCES

1. Aldridge KE, Kogos C, Sanders CV, et al. Comparison of rapid identification assays for *Staphylococcus aureus*. J Clin Microbiol 1984;19:703–704.

2. Almeida RJ, Jorgensen JH. Identification of coagulase-negative staphylococci with the API Staph-IDENT system. J Clin Microbiol 1983;18:254–257.

3. Almeida RJ, Jorgensen JH, Johnson JE. Evaluation of the AutoMicrobic system gram-positive identification card for species identification of coagulase-negative staphylococci. J Clin Microbiol 1983;18:438–439.

4. Archer GL. *Staphylococcus epidermidis* and other coagulase-negative staphylococci. In: Mandell GL, Bennett JE, eds. Principles and practice of infectious diseases. New York, Churchill Livingstone, 1990:1511–1518.

5. Baddour LM, Barker LP, Christensen GD, et al. Phenotypic variation of *Staphylococcus epidermidis* in infection of transvenous endocardial pacemaker electrodes. J Clin Microbiol 1990;28:676–679.

6. Baker JS. Comparison of various methods for differentiation of staphylococci and micrococci. J Clin Microbiol 1984;19:875–879.

7. Baker JS, Borman MA, Boudreau DH. Evaluation of various rapid agglutination methods for the identification of *Staphylococcus aureus*. J Clin Microbiol 1985;21:726–729.

8. Barlow JF, Vogele KA, Dzintars PF. Septicemia with *Stomatococcus mucilaginosus*. Clin Microbiol Newsl 1986;8:22.

9. Bergan T, Kocur M. *Stomatococcus mucilaginosus* gen. nov., sp. nov., emend. rev., a member of the family Micrococcaceae. Int J Syst Bacteriol 1982; 32:374–377.

10. Bergan T, Kocur M. Genus II. *Stomatococcus*. In: Sneath PHA, Nair NS, Holt JG, eds. Bergey's manual of systematic bacteriology. Vol 2. Baltimore, Williams & Wilkins, 1986:1008–1010.

11. Bergdoll MS, Schlievert PM. Toxic shock syndrome toxin. Lancet 1984;2:691.

12. Carney DN, Fossieck BE, Parker RH, et al. Bacteremia due to *Staphylococcus aureus* in patients with cancer: report on 45 cases and a review of the literature. Rev Infect Dis 1982;4:1–12.

13. Christensen GD, Parisi JT, Bisno AL, et al. Characterization of clinically significant strains of coagulase-negative staphylococci. J Clin Microbiol 1983;18:258–269.

14. Coudron PE, Markowitz SM, Mohanty LB, et al. Isolation of *Stomatococcus mucilaginosus* from drug user with endocarditis. J Clin Microbiol 1987;25:1359–1363.

15. Curry JC, Borovian GE. Selective medium for distinguishing micrococci from staphylococci in the clinical laboratory. J Clin Microbiol 1976;4:455–457.

16. Devriese LA, Hajek V, Oeding P, et al. *Staphylococcus hyicus* (Sompolinsky 1953) comb. nov. and *Staphylococcus hyicus* subsp. *chromogenes* subsp. nov. Int J Syst Bacteriol 1978;28:482–490.

17. Devriese LA, Poutrel B, Kilpper-Balz R, et al. *Staphylococcus gallinarum* and *Staphylococcus caprae*, two new species from animals. Int J Syst Bacteriol 1983;33:480–486.

18. Doern GV. Evaluation of a commercial latex agglutination test for identification of *Staphylococcus aureus*. J Clin Microbiol 1980;12:641–643.

19. Eisenberg ES, Ambalu M, Szylagi G, et al. Colonization of the skin and development of peritonitis due to coagulase-negative staphylococci in patients undergoing peritoneal dialysis. J Infect Dis 1987;156:478–482.

20. Falk D, Guering SJ. Differentiation of *Staphylococcus* and *Micrococcus* spp. with the Taxo A bacitracin disk. J Clin Microbiol 1983;18:719–720.

21. Faller A, Schleifer KH. Modified oxidase and benzidine tests for separation of staphylococci and micrococci. J Clin Microbiol 1981;13:1031–1035.

22. Freney J, Brun Y, Bes M, et al. *Staphylococcus lugdunensis* sp. nov. and *Staphylococcus schleiferi* sp. nov., two species from human clinical specimens. Int J Syst Bacteriol 1988;38:168–172.

23. Gill VJ, Selepak AT, Williams EC. Species identification and antibiotic susceptibilities of coagulase-negative staphylococci isolated from clinical specimens. J Clin Microbiol 1983;18:1314–1319.

24. Goldstein J, Schulman R, Kelley E, et al. Effect of different media on determination of novobiocin resistance for differentiation of coagulase-negative staphylococci. J Clin Microbiol 1983;18:592–595.

25. Gregson DB, Low DE, Skulnick M, et al. Problems with rapid agglutination of *Staphylococcus aureus* when *Staphylococcus saprophyticus* is being tested. J Clin Microbiol 1988;26:1398–1399.

26. Gudding R. Differentiation of staphylococci on the basis of nuclease properties. J Clin Microbiol 1983;18:1098–1101.

27. Hajek V. *Staphylococcus intermedius*, a new species isolated from animals. Int J Syst Bacteriol 1976;26:401–408.

28. Hamory BH, Parisi JT. *Staphylococcus epidermidis*: a significant nosocomial pathogen. Am J Infect Control 1987;15:59–74, 1987

29. Hebert GA. Hemolysins and other characteristics that help differentiate and biotype *Staphylococcus lugdunensis* and *Staphylococcus schleiferi*. J Clin Microbiol 1990;28:2425–2431.

30. Hovelius B, Mardh PA. *Staphylococcus saprophyticus* as a common cause of urinary tract infections. Rev Infect Dis 1984;6:328–337.

31. Igimi S, Kawamura S, Takahashi E, et al. *Staphylococcus felis*, a new species from clinical specimens from cats. Int J Syst Bacteriol 1989;39:373–377.

32. Jean-Pierre H, Darbas H, Jean-Roussenq, et al. Pathogenicity in two cases of *Staphylococcus schleiferi*, a recently described species. J Clin Microbiol 1989;27:2110–2111.

33. Jungkind DJ, Torhan NJ, Korman KE, et al. Comparison of two commercially available test methods with conventional coagulase tests for identification of *Staphylococcus aureus*. J Clin Microbiol 1984;19:191–193.

34. Karchmer AW, Archer GL, Dismukes WE. *Staphylococcus epidermidis* causing prosthetic valve endocarditis: microbiologic and clinical observations as guides to therapy. Ann Intern Med 1983;98:447–455.

35. Kilpper-Balz R, Schleifer KH. Transfer of *Peptococcus saccharolyticus* (Foubert and Douglas) to the genus *Staphylococcus: Staphylococcus saccharolyticus* (Foubert and Douglas) comb. nov. Zentralbl Bakteriol Parasitenkd Infektionskr Hyg 1981;2:324–331.

36. Kloos WE, Schleifer KH. Isolation and characterization of staphylococci from human skin. II. Description of four new species: *Staphylococcus warneri, Staphylococcus capitis, Staphylococcus hominis*, and *Staphylococcus simulans*. Int J Syst Bacteriol 1975;25:62–79.

37. Kloos WE, Schleifer KH. Simplified scheme for routine identification of human *Staphylococcus* species. J Clin Micobiol 1975;1:82–87.

38. Kloos WE, Schleifer KH. *Staphylococcus auricularis* sp. nov.: an inhabitant of the human external ear. Int J Syst Bacteriol 1983;33:9–14.

39. Kloos WE, Schleifer KH. Genus IV. *Staphylococcus* Rosenbach 1984, 19[AL] (Nom. Cons. Opin. 17 Jud. Comm. 1958, 163). In: Sneath PHA, Mair NS, Sharpe ME, Holt JG, eds. Bergey's manual of systematic bacteriology. Baltimore, Williams & Wilkins, 1986;2:1013–1035.

40. Kloos WE, Schleifer KH, Smith RF. Characterization of *Staphylococcus sciuri* sp. nov. and its subspecies. Int J Syst Bacteriol 1976;26:22–37.

41. Kocur M. Genus I. *Micrococcus*. In: Sneath PHA, Nair NS, Holt JG, eds. Bergey's manual of systematic bacteriology. Baltimore, Williams & Wilkins, 1986;2:1003–1008.

42. Kocur M. Genus III. *Planococcus*. In: Sneath PHA, Nair NS, Holt JG, eds. Bergey's manual of systematic bacteriology. Baltimore, Williams & Wilkins, 1986;2:1011–1013.

43. Landau W, Kaplan RL. Room temperature coagulase production by *Staphylococcus aureus* strains. Clin Microbiol Newsl 1980;2:10.

44. Langlois BE, Harmon RJ, Akers K, et al. Comparison of methods for determining DNase and phosphatase activities by staphylococci. J Clin Microbiol 1989;27:1127–1129.

45. Males BM, Bartholomew WR, Amsterdam D. *Staphylococcus simulans* septicemia in a patient with chronic osteomyelitis and pyoarthritis. J Clin Microbiol 1985;21:255–257.

46. Myrick BA, Ellner PD. Evaluation of the latex slide agglutination test for identification of *Staphylococcus aureus*. J Clin Microbiol 1982;15:275–277.

47. Pennell DR, Rott-Petri JA, Kurzynski TA. Evaluation of three commercial agglutination tests for the identification of *Staphylococcus aureus*. J Clin Microbiol 1984;20:614–617.

48. Pinsky RL, Piscitelli V, Patterson JE. Endocarditis caused by relatively penicillin-resistant *Stomatococcus mucilaginosus*. J Clin Microbiol 1989;27:215–216.

49. Poirier LP, Gaudreau CL. *Stomatococcus mucilaginosus* catheter-associated infection with septicemia. J Clin Microbiol 1989;27:1125–1126.

50. Ponce de leon S, Wenzel RP. Hospital-acquired bloodstream infections with *Staphylococcus epidermidis*: review of 100 cases. Am J Med 1984;77:639–644.

51. Prag J, Kjoller E, Espersen F. *Stomatococcus mucilaginosus* endocarditis. Eur J Clin Microbiol 1985;4:422–424.

52. Relman DA, Ruoff K, Farraro MJ. *Stomatococcus mucilaginosus* endocarditis in an intravenous drug abuser. J Infect Dis 1987;5:1080–1082.

53. Schleifer KH, Fischer U. Desription of a new species in the genus *Staphylococcus: Staphylococcus carnosus*. Int J Syst Bacteriol 1982;32:153–156.

54. Schleifer KH, Geyer U, Kilpper-Balz R, et al. Elevation of *Staphylococcus sciuri* subsp. *lentus* (Kloos et al.) to species status: *Staphylococcus lentus* (Kloos et al.) comb. nov. Syst Appl Microbiol 1983;4:382–387.

55. Schleifer KH, Kilpper-Balz R, Devriese LA. *Staphylococcus arlettae* sp. nov., *S. equorum* sp. nov., and *S. kloosii* sp. nov.: three new coagulase-negative, novobiocin-resistant species from animals. Syst Appl Microbiol 1984;5:501–509.

56. Schleifer KH, Kloos WE. Isolation and characterization of staphylococci from human skin: I. Amended descriptions of *Staphylococcus epidermidis* and *Staphylococcus saprophyticus* and descriptions of

three new species: *Staphylococcus cohnii, Staphylococcus haemolyticus*, and *Staphylococcus xylosus*. Int J Syst Bacteriol 1975;25:50–61.

57. Schlievert PM, Shands KN, Dan BB, et al. Identification and characterization of an exotoxin from *Staphylococcus aureus* associated with toxic shock syndrome. J Infect Dis 1981;143:509–516.

58. Schwalbe RS, Stapleton JT, Gilligan PH. Emergence of vancomycin resistance in coagulase-negative staphylococci. N Engl J Med 1987;316:927–931.

59. Schwalbe RS, Ritz WJ, Verma PR, et al. Selection for vancomycin resistance in clinical isolates of *Staphylococcus haemolyticus*. J Infect Dis 1990;161:45–51.

60. Sewell CM, Clarridge JE, Young EJ, et al. Clinical significance of coagulase-negative staphylococci. J Clin Microbiol 1982;16:236–239.

61. Talen DA, Staatz D, Staatz A, et al. *Staphylococcus intermedius* in canine gingiva and canine-inflicted wound infections: a newly recognized zoonotic pathogen. J Clin Microbiol 1989;27:78–81.

62. Tu KK, Palutke WA. Isolation and characterization of a catalase-negative strain of *Staphylococcus aureus*. J Clin Microbiol 1976;3:77–78.

63. Varaldo PE, Kilpper-Balz R, Biavasco F, et al. *Staphylococcus delphini* sp. nov., a coagulase-positive species isolated from dolphins. Int J Syst Bacteriol 1988;38:436–439.

64. Veach LA, Pfaller MA, Bennett M, et al. Vancomycin resistance in *Staphylococcus haemolyticus* causing colonization and bloodstream infection. J Clin Microbiol 1990;28:2064–2068.

65. von Rheinbaben KE, Hadlock RM. Rapid distinction between micrococci and staphylococci with furazolidone agar. Antonie von Leeuwenhoek J Microbiol Serol 1981;47:41–51.

66. Wade JC, Schimpf SC, Newman KA. *Staphylococcus epidermidis*: an increasing cause of infection in patients with granulocytopenia. Ann Intern Med 1982;96:1–10.

67. Waldvogel FA. *Staphylococcus aureus* (including toxic shock syndrome). In: Mandell GL, Douglas RG Jr, Bennett JE, eds. Principles and practice of infectious diseases. 3rd ed. New York, Churchill Livingstone, 1990:1489–1510.

68. Westblom TU, Gorse GJ, Milligan TW, et al. Anaerobic endocarditis caused by *Staphylococcus saccharolyticus*. J Clin Microbiol 1990;28:2818–2819.

69. Winston DJ, Dudnick DV, Chapin M, et al. Coagulase-negative staphylococcal bacteremia in patients receiving immunosuppressive therapy. Arch Intern Med 1983;143:32–36.

70. Woolfrey BF, Lally RT, Ederer MN. An evaluation of three rapid coagglutination tests: Sero-STAT-Staph, Accu-Staph, and Staphyloslide for differentiating *Staphylococcus aureus* from other species of staphylococci. Am J Clin Pathol 1984;81:345–348.

9

Streptococci and Streptococcus-Like Bacteria

THE FAMILY STREPTOCOCCACEAE: TAXONOMY AND CLINICAL SIGNIFICANCE

In traditional and clinically useful taxonomic schemes, the streptococci belong to the Streptococcaceae. These organisms are gram-positive, catalase-negative bacteria that tend to grow in pairs and chains. The detection of cytochrome enzymes with the catalase test distinguishes members of the Micrococcaceae (catalase-positive) from the members of the Streptococcaceae (catalase-negative). Significant changes have occurred in the taxonomy of the group D streptococci, with the creation of the new genus *Enterococcus* and the description of several new enterococcal species.[50]

In *Bergey's Manual of Systematic Bacteriology*, the Streptococcaceae are divided into 10 species, including *Streptococcus*[48] (Table 9-1). Since the publication of *Bergey's Manual*, several modifications concerning the taxonomy of the streptococci and *Streptococcus*-like bacteria have been proposed and adopted:

1. Members of the genus *Peptococcus* have been incorporated into the genus *Peptostreptococcus*, with the exception of one species, *Peptococcus niger*.[40]
2. On the basis of DNA–ribosomal RNA hybridization studies, the genus *Streptococcus* has been subdivided into three groups[57]: The genus *Streptococcus*, in the strict sense, comprises most of the various species, including the pyogenic

streptococci, the viridans streptococci, and the pneumococci. The genus *Enterococcus* includes the former group D enterococci, and the genus *Lactococcus* (lactic acid streptococci) includes the streptococci that carry the Lancefield group N antigen.
3. The number of separate species assigned to the genus *Enterococcus* has expanded to 12. These are discussed later.

The genera listed in Table 9-1 can also be placed into a useful taxonomic framework for the clinical laboratory on the basis of their growth requirements regarding atmospheric oxygen. In this chapter the focus is on those organisms listed in group 1.

Group 1: Facultative Anaerobes
Streptococcus
Enterococcus
Aerococcus
Leuconostoc
Pediococcus
Gemella
Lactococcus

Group 2: Strict Anaerobes
Peptococcus
Peptostreptococcus
Ruminococcus
Coprococcus
Sarcina

General Characteristics of Streptococci

Streptococci are facultative anaerobes, and, in fact, some strains will grow better under anaerobic conditions. Many isolates are also stimulated by increased CO_2. Medically important streptococci, enterococci, and aerococci are *homofermentative*, meaning that the sole product of glucose fermentation is lactic acid.

The streptococci can be grouped according to the *Lancefield grouping system*. The β-hemolytic streptococci encompass several human, animal, and environmental strains.[57] The antigens detected in the Lancefield grouping system are either cell wall polysaccharides (as in the human group A, B, C, F, and G streptococci) or cell wall lipoteichoic acids (group D streptococci and *Enterococcus* species).

Table 9-1
Streptococcal Nomenclature in *Bergey's Manual of Systematic Bacteriology*

Family Deinococcaceae
   Genus *Deinococcus*
Other Genera (Family Streptococcaceae?)
   Genus *Streptococcus*
   Genus *Aerococcus*
   Genus *Leuconostoc*
   Genus *Pediococcus*
   Genus *Peptococcus*
   Genus *Peptostreptococcus*
   Genus *Gemella*
   Genus *Ruminococcus*
   Genus *Coprococcus*
   Genus *Sarcina*

Pathogenic streptococci have several characteristics that contribute to their virulence. Group A, β-hemolytic streptococci (*S. pyogenes*) possess cell surface antigens (*M proteins*) that render the organisms resistant to phagocytosis by leukocytes.[4] Group A streptococci also produce two hemolysins: streptolysin O and streptolysin S. *Streptolysin O* is oxygen labile, antigenic, inhibited by cholesterol, and toxic to a variety of cell types, including leukocytes, monocytes, and cultured cells. Streptolysin O is also produced by some group C and group G streptococci. Measurement of antibodies against streptolysin O (ASO titers) in serum is useful for retrospective detection of recent streptococcal infections. *Streptolysin S* is oxygen stable, nonantigenic, and also toxic to a variety of cell types. These organisms also produce deoxyribonucleases, hyaluronidase, streptokinase, amylase, and esterase. The contribution of these enzymes and toxins to infection is uncertain.

The pathogenicity of *S. pneumoniae* is related primarily to the *polysaccharide capsule* of the organism, with encapsulated organisms being more virulent than nonencapsulated organisms. There are 84 capsular types of *S. pneumoniae*; 23 of these types account for over 88% of pneumococcal bacteremia and meningitis.[39]

Group A β-Hemolytic Streptococci

Group A β-hemolytic streptococci, transmitted from person to person through the respiratory route, cause pharyngitis, tonsillitis, sinusitis, otitis media, cervical adenitis, pyoderma, lymphadenitis, impetigo, erysipelas, cellulitis, bacteremia, osteomyelitis, arthritis, and endocarditis. This infection is characterized by a severe sore throat, with malaise, fever, and headache. The posterior pharynx is usually inflamed and swollen, and a grayish white exudate may be present on the tonsils. Rare cases of meningitis and pneumonia have also been reported.[4] Up to 25% of persons with streptococcal pharyngitis may become asymptomatic carriers of the organisms after treatment. Of concern in the management of group A pharyngitis, are the well-studied "nonsuppurative" complications of group A streptococcal infections, rheumatic fever, and glomerulonephritis.[4] Rheumatic fever, which can occur 1 to 5 weeks after acute pharyngitis, is a multisystemic collagen vascular disease characterized by carditis, polyarthritis, subcutaneous nodules, and erythema marginatum (rash). Although the course is self-limited, chronic or progressive damage to the heart valves may occur. Poststreptococcal glomerulonephritis is an inflammatory disease of the renal glomerulus that may occur as soon as 10 days after pharyngitis or more than 3 weeks after skin infections. It is associated with diffuse glomerular lesions, hypertension, hematuria, and proteinuria.

Severe group A streptococcal infections associated with a toxic shock–like syndrome, with presentations similar to those found in patients with classic staphylococcal toxic shock syndrome, have also been described.[11,59] These clinical characteristics include hypotension, renal dysfunction, hypoalbuminuria, thrombocytopenia, hypocalcemia, and respiratory failure.

Group B β-Hemolytic Streptococci (*S. agalactiae*)

Group B β-hemolytic streptococci are a major cause of disease in the perinatal and the neonatal periods.[17,53] Females become colonized with the organism in the vagina and the rectum, and asymptomatic vaginal colonization is found in 5% to 35% of pregnant women.[33] Among colonized pregnant women, 40% to 70% of their infants acquire the identical group B strain either in utero or during delivery. Among the colonized infants, disease may occur in 2 to 5 infants per 1000 live births.

Group C β-Hemolytic Streptococci

Streptococcus equisimilis, the most common human group C isolate, has been recovered from the pharynges of carriers and from those with exudative pharyngitis and tonsillitis. It has also caused several other human infections, including sepsis in neutropenic hosts, puerperal sepsis, cellulitis, necrotizing fasciitis, pneumonia, epiglottitis, empyema, bacteremia, meningitis, brain abscess, osteomyelitis, septic arthritis, and endocarditis.[1,36,45,54,58] Outbreaks of human pharyngitis caused by *S. zooepidemicus* traced to ingestion of unpasteurized cow's milk and contaminated homemade cheese have been reported.[49] Cases of poststreptococcal pharyngitis secondary to *S. zooepidemicus* have also been reported.[2]

Group D Streptococci
(*S. bovis* and *S. equinus*)

Group D streptococci possess the group D lipoteichoic acid antigen in their cell walls. Although these organisms are β-hemolytic on rabbit blood agar, they are usually α-hemolytic or nonhemolytic on the sheep blood agar used routinely in clinical laboratories. Some former group D species are predominant normal inhabitants of the human gastrointestinal tract and were termed *enterococci*, while other species that possess the group D antigen and comprise only a small part of the normal enteric flora were termed *nonenterococci*.

Enterococcal species are now placed in the separate genus *Enterococcus*, while the group D streptococci now includes only two species, *Streptococcus bovis* and *Streptococcus equinus*.[50,56] The practical consideration behind the division of these organisms into two groups was that the enterococci are generally more resistant to penicillin, cephalosporins, and the aminoglycosides than the nonenterococcal group D streptococci.[18,28] Isolation of *S. bovis* has been associated with carcinoma of the colon in humans. The organism may be recovered from both feces and blood in patients with colonic carcinoma, and this association has been confirmed in several clinical studies.[35,52] Recovery of this organism from the blood should provoke a search for gastrointestinal lesions of carcinoma. This organism has also been involved in cases of meningitis, urinary tract infections, and endocarditis.

Group F β-Hemolytic Streptococci

These organisms have the species name *S. anginosus* (or *S. milleri* in the British taxonomic scheme). Group F streptococci characteristically grow as "minute colonies" on agar media. Group F β-hemolytic streptococci are recognized causes of severe suppurative infections, including cellulitis, deep tissue abscesses, bacteremia, osteomyelitis, and endocarditis.[43,51]

Group G β-Hemolytic Streptococci

Group G streptococci constitute a part of the normal human gastrointestinal, vaginal, oropharyngeal, and skin flora. Infections caused by this organism include pharyngitis, otitis media, pleuropulmonary infection, cellulitis, septic arthritis, septic thrombophlebitis, bacteremia, endocarditis, and meningitis.[61,63]

Streptococcus pneumoniae

The pneumococcus is the major cause of community-acquired bacterial pneumonia.[41] The organism may be harbored in the upper respiratory tract of 5% to 10% of adults, although carriage rates greater than 60% have been reported in closed populations. In the appropriate host, the organism gains access to the alveolar spaces and eventually causes a lobar pneumonia with consolidation and bacteremia. Complications of pneumococcal pneumonia include lung abscess, pericardial infections, empyema, and pleural effusions. This organism is also the most frequent cause of otitis media with bacteremia in children and is the second most common cause of bacterial meningitis.[34,53] *S. pneumoniae* also causes sinusitis, mastoiditis, arthritis, peritonitis, and endocarditis. Pneumococci are infrequent causes of arthritis and peritonitis.

Viridans Streptococci

The viridans group of streptococci includes several species of α-hemolytic and nonhemolytic streptococci, most of which comprise part of the normal upper respiratory tract flora (Table 9-2). These organisms are the most frequent streptococcal isolates from cases of subacute bacterial endocarditis[27] and, in this setting, may be isolated from multiple sets of blood cultures. Viridans streptococci may also be isolated on occasion from other serious infections, such as meningitis, particularly in compromised hosts.[3,44,60] The taxonomy of this group of organisms, comparing the British and Centers for Disease Control classifications, is evolving as shown in Table 9-2, including an indication of the "current" status of the individual species.

One group, known as nutritionally variant streptococci, are viridans streptococci that require thiol compounds, cysteine, or the active form of vitamin B_6—pyridoxal or pyridoxamine—for growth in media.[8] These isolates have variously been called nutritionally variant, nutritionally deficient, thiol-requiring, pyridoxal-requiring, and "satelliting" streptococci.[55] With the use of media supplemented with pyridoxal, a taxonomic relationship was suggested to exist between nutritionally variant streptococci *S. mitis*, and *S. sanguis* II.[9] These streptococci have been recovered primarily from patients with endocarditis, although isolates from other sites (eg, respiratory tract, vaginal discharge, conjunctivae, cutaneous wounds, pleural fluid, middle ear aspirates, brain abscess,

Table 9-2
Classification of the Viridans Streptococci

BRITISH SCHEME	CDC SCHEME	CURRENT TAXONOMIC STATUS
S. mitior (glucan +/−)	*S. mitis*	*S. mitis* (retained, with suggestions for a new type strain [*S. oralis*?])
S. sanguis	*S. sanguis* I *S. sanguis* II	*S. sanguis* (genetic groups 1 and 2) Genetically the same as *S. mitis*
S. salivarius	*S. salivarius*	*S. salivarius*
S. milleri	*S. intermidius* *S. constellatus*	*S. anginosus* or *S. intermedius* *S. anginosus* or *S. constellatus*
S. mutans	*S. mutans*	"*S. mutans* group" *S. mutans* *S. rattus* *S. cricetus* *S. sobrinus* *S. ferus* *S. macacae* *S. downei*
S. acidominimus	*S. acidominimus*	*S. acidominimus*
Pyridoxal-dependent streptococci	Not included	*S. defectivus, S. adjacens*
S. pneumoniae	Not included	Not included
Not included	Not included	*S. bovis, S. bovis* variant *S. equinus*
Not included	*S. morbillorum*	*Gemella morbillorum*
Not recognized	*S. uberis/para-uberis*	*S. uberis* *S. vestibularis* (new oral species) "*S. oralis*" (same as *S. mitis*?) "*S. gordonii*" (proposed species)

pancreatic abscess) have also been reported.[6,9] It is, therefore, essential that the microbiologist know when to suspect such isolates and how to go about recovering them from clinical specimens.

Enterococcus Species

The enterococci are found as normal flora in the gastrointestinal tracts of humans and animals. They are becoming increasingly important agents of human disease, largely because of their resistance to antimicrobial agents to which other streptococci are generally susceptible.[2,42] Enterococci rank third as agents of nosocomial infections.[10] *Enterococcus* species are important agents in endocarditis, bacteremia, intraabdominal and pelvic infections, urinary tract infections, wound and soft tissue infections, and neonatal sepsis.[28,38] Because of their resistance to penicillins and cephalosporins of several generations, and the acquisition of high-

level resistance to aminoglycosides, these bacteria are often involved in serious superinfections among patients receiving these antimicrobial agents.[46]

Streptococcus-Like Species

Aerococcus species, *Pediococcus* species, *Leuconostoc* species, and *Gemella* species are other *Streptococcus*-like organisms that may occasionally be recovered from human sources and may be encountered as unknowns in proficiency survey programs. These organisms have economic importance because of their use in the dairy and pickling industries and in winemaking. In recent years, these organisms have been isolated from human infections, most of which occurred in immunocompromised hosts.[7,29] In contrast to other *Streptococcus*-like bacteria, *Leuconostoc* species are resistant to vancomycin, which is a helpful laboratory identifying feature.

IDENTIFICATION OF STREPTOCOCCI AND *STREPTOCOCCUS*-LIKE BACTERIA

Direct Gram-Stained Smears

Gram-stained smears of clinical specimens that yield streptococci on culture generally show gram-positive or gram-variable cocci arranged in pairs and chains. Chains of cells in both specimens and broth cultures tend to appear as chains of pairs of cells rather than as chains of individual cells. Individual cell shapes range from those that resemble diplococci to those that are coccobacillary or coryneform, and this morphology is often observed on smears from broth cultures and from solid media as well. Viridans streptococci, in particular, tend to have more elongated individual cells. *S. pneumoniae* will most often appear as pairs of lanceolate cells. On smears of specimens yielding mucoid, heavily encapsulated strains, the capsule may appear as a pink halo or as a nonstaining area surrounding the cells in relief against a pink background surrounding the organism.

Culture Media

Specimens that may be expected to yield streptococci on culture should be plated onto a suitable blood-containing medium that has a peptone base rich enough to support these fastidious organisms. The agar base medium should be a peptone infusion medium (eg, tryptic soy, proteose peptone, Todd-Hewitt) without added carbohydrates. Although the colonies generally are larger on glucose-containing media (eg, Columbia base medium) after 24 hours, acid produced from glucose utilization inactivates the streptolysin S of group A streptococci and may interfere with the interpretation of the hemolytic qualities of the organism. Sheep blood is added to the basal medium at a 5% concentration as the indicator cells for hemolysis. Lower concentrations of blood in the media make the hemolytic reaction difficult to discern, while higher concentrations may obscure hemolysis entirely. On sheep blood agar, streptococci belonging to groups A, B, C, F, and G are β-hemolytic while most *Enterococcus* species and group D streptococci are α-hemolytic or nonhemolytic.

Sheep blood agar can be made selective for the recovery of group A streptococci from throat cultures by adding trimethoprim (1.25 μg/mL) and sulfamethoxazole (23.75 μg/mL).[16,43] Much of the normal flora of the oropharynx (eg, viridans streptococci, micrococci, staphylococci, and neisseriae) will be inhibited on this medium. Use of this selective medium enhances recovery of group A and B streptococci and allows visualization of β-hemolysis without the "background" of other organism growth.

Hemolysis on Blood Agar

Four types of hemolysis may be produced by streptococci on sheep blood agar. Observation and correct interpretation of the hemolytic properties of streptococci is important, since the performance of subsequent tests is predicated on this initial evaluation.

α-*Hemolysis*: Partial lysis of the erythrocytes surrounding a colony, causing a gray-green or brownish discoloration in the media.

β-*Hemolysis*: Complete lysis of the red blood cells surrounding a colony, causing a clearing of blood from the medium.

γ-*Hemolysis*: No hemolysis and, consequently, no color change of the medium surrounding a colony. Organisms showing no hemolysis are generally termed *nonhemolytic* rather than γ-hemolytic.

α-*Prime or wide-zone α-hemolysis*: A small zone of intact erythrocytes immediately adjacent to the colony, with a zone of complete red blood cell hemolysis surrounding the zone of intact erythrocytes. This type of hemolysis may be confused with β-hemolysis.

Hemolysis is best observed by examining colonies grown under anaerobic conditions or by inspecting subsurface colonies in pour plates or streak-stab plates, since, in the case of group A streptococci, maximal activity of both the oxygen-labile (SLO) and oxygen-stable (SLS) hemolysins is only observed under anaerobic conditions. This can be easily accomplished by the "streak-and-stab" technique, in which the agar is stabbed in several places to force some of the inoculum under the agar, hence creating a relatively anaerobic environment. Plates should be incubated at 35°C in air or in 5% to 7% CO_2.

Nonculture Techniques

Nonculture techniques for direct detection of group A streptococci on throat swab specimens are in wide use in both clinical laboratories and physicians' offices. These techniques include nitrous acid or enzymatic extraction of the swab followed by an antigen detection step. Most available kits use latex agglutination or enzyme immunoassay methods for antigen detection.[30,47] Although the specificity of these kits is high (usually greater than 98%), the sensitivities of the various kits for group A streptococcal detection vary widely (60% to 95%). If such a system is employed in the laboratory, it may be prudent to collect double swabs from patients, with culture only being performed on specimens yielding negative direct detection results.

Colony Morphology and Catalase Testing

The following colony descriptions of the several streptococci and *Streptococcus*-like organisms are characteristic on blood agar after 18 to 24 hours of incubation:

1. Group A streptococci are about 0.5 mm in diameter, are translucent or transparent, have a smooth or matte surface, and are surrounded by a zone of β-hemolysis two to four times the diameter of the colony.
2. Groups C and G also have a similar appearance.
3. Group B streptococci form larger colonies with comparatively smaller zones of hemolysis, which is generally softer and less obvious. Up to 11% of group B streptococci may be non-hemolytic.
4. Group D streptococcal colonies are usually larger than those of group A (0.5 to 1 mm), are usually gray and smooth, have an entire edge, and are α-hemolytic.
5. Group F streptococci form extremely small colonies, called minute colonies, surrounded by a large, florid zone of β-hemolysis.
6. *S. pneumoniae* displays a spectrum of colony types from rough (nonencapsulated) to smooth (encapsulated). In all cases, these colonies are generally surrounded by a large zone of intense green α-hemolysis. The central portion of

rough colonies may collapse, giving the characteristic "checker" or "nail-head" colonies.
7. Colonies of *Aerococcus*, *Pediococcus*, *Gemella*, *Leuconostoc*, and the facultative *Lactobacillus* species strongly resemble viridans streptococci or group D streptococci in their appearance, and they are either α-hemolytic or nonhemolytic.

In brief, these organisms are also catalase-negative; some are intrinsically resistant to vancomycin and related cyclic glycopeptide antibiotics (eg, ristocetin, aracidin, and teicoplanin), a clue by which they may be suspected. These look-alike organisms may be differentiated from *Streptococcus* and *Enterococcus* species, and from one another with the tests shown in Table 9-3 and Figure 9-1.[22,25,32]

Presumptive Identification of Streptococci

β-Hemolytic streptococci, pneumococci, group D streptococci, and enterococci are definitively identified using serologic procedures that detect either the Lancefield group antigens (groups A, B, C, D, F, and G) or the capsular polysaccharide antigens (*S. pneumoniae*) of the organisms. Species identification of group D streptococci, *Enterococcus* species, and the viridans streptococci is done primarily by biochemical, physiologic, and enzymatic tests. Many laboratories, however, use a handful of *presumptive* tests that correlate highly with the serologic methods yet are less expensive to perform (Table 9-4).

Susceptibility to Bacitracin

The bacitracin susceptibility test is used for the presumptive identification of group A β-hemolytic streptococci. Group A streptococci are susceptible to relatively low concentrations of bacitracin; thus, the test can be used to differentiate this group from other β-hemolytic streptococci that are resistant. The test is performed by placing a 0.04-unit bacitracin disk on an agar plate in an area where a colony suspected of being group A *Streptococcus* has been inoculated. Any zone of inhibition around the disk is interpreted as a presumptive identification for group A streptococci.

Table 9-3
Characteristics of Gram-Positive, Catalase-Negative Cocci and Coccobacilli

GENUS	VANCOMYCIN	GAS FROM GLUCOSE	BILE-ESCULIN HYDROLYSIS	PYR	GROWTH IN 6.5% NaCl	GROUP D ANTIGEN	GROWTH AT 10°C	GROWTH AT 45°C	ARGININE HYDROLYSIS	LEUCINE AMINOPEPTIDASE
Streptococcus	S	−	V	−	−	−	−	V	V	+
Enterococcus	S	−	+	+	+	+	V	+	V	+
Lactococcus	S	−	V	V	V	−	+	V	−	+
Aerococcus	S	−	V	+	+	−	−	−	V	−
Gemella	S	−	−	V	−	−	−	−	−	+
Leuconostoc	R	+	+	−	V	V	V	−	−	−
Pediococcus	R	−	+	−	V	+	−	V	V	+
Lactobacillus	R	V	V	−	V	V	+	V	V	V

S, susceptible; R, resistant; +, most strains positive; −, most strains negative; V, variable reaction.

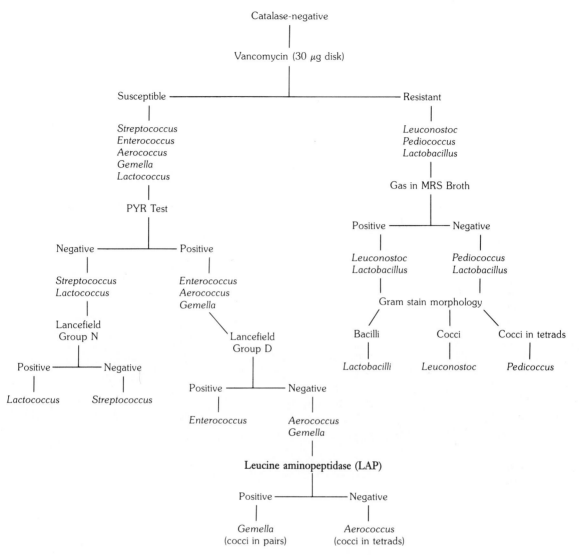

Figure 9-1. Flow chart for differentiation of streptococci and *Streptococcus*-like bacteria. (Adapted from Carey RB. The crazy cocci. Presentation at South Central Association for Clinical Microbiology Spring Meeting, Louisville, KY, 1990)

Susceptibility to Trimethoprim-Sulfamethoxazole

The trimethoprim-sulfamethoxazole susceptibility test is performed similar to the bacitracin test and is used to distinguish groups A and B streptococci from other β-hemolytic streptococci. When used in conjunction with the bacitracin test, the trimethoprim-sulfamethoxazole susceptibility test helps to screen out those non-A, non-B streptococci that may be susceptible to bacitracin, since both group A and B strains are resistant to tri-

methoprim-sulfamethoxazole while groups C, F, and G are susceptible to this combined agent.

CAMP Test

The CAMP test (named for Christie, Atkins, and Munch-Petersen) is used to presumptively identify group B streptococci. The hemolytic activity of the β-hemolysin produced by most strains of *Staphylococcus aureus* is enhanced by an extracellular protein produced by group B streptococci. Interaction of

Table 9-4
Presumptive Identification of Clinically Significant Streptococci

ORGANISM	HEMOLYSIS	BACITRACIN	TRIMETHOPRIM-SULFAMETHOXAZOLE	CAMP TEST	HYDROLYSIS OF Hippurate	PYR	BILE-ESCULIN HYDROLYSIS	GROWTH IN 6.5% NaCl	OPTOCHIN	BILE SOLUBILITY
Group A	β	+	−	−	−	+	−	−	−	−
Group B	β, none	−	−	+	+	−	−	V	−	−
Groups C, F, and G	β	V	+	−	−	−	−	−	−	−
Group D *Enterococcus*	α, β, none	−	−	−	V	+	+	+	−	−
Group D not *Enterococcus*	α, none	−	+	−	−	−	+	−	−	−
Viridans streptococci	α, none	V	+	−	V	−	V	−	−	−
Pneumococcus	α	V	+	−	−	−	−	−	+	+

+, positive reaction or susceptible; −, negative reaction or resistant; V, variable reaction.

the β-hemolysin with this factor causes "synergistic hemolysis," which is easily observed on a blood agar plate. To perform the test, a streak of a β-hemolysin–producing *Staphylococcus aureus* strain (ATCC #25923) is inoculated onto a blood agar plate and a single streak of the organism to be identified is streaked perpendicular to, but not touching, the staph streak. The plate is then incubated at 35°C overnight in normal atmosphere or in 5% CO_2. During growth, group B streptococci secrete a protein called the CAMP factor. This appears as an arrowhead-shaped area of increased hemolysis in the area where the two streaks of growth are closest.[14]

Hydrolysis of Sodium Hippurate

Group B streptococci are also able to hydrolyze hippurate to its components, glycine and benzoic acid. After overnight incubation of hippurate broth inoculated with the unknown organism, ferric chloride reagent (0.2 mL; $FeCl_3 \cdot 6H_2O$, 12 g, in 100 mL 2% aqueous hydrochloride) is then added to the supernatant (0.8 mL). The persistence of a heavy precipitate after 10 minutes indicates a positive test. Alternatively, ninhydrin reagent may be added to the supernatant to detect free glycine;[31] the formation of a deep blue color is positive.

Hydrolysis of L-Pyrrolindonyl-β-Naphthylamide (PYR)

PYR hydrolysis is a presumptive test for both group A and group D enterococcal streptococci.[24] It replaces the bacitracin test and the salt tolerance test for group A streptococci and *Enterococcus* species, respectively. This test is highly sensitive and specific for group A streptococci and *Enterococcus*. Several adaptations of the PYR hydrolysis test are commercially available and provide rapid results (15 minutes or less).[62] Other organisms (eg, some lactococci, *Aerococcus*, *Gemella*, and the nutritionally variant streptococci) are also PYR-positive.

Bile-Esculin Test

The bile-esculin test, based on the ability of certain bacteria, notably the group D streptococci and *Enterococcus* species, to hydrolyze esculin in the presence of 40% bile, is used for the presumptive

identification of *Enterococcus* species and group D streptococci (*S. bovis*). The test is generally performed on an agar slant or in a plate that contains bile-esculin medium. Any blackening of the agar in the plate indicates a positive test result. Rare group D strains may require 48 hours of incubation before hydrolysis is apparent.

Salt Tolerance Test (6.5% NaCl Broth)

The salt tolerance test, based on the ability of an organism to grow in 6.5% NaCl, separates *Enterococcus* species from group D nonenterococcal *S. bovis*. The organism to be identified is inoculated into an infusion-based agar or broth containing 6.5% NaCl. After overnight incubation, the medium is observed for the presence of growth. *Enterococcus* species will be salt tolerant; *S. bovis* will not grow.

Susceptibility to Ethyl Hydrocupreine Hydrochloride (Optochin)

Ethylhydrocupreine hydrochloride (optochin), a quinine derivative, at the very low concentration of 5 μg/mL or less, selectively inhibits the growth of *S. pneumoniae*. Thus, susceptibility to optochin is used to differentiate *S. pneumoniae* from the other viridans streptococci. To perform the test, a few colonies are subcultured to another blood agar plate and are streaked as a lawn. An optochin disk (TAXO P disk, Becton Dickinson Microbiology Systems, Cockeysville, MD) is placed on the inoculum, and the plate is incubated overnight at 35°C in a 5% CO_2 or air atmosphere. A zone of 14 mm or greater around the 6-mm disk indicates susceptibility to optochin and identifies the organism as *S. pneumoniae*.

Bile Solubility Test

The bile solubility test is another test for identification of *S. pneumoniae*. The test can be performed on a broth or saline suspension of the organism or directly on a plate. In the tube test, clearing of the 10% deoxycholate suspension after inoculation of the unknown organism and incubation for 3 hours indicates lysis of the bacterial cells and identifies the organism as *S. pneumoniae*. For the plate test, a drop of 2% sodium deoxycholate is placed directly on a few isolated colonies of the organism, and the plate is incubated at 35°C, without inverting, for 30 minutes. *S. pneumoniae* colonies will lyse and disappear, leaving only the area of hemolysis. Alternatively, the broth test can be performed by making a suspension of the organism to be tested in a solution of 10% sodium deoxycholate and observing for clearing after 15 to 30 minutes of incubation at 35°C.

Commercial Presumptive Tests

Commercially available triplates are available for the presumptive identification of β-hemolytic streptococcal groups A and B, the group D streptococci, and *Enterococcus* species. The Strep-ID Tri-Plate (Remel Laboratories, Lenexa, KS) contains three compartments: a sheep blood agar quadrant for assessment of hemolysis and performance of the CAMP and trimethoprim-sulfamethoxazole tests, a bile-esculin agar quadrant, and a PYR medium quadrant. After inoculation and overnight incubation, the tests are interpreted as shown in Table 9-5.

Serologic Identification of Streptococci

Based on the pioneering work of Rebecca Lancefield, the serologic classification of human streptococci is based on the detection of the group-specific carbohydrate antigen from the cell wall of the organism.[37] The various techniques by which serologic identification of streptococci may be accomplished include the following:

- The capillary precipitin test, the method used by Lancefield, in which the extracted antigen is layered over group-specific antisera in a capillary tube and the formation of a precipitin reaction at the extract–antiserum interface provides the group designation of the organism
- Coagglutination, in which visible agglutination of the staphylococcal cells coated with a specific antiserum provides the group designation of the organism
- Latex agglutination, in which polystyrene latex beads are used as the carriers for the group-specific antisera that are reacted with the organism extract, with visible agglutination of the latex particles serving as a positive test[5,13,21]

Several commercial kits, based on coagglutination and latex techniques, are available.

Quellung Test

The quellung test may employ a serum pool as well as type-specific antisera. A light suspension of the organism is prepared in saline, and a loopful of this suspension is mixed with a loopful of antiserum and a loopful of methylene blue on a glass slide. A glass coverslip is applied, and the slide is incubated at room temperature for 10 minutes. The slide is examined under the high dry objective and under oil immersion, with decreased light. Because of a microprecipitin reaction occurring on the surface of the organism, the refractive index of the capsule

Table 9-5
Interpretation of Test Reactions in the Strep-ID TRI Plate

ORGANISM	HEMOLYSIS	CAMP TEST	PYR	BILE-ESCULIN HYDROLYSIS
Presumptive group A	β	−	+	−
Presumptive group B	β, none	+	−	−
Not groups A or B	β	−	−	−
Enterococcus species	α, β, none	−	+	+
Group D *Streptococcus*	α, none	−	−	+
Viridans streptococci	α, none	−	−	−/W+

+, *positive reaction;* −, *negative reaction; S, susceptible; R, resistant;* −/W+, *occasional weak positive reaction for some isolates.*

changes and takes on a swollen, more visible appearance as a halo around the blue-stained bacterial cells if the bacterial strain being tested is complementary to the antisera being used.

Identification of *Enterococcus* Species

Identification of *Enterococcus* species is accomplished by biochemical and physiologic tests. Only about 80% of *Enterococcus* species react with antiserum against Lancefield group D by capillary precipitin or latex agglutination (ie, Murex Diagnostics, Norcross, GA).[50] All *Enterococcus* species hydrolyze esculin in the presence of bile, grow in broth containing 6.5% NaCl, and are PYR-positive.[24] Facklam and Collins[30] have proposed a stepwise method for identifying *Enterococcus* species. Isolates that fit the criteria listed earlier are inoculated into several test media and are divided into three groups based on those reactions. Individual species within each group are further differentiated into separate species on the basis of additional tests or characteristics. A flow chart for identifying *Enterococcus* species based on the work of Facklam and Collins[20] is shown in Figure 9-2. This identification scheme is performed with conventional biochemicals.

Identification of the Viridans Streptococci

The viridans streptococci other than *S. pneumoniae* encompass several species of α-hemolytic and nonhemolytic organisms (Table 9-6). Unlike the human β-hemolytic streptococci, these organisms, with the exception of *S. bovis, S. bovis* variants, and *S. equinus*, lack specific Lancefield serologic group antigens, although some may carry antigens that cross-react with these antisera. Unlike the pneumococci, they are optochin resistant and bile insoluble. Under certain circumstances, it may be clinically helpful to identify these organisms. The conventional method for identifying the viridans streptococci, like that for the staphylococci, is cumbersome and time consuming. The scheme proposed by Facklam in 1977 has been extensively modified, and Table 9-6 presents an amalgamation of identification characteristics for human viridans streptococcal isolates.[12,19,25,26]

Kit Systems for Identifying Streptococci

The development of kit systems that incorporate similar types of physiologic and enzymatic tests for streptococcal identification have been of great help in species identification of the viridans streptococci, *Enterococcus* species, and the group D streptococci. The biochemical reactions included in the kit systems are used to generate an organism biotype number that corresponds to the organism's identity. Although these systems include the β-hemolytic streptococci in their data bases, these organisms are best handled using other methods, such as the presumptive tests described earlier or the rapid streptococcal grouping kits that are available. Full descriptions of the following commercial systems for the identification of streptococci can be found by referring to the manufacturers' product inserts:

- API Rapid STREP (bioMérieux Vitek, Inc, Hazelwood, MO)
- RapID STR (Innovative Diagnostics, Inc, Norcross, GA)
- Vitek Gram Positive Identification (GPI) Card (bioMérieux Vitek Systems, Inc, Hazelwood, MO)
- API 20S (bioMérieux Vitek, Inc, Hazelwood, MO)
- Minitek Gram-Positive Kit (Becton Dickinson Microbiology Systems, Cockeysville, MD)

Microtiter format systems for streptococcal identification are available from American MicroScan (Sacramento, CA) and from MicroMedia (San Jose, CA), but these have not been evaluated.

Identification of Minute Colony Streptococci

Minute colony streptococci form very small colonies on blood agar and may be α-hemolytic, β-hemolytic, or nonhemolytic. β-Hemolytic isolates may carry group A, C, F, or G antigens or may be nongroupable.[51] As mentioned previously, these organisms are called *S. anginosus* regardless of group reactivity. α-Hemolytic or nonhemolytic strains are identified as *S. intermedius* or *S. constellatus*. The API Rapid STREP and the RapID STR kits will identify these organisms.

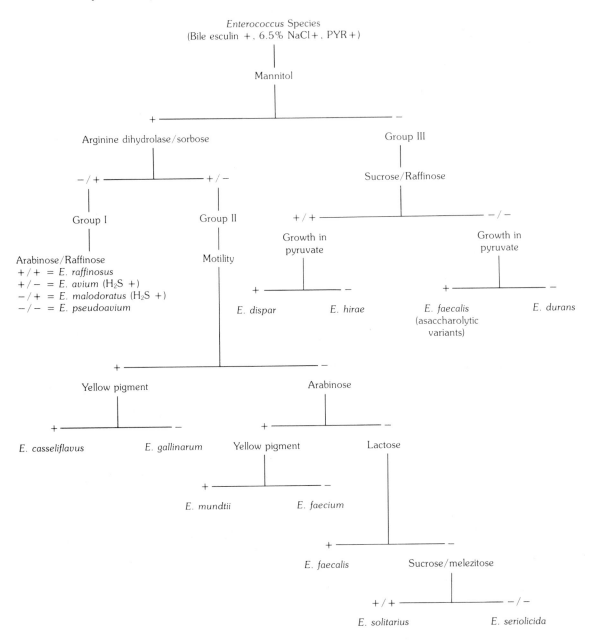

Figure 9-2. Flow chart for biochemical identification of *Enterococcus* species. (After Facklan RR, Collins MD. Identification of *Enterococcus* species isolated from human infections by a conventional test scheme. J Clin Microbiol 1989;27:731–734)

Isolation and Identification of Nutritionally Variant Streptococci

These organisms should be suspected when direct Gram stains of specimens or of positive blood cultures show streptococcal organisms that fail to grow on subsequent culture or subculture. Commercial blood culture medium does contain pyridoxal and will support the growth of these organisms. Subculture onto blood agar, and the placement of a staphylococcal streak as is done in the satellite test for *Haemophilus* species, will allow growth of the nutritionally variant streptococci adjacent to the staph streak. Alternatively, disks impregnated with py-

Table 9-6
Biochemical Characteristics of the Viridans Streptococci

| SPECIES | HEMO-LYSIS | ARGININE DIHYDRO-LASE | ESCU-LIN | VOGES-PROS-KAUER | ALKALINE-PHOS-PHATASE | β-GLUC-URONIDASE | ACID PRODUCTION FROM | | | | | | | | H_2O_2 |
							Mann-itol	Sor-bitol	Raffi-nose	Inulin	Treha-lose	Sali-cin	Starch	Glyco-gen	
S. sanguis 1	α	+	+	−	+	−	−	−	V	V	+	+	−	−	+
S. sanguis 2	α	+	+	−	−	−	−	V	V	V	+	+	+	−	+
S. salivarius	γ	−	+	+	V	−	−	−	+	+	V	+	V	−	−
S. mitis	α	−	−	−	V	−	−	−	V	−	V	V	V	−	+
S. mutans	α, γ	−	+	+	−	−	+	+	+	+	+	+	−	−	−
S. vestibularis	α	−	+	V	V	NA	−	−	−	−	V	+	−	−	+
S. acidominimus	α	V	−	−	V	V	V	−	−	−	V	−	−	−	NA
S. uberis	α, γ	+	+	+	+	−	+	+	−	+	+	−	−	−	NA
"S. oralis"	α	−	−	−	+	−	−	−	V	−	V	V	−	−	+
S. constellatus	α, γ	+	+	+	+	−	V	−	V	−	V	V	V	V	V
S. intermedius	α, γ	+	+	+	+	−	−	−	−	−	+	+	+	+	−
S. anginosus	α, γ, β	+	+	+	+	−	V	−	V	−	+	+	V	+	V

+, most strains positive; −, most strains negative; V, variable reaction; NA, data not available.

213

ridoxal may also be placed on the subculture plate with subsequent growth of the organisms appearing as satellite colonies surrounding the disk.

Recognition and Identification of *Aerococcus, Leuconostoc, Pediococcus,* and *Gemella* Species

Aerococci closely resemble the viridans streptococci or enterococci. They are usually α-hemolytic. Some strains may also be bile-esculin– and PYR-positive. Most strains also grow in broth containing 6.5% NaCl. Characteristics of the aerococci that help to differentiate them from group D enterococci and other *Streptococcus*-like organisms are listed in Table 9-3. These organisms are vancomycin susceptible, like streptococci, lactococci, and most enterococci, but, unlike these other organisms, are leucine aminopeptidase-negative. In addition, these organisms characteristically appear as tetrads on Gram-stained smears. The Rapid STREP and the RapID-STR kits are able to identify these organisms reliably.[23,64]

Although only a single species, *A. viridans,* is formally recognized, a second "genospecies" has been described on the basis of DNA hybridization studies.[15]

Leuconostoc species are gram-positive cocci that are recognized by their resistance to vancomycin and the production of gas from glucose (see Table 9-3 and Fig. 9-1) This latter property is best determined in MRS (Mann-Rogosa-Sharpe) broth (Difco Laboratories, Detroit, MI) overlaid with sterile petrolatum. The formation of bubbles under the petrolatum seal indicates gas production and confirms their heterofermentative metabolism. The eight *Leuconostoc* species are further identified by a battery of biochemical tests.

Pediococcus species are also vancomycin-resistant gram-positive cocci. They are generally homofermentative like the streptococci and, unlike *Leuconostoc* species, they do not produce gas from glucose in MRS broth. The organisms appear as gram-positive cocci in pairs, clusters, and tetrads, and they are catalase-negative. Growth occurs over a temperature range of 25° to 50°C. On plates, they resemble viridans streptococci in their colony morphology. They may be confused with group D streptococci or enterococci because they are positive for bile-esculin hydrolysis, they possess the Lancefield group D antigen, and some strains grow in the presence of 6.5% NaCl. Pediococci are not PYR-positive.

There are two species in the genus *Gemella*—*G. themolysans* and *G. morbillorum.*[48] As mentioned previously, *G. morbillorum* was formerly called *Streptococcus morbillorum* and was classified with the viridans streptococci. *Gemella* species are α-hemolytic or nonhemolytic on sheep blood agar and resemble colonies of viridans streptococci. Because of their thin cell walls, these bacteria easily decolorize on Gram staining and may appear as gram-negative cocci in pairs, tetrads, clusters, and short chains. The individual cells in these arrangements may show considerable variations in size. Because of limited numbers of clinical isolates, the performance of kit systems for identifying these bacteria cannot be assessed critically, although they are included in the data bases of both the Vitek GPI card and the API Rapid STREP system.

REFERENCES

1. Arditi M, Shulman ST, Davis AT, et al. Group C beta-hemolytic streptococcal infections in children: nine pediatric cases and review. Rev Infect Dis 1989;11:34–45.
2. Barnham M, Thornton TJ, Lange K. Nephritis caused by *Streptococcus zooepidemicus* (Lancefield group C). Lancet 1983;1:945–946.
3. Bignardi GE, Issacs D. Neonatal meningitis due to *Streptococcus mitis.* Rev Infect Dis 1989;11:86–88.
4. Bisno AL. *Streptococcus pyogenes.* In: Mandell GL, Douglas RG Jr, Bennett JE, eds. Principles and practice of infectious diseases. 3rd ed. New York, Churchill Livingstone, 1990:1519–1528.
5. Bixler-Forell E, Martin WJ, Moody MD. Clinical evaluation of the improved Streptex method for grouping streptococci. Diagn Microbiol Infect Dis 1984;2:113–118.
6. Bouvet A, Grimont F, Grimont PAD. *Streptococcus defectivus* sp. nov. and *Streptococcus adjacens* sp. nov., nutritionally variant streptococci from human clinical specimens. Int J Syst Bacteriol 1989;39:290–294.
7. Buu-hoi A, Branger C, Acar JF. Vancomycin-resistant streptococci or *Leuconostoc* sp. Antimicrob Agents Chemother 1985;28:458–460.
8. Carey RB. Vitamin B6–dependent *Streptococcus mitior (mitis).* J Infect Dis 1975;131:722–726.
9. Carey RB, Gross KC, Roberts RB. Vitamin B6–dependent *Streptococcus mitior (mitis)* isolated from

patients with systemic infections. J Infect Dis 1975;131:722–726.

10. Chenoweth C, Schaberg D. The epidemiology of enterococci. Eur J Clin Microbiol Infect Dis 1990;9:80–89.

11. Cone LA, Woodard DR, Schlievert PM, et al. Clinical and bacteriologic observations of a toxic shock–like syndrome due to *Streptococcus pyogenes*. N Engl J Med 1987;317:146–149.

12. Coykendall AL. Classification and identification of the viridans streptococci. Clin Microbiol Rev 1989;2:315–328.

13. Daly JA, Seskin KC. Evaluation of rapid, commercial latex techniques for serogrouping beta-hemolytic streptococci. J Clin Microbiol 1988;26: 2429–2431.

14. Darling CL. Standardization and evaluation of the CAMP reaction for the prompt, presumptive identification of *Streptococcus agalactiae* (Lancefield group B) in clinical material. J Clin Microbiol 1975;1:171–174.

15. DeMan JC, Rogosa M, Sharpe ME. A medium for the cultivation of lactobacilli. J Appl Microbiol 1960;23:130–135.

16. Dykstra MA, McLaughlin JC, Bartlett RC. Comparison of media and techniques for detection of group A streptococci in throat swab specimens. J Clin Microbiol 1979;9:236–238.

17. Edwards MS, Baker CJ. *Streptococcus agalactiae* (group B streptococcus). In: Mandell GL, Douglas RG Jr, Bennett JE, eds. Principles and practice of infectious diseases. 3rd ed. New York, Churchill Livingstone, 1990:1554–1563.

18. Eliopoulos GM, Eliopoulos CT. Therapy of enterococcal infections. Eur J Clin Microbiol Infect Dis 1990;9:118–126.

19. Ezaki T, Facklam RR, Takeuchi N, et al. Genetic relatedness between the type strain of *Streptococcus anginosus* and minute colony forming beta hemolytic streptococci carrying different Lancefield grouping antigens. Int J Syst Bacteriol 1986;36: 345–347.

20. Facklam RR, Collins MD. Identification of *Enterococcus* species isolated from human infections by a conventional test scheme. J Clin Microbiol 1989; 27:731–734.

21. Facklam RR, Cooksey RC, Wortham EC. Evaluation of commercial latex agglutination reagents for grouping streptococci. J Clin Microbiol 1979;10: 641–646.

22. Facklam R, Hollis D, Collins MD. Identification of gram-positive coccal and coccobacillary vancomycin-resistant bacteria. J Clin Microbiol 1989;27:724–730.

23. Facklam RR, Rhoden DL, Smith PB. Evaluation of the Rapid Strep system for identification of clinical isolates of *Streptococcus* species. J Clin Microbiol 1984;20:894–898.

24. Facklam RR, Thacker LG, Fox B, et al. Presumptive identification of streptococci with a new test system. J Clin Microbiol 1982;15:987–990.

25. Fertally SS, Facklam R. Comparison of physiologic tests used to identify non-beta-hemolytic aerococci, enterococci, and streptococci. J Clin Microbiol 1987;25:1845–1850.

26. French GL, Talsania H, Charlton JRH, et al. A physiological classification of the viridans streptococci by use of the API-20 STREP system. J Med Microbiol 1989;28:275–286.

27. Gallis HA. Viridans and beta-hemolytic (nongroup A, B, and D) streptococci. In: Mandell GL, Douglas RG Jr, Bennett JE, eds. Principles and practice of infectious diseases. 3rd ed. New York, Churchill Livingstone, 1990:1563–1572.

28. Gullberg RM, Homann SR, Phair JP. Enterococcal bacteremia: analysis of 75 episodes. Rev Infect Dis 1989;11:74–85.

29. Hamilton JR. Comparison of Meritec-Strep with Streptex for direct colony grouping of beta-hemolytic streptococci from primary isolation and subculture plates. J Clin Microbiol 1988;26:692–695.

30. Hoffmann S. Detection of group A streptococcal antigen from throat swabs with five diagnostic kits in general practice. Diagn Microbiol Infect Dis 1990;13:209–215.

31. Hwang M, Ederer GM. Rapid hippurate hydrolysis method for presumptive identification of group B streptococci. J Clin Microbiol 1975;1: 114–115.

32. Isenberg HD, Vellozi EM, Shapiro J, et al. Clinical laboratory challenges in the recognition of *Leuconostoc* spp. J Clin Microbiol 1988;26:479–484.

33. Jones DE, Friedl EM, Kanarek KS, et al. Rapid identification of pregnant women heavily colonized with group B streptococci. J Clin Microbiol 1983;18:558–560.

34. Klein JO. The epidemiology of pneumococcal disease in infants and children. Rev Infect Dis 1981; 3:246–253.

35. Klein RS, Recca RA, Catalano MT, et al. Association of *Streptococcus bovis* with carcinoma of the colon. N Engl J Med 1977;296:800–802.

36. Kuskie MR. Group C streptococcal infections. Pediatr Infect Dis J 1987;6:856–859.

37. Lancefield RC. A serological differentiation of human and other groups of beta-hemolytic streptococci. J Exp Med 1933;57:571–595.

38. Lewis CM, Zervos MJ. Clinical manifestations of enterococcal infection. Eur J Clin Microbiol Infect Dis 1990;9:111–117.

39. Lieberman JM, Greenberg DP, Ward JI. Prevention of bacterial meningitis: vaccines and chemo-

prophylaxis. Infect Dis Clin North Am 1990;4: 703–729.

40. Ludwig W, Weizenegger M, Kilpper-Balz R, et al. Phylogenetic relationships of anaerobic streptococci. Int J Syst Bacteriol 1988;38:15–18.

41. Mufson MA. *Streptococcus pneumoniae*. In: Mandell GL, Douglas RG Jr, Bennett JE, eds. Principles and practice of infectious diseases. 3rd ed. New York, Churchill Livingstone, 1990:1539–1550.

42. Murray BE. The life and times of the enterococcus. Clin Microbiol Rev 1990;3:46–65.

43. Murray HW, Gross KC, Masur H, et al. Serious infections caused by *Streptococcus milleri*. Am J Med 1978;64:759–764.

44. Nachamkin I, Dalton HP. The clinical significance of streptococcal species isolated from cerebrospinal fluid. Am J Clin Pathol 1983;79:195–199.

45. Ortel TL, Kallianos J, Gallis HA. Group C streptococcal arthritis: case report and review. Rev Infect Dis 1990;12:829–837.

46. Patterson JE, Zervos MJ. High level gentamicin resistance in *Enterococcus*: microbiology, genetic basis, and epidemiology. Rev Infect Dis 1990;12: 644–652.

47. Radetsky M, Wheeler RC, Roe MH, et al. Comparative evaluation of kits for rapid diagnosis of group A streptococcal disease. Pediatr Infect Dis 1985;4:274–281.

48. Reyn A. Genus *Gemella* Berger 1960, 253[AL]. In: Sneath PHA, Mair NS, Sharpe ME, eds. Bergey's manual of systematic bacteriology. Baltimore, Williams & Wilkins, 1986;2:1081–1082.

49. Rudensky B, Isacsohn M. Beta hemolytic group C streptococci and pharyngitis. Rev Infect Dis 1989; 11:668.

50. Ruoff KL. Recent taxonomic changes in the genus *Enterococcus*. Eur J Clin Microbiol Infect Dis 1990;9:75–79.

51. Ruoff KL, Kunz LJ, Ferraro MJ. Occurrence of *Streptococcus milleri* among beta-hemolytic streptococci isolated from clinical specimens. J Clin Microbiol 1985;22:149–151.

52. Ruoff KL, Miller SI, Garner CV, et al. Bacteremia with *Streptococcus bovis* and *Streptococcus salivarius*: clinical correlates of more accurate identification of isolates. J Clin Microbiol 1989;27:305–308.

53. Saez-Llorens X, McCracken GH. Bacterial meningitis in neonates and children. Infect Dis Clin North Am 1990;4:623–644.

54. Salata RA, Lerner PI, Shlaes DM, et al. Infections due to Lancefield group C streptococci. Medicine (Balt) 1989;68:225–239.

55. Schiller NL, Roberts RB. Vitamin B$_6$ requirements of nutritionally variant *Streptococcus mitior*. J Clin Microbiol 1982;15:740–743.

56. Schleifer KH, Kilpper-Balz R. Transfer of *Streptococcus faecalis* and *Streptococcus faecium* to the genus *Enterococcus* nom. rev. as *Enterococcus faecalis* comb. nov. and *Enterococcus faecium* comb. nov. Int J Syst Bacteriol 1984;34:31–34.

57. Schleifer KH, Kilpper-Balz R. Molecular and chemotaxonomic approaches to the classification of streptococci, enterococci, and lactococci: a review. Syst Appl Microbiol 1987;10:1–9.

58. Stamm AM, Cobbs CG. Group C streptococcal pneumonia: report of a fatal case and review of the literature. Rev Infect Dis 1980;2:889–898.

59. Stevens DL, Tanner MH, Winship J, et al. Severe group A streptococcal infections associated with a toxic shock–like syndrome and scarlet fever toxin A. N Engl J Med 1989;321:1–7.

60. Swenson FJ, Rubin SJ. Clinical significance of viridans streptococci isolated from blood cultures. J Clin Microbiol 1982;15:725–727.

61. Watsky KL, Kollisch N, Densen P. Group G streptococcal bacteremia: the clinical experience at Boston University Medical Center and a critical review of the literature. Arch Intern Med 1985;145: 58–61.

62. Yajko DM, Lawrence J, Nassos P, et al. Clinical trial comparing bacitracin with Strep-A-Chek for accuracy and turnaround time in the presumptive identification of *Streptococcus pyogenes*. J Clin Microbiol 1986;24:431–434.

63. Yanelli B, Gurevich I, Schoch PE, et al. Group G streptococcal bacteremia. Clin Microbiol Newsl 1987;9:86–87.

64. You MS, Facklam RR. New test system for identification of *Aerococcus*, *Enterococcus*, and *Streptococcus*. J Clin Microbiol 1986;24:607–611.

10

The Aerobic Gram-Positive Bacilli

Clinical microbiologists must be able to isolate and must learn to recognize the various commonly encountered aerobic and facultatively anaerobic gram-positive bacilli. They must also become familiar with the key differential characteristics that differentiate the species of classic medical importance (Table 10-1) from those that are rarely, if ever, pathogenic for humans. Gram-positive bacilli should be identified to the species level when their presence in clinical specimens carries potential clinical significance. Thus, isolates from body fluids other than urine (eg, blood, cerebrospinal fluid, pleural fluid) should be identified. Species identifications, however, are required for isolates recovered from specimens properly selected and collected from infected sites of immunocompromised patients. These specimens frequently contain *Corynebacterium jeikeium* or other *Corynebacterium* species that may be resistant to multiple antibiotics.

The virulence of the gram-positive bacilli is highly variable. For example, *Bacillus anthracis* is one of the most highly pathogenic microorganisms known to humans (see Table 10-1). Most gram-positive bacilli isolated in hospital laboratories are of the genera *Bacillus*, *Corynebacterium*, and *Lactobacillus*. Many of these isolates (eg, *Bacillus cereus*, other *Bacillus* species, and various *Corynebacterium* species other than *C. diphtheriae*) are common laboratory contaminants. On the other hand, certain stains have the potential to be opportunistic pathogens, capable of producing disease only in persons with compromised host resistance related to underlying disorders. Thus, in the setting of an immunocompromised patient who has clinical signs of sepsis, the finding of a *Bacillus* species other than *B. anthracis* or a *Corynebacterium* species other than *C. diphtheriae* in two or more sets of positive blood cultures may be highly clinically significant rather than representative of contamination.

ENDOSPORE-FORMING AEROBIC OR FACULTATIVELY ANAEROBIC BACILLI

The Genus *Bacillus*

The genus *Bacillus*, the type genus of the family Bacillaceae, currently comprises more than 60 species of aerobic or facultatively anaerobic gram-positive bacilli that produce endospores (Color Plate 10-1*A*). They are ubiquitous, inhabiting soil,

water, and airborne dust. Some species may be part of the normal intestinal microbiota of humans and other animals.

Diseases Caused by *Bacillus* Species

Anthrax

Although anthrax is rare in the United States, principally because the disease has been controlled in animals, it remains enzootic in certain foreign countries (eg, Turkey, Iran, Pakistan, and Sudan).[43] Anthrax is primarily a disease of herbivorous animals and can be transmitted to humans by direct contact with certain animal products, principally wool and hair. Anthrax spores can remain infectious for decades. Spore contamination in these materials has been the source of isolated outbreaks and poses a continuing threat in different geographic regions as the infective material is spread between fields.[43] Human anthrax infections have usually been encountered as an occupational disease of veterinarians, agricultural workers, and others who handle animals and animal products.[75]

About 95% of human cases of anthrax are cutaneous infections, beginning 1 to 5 days after contact with the infected materials as a small, pruritic, nonpainful papule at the site of inoculation. The papule then develops into a hemorrhagic vesicle, which ultimately ruptures, leading to a slow-healing painless ulcer that is covered with a black eschar surrounded by edema. In contrast to the 20% mortality in untreated cutaneous anthrax, inhalation anthrax, a severe hemorrhagic mediastinal adenitis resulting from inhalation of anthrax spores, is almost always fatal. Meningitis may also complicate both cutaneous and inhalation forms of the disease. Fortunately, inhalation anthrax is more rare than cutaneous anthrax. A third form of the disease, gastrointestinal anthrax, has not been reported in the United States but is found in developing nations. Penicillin is usually the drug of choice for the treatment of anthrax; tetracycline is an acceptable alternative.

Bacillus cereus Food Poisoning

Food poisoning caused by *B. cereus*, a toxin-mediated disease, rather than infection, has been increasing in frequency in recent years.[8,73] Two toxins are responsible for clinical illness: an emetic toxin that causes vomiting and an enterotoxin that is associated with diarrhea. The emetic or vomiting

Table 10-1
Some Diseases of Humans Caused by, or Associated With, Aerobic and Facultatively Anaerobic Gram-Positive Rods

DISEASE	SPECIES OR GROUP OF ORGANISMS	MAJOR BODY SITES INVOLVED AND ASSOCIATED DISORDERS
Anthrax	*Bacillus anthracis*	Skin, rarely lungs, more rarely intestinal tract
Actinomycosis	*Actinomyces israelii* and *A. naeslundii* are the most common species. (They include obligate anaerobes and facultative anaerobes)	Cervicofacial, thoracic, intra-abdominal, and intrauterine
Actinomycetoma	*Actinomadura madurae, A. pelletieri, Nocardia asteroides, N. brasiliensis, Nocardiopsis dassonvillei, Streptomyces somaliensis*, others	Body surfaces, especially feet, legs, and upper extremities
Diphtheria	*Corynebacterium diphtheriae*	Infections localized to throat, occasionally nose, and rarely wounds. Local production of toxin causes systemic disease.
Endocarditis	*Corynebacterium jeikeium* and other "nondiphtheria" *Corynebacterium* species, *Listeria monocytogens*, "Nonanthrax" *Bacillus* species, *Lactobacillus* species, *Erysipelothrix rhusiopathiae, Kurthia bessonii, Oerskovia turbata*	Infection of the heart valves by gram-positive rods is rare and usually occurs on prosthetic valves or scarred (fibrotic) valves
Erysipeloid	*Erysipelothrix rhusiopathiae*	Usually skin (especially fingers or hand), but patient may also have septicemia, arthritis, or endocarditis
Food-borne gastroenteritis	*Bacillus cereus*	Gastrointestinal tract
Hypersensitivity pneumonitis	*Thermoactinomyces vulgaris, Micropolyspora faeni, Saccharomonospora viridis*	Lung
Listeriosis	*Listeria monocytogenes*	Food-borne gastroenteritis
		Asymptomatic carriers (intestinal)
		Septicemia (pregnant, newborn, and immunosuppressed patients)
		Granulomatosis infantiseptica (transplacental infection and abortion?)
		Meningitis (cerebritis, meningoencephalitis) Focal lesions (skin lesions, conjunctivitis, lymphadenitis, endocarditis, peritonitis, osteomyelitis, pneumonitis, brain abscess)
Leprosy	*Mycobacterium leprae*	Skin
Mycobacterioses (and tuberculosis)	Various species of *Mycobacterium*, including *M. tuberculosis, M. avium* complex, and others	Lungs, lymph nodes, skin, gastrointestinal tract
Nocardiosis	*Nocardia asteroides*; rarely *N. brasiliensis, N. caviae, N. farcinica*	Lungs most common; also, disseminated form may involve lung, central nervous system, kidney, and other sites. Superficial form involves skin, especially of extremities.
Miscellaneous infections	*Corynebacterium jeikeium*	Septicemia caused by multiple antibiotic–resistant organisms in immunocompromised patients, endocarditis, pneumonia, wound infections
	Corynebacterium group D2	Alkaline-encrusted cystitis, urinary tract infections with multiple antibiotic–resistant bacteria

(continued)

Table 10-1 (continued)

DISEASE	SPECIES OR GROUP OF ORGANISMS	MAJOR BODY SITES INVOLVED AND ASSOCIATED DISORDERS
Miscellaneous infections	"Corynebacterium ulcerans"	Pharyngitis following consumption of raw milk; diphtheria-like disease
	Corynebacterium pseudodiphtheriticum	Endocarditis (prosthetic valve), pneumonia, lung abscess, lymphadenopathy, urinary tract infections
	Corynebacterium aquaticum	Rare cases of meningitis, urinary tract infection, peritonitis, bacteremia
	Corynebacterium minutissimum	Rare cases of erythrasma (a superficial skin infection) and septicemia
	Arcanobacterium hemolyticum	Pharyngitis sometimes with diphtheria-like pseudomembranes, wound infections, septicemia
	Actinomyces pyogenes	Skin infections, septicemia, endocarditis, pneumonia
	Rhodococcus equi	Bronchopneumonia in horses; most infections in humans follow exposure to livestock; isolates commonly from patients with acquired immunodeficiency syndrome, pneumonia, bacteremia; osteomyelitis; wounds

syndrome has been associated with a heat-stable toxin of *B. cereus*. This syndrome clinically resembles staphylococcal food poisoning; symptoms of nausea and vomiting usually develop 1 to 6 hours after ingesting food that contains the toxin. Patients usually recover 6 to 24 hours after the onset of symptoms. Most outbreaks of the emetic syndrome have been associated with consuming fried rice prepared in Oriental restaurants.[11]

The diarrheal syndrome with symptoms of abdominal pain and watery diarrhea, caused by a heat-labile toxin, resembles *Clostridium perfringens* food poisoning clinically and has an average incubation time of 10 to 12 hours. Recovery of organisms in culture is usually within 12 hours after onset of symptoms. Implicated foods associated with the diarrheal syndrome have included poultry, cooked meats, mashed potatoes, various soups, and desserts.

Opportunistic Infections

Serious opportunistic infections, associated with significant morbidity and mortality, have been caused by a variety of *Bacillus* species, including septicemia, endocarditis, osteomyelitis, myonecrosis simulating clostridial gas gangrene (involving *B. cereus*),

rotizing fascitis, bronchopneumonia, necrotizing pneumonia, empyema, meningitis, peritonitis, and endophthalmitis.[7,26,54,67,74,75] In addition to *B. cereus*, the *Bacillus* species that may be clinically significant occasionally, and viewed as potential opportunistic pathogens, include *B. subtilis*, *B. sphaericus*, *B. megaterium*, *B. pumilus*, *B. circulans*, *B. licheniformis*, *B. mycoides*, *B. macerans*, *B. coagulans*, and *B. thuringiensis*. Life-threatening infections caused by these organisms commonly occur in a variety of conditions—parenteral drug abuse, operative procedures, hemodialysis, posttraumatic wounds, burns, immunosuppression, and other predisposing factors. Granulocytopenic bone marrow transplant and other organ transplant recipients, patients receiving corticosteroids, and patients being treated with various antineoplastic chemotherapeutic agents are examples of patients who appear to have the highest risk.

Clues that may aid in determining whether a given isolate is clinically significant include the following[48]:

1. Presence of *Bacillus* colonies (of the species that has questionable significance) on the streak lines of agar plate cultures (and not outside the streaks)
2. Isolation of the same species from two or more

blood culture specimens (collected from different venipuncture sites)

3. Repeated isolation of the identical species from other normally sterile sites
4. The presence of morphologic forms, suggestive of the organism that was isolated, along with acute inflammatory cells, in a direct smear of the specimen that was culture-positive
5. Clinical evidence of infection in a compromised patient, such as a parenteral drug-abuser or an immunosuppressed individual, that is not explained by infection with another etiologic agent

Therefore, close communication between the microbiologist and the clinician is required to determine the clinical significance of isolates of *Bacillus* species on a case-by-case basis.

Specimen Collection and Processing for Culture

Anthrax

If anthrax is suspected, the state public health laboratory and the Centers for Disease Control and Prevention (CDC) in Atlanta, Georgia (telephone: [404] 639-3311), should be notified immediately. Laboratory safety is of utmost importance when working with any material believed to contain *B. anthracis*.[43] All specimens and cultures should be processed and examined with great care in a biologic safety cabinet.[22] Every precaution should be taken to avoid the production of aerosols of the infected material. Laboratory personnel should wear protective coats or gowns, masks, and surgical gloves when processing the samples. This safety apparel should be autoclaved before it is reused, or it should be discarded. When the work is finished, all surfaces in the biologic safety cabinet and laboratory workbenches must be decontaminated with 5% hypochlorite or 5% phenol and all instruments used for processing the specimen must be autoclaved.

In cutaneous anthrax infections, specimens to collect include swab samples of the serous fluid of vesicles or of material beneath the edge of the black eschar, plus three sets of blood cultures (drawn before administration of antimicrobial agents). With inhalation anthrax, a sputum sample and blood cultures (also three sets) should be obtained. If gastrointestinal anthrax is suspected, gastric as-

pirates, feces, or food may be cultured, along with blood cultures.

Bacillus cereus Food Poisoning

Epidemiologically implicated food should be collected when *B. cereus* food poisoning is suspected. Sufficient specimen sample to perform all the laboratory studies required (eg, 25 to 50 g) should be collected. Refrigeration in a clean, sealed, leakproof container should be done if storage is required. The specimen may be shipped to the state health department laboratory or to the CDC (as per their instructions) after consultation with authorities at these agencies. Because *B. cereus* may be a commensal in the large intestine, stool specimens usually provide inadequate information to implicate *B. cereus* as the cause of food poisoning. Several outbreaks have been reported by the CDC.[11-13] The emetic form of the disease clinically resembles staphylococcal food poisoning; symptoms of nausea and vomiting usually develop 1 to 6 hours after ingesting food that contains the toxin. Patients usually recover 6 to 24 hours after the onset of symptoms.

Other *Bacillus* Species Infections

No special collection and handling procedures, beyond those recommended in Chapter 1, are required. These organisms usually grow well on the blood agar routinely used in clinical laboratories, and special procedures are not required.

Isolation and Identification of *Bacillus* Species

Bacillus anthracis

Bacillus anthracis cells are large, gram-positive bacilli, measuring 1 to 1.3 μm by 3 to 10 μm, with square or concave ends. Ovoid, subterminal endospores that do not cause any significant swelling of the cells may be observed. The spores appear as unstained areas within the bacterial cells in Gram-stained preparations.

Bacillus anthracis grows well on ordinary blood agar within 18 to 24 hours at 35°C. Typically, the colonies are flat and irregular, are 4 to 5 mm in diameter, and have a slightly undulate margin when grown on heart infusion blood agar. The organism is not hemolytic on sheep agar plate (SAP), a helpful feature in differentiating *B. anthracis* from α- or β-hemolytic isolates of other

Bacillus species. Under the dissecting microscope, numerous undulated outgrowths consisting of long filamentous chains of bacilli may be seen (so-called Medusa-head appearance).

The biochemical characteristics that aid in differentiating *B. anthracis* from other species of *Bacillus* are shown in Table 10-2.

Bacillus cereus and Other *Bacillus* Species

Colonies of *B. cereus*, after overnight growth on SAP or phenylethyl alcohol (PEA) plates, are frequently surrounded by a large zone of β-hemolysis. *B. cereus* colonies are variable in size, depending on growth conditions, but are often 3 to 8 mm in diameter, raised, and irregular, with a grayish to greenish frosted-glass appearance and undulate margins (see Color Plate 10-1*B*). Most strains do not grow on MacConkey agar; rare strains that do grow may be mistaken for a gram-negative *Bacillus* unless a Gram stain is performed to avoid this error. The key biochemical characteristics by which *B. cereus* can be suspected are the following:

- Motility-positive
- Lecithinase-positive
- Gelatin hydrolysis–positive
- Production of acid from:
  - Glucose
  - Maltose
  - Salicin

Colonies that are larger and have hairy, rhizoid, rootlike outgrowths from the colony margin, which spread over the surface of the agar, should suggest *B. mycoides* (formerly *B. cereus* var. *mycoides*), which is a nonmotile species. The colonies of many other *Bacillus* species encountered clinically are also commonly β-hemolytic; they tend to be large with a frosted-glass appearance initially, but may become opaque, and their colors vary.[33,69] Colonies of *B. licheniformis* are leathery, irregular, and flat with undulate or rhizoid edges (a case of sepsis has been reported by Sugar and McCloskey).[72] Some species form smooth colonies that resemble colonies of Enterobacteriaceae; others are mucoid and spreading, simulating *Pseudomonas aeruginosa*. Catalase is produced by most species, and sporulation is not inhibited by aerobic incubation, positive characteristics that aid in distinguishing *Bacillus* from *Clostridium* (see Chapter 11). Figure 10-1 is an algorithm that can facilitate the identification of the various *Bacillus* species using several biochemical characteristics that have been selected from published identification charts.

MORPHOLOGICALLY REGULAR NON–SPORE-FORMING RODS

The cells of organisms discussed under this subheading tend to be more regular in shape than the cells of bacteria discussed under the subheading Irregular or Coryneform Non–Spore-Forming Rods. Although three additional genera, *Brochothrix*, *Caryophanon*, and *Renibacterium*, are included in this category, and may be important to clinical microbiologists involved in environmental work (eg, as part of an epidemiologic investigation), they will not be discussed further here since they are rarely encountered in clinical laboratories. The discussion is limited to the genera *Listeria*, *Erysipelothrix*, *Lactobacillus*, and *Kurthia*.

Listeria Monocytogenes

Of the 10 species within the genus *Listeria*, only *L. monocytogenes* and *L. ivanovii* (formerly called *L. bulgarica* and *L. monocytogenes* serovar 4) are associated with disease in humans. *L. monocytogenes*, a known human pathogen, is the clinically important species most commonly encountered in clinical laboratories; the pathogenicity of *L. ivanovii* for humans is uncertain. *L. monocytogenes* is found in a wide variety of habitats, including the normal microbiota of healthy ferrets, chinchillas, and ruminants and the gastrointestinal tract of asymptomatic humans; environmental sources include river water, sewage, soil, silage, fertilizers, and decaying vegetation.[9,64,77] This bacterium has been isolated from the feces of many species of warm-blooded and cold-blooded animals, including fish, from milk and milk products (both unpasteurized and pasteurized) and from various plants and vegetables (eg, cabbage and coleslaw).[6,27,36,37,59–61] About 1% to 15% of healthy humans are asymptomatic intestinal carriers of *L. monocytogenes*.[9,63]

Epidemiologic and Clinical Aspects

Listeria monocytogenes causes meningoencephalitis in cattle and sheep and causes stillbirths in a variety

Table 10-2
Differentiation of *Listeria* and *Erysipelothrix* From Certain Other Organisms That May Be Similar Morphologically*

ORGANISM	CELLULAR MORPHOLOGY	STRICT AEROBE	β-HEMOLYSIS	CATALASE	MOTILITY	H₂S/TSI	ESCULIN	FERMENTATION OF			OTHER CHARACTERISTICS
								Glucose	Mannitol	Salicin	
Listeria monocytogenes	Short, thin, coccobacillary to diphtheroidal	−	+	+	+ (25°C)	−	+	+	−	+	"Umbrella" growth in stab culture; translucent colonies
Erysipelothrix rhusiopathiae	Same as above but may form long filaments	−	−	−	−	+	−	+	−	−	"Bottle brush" growth in stab culture
Lactobacillus species	Long, slender to short coccobacilli; chain formation common	−	−	−	−	−	−	+	+ or −	+ or −	"Good growth" on tomato juice agar
Kurthia species	Long, parallel chains of rods (0.8 to 1.2 mm wide × 2 to 4 mm long); old cultures contain coccoid cells formed by fragmentation of rods	+	−	+	+	− (or V)	−	−	−	−	"Bird-feather" growth in stab culture; rhizoid colonies
Corynebacterium species	Medium size, diphtheroidal	V	V	+	−	−	−	+	+	−	Opaque colonies
C. jeikeium (group JK)	Pleomorphic, short coccobacilli and long bacillary forms	−	−	+	−	−	−	+	−	−	Opaque colonies
Enterococcus species	Long to short chains of cocci; produce rodlike cells under some conditions	−	V	−	−	−	+				Both *L. monocytogenes* and *Enterococcus* species grow in 6.5% NaCl
Group B *Streptococcus*	Long to short chains of cocci; produce rodlike cells under some conditions	−	+	−	−	−	−				Both *L. monocytogenes* and group B streptococci may be CAMP + organisms that may be similar morphologically

+, 90% or more strains positive; V, 11%–89% strains positive; −, 1%–10% strains positive.

*Other bacteria that can be confused with those included in this table are Propionibacterium and Actinomyces species, because some of these organisms grow in 5% to 10% CO₂, or in air. Their identification is discussed in Chapter 11. The identification of obligate aerobes that produce long, branching filaments, such as Nocardia, Streptomyces, and Actinomadura species, is discussed in the last section of this chapter.

(Data from Hollis DG, Weaver RE. Gram-positive organisms: a guide to identification. Atlanta, Centers for Disease Control, 1981; Keddie RM, Shaw S. Kurthia: genus Kurthia Trevisan 1885, 92AL Nom. cons. Opin. 13 Jud. Comm. 1954, 152. In: Sneath PHA, Mair NS, Sharpe ME, Holt JG, eds. Bergey's manual of systematic bacteriology. Baltimore, Williams & Wilkins, 1986;2:1255–1258.)

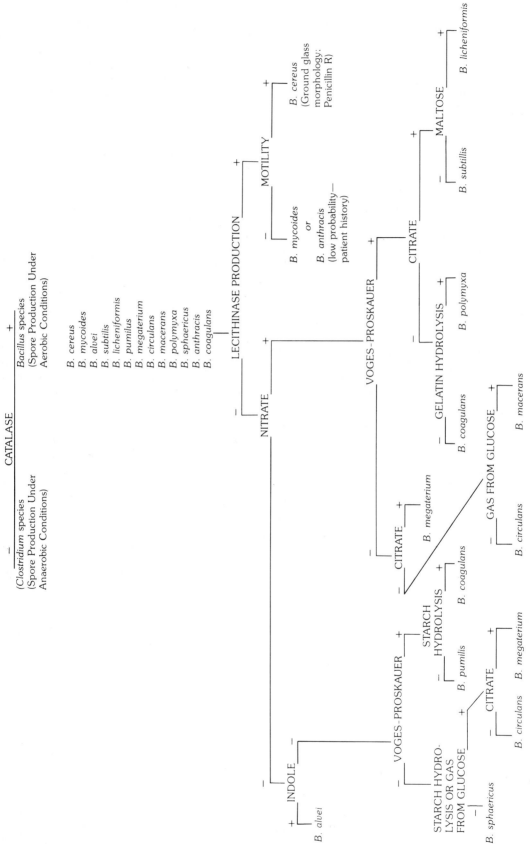

Figure 10-1. Flow chart for identification of *Bacillus* species.

of animals. The organism is not commonly encountered in hospital diagnostic microbiology laboratories. In humans, it most commonly causes infectious disease in pregnant women, stillbirths, and infections in neonates, immunocompromised patients, and elderly persons. During the 1980s several outbreaks of listeriosis were associated with the ingestion of commercial food products as well as noncommercially prepared foods.[27,48,59–61,63]

Other possible modes of transmission include one report of infection after direct contact with infected calves, resulting in skin infections in veterinarians.[10] The suggestion that *L. monocytogenes* can be transmitted sexually has not been substantiated.[63] Other possible sources of the organism have been reviewed elsewhere.[4,63]

Pregnant women and their fetuses are high on the list of persons developing listerosis. During pregnancy, infections have occurred more often in the third trimester. The pregnant patient usually has a transient illness with nonspecific, mild to moderate symptoms, including fever, headache, vomiting (and possibly other gastrointestinal complaints) and may mention that she has back pain. The symptoms and signs are often self-limiting, and the patient may not request treatment. Fetuses acquire their infection in utero from the mother, resulting in stillbirth, septicemia, or meningitis.[25,45] Ascending infection from direct extension from the vagina to the uterus remains another possibility suggested in the older literature.[4,36,59,60]

Among the other factors that have predisposed persons to listeriosis less frequently are alcoholism, cirrhosis, hemochromatosis (in which there is increased iron), ulcerative colitis, and asthma. Other immunologic conditions, including the acquired immunodeficiency syndrome, have been less commonly associated with listeriosis.[4,41] It is likely, but not proven, that bacteremia in the mother, resulting from *Listeria* enteritis (or local invasion of the intestinal epithelium) may extend to transplacental infection.

Collection, Transport, and Processing of Specimens for Culture

Cerebrospinal fluid, blood, amniotic fluid, placenta, genital tract specimens, stool specimens (which are preferred rather than rectal swabs), or other materials for culture are collected, transported, and processed as outlined in Chapter 1. Because *L. monocytogenes* may be difficult to isolate from certain clinical specimens, particularly from tissues removed at surgery or at autopsy, a cold enrichment technique has been recommended.[35] This involves mixing contaminated materials with trypticase soy broth or alternatively with tryptose broth, at a ratio of one part specimen with nine parts broth. The specimen–broth combination is then held at a low temperature (4°C) for several days to 2 months and is subcultured onto solid media at frequent intervals until recovery has been accomplished.

Microscopic Examination of Smear Preparations

Listeria monocytogenes is a non–spore-forming, short, gram-positive bacillus with cells varying from 0.4 to 0.5 μm by 1 to 2 μm. It is somewhat smaller than other species of aerobic gram-positive bacilli. The cells are coccobacillary; on occasion, diplobacilli occurring in short chains may be observed (see Color Plate 10-1*C*). If the Gram-stained preparation is over-decolorized, the bacterial cells of *L. monocytogenes* may appear gram-negative and can be confused with *Haemophilus* species. In other smear preparations, the organisms may assume the pleomorphic, palisade forms of diphtheroids.

Primary Isolation and Cultural Characteristics

On sheep blood agar (SAP) (or colistin and nalidixic acid [CNA] plates) incubated at 35°C for 24 hours in ambient air, the growth is generally light. Growth may also be obtained on SAP plates incubated in 5% to 10% CO_2 or anaerobically. The colonies are small, translucent, and gray, and most strains produce a narrow zone of β-hemolysis around the colonies (see Color Plate 10-1*D*). On occasion, this β-hemolysis may be confused with that produced by β-hemolytic streptococci (particularly group B streptococci) and a Gram stain should always be performed when this type of colony is recovered in cultures of cerebrospinal fluid, blood, or vaginal secretions. Additional characteristics by which *L. monocytogenes* may be identified are as follows:

- Catalase-positive
- Optimal motility at 25°C (subsurface umbrella pattern; see Color Plate 10-1*E*)

- Growth at 4°C
- Narrow zone of β-hemolysis on blood agar
- Production of acid from:
  - Glucose
  - Trehalose
  - Salicin
- Esculin hydrolysis–positive
- Hydrogen sulfide–negative

The results of these reactions are compared with *Erysipelothrix* and other gram-positive bacilli and are listed in Table 10-2.

Erysipelothrix rhusiopathiae

Erysipelothrix rhusiopathiae, the only species of this genus, is rarely encountered in most clinical laboratories. The organism is widely distributed in nature and has been isolated from soil, food, and water, presumably contaminated by infected animals. Various animal hosts have been found for this organism, including cattle, horses, dogs, rodents, poultry, other birds, several species of fish, and shellfish. It has been isolated from the gastrointestinal tracts of healthy swine; domestic pigs are believed to be the major reservoir.[56]

Human Diseases Caused by *Erusipelothrix rhusiopathiae*

In humans, the organism causes a cutaneous inflammatory disease, usually of the hands and fingers, called erysipeloid.[49] Erysipeloid is largely an occupational disease of persons who handle meat, poultry, fish, or crustaceans. The organism is believed to enter the skin through minor abrasions, scratches, or punctures, leading to raised, erythematous areas of inflammation of the hands and fingers. The lesions are painful and tend to spread peripherally while the central areas fade. The organism is able to survive for long periods of time outside the animal body in the soil and is not killed by salting, smoking, or pickling procedures used for the preservation of meats. In rare instances, severe systemic infection of humans occur with manifestations of septicemia and endocarditis.

The treatment and antimicrobial susceptibility of *E. rhusiopathiae* infection has been reviewed in more detail elsewhere.[32,49,56] Most isolates are highly susceptible to penicillin G (the drug of choice), ampicillin, methicillin/nafcillin, and cephalothin.

Collection and Processing of Clinical Specimens for Culture

In patients with clinical erysipeloid, it is best to obtain a biopsy through the full thickness of the infected skin at the advancing margin of the lesion. The skin surface should be first cleansed and disinfected with alcohol and povidone-iodine before the biopsy procedure. Blood specimens should be obtained in suspected cases of endocarditis or septicemia.

Selective media are not required for the isolation of the organism from skin or tissue aspirates, provided that the skin surface is properly decontaminated during collection. The organism grows well on routinely used blood agar media. Cutaneous biopsy specimens should be placed in an infusion broth containing 1% glucose and incubated aerobically under 5% to 10% CO_2 at 35°C. The broth is then subcultured to a routine blood agar plate at 24-hour intervals.

Laboratory Identification of *Erysipelothrix rhusiopathiae*

Both smooth and rough colonies develop on blood agar. The smooth colonies are smaller, measuring 0.5 to 1 mm in diameter, and are convex, circular, and transparent (see Color Plate 10-1*F*). The larger rough colonies show a matte surface with a fimbriated edge. Greenish discoloration of the blood medium adjacent to the colonies may be seen after prolonged incubation. Cells from smooth colonies typically appear as short, slender, straight, or slightly curved gram-positive bacilli, measuring 0.2 to 0.4 μm by 1 to 2.5 μm (see Color Plate 10-1*G*). There is also a tendency for the cells to form long filaments (4 to 15 μm long).

Erysipelothrix rhusiopathiae is nonmotile, does not produce catalase, and produces either α-hemolysis or no hemolysis on blood agar, which helps to distinguish it from *Listeria*. The important biochemical characteristics for the identification of *E. rhusiopathiae* are listed in Table 10-2. The ability of this organism to produce hydrogen sulfide in Kligler iron agar (KIA) or triple sugar iron (TSI) agar is a helpful feature for separating it from other gram-positive bacilli (see Color Plate 10-1*H*). The "bottle brush" extension laterally from the streak line in soft gelatin agar is also a helpful characteristic in identifying *E. rhusiopathiae* (see Color Plate 10-1*H*). *E. rhusiopathiae* is also among a small group of gram-positive organisms that is resistant to vancomycin, which underscores the need for prompt identification of gram-positive bacilli.

The Genus *Lactobacillus*

The genus *Lactobacillus* consists of non–spore-forming, gram-positive bacilli that are classified in the family Lactobacillaceae. The genus is defined in part by the metabolic products produced, and most species are homofermentative, that is, they form lactic acid from glucose as the major fermentation product. Heterofermentative species may be encountered that produce about 50% lactic acid and varying amounts of CO_2, acetic acid, and ethanol from glucose. Lactobacilli are widely distributed in nature and are ubiquitous in humans. They inhabit the mouth, gastrointestinal tract, vagina, and other sites.

Diseases Caused by Lactobacilli

Lactobacilli are commonly encountered in the clinical laboratory as an important component of the human indigenous flora, as commensals, or as isolates of little or doubtful significance. They have rarely been implicated in clinically significant bacteremia, pneumonia, endocarditis, meningitis, and focal or localized infections.[23,65]

Laboratory Identification of Lactobacilli

The lactobacilli are non–spore-forming, rod-shaped bacteria, varying from long and slender forms to short coccobacilli, at times producing short chains. Pleomorphic forms are at times encountered with some tendency to form palisades. Most species are nonmotile. The lactobacilli are generally grown on blood agar and chocolate agar media. Good growth is also obtained on Rogosa's selective tomato juice agar medium (LBS medium, Becton Dickinson Microbiology Systems, Cockeysville, MD), which has an acid *p*H. Additional characteristics for differentiating the lactobacilli from other species of gram-positive bacilli are shown in Table 10-2. The negative catalase reaction, the production of major quantities of lactic acid (as determined by gas–liquid chromatography), and the lack of lateral outgrowth from the stab line in a gelatin tube are among the most helpful differentiating features. The use of en-

riched thioglycolate broth is helpful to allow differentiation of lactobacilli from streptococci; the latter form chains of cocci. Most strains of lactobacilli are also resistant to vancomycim.[30]

The Genus *Kurthia*

Kurthia bessonii has been recovered from blood cultures and excised aortic valve tissue of a patient with endocarditis. As referred to by Pancoast and colleagues,[52] isolates of this species in the past have been from feces, a pilonidal cyst, sputum, and an eye. Members of this species are motile by peritrichous flagella, non–spore-forming, gram-positive, not acid-fast, obligately aerobic, catalase-positive, and oxidase-negative, and they neither reduce nitrate nor produce acid from carbohydrates (see Table 10-2).

IRREGULAR OR CORYNEFORM NON–SPORE-FORMING BACILLI

Corynebacterium Classification

The genus *Corynebacterium* includes a heterogenous group of bacteria of uncertain family affiliation. The type species is *C. diphtheriae*. Characteristics that members of this genus have in common include (1) gram-positive pleomorphic bacilli; (2) lack of endospore formation; (3) snapping when cells divide, which results in the resemblance to Chinese letters; (4) aerobic or facultatively anaerobic metabolism; (5) positive reaction for catalase; and (6) positive reaction for cytochrome oxidase.[5,18,69,78] Among several shifts in taxonomy and name changes among the corynebacteria that are of importance in clinical laboratory practice include shift of the organism formerly called *C. haemolyticum* to a new genus, *Arcanobacterium haemolyticum*[17]; *C. pyogenes* is now in the genus *Actinomyces*,[16] and organisms formerly classified as *C. equi* are currently in the genus *Rhodococcus* as *R. equi*.[31] The organisms formerly referred to as CDC group JK are now *Corynebacterium jeikeium*.[38]

Habitat

The corynebacteria are widely distributed in nature and are commonly found in the soil and water.

They reside on the skin and mucous membranes of man and other animals. Except for *C. diphtheriae*, *Corynebacterium* species are usually regarded as contaminants when recovered in the clinical laboratory. On the other hand, the repeated isolation of *Corynebacterium* species from blood, cerebrospinal fluid, and other body fluids that are normally sterile suggests that the organism may be the cause of an infectious process. *C. diphtheriae* infection usually involves the upper respiratory tract, but this species has also been recovered from wounds, the skin of infected persons, and the oropharynx of healthy carriers. This species is not found in animals.

Diseases Caused by *Corynebacterium* Species

DIPHTHERIA. Diphtheria is an acute, contagious, febrile illness caused by *C. diphtheriae*.[5] The disease is characterized by a combination of local inflammation with pseudomembrane formation in the oropharynx and damage to the heart and peripheral nerves caused by the action of a potent exotoxin. *C. diphtheriae* is spread primarily by convalescent and healthy carriers by means of the respiratory route. During infection, *C. diphtheriae* grows in the nasopharynx or elsewhere in the upper respiratory tract and elaborates an exotoxin that causes necrosis and superficial inflammation of the mucosa. A grayish pseudomembrane is formed, which is an exudate composed of neutrophils, necrotic epithelial cells, erythrocytes, and numerous bacteria embedded in a meshwork of fibrin. The organisms do not invade the submucosal tissue. The exotoxin produced locally in the throat is absorbed through the mucosa and is carried in the circulation to distant organs. The major sites of action of the toxin are the heart and peripheral nervous system, although other organs and tissues may be affected as well.

Diphtheria toxin is produced only by strains of *C. diphtheriae* that have been infected by a specific bacteriophage called β-phage. Nontoxigenic strains of *C. diphtheriae* are commonly isolated from carriers, particularly during a diphtheria outbreak. Such strains may cause pharyngitis but do not produce the systemic manifestations of diphtheria. Therefore, the laboratory confirmation of diphtheria includes not only recovery of the organism in culture but also animal testing for toxigenic effects. *C. ulcerans*, recovered on occasion from the throat of persons with a diphtheria-like disease can also elaborate diphtheria-like toxin. Some strains of *C. ulcerans* elaborate a second toxic substance that is not an exotoxin.

Selection, Collection, and Transport of Clinical Specimens for Culture. When diphtheria is suspected clinically, a cotton swab should be rubbed vigorously over any inflammatory lesion to obtain suitable material for laboratory examination. Nasopharyngeal specimens, not material from the anterior nares, should be submitted for culture in addition to the throat swab. If the swab cannot be transported immediately to the laboratory, the specimen should be inoculated directly on the Löffler's serum medium or tellurite medium, as described later. If the personnel working in a given laboratory are not experienced in the recovery and identification of *C. diphtheriae*, the specimens should be sent to a reference laboratory such as a state health department laboratory. Such specimens should be shipped dry in packets or tubes containing a desiccant such as silica gel.[18,78]

Cultural Characteristics of *C. diphtheriae*. Primary recovery of *C. diphtheriae* from clinical specimens requires the use of selective and nonselective culture media. As outlined in Figure 10-2, the following media are recommended:

- Blood agar plate (screen for the presence of group A, β-hemolytic streptococci, which can simulate diphtheria pharyngitis in some cases)
- A slant of Löffler's serum medium. Löffler's serum medium may be used both for the direct recovery of species of *Corynebacterium* from clinical specimens and for the subculture of colonies suspicious for *C. diphtheriae* to tellurite media. Growth on Löffler's medium is used to enhance the granule formation as seen in methylene blue stains to demonstrate the characteristic cellular morphology of *C. diphtheriae*.
- Medium containing potassium tellurite (Tinsdale agar or cystine-tellurite blood agar). Potassium tellurite inhibits the growth of most of the normal flora of the upper respiratory tract, allowing *C. diphtheriae* and other saprophytic corynebacteria to grow. All corynebacteria produce grayish black colonies on tellurite media after 24 to 48 hours of incubation at 35°C.

Tests for Toxigenicity. Nontoxigenic strains of *C. diphtheriae* may be carried in a person's throat or nasopharynx; therefore, for epidemiologic and

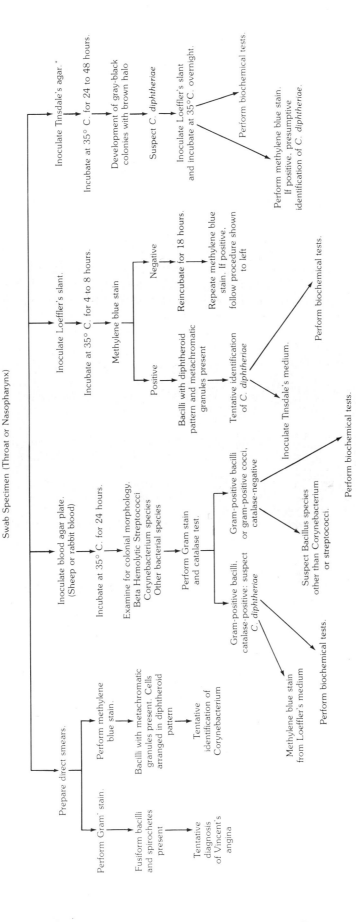

Swab Specimen (Throat or Nasopharynx)

Prepare direct smears.

Perform methylene blue stain.

Bacilli with metachromatic granules present. Cells arranged in diphtheroid pattern

Tentative identification of Corynebacterium

Perform Gram stain.

Fusiform bacilli and spirochetes present

Tentative diagnosis of Vincent's angina

Inoculate blood agar plate. (Sheep or rabbit blood)

Incubate at 35° C. for 24 hours.

Examine for colonial morphology. Beta Hemolytic Streptococci Corynebacterium species Other bacterial species

Perform Gram stain and catalase test.

Gram-positive bacilli. catalase-positive: suspect C. diphtheriae

Methylene blue stain from Loeffler's medium

Perform biochemical tests.

Gram-positive bacilli or gram-positive cocci, catalase-negative

Suspect Bacillus species other than Corynebacterium or streptococci.

Inoculate Tinsdale's medium.

Perform biochemical tests.

Inoculate Loeffler's slant.

Incubate at 35° C. for 4 to 8 hours.

Methylene blue stain

Positive

Bacilli with diphtheroid pattern and metachromatic granules present

Tentative identification of C. diphtheriae

Inoculate Tinsdale's medium.

Perform biochemical tests.

Negative

Reincubate for 18 hours.

Repeat methylene blue stain. If positive, follow procedure shown to left

Inoculate Tinsdale's agar. *

Incubate at 35° C. for 24 to 48 hours.

Development of gray-black colonies with brown halo

Suspect C. diphtheriae

Inoculate Loeffler's slant and incubate at 35°C. overnight.

Perform biochemical tests.

Perform methylene blue stain. If positive, presumptive identification of C. diphtheriae.

*Use within 3 days of preparation.

Figure 10-2. Schema for specimen processing in the laboratory diagnosis of diphtheria.

clinical reasons, the definitive laboratory identification of pathogenic strains must include tests for toxigenicity. In vivo and in vitro methods are available, and one or the other may be performed.[3,78]

Other *Corynebacterium* Species and Related Bacteria

Coryneform bacteria other than *C. diphtheriae* are frequently isolated from a variety of clinical specimens. They should be identified (see Tables 10-2 and 10-3) to the genus level and, if clinically relevant, to the species level when isolated in pure culture; when isolated from blood, cerebrospinal fluid, and other usually sterile body fluids; when isolated repeatedly from specimens; when isolated in high number (eg, more than 10,000 colony-forming unitsper milliliter of urine with no more than one other organism present); or when isolated as the predominant organism from a mixed infection.[15,18,19] In addition, yellow (possible *Oerskovia* species) or salmon-pink (possible *Rhodococcus* species) colonies and colonies with hemolysis (possible *Arcanobacterium haemolyticum*, *Actinomyces pyogenes* or *Listeria monocytogenes*) should be picked for identification. If Tables 10-2 and 10-3 are used for differentiation, biochemical tests should be done using enteric fermentation base containing Andrade or bromcresol purple indicator.[42] The addition of 1 to 2 drops of sterile rabbit serum to the biochemical test media is necessary to promote the activity of several species.

Commercial packaged kit systems are also available for the rapid differentiation of corynebacteria: Rapid Identification Method (RIM; Austin Biological Laboratories, Inc, Austin, TX), the API Rapid Coryne Strip (bioMérieux Vitek, Hazelwood, MO), and the Minitek System (Becton Dickinson Microbiology Systems, Cockeysville, MD).[29,34,40,66] Although these approaches showed promise for recognition of the JK group (now *C. jeikeium*) or the D-2 group isolates, and might be devised to provide some supplemental tests, it cannot be recommended that they be used to replace the conventional test system of Hollis and Weaver (see Table 10-3).

Corynebacterium jeikeium (Formerly CDC Group JK)

In 1976, four cases of life-threatening septicemia in immunocompromised patients caused by a cor-

yneform bacterium that was highly resistant to multiple antibiotics were reported. Subsequently, similar organisms were isolated from blood of oncology patients, caused bacteremia in 32 of 284 marrow transplant patients,[71] were seen in an outbreak setting,[55] and caused septicemia in even an immunocompetent patient.[21]

Corynebacterium jeikeium organisms are pleomorphic, nonmotile, non–spore-forming, gram-positive rods that vary from short coccobacilli to long bacillary forms. Colonies are punctate, smooth, and whitish on sheep blood agar after 18 to 24 hours of incubation in a 5% to 10% CO_2 incubator at 30°C. A negative test for nitrate reduction, negative urease test, and acid production from glucose, plus resistance to many antibiotics, are key characteristics of this organism. Further characteristics are given in Tables 10-2 and 10-3.

CDC *Corynebacterium* Group D-2

CDC *Corynebacterium* group D-2 is isolated from patients with alkaline-encrusted cystitis and other urinary tract infections.[1,62,70] Similar to *C. jeikeium*, the resistance of these organisms to multiple antimicrobial agents is noteworthy.

Corynebacterium ulcerans

Corynebacterium ulcerans produces mastitis in cattle. *C. ulcerans* infections have presented as a pharyngitis or as a diphtheria-like illness usually after ingestion of infected raw milk.[53] Pseudomembrane formation with toxic involvement of the central nervous system or heart similar to diphtheria has been reported,[53] caused by strains that also carry the β-phage or a related phage.

Corynebacterium pseudotuberculosis

Infections in humans are extremely rare. Most infections have occurred in persons who developed a suppurative granulomatous lymphadenitis after contact with animals. Cases of diphtheria caused by *C. pseudotuberculosis* have not been reported.

Corynebacterium xerosis

A common commensal that colonizes the normal human skin, nasopharynx and conjunctival sac, *C. xerosis* rarely causes infections, which include endo-

(*text continues on page 234*)

Table 10-3
Some Differential Characteristics of Coryneform Bacteria and Their Allies That May Be Encountered in Clinical Specimens

ORGANISM	CATA-LASE	MOTIL-ITY	NI-TRATE REDUC-TION	UREASE	GELATIN HYDRO-LYSIS	CARBOHY-DRATE FERMEN-TATION*	ACID FROM: GLU-COSE	Xy-lose	Mann-itol	Lac-tose	Suc-rose	Mal-tose	MAJOR ACID META-BOLIC PROD-UCTS	PYRA-ZIN-AMI-DASE	OTHER CHARACTER-ISTICS
C. diphtheriae	+	–	+(–)	–	–	+	+	–	–	–	–	+	AFP(L)	–	
C. ulcerans	+	–	–	+	–37°C +25°C	+	+	–	–	–	V	+		–	
C. xerosis	+	–	+	–	–	+	+	–	–	–	+	+		+	
C. bovis	+	–	–	–	–	+	+	–	–	–	–	–	AL	+	ONPG positive
C. minutissimum	+	–	–	–	–	+	+	–	–	–	+	+		+	
Arcanobacterium haemolyticum (C. haemolyticm)	–	–	–	–	–	+	+	–	–	+	V	+			β-hemolytic
Actinomyces pyogenes (C. pyogenes)	–	–	–	–	+	+	+	+	V	+	V	V	AL		β-hemolytic
C. renale	+	–	–	+	–	+	+	–	–	–	–	–	L	+	
C. striatum	+	–	+	–	–	+	+	–	–	–	+	–		+	

Table 10-3 (continued)

ORGANISM	CATA-LASE	MOTIL-ITY	NI-TRATE REDUC-TION	UREASE	GELATIN HYDRO-LYSIS	CARBOHY-DRATE FERMEN-TATION*	ACID FROM						MAJOR ACID META-BOLIC PROD-UCTS	PYRA-ZIN-AMI-DASE	OTHER CHARACTER-ISTICS
							GLU-COSE	Xy-lose	Mann-itol	Lac-tose	Suc-rose	Mal-tose			
C. pseudotuber-culosis	+	−	+(−)	+	−	+	+	−	−	−	−	+	AFP	−	
C. kutscheri	+	−	+	+	+	+	+	−	−	−	+	+	PL	+	
C. pseudodiph-theriticum	+	−	+	+	−	−	−	−	−	−	−	−		+	
C. aquaticum	+	+	−(+)	−	v	−	+d	v	v	v	+	+			
Rhodococcus equi (C. equi)	+	−	v	v	−	−	v	v	v	−	+	v			Salmon-pink colonies
C. matruchotii (Bacterionema ma-truchotii)	+	−	v	−	−	+	v	−	v	−	v	v			"Whip-han-dle" forms
Oerskovia turbata	+	+	v	v	+	+	+	+	−	v	+	+			Xanthine hy-drolysis—negative; yellow colonies
O. xanthineolytica	+	+	+	v	+	+	+	+	−	v	+	+			Xanthine hy-drolysis—positive; yel-low colonies

											Golden yellow pigment
Brevibacterium acetylicum	+	+	v	−	v	+	+	+	−	+	+
Rothia dentocariosa	−	+	−	+	v	+	+	−	−	+	+
Mycobacterium fortuitum	−	−	v	v	v	−	−	v	−	−	−
Corynebacterium jeikeium (group JK)	+*	−	−	−	−	+	+	−	−	v	ONPG-negative
Corynebacterium group D-2	+	+	+(−)	+	v	−	−	−	−	−	−
Corynebacterium group A-4	+	v	v	−	v	+	+	+	+	+	+
Corynebacterium group G-2	+	−	−	−	+	+	+	−	−	+	v
Corynebacterium Group E (aerotolerant *Bifidobacterium adolescentis?*)	−	−	−	−	−	+	+	−	v	+	+

+, positive reaction; −, negative reaction; A, acetic; F, formic, P, propionic, L, lactic acids; d, oxidative reaction; ONPG, ortho-nitrophenyl-β-D-galactopyranoside; reactions in parenthesis are reactions recorded for a minority of cultures.

*Carbohydrate fermentation tests performed in peptone-meat extract broth fermentation base.

[Data from Hollis DG, Weaver RE. Gram-positive organisms: a guide to identification. Atlanta, Centers for Disease Control, 1981; Reddy CA, Kao M. Value of acid metabolic products in identification of certain corynebacteria. J Clin Microbiol 1978; 7:428–433; Riley PS, Hollis DGH, Uttev GV, et al. Characterization and identification of 95 diphtheroid (group JK) cultures isolated from clinical specimens. J Clin Microbiol 1979; 9:418–424; Sulea IT, Pollice MC, Barksdale L. Pyrazine carboxylamidase activity in Corynebacterium. Int J System Bacteriol 1980;30:466–472; and Weaver RE, Tatum HW, Hollis DG. The identification of unusual pathogenic gram-negative bacteria. Atlanta, Centers for Disease Control, 1974:1–12.]

carditis, clinically significant bacteremia, wound infections, and pneumonia.[19]

Corynebacterium pseudodiphtheriticum

Corynebacterium pseudodiphtheriticum is commonly encountered in the human oropharynx as a member of the normal flora and has been a rare cause of prosthetic value endocarditis, lung abscess in a patient with acquired immunodeficiency syndrome–related complex, pneumonia, urinary tract infection in a kidney transplant patient, suppurative lymphadenopathy, septic arthritis, and vertebral osteomyelitis.[2,19,44,47,50]

Corynebacterium minutissimum

Corynebacterium minutissimum is thought to be the causative agent of erythrasma, a superficial skin infection characterized by small, brown-red macular areas between the toes, between the fingers, and in the axillae.[19] Three anecdotal cases of infections other than erythrasma in humans have been reported.

Corynebacterium striatum

Corynebacterium striatum is a normal inhabitant of the skin and the anterior nares. Only two cases of pleuropulmonary infection have been reported.[19]

Arcanobacterium haemolyticum (Formerly Corynebacterium haemolyticum)

Arcanobacterium haemolyticum is morphologically similar to *C. diphtheriae* and has been recovered from patients with symptomatic pharyngitis, occasionally accompanied by a cutaneous rash and sometimes with pseudomembranes on the pharynx and tonsils and submandibular lymphadenopathy.[17]

Gardnerella vaginalis

Gardnerella is gram-negative to weakly gram-positive. Because of the variable Gram stain reactions, the organism currently designated *Gardnerella vaginalis* was previously included in the genera *Corynebacterium* and *Haemophilus*. Culture of *G. vaginalis* is best accomplished using semiselective media, most commonly either human blood bilayer Tween agar (HBT agar) or "V" agar. Both are commercially available. Cultures usually take longer than 24 hours to grow, with tiny, β-hemolytic colonies appearing on one of the human blood–containing selective media after 48 to 72 hours of incubation. Presumptive identification of an unknown isolate may be sufficient in most clinical settings and can be made based on the typical cellular morphology described earlier, by finding small gram-variable coccobacilli in Gram stains, and by demonstrating the lack of oxidase and catalase reactivity. *G. vaginalis* is associated with bacterial vaginosis but can also be isolated from women without any signs or symptoms of infection. The infection can be suspected from the production of a discharge with an offensive odor. The observation in stained smears of vaginal secretions of large numbers of squamous epithelial cells heavily colonized with surface pleomorphic bacilli is one accepted method for making a presumptive diagnosis.

Another nonculture method for making a presumptive diagnosis is based on the liberation of a fishlike odor when a drop of 10% potassium hydroxide is added to the vaginal fluid from patients with *G. vaginalis* infections (the so-called whiff test). This reaction reflects high concentrations of amines found in the vaginal secretions of symptomatic women but not in those of normal women. The production of these amines at a more basic *p*H also explains why women with *G. vaginalis* vaginosis particularly complain of foul-smelling vaginal discharge after intercourse, since the seminal ejaculate is alkaline. In fact, *G. vaginalis* vaginosis is considered a sexually transmitted disease since the organism can be recovered in high concentrations from male sexual partners or females who incur reinfection after successful treatment of previous infections. The differential characteristics by which each of these *Corynebacterium* species can be identified in the laboratory are listed in Table 10-4.

NOCARDIOFORMS AND AEROBIC ACTINOMYCETES

The aerobic actinomycetes are commonly termed *nocardioform*, a term that is used simply for convenience and is as imprecise a term as *coryneform* or *diphtheroid*. *Nocardia* species serve as the point of reference for this group, which includes organisms belonging to several closely related genera, including *Streptomyces, Nocardiopsis, Actinomadura, Rhodococcus, Oerskovia,* and *Dermatophilus. Streptomyces* and *Actinomadura* species resemble *Nocardia* species in many cultural characteristics, but they differ in that they form a specialized aerial mycelium that produces spores, often in chains, rather than a substrate mycelium that undergoes fragmentation. Organisms in the genus *Nocardiopsis* produce a substrate mycelium that fragments on aging into bacillary and coccoid elements in addition to an aerial mycelium that produces long chains of coccoid spores. *Dermatophilus* species produce a rudimentary substrate mycelium that eventually becomes both longitudinally and transversely septate, ultimately fragmenting into motile "spores." There is overlap morphologically and phylogenetically with the coryneform bacteria and the anaerobic actinomycetes (eg, *Actinomyces, Propionibacterium,* and *Bifidobacterium*).

These organisms can be presumptively recognized in the laboratory because they form glabrous, tough, adherent, waxy or chalky colonies that grow after 3 days to 2 weeks of incubation. Tan, pink, orange, or gray pigments may be observed. The odor of a musty basement or freshly turned soil is another clue by which they can be recognized. The optimum temperature for growth is 30° to 36°C, both in the CO_2 incubator (as for the culture of mycobacteria) or in ambient air (as in the incubator used for fungal cultures). They grow well on culture media such as Löwenstein-Jensen and Middlebrook synthetic agars and on most fungal recovery media that are free of cyclohexamide. All species are gram-positive, although *Nocardia* species, in particular, tend to stain with a beaded, gram-variable pattern.

An overview of the physiologic and biochemical characteristics by which species identifications can be made is found in Table 10-4. Only *Nocardia,* Streptomyces, and *Rhodococcus* species are discussed here.

The Genus *Nocardia*

Epidemiologic, Clinical, and Pathologic Aspects

Nocardiosis is an infectious disease most commonly caused by *Nocardia asteroides* (over 90% of cases), less commonly by *N. brasiliensis* and *N.*

otitidiscaviarum (formerly *N. caviae*),[20,46,57,68] and even less frequently by *N. farcinica.* The nocardioforms and aerobic actinomycetes are widely distributed in terrestrial and aquatic ecosystems throughout the world. *N. asteroides* is found normally in soil, compost, and other forms of decaying vegetation. *N. brasiliensis,* which also has a worldwide distribution in soil, is present in many areas of North and South America (including the United States) but is highly endemic in parts of Brazil, Central America, and Mexico.[68] Because foods may be contaminated with *Nocardia* species, gastric cultures are not clinically relevant specimens to attempt to isolate *Nocardia* from patients. In addition, *N. asteroides* has been isolated from various diseased animals, including cattle and fish, and, as referred to by Rippon,[57] has been isolated from normal human skin.

Nocardia asteroides is an opportunistic pathogen in persons whose host defenses are compromised (eg, patients with leukemia, malignant lymphoma, solid tumors, asthma, bronchiectasis, tuberculosis, chronic obstructive pulmonary disease, hemochromatosis, ulcerative colitis, alcoholism, and cirrhosis; those receiving long-term corticosteroids and renal and cardiac transplant recipients seem to be particularly at risk).[20,57] Yet, many persons with nocardiosis have no known underlying impairment in their host defenses.[20,46]

Nocardiosis is an acute, subacute, or chronic disease that usually begins in the respiratory tract. It is acquired by inhalation of airborne conidia from the soil or other environmental sources, which results in a primary pneumonitis. Manifestations include fever, a cough productive of mucopurulent sputum, and nonresolving infiltrates of varying appearance on a chest radiograph. Progressive bronchopneumonia, localized infiltrates, diffuse infiltrates, extensive consolidation, single or multiple abscesses, pleural effusions, empyema, and sinus tracts with involvement of the chest wall are the various modes of infection reported. From the lungs, hematogenous (bloodstream) dissemination of the organisms occurs in about half of patients, and disseminated infection can involve virtually any organ.[20,46]

Traumatic implantation of the organism into the deep subcutaneous tissue may result in an indolent condition called *actinomycotic mycetoma,* a term that distinguishes this condition from the eumycotic ("true") mycetomas caused by certain species of

Table 10-4
Biochemical and Physiologic Tests for the Identification of Medically Important Aerobic Actinomycetes

ORGANISM	MODIFIED ACID FAST	LYSO-ZYME	DECOMPOSITION OF				UREASE	GELATIN HYDRO-LYSIS	ACID PRODUCED FROM			NITRATE REDUC-TION
			Casein	Tyrosine	Xanthine	Hypo-zanthine			Lactose	Xylose	Arabi-nose	
Nocardia asteroides	+	R	−	−	−	−	+	−	−	−	−	+
Nocardia brasiliensis	+	R	+	+	−	+	+	+	−	−	−	+
Nocardia otitidiscaviarum (N. caviae)	+	R	−	−	+	+	+	−	−	−	−	+
Nocardia transvaliensis	+	R	−	+	−	+	+	−	−	−	−	+
Nocardia coeliaca	+	S	−	V	+	+	+	NA	+	+	+	−
Actinomadura madurae	−	S	+	+	−	+	−	+	+	+	+	+
Actinomadura pelletieri	−	S	+	+	−	+	−	+	−	−	−	+
Streptomyces somaliensis	−	S	+	+	−	−	−	+	−	−	−	−
Streptomyces griseus	−	S	+	+	+	+	V	+	−	−	−	−
Streptomyces albus	−	S	+	+	+	+	+	+	−	−	−	−
Nocardiopsis dassonvillei	−	S	+	+	+	+	+	+	−	+	+	+
Streptomyces species	−	S	+	+	+	+	V	+	V	V	V	V

+, positive; −, negative; V, variable; R, resistant; S, susceptible; NA, not available.

"true" fungi. The lesions caused by these organisms may become extensive, consisting of suppurating abscesses, granulomas, and the formation of sinus tracts. Some patients may develop a lymphocutaneous syndrome that simulates sporotrichosis.[57] Granules or grains may be observed in the purulent exudate, the size, shape, and color of which may suggest a specific etiology.

The delicate, branching, filamentous rods of *Nocardia* species can be seen with Gram stain and with modified Kinyoun acid-fast stain (in which destaining is done with 1% aqueous hydrogen sulfate, instead of the usual acid alcohol that is used in the Ziehl-Neelsen method). The Fite-Ferraco acid-fast stain is recommended for paraffin sections.[24] With these stains, *Nocardia* are acid-fast (or "partially acid-fast"). *Mycobacterium* species are strongly acid-fast, while *Actinomyces israeli* and the other anaerobic actinomycetes are not acid-fast (see Table 10-4).

Primary Isolation of *Nocardia* and Other Aerobic Actinomycetes

Nocardia asteroides and other *Nocardia* species are aerobic organisms that grow on a variety of ordinary media, including blood agar, brain heart infusion agar, and Sabouraud dextrose agar without antibiotics and antifungal agents (eg, they are inhibited by chloramphenicol, penicillin, streptomycin, and cyclohexamide). *N. asteroides* grows well at 25°C, at 35° to 37°C, and at 42° to 45°C. Incubation at 42° to 45°C permits growth of *N. asteroides* while many other bacteria will be inhibited. Growth on ordinary laboratory media may take from 4 days to 6 weeks of incubation. Growth is enhanced by incubation in 10% CO_2.

Nocardia asteroides can survive the usual N-acetylcysteine digestion procedure (without sodium hydroxide) that is done on sputum or bronchial washings.[51] Cultures of sputum and bronchial washings for isolation of *Nocardia* (when nocardiosis is suspected) should be done both before and after the digestion procedure. Some strains grow well on the media that are used for primary isolation of mycobacteria (eg, Middlebrook 7H1O or Löwenstein-Jensen media).

Laboratory Identification of *Nocardia* Species

The laboratory identification of *Nocardia* species can be made using the following criteria. The typical colonies of *Nocardia* are dry to chalky, usually heaped or folded, and range from yellow to gray-white. *Nocardia* species are more commonly some shade of yellow or orange. The colonies usually have a pungent musty-basement odor. A Gram stain of a portion of a suspected colony shows delicate, branching filaments no more than 1 μm in diameter. *Nocardia* species are partially acid-fast (ie, they do not decolorize when treated with 1% hydrogen sulfate or 3% hydrochloric acid instead of the more active acid-alcohol decolorizer used in the Ziehl-Neelsen or Kinyoun stains), whereas the related species mentioned earlier are not partially acid-fast. Emerging technologies for the direct detection of *Nocardia* species in clinical specimens include enzyme immunoassay techniques and the use of monoclonal antibodies and recombinant DNA probes.[3]

Growth in the presence of lysozyme is useful in identifying *Nocardia* species (see Table 10-4), particularly those strains that are not acid-fast. All *Nocardia* species are resistant to lysozyme and will grow in its presence in 5 to 20 days. A control tube of glycerol broth without lysozyme and both positive and negative controls should be performed with each test.

HYDROLYSIS OF CASEIN, XANTHINE, AND TYROSINE AGARS. The differential ability of the various *Nocardia* species, and the related aerobic actinomycetes to hydrolyze casein, xanthine, and tyrosine is one of the mainstays of making identifications in most clinical laboratories. The patterns of reactions are shown in Table 10-5. The differential plates are inoculated with the unknown organism for up to 2 weeks at 30°C and observed for hydrolysis (clearing of the medium around the colonies).

The Genus *Streptomyces*

Streptomyces species are environmental organisms of the soil that have significant importance in the industrial and pharmaceutical fields. A few species cause human infections and have been isolated from sputum, other respiratory tract specimens, superficial wounds, skin, and other specimens. *S. somaliensis* causes actinomycotic mycetoma, primarily in natives of Somalia, Kenya, Senegal, Chad, India, and Mexico. Grains from mycetoma lesions are large (2 to 4 mm) and yellow-brown. *S. griseus*, an organism causing subcutaneous mycetomas in felines and dolphins, also has been recovered from human mycetomas.

Streptomyces species typically form dry, chalky gray-white colonies that emit a pungent musty-basement odor. Beaded, branching, gram-positive filaments are observed microscopically, but the partial acid-fast stain is negative. *Streptomyces* species are sensitive to lysozyme, typically rapidly hydrolyze casein (see Table 10-4), and more slowly hydrolyze xanthine and tyrosine. In contrast to *Nocardia* species, *Streptomyces* species do not reduce nitrate to nitrites.

The Genus *Rhodococcus*

Rhodococcus equi was previously known as *Corynebacterium equi*. It has also been called *Mycobacterium rhodochrous* and has been referred to as the rhodochrous complex.[31] The organism does not form aerial hyphae. On blood and chocolate agars the colonies are smooth and glistening, resembling *Klebsiella* species early on. They will grow on CNA agar but not on MacConkey agar. One clue to their identification is the appearance of a salmon-pink or coral pigment on prolonged incubation, particularly on chocolate agar at room temperature. On microscopic examination, diphtheroid gram-positive rods show traces of branching in early stages of growth. Like other *Rhodococcus* and *Nocardia* species, the rod-shaped cells fragment into coccoid cells.[31] Like *Nocardia* species, *Rhodococcus* species may be partially acid-fast using the modified Kinyoun stain. Detailed differential characteristics of *R. equi* and *R. aurantiacus* are listed in Table 10-4.

Rhodococcus equi is the cause of pulmonary disease in foals and other domestic animals. Since 1967, a few human infections have been reported. Human infections are believed to result from contact with animal carriers (eg, cattle, pig, horses, cattle manure), presumably through a respiratory route.[76] The rhodococci are widely distributed in soil and may account for the source of infection in persons who do not recall animal contacts. Human infections most commonly occur in the immunocompromised, primarily those with defects in cell-mediated immunity; in patients with lymphoma, Hodgkin's disease, leukemia, and the acquired immunodeficiency syndrome; and in recipients of organ transplants.[58,76] Hematogenous spread to distant organs occasionally occurs, and

the organism may be recovered from these isolated infected sites. Isolates are frequently resistant to penicillins and cephalosporins, while most strains are susceptible to erythromycin, chloramphenicol, vancomycin, and the aminoglycosides.

Susceptibility of *Nocardia* Species and Related Bacteria to Antimicrobial Agents

The drugs of choice for treatment of nocardiosis, even in immunosuppressed patients, are still the sulfonamides (eg, sulfadiazine, sulfisoxazole, and triple-sulfonamide combinations). Despite considerable initial enthusiasm about treatment with the trimethoprim-sulfamethoxazole combination, there have been reports of treatment failure and relapses, and trimethoprim-sulfamethoxazole may not be as effective as a single sulfonamide used alone.[46,57]

REFERENCES

1. Aguado JM, Ponte C, Soriano F. Bacteriuria with a multiply resistant species of *Corynebacterium* (*Corynebacterium* group D2): an unnoticed cause of urinary tract infection. J Infect Dis 1987;156:144–150.

2. Andavolu RH, Jagadha V, Lue Y, et al. Lung abscess involving *Corynebacterium pseudodiphtheriticum* in a patient with AIDS-related complex. NY State J Med 1986;86:594–596.

3. Angeles AM, Sugar AM. Rapid diagnosis of nocardiosis with an enzyme immunoassay. J Infect Dis 1987;155:292–296.

4. Armstrong D. *Listeria monocytogenes*. In: Mandell GL, Douglas RG Jr, Bennett JE, eds. Principles and practice of infectious diseases. 3rd ed. New York, Churchill Livingstone, 1990:1587–1593.

5. Barksdale L. *Corynebacterium diphtheriae* and its relatives. Bacteriol Rev 1970;34:378–422.

6. Barza M. Listeriosis and milk. N Engl J Med 1985; 312:438–440.

7. Bekemeyer WB, Zimmerman GA. Life-threatening complications associated with *Bacillus cereus* pneumonia. Am Rev Respir Dis 1985;131:466–469.

8. Berg R, Chmel H, Mayo J, Armstrong D. *Corynebacterium equi* infection complicating neoplastic disease. Am J Clin Pathol 1977;68:73–77.

9. Bojsen-Moller J. Human listeriosis: diagnostic, epidemiologic and clinical studies. Acta Pathol Microbiol Scand [B] (Suppl) 1972;229:72–92.

10. Cain DB, McCann VL. An unusual case of cutaneous listeriosis. J Clin Microbiol 1986;23:976–977.

11. Centers for Disease Control. *Bacillus cereus* — Maine. MMWR 1986;35:408–410.

12. Centers for Disease Control. CDC surveillance summaries. MMWR 1986;35(155).

13. Centers for Disease Control. CDC surveillance summaries. MMWR 1990;39(No. SS-1).

14. Centers for Disease Control. Listeriosis outbreak associated with Mexican-style cheese — California. MMWR 1985;34:357–359.

15. Clarridge JE, Weissfeld AS. Aerobic asporogenous gram-positive bacilli. Clin Microbiol Newsl 1984; 6:115–119.

16. Collins MD, Jones D. Reclassification of *Corynebacterium pyogenes* (Glage) in the genus *Actinomyces*, as *Actinomyces pyogenes* comb. nov. J Gen Microbiol 1982;128:901–903.

17. Collins MD, Jones D, Schofield GM. Reclassification of *Corynebacterium haemolyticum* (MacLean, Liebow and Rosenberg) in the genus *Arcanobacterium* gen. nov. as *Arcanobacterium haemolyticum* nom. rev., com. nov. J Gen Microbiol 1982;128: 1274–1281.

18. Coyle MB, Holis DB, Groman NB. *Corynebacterium* spp. and other coryneform organisms. In: Lennette EH, Balows lAW, Hausler WJ Jr, et al, eds. Manual of clinical microbiology. 4th ed. Washington, DC, American Society for Microbiology, 1985:193–204.

19. Coyle MB, Lipsky BA. Coryneform bacteria in infectious disease: clinical and laboratory aspects. Clin Microbiol Rev 1990;3:227–246.

20. Curry WA. Human nocardiosis: a clinical review with selected case reports. Arch Intern Med 1980; 140:818–826.

21. Dan J. *Corynebacterium* group JK septicemia: community-acquired infection in an apparently immunocompetent patient. Isr J Med Sci 1984;20: 1107–1108.

22. Doyle RJ, Keller KF, Ezzel JW. *Bacillus*. In: Lennette EH, Balows AW, Hausler WJ Jr, et al, eds. Manual of clinical microbiology. 4th ed. Washington, DC, American Society for Microbiology, 1985:211–215.

23. Du et Naude W, Swanepoel A, Bohmer RH, Bolding E. Endocarditis caused by *Lactobacillus casei* subspecies *rhamnosus*: a case report. S Afr Med J 1988;73:612–614.

24. Emmons CW, Binford CH, Utz JP, Kwon-Chung KJ. Medical mycology. 3rd ed. Philadelphia, Lea & Febiger, 1977.

25. Evans JR, Allen AC, Stinson DA, et al. Perinatal listeriosis: report of an outbreak. Pediatr Infect Dis 1985;4:237–241.

26. Farrar WE. Serious infections due to "non-pathogenic" organisms of the genus *Bacillus*: review of their status as pathogens. Am J Med 1963;34: 134–141.

27. Fleming DW, Cochi SL, MacDonald KL. Pasteurized milk as a vehicle of infection in an outbreak of listeriosis. N Engl J Med 1985;312: 404–407.

28. Fraser DT, Weld CB. The intracutaneous "virulence test" for *Corynebacterium diphtheriae*. Trans R Soc Can 1926;10(Section V):343–345.

29. Freney J, Duperron MT, Courteier C, Hansen W, Allard F, Boeufgras JM, Monget D, Fleurette J. Evaluation of API Coryne in comparsion with conventional methods for identifying Coryneform bacteria. J Clin Microbiol 1991;29:38–41.

30. Golledge C. Vancomycin-resistant lactobacilli. J Hosp Infect 1988;11:292–295.

31. Goodfellow M, Alderson G. The actinomycete genus *Rhodococcus*: a home for the *rhodocrous* complex. J Gen Microbiol 1977;108:99–122.

32. Gorby GL, Peacock JE Jr. *Erysipelothrix rhusiopathiae* endocarditis: microbiologic, epidemiologic, and clinical features of an occupational disease. Rev Infect Dis 1988;10:317–325.

33. Gordon RE, Haynes WC, Pang CN-N. The genus *Bacillus*. US Department of Agriculture, Agriculture Handbook No. 427, 1973.

34. Grasnick AE, Bruckner DA. Comparison of rapid identification method and conventional substrates for identification of *Corynebacterium* Group JK isolates. J Clin Microbiol 1987;25:1111–1112.

35. Gray NL, Killinger AH. *Listeria monocytogenes* and listeric infections. Bacteriol Rev 1966;30:309–381.

36. Hayes PS, Feeley JC, Graves LM, et al. Isolation of *Listeria monocytogenes* from raw milk. Appl Environ Microbiol 1986;51:438–440.

37. Ho JL, Shands KN, Friedland G, et al. An outbreak of type 4b *Listeria monocytogenes* infection involving patients from eight Boston hospitals. Arch Intern Med 1986;146:520–524.

38. Jackman PJH, Pitcher DG, Pelczynska S, Borman P. Classification of corynebacteria associated with endocarditis (group JK) as *Corynebacterium jeikeium* sp. nov. Syst Appl Microbiol 1987;9:83–90.

39. Keddie RM, Shaw SL. Genus *Kurthia* Trevisan 1885, 92[AL] Nom. cons. Opin. 12 Jed. Comm. 1954, 152 In: Sneath PHA, Mair NS, Sharpe Me, et al, eds. Bergey's manual of systematic bacteriology, vol 2. Baltimore, Williams & Wilkins, 1986:1255.

40. Kelly MC, Smith ID, Anstey RJ, Thornley JH, Rennie RP. Rapid identification of antibiotic-resistant corynebacteria with the API 20S system. J Clin Microbiol 1984;19:245–247.

41. Koziol K, Rielly KS, Bonin RA, et al. *Listeria monocytogenes* meningitis in AIDS. Can Med Assoc J 1986;135:43–44.

42. Krech T, Hollis DG. *Corynebacterium* and related organisms. In: Balows A, Hausler WJ Jr, Herrmann KL, Isenberg HD, Shadomy HJ, eds. Manual of clinical microbiology. 5th ed. Washington, DC, American Society for Microbiology, 1991: 277–286.

43. Laforce MF. *Bacillus anthracis* (anthrax). In: Mandell GL, Douglas RG Jr, Bennett JE, eds. Principles and practice of infectious diseases. 3rd ed. New York, Churchill Livingstone, 1990:1593–1595.

44. Larocco M, Robinson C, Robinson A. *Corynebacterium pseudodiphtheriticum* associated with suppurative lymphadenitis. Eur J Clin Microbiol 1987;6:79.

45. Lennon D, Lewis B, Mantell C, et al. Epidemic perinatal listeriosis. Pediatr Infect Dis 1984;3: 30–34.

46. Lerner PI. *Nocardia* species. In: Mandell GL, Douglas RG Jr, Bennett JE, eds. Principles and practice of infectious diseases. 3rd ed. New York, Churchill Livingstone, 1990:1926–1932.

47. Linder PS, Hardy DJ, Murphy TF. Endocarditis due to *Corynebacterium pseudodiphtheriticum*. NY State J Med 1986;86:102–104.

48. Linnan MJ, Mascola L, Lou XD, et al. Epidemic listeriosis associated with Mexican-style cheese. N Engl J Med 1988;319:823–828.

49. McClain JB. *Erysipelothrix rhusiopathiae*. In: Mandell GL, Douglas RG Jr, Bennett JE, eds. Principles and practice of infectious diseases. 3rd ed. New York, Churchill Livingstone, 1990:1599–1600.

50. Miller RA, Rompalo A, Coyle MB. *Corynebacterium pseudodiphtheriticum* pneumonia in an immunologically intact host. Diagn Microbiol Infect Dis 1986;4:165–171.

51. Murray PR, Neeren RL, Niles AC. Effect of decontamination procedures on recovery of *Nocardia* spp. J Clin Microbiol 1987;25:2010–2011.

52. Pancoast SJ, Ellner PD, Jahre HA, et al. Endocarditis due to *Kurthia bessonii*. Ann Intern Med 1979;90:936–937.

53. Pers C. Infection due to "*Corynebacterium ulcerans,*" producing diphtheria toxin. Acta Path Microbiol Immunol Scand 1987;95:361–362.

54. Poretz DM. Other *Bacillus* species. In: Mandell GL, Douglas RG Jr, Bennett JE, eds. Principles and practice of infectious diseases. 2nd ed. New York, John Wiley & Sons, 1985:1184.

55. Quinn JP, Arnow PM, Weil D, et al. Outbreak of JK diphtheroid infections associated with environmental contamination. J Clin Microbiol 1984;19: 668–671.

56. Reboli A, Farrar WE. *Erysipelothrix rhusiopathiae*: an occupational pathogen. Clin Microbiol Rev 1989;2:354–359.

57. Rippon JSW. Nocardosis. In: Medical mycology: the pathogenic fungi and the pathogenic actinomycetes. Philadelphia, WB Saunders, 1988: 53–68.

58. Sane DC, Durack DT. Infection with *Rhodococcus equi* in AIDS. N Engl J Med 1986;314:56–57.

59. Schlech WF. Listeriosis: new pieces to an old puzzle. Arch Intern Med 1986;146:459–460.

60. Schlech WF. New perspectives on the gastrointestinal mode of transmission in invasive *Listeria monocytogenes* infection. Clin Invest Med 1984;7: 321–324.

61. Schlech WF III, Lavinge PM, Bortolussi RA, et al. Epidemic listeriosis: evidence for transmission by food. N Engl J Med 1983;308:203–206.

62. Schoch PA, Ferragamo MA, Cunha BA. *Corynebacterium* group D2 pyelonephritis. Urology 1987;29: 66–67.

63. Schuchat A, Swaminathan B, Broome CV. Epidemiology of human listeriosis. Clin Microbiol Rev 1991;4:169–183.

64. Seeliger HPR, Jones D. Genus *Listeria* Pirie 1940, 383[AL]. In: Sneath PHA, Mair NS, Sharpe ME, et al, eds. Bergey's manual of systemic bacteriology. Baltimore, Williams & Wilkins, 1986:1235–1245.

65. Sharpe ME, Hill LR, LaPage SP. Pathogenic lactobacilii. J Med Microbiol 1973;6:281–286.

66. Slifkin M, Gil GM, Engwall C. Rapid identification of Group JK and other corynebacteria with the Minitek system. J Clin Microbiol 1986;24: 177–180.

67. Sliman R, Rehm S, Shales DS. Serious infections caused by *Bacillus* species. Medicine 1987;66: 218–223.

68. Smego RA, Gallis HA. The clinical spectrum of *Nocardia brasiliensis* infection in the United States. Rev Infect Dis 1984;6:164–180.

69. Sneath PHA. Endospore-forming gram-positive rods and cocci. In: Sneath PHA, Mair NS, Sharpe ME, eds. Bergey's manual of systematic bacteriology. Baltimore, Williams & Wilkins, 1986: 1104–1105.

70. Soriana F, Fernandez-Roblas R. Infections caused by antibiotic-resistant *Corynebacterium* group D2. Eur J Clin Microbiol Infect Dis 1988;7:337–341.

71. Stamm WE. Other corynebacteria. In: Mandell GL, Douglas RG Jr, Bennett JE, eds. Principles and practice of infectious diseases. 2nd ed. New York, John Wiley & Sons, 1985:1174–1177.

72. Sugar AM, McCloskey RV. *Bacillus licheniformis* sepsis. JAMA 1977;238:1180–1181.

73. Terranova W, Blake PA. *Bacillus cereus* food poisoning. N Engl J Med 1978;298:143–144.

74. Tuazon CU, Murray HW, Levy C, et al. Serious infections from *Bacillus* spp. JAMA 1979;241: 1137–1140.

75. Turnbull PCB, Kramer JM. *Bacillus*. In: Balows A, Hausler WJ Jr, Herrmann KL, Isenberg HD, Shadomy HJ, eds. Manual of clinical microbiology. 5th ed. Washington, DC, American Society for Microbiology, 1991:296–303.

76. Van Etta LL, Filice GA, Ferguson RM, et al. *Corynebacterium equi*: a review of 12 cases of human infection. Rev Infect Dis 1983;5:1012–1018.

77. Watkins J, Sleath KP. Isolation and enumeration of *L. monocytogenes* from sewage, sewage sludge, and river water. J Appl Bacteriol 1981;50:1–9.

78. Wiggins GL, Sottnek FO, Hermann G. Diphtheria and other corynebacterial infections. In: Balows A, Hausler WJ Jr, eds. Diagnostic procedures for bacterial, mycotic and parasitic infections. 6th ed. Washington, DC, American Public Health Association, 1981.

11

The Anaerobic Bacteria

RELATIONSHIPS OF BACTERIA TO OXYGEN

The *obligately anaerobic bacteria* are those bacteria that grow in the absence of free oxygen but fail to multiply in the presence of oxygen on the surface of nutritionally adequate solid media incubated in room air or in a CO_2 incubator (containing 5% to 10% CO_2 in air). Most anaerobes identified in the clinical laboratory grow initially on anaerobe blood agar, or on one of the selective anaerobic media, or in an enrichment broth incubated anaerobically, but not on blood agar or chocolate agar plates incubated aerobically or in a CO_2 incubator.

Obligate aerobes, including species of *Micrococcus* and *Pseudomonas*, require molecular oxygen as a terminal electron acceptor, resulting in the formation of water, and do not obtain energy by fermentative pathways. Molecular oxygen varies in its toxicity to different species of anaerobic bacteria and is not a terminal electron acceptor for the anaerobic bacteria. In general, the clinically important anaerobes obtain their energy through fermentative pathways, in which organic compounds such as organic acids, alcohols, and other products serve as final electron acceptors.

Anaerobes are divided into two major groups: the obligate anaerobes (defined previously) and the aerotolerant anaerobes. The obligate anaerobes have been further subdivided into two groups based on their ability to grow in the presence of or to tolerate oxygen. *Strict obligate anaerobes* are not capable of growth on agar surfaces exposed to O_2 levels above 0.5%. Atmospheric oxygen is highly toxic for these organisms for reasons that are not entirely known. Examples of these bacteria include *Clostridium haemolyticum*, and *C. novyi* type B. The *moderate obligate anaerobes* are bacteria that can grow when exposed to oxygen levels ranging from about 2% to 8% (average 3%). Examples of these

bacteria include the *Bacteroides fragilis* group, *Fusobacterium nucleatum*, and *Clostridium perfringens*.[62]

The term *aerotolerant anaerobe* describes those anaerobic bacteria that will show limited or scant growth on agar in room air or in a 5% to 10% CO_2 incubator but show good growth under anaerobic conditions. Examples of these bacteria include *Clostridium carnis*, *C. histolyticum*, and *C. tertium*. Most of the anaerobes isolated from properly selected and collected specimens fit into the moderate obligate anaerobe category. These organisms are more tolerant to the toxic effects of oxygen than the strict obligate anaerobes but are still killed by oxygen, unless anaerobic conditions are maintained during specimen collection and transport to the laboratory and during processing of specimens and isolation and identification.

The *facultative anaerobes* (eg, *Escherichia coli* and *Staphylococcus aureus*) grow under either aerobic or anaerobic conditions. They use oxygen as a terminal electron acceptor or, less efficiently, can obtain their energy through fermentation reactions under anaerobic conditions.[18]

The *microaerophiles* require oxygen as a terminal electron acceptor, yet do not grow on the surface of solid media in an aerobic incubator (21% O_2) and grow minimally if at all under anaerobic conditions. An example of a microaerophile is *Campylobacter jejuni*, which grows optimally in 5% O_2 (the incubation environment for recovering this organism in clinical laboratories usually contains 5% O_2, 10% CO_2, and 85% N_2).

Oxygen Tolerance

The strict obligate anaerobes are killed when exposed to atmospheric oxygen on the open laboratory bench for 10 minutes or longer. On the other hand, most of the moderate obligate anaerobes encountered in human infections tolerate exposure to oxygen for longer times. The reasons why anaerobes vary in their tolerance to oxygen are probably multiple, but one idea is that the oxygen tolerance of many moderate obligate anaerobes depends on their production of superoxide dismutase, catalase, and possibly peroxidase enzymes, which are protective against toxic oxygen reduction products, including the negatively charged superoxide radical (O_2^-), hydrogen peroxide (H_2O_2), free hydroxyl radicals (OH •), and other toxic oxygen reduction products.[18,81,95,101]

Oxidation-Reduction Potential

The oxidation-reduction potential (abbreviated "redox" potential or Eh) of a culture medium, expressed in millivolts, can be measured by using a platinum wire electrode, along with a standard reference electrode connected to a pH meter. Redox potential is affected by pH and is commonly expressed at pH 7 as Eh. Reducing agents, such as thioglycolate and L-cysteine may be added to anaerobic transport media and to certain culture media to help maintain reduced conditions (or a low Eh) in the medium. A positive redox potential (eg, as indicated by pink color of resazurin indicator in certain media or a blue color of methylene blue indicator in other media) means that the medium is oxidized.

What is the relative significance of the redox potential versus atmospheric oxygen in relation to survival and growth of anaerobic bacteria? The elimination of oxygen from the cultural environment, to avoid oxygen toxicity, is probably more important than the establishment of a low redox potential.[101] Accordingly, the rapid achievement and maintenance of a low oxygen tension, or the absence of oxygen, is an essential requirement for the successful cultivation of anaerobes in modern anaerobic systems (eg, anaerobic jars and glove boxes used for incubation of anaerobes in the clinical laboratory).

HABITATS

Anaerobic bacteria are widespread in soil, marshes, lake and river sediments, oceans, sewage, foods, and animals. In humans, anaerobic bacteria normally are prevalent in the oral cavity around the teeth; in the gastrointestinal tract, especially in the colon, where they outnumber coliforms by at least 1000:1; in the orifices of the genitourinary tract; and on the skin.[35,89] Most of these anaerobic habitats have both a low oxygen tension and reduced Eh resulting from the metabolic activity of microorganisms that consume oxygen through respiration.[18] If the oxygen is not replaced, anaerobic conditions are maintained in the environment.

A brief summary of commonly encountered anaerobes in the normal flora of the human body is given in the list that follows:

Oral Cavity and Upper Respiratory Passages
Pigmented *Prevotella* spp.; *Porphyromonas* spp.
Nonpigmented *Prevotella* spp. (especially *P. oralis*)
Bacteroides spp. (eg, *B. ureolyticus*)
Fusobacterium spp. (especially *F. nucleatum*)
Peptostreptococcus spp. (anaerobic streptococci)
Veillonella spp.
Actinomyces spp. and *Propionibacterium* spp.

Stomach (During Fasting)
Lactobacilli

Small Intestine (Proximal Portion)
Streptococci
Lactobacilli

Large Bowel (and Terminal Ileum)
Bacteroides fragilis group
Porphyromonas spp.
Fusobacterium spp.
Anaerobic cocci—many species
Clostridium spp.
Eubacterium spp.
Bifidobacterium spp.
Propionibacterium spp.

Genitourinary Tract: Vagina and Cervix
Pigmented *Prevotella* spp; *Porphyromonas* spp.
Nonpigmented *Prevotella*
Bacteroides spp.
Peptostreptococcus spp.
Clostridium spp.
Veillonella spp.
Lactobacillus
Eubacterium
Propionibacterium

Urethra (Male and Female)
Propionibacterium spp.
Peptostreptococcus spp.
Bacteroides (*Prevotella*)
Fusobacterium

Skin
Propionibacterium spp.
Peptostreptococcus spp.

CLASSIFICATION AND NOMENCLATURE

The anaerobes include essentially all morphologic forms of bacteria. Based on their ability to form spores and on the morphologic characteristics observed in Gram-stained preparations, the anaerobic bacteria are broadly classified as shown in Table 11-1. Several of the genera in this table are found only in nonpathogenic habitats and have not been shown to occur in diseases of humans. Most of these genera are not discussed further here.

HUMAN INFECTIONS

Anaerobic infections in humans and various animals can involve virtually any organ when conditions are suitable. Some of the more commonly involved sites are shown in Figure 11-1. Based on other reports in the literature, the relative incidence of anaerobes in infections is listed in Table 11-2.[14,32]

Most deep-seated abscesses and necrotizing lesions involving anaerobes are polymicrobial and may include obligate aerobes, facultative anaerobes, or microaerophiles as concomitant microorganisms.[32] These microorganisms, acting in concert with trauma, vascular stasis, or tissue necrosis, lower the oxygen tension and the oxidation-reduction potential in tissues, and provide favorable conditions for obligate anaerobes to multiply. Historically, infections and diseases involving anaerobes from exogenous sources are the ones that have been best known:

- *Clostridium difficile* hospital-acquired (nosocomial) diarrhea
- Food-borne botulism
- Infant botulism
- Wound botulism
- *Clostridium perfringens* gastroenteritis
- Myonecrosis (gas gangrene)
- Tetanus
- Crepitant cellulitis
- Benign superficial infections

- Infections after animal or human bites
- Septic abortion

Within the past few decades, however, endogenous anaerobic infections have become far more common. There are two probable explanations. One is that laboratory recovery of anaerobic bacteria has improved so that endogenous infections are no longer misdiagnosed or overlooked as they were in the past. The other is that a larger proportion of the patient population is receiving immunosuppressive drugs for malignancy and other disorders, resulting in compromised host resistance.[32] Primary anaerobic infections easily become established in areas of tissue damage, and bacteremia, metastatic spread of bacteria with formation of distant abscesses, and a progressive chain of events, sometimes resulting in a fatal outcome, may occur. The more common endogenous anaerobic infections are listed below:

- Abscess of any organ
- Actinomycosis
- Antibiotic-associated diarrhea and colitis
- Aspiration pneumonia
- Complications of appendicitis or cholecystitis
- Crepitant and noncrepitant cellulitis
- Clostridial myonecrosis
- Dental and periodontal infections
- Endocarditis
- Meningitis, usually after brain abscess
- Necrotizing pneumonia
- Osteomyelitis
- Otitis media
- Peritonitis
- Septic arthritis
- Sinusitis
- Subdural empyema
- Tetanus
- Thoracic empyema

It is essential to isolate and identify anaerobic bacteria because (1) these infections are associated with high morbidity and mortality, and (2) the treatment of the infection varies with the bacterial species involved. Antibiotic therapy for certain anaerobic infections is different from that used for many infections caused by aerobic or facultatively anaerobic bacteria.[33] Prompt surgical intervention, including debridement of necrotic tissue or amputation of a limb, may be of extreme importance,

Table 11-1
Classification of the Genera of Anaerobic Bacteria

Spores Formed

Gram-positive bacilli
*Clostridium**
Desulfotomaculum

Spores Not Formed

Gram-positive bacilli
Acetobacterium
*Actinomyces**
*Arcanobacterium**
*Bifidobacterium**
*Eubacterium**
Lachnospira
*Lactobacillus**
Methanobacterium
*Propionibacterium**

Gram-positive cocci
Coprococcus
Gemmiger
Peptococcus
*Peptostreptococcus**
Ruminococcus
Sarcina
*Staphylococcus**
*Streptococcus**
*Gemella**

Gram-negative bacilli (curved, spiral, and spirochete forms are included)
Acetivibrio
Anaerovibrio
Anaerorhabdus
Anaerobiospirillum
Anaerobacter
*Bacteroides**
*Bilophila**
Borrelia
Butyrivibrio†
Capnocytophaga
Capsularis
*Campylobacter**
Centipeda
Cristispira
Desulfobacter
Desulfobulbus

Gram-negative bacilli (*continued*)
Desulfococcus
Desulfosarcina
Desulfomonas
Desulfuromonas
Desulfovibrio
Dichelobacter
Fibrobacter
*Fusobacterium**
Helicobacter
Ilyobacter
Leptotrichia
Megamonas
Mitsuokella
*Mobiluncus**
Pelobacter
Pectinatus
*Prophyromonas**
*Prevotella**
Propionigenium
Propionispira
Rikenella
Roseburia
Ruminobacter
Sebaldella
Selenomonas
Serpula
Spirochaeta
Succinimonas
Succinivibrio
Tissierella
Treponema
Wolinella

Gram-negative cocci
Acidaminococcus
Megasphaera
*Veillonella**

In most properly collected clinical specimens, only the genera indicated with asterisks need to be considered by the clinical microbiologist. On rare occasions, however, serious illness may involve Anaerobiospirillum, Succinivibrio, Wolinella, or one of the other genera here that are not listed in Table 11-3.

†Butyrivibrio *is discussed with the gram-negatives in volume 1 and with the irregular non–spore-forming gram-positive anaerobic rods in volume 2 of* Bergey's. Butyrivibrio *cells stain either negative or weakly positive with the Gram stain, but the cell wall is structurally gram-positive.*

(Adapted and modified from Bergey's manual of systemic bacteriology[60,91] and from various recent publications [volumes 34 to 43 of the International Journal of Systemic Bacteriology contain numerous publications related to recent changes in anaerobe taxonomy]).

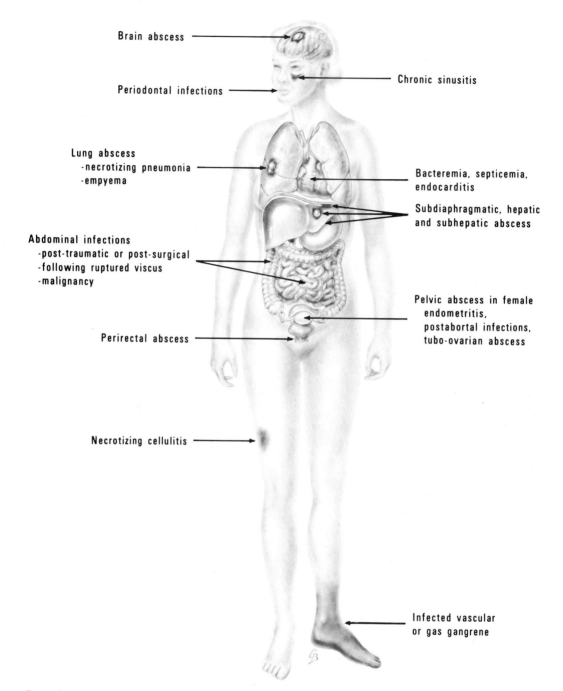

Figure 11-1. Common locations of infections involving anaerobic bacteria.

Table 11-2
Incidence of Anaerobes in Infections

TYPE OF INFECTION	INCIDENCE (%)
Aspiration pneumonia, lung abscess, necrotizing pneumonia	85–93
Bacteremia	9–20
Brain abscess	60–89
Dental infection, chronic sinusitis	50–100
Thoracic empyema	76
Intraabdominal/pelvic sepsis	60–100
Miscellaneous soft tissue infections	
Breast abscess	83
Postappendectomy and elective colon surgery wounds	79–95
Cutaneous abscesses	60
Nonclostridial crepitant cellulitis	75
Pilonidal sinus	73
Diabetic foot ulcers, infected diabetic gangrene	63–85
Urinary tract infection	1

(Modified from Finegold SM, George WL, eds. Anaerobic infections in humans. San Diego, CA, Academic Press, 1989; and Bartlett JG. Anaerobic bacteria: general concepts. In: Mandell GL, Douglas RB Jr, Bennett JE, eds. Principles and practices of infectious diseases. 3rd ed. New York, Churchill Livingstone, 1990: 1828–1842.)

particularly in cases of clostridial gas gangrene or in loculated abscesses in which antibiotics may be ineffective until the exudate is drained.

Before the mid 1960s, clostridial infections predominated; at present, 85% of anaerobes isolated from properly selected clinical specimens are accounted for by *Bacteroides*, *Prevotella*, *Porphyromonas*, *Fusobacterium*, *Peptostreptococcus* species, and the gram-positive, non–spore-forming bacilli (Table 11-3).

ISOLATION OF ANAEROBIC BACTERIA

The steps involved in the laboratory diagnosis of anaerobic infections are similar to those described in Chapter 1. It is particularly important that attention be paid to the proper selection, collection, and transport of clinical specimens for recovering anaerobic bacteria. The processing of specimens, selection of media, inoculation and incubation methods, and inspection of positive cultures are laboratory procedures that must be carefully qual-

ity controlled. Failure to perform any one step correctly may lead to erroneous results, thus creating the potential to supply misinformation to the physician.

Since Chapter 1 covers each of these steps, only a few comments pertaining specifically to the anaerobic bacteria are included here.

Selection of Specimens for Culture

With few exceptions, all materials collected from sites not harboring an indigenous flora, such as body fluids other than urine, exudates from deep abscesses, transtracheal aspirates or direct lung aspirates, and tissue biopsy specimens, should be cultured for anaerobic bacteria.[5] Since anaerobes normally inhabit the skin and mucous membranes as part of the normal indigenous flora, the specimens in the list in Table 11-4 are virtually always unacceptable for anaerobic culture because the results cannot be interpreted.

Collection and Transport of Specimens

Wounds, Abscesses, Body Fluids

When collecting specimens from mucous membranes or the skin, stringent precautions must be taken to decontaminate the surface properly. An alcohol scrub followed by 10% povidone-iodine (Betadine) is satisfactory provided that the povidone-iodine is allowed to remain on the skin for at least 2 minutes before the specimen is collected.

A needle and syringe should be used whenever possible for collecting specimens for anaerobic culture. Collection of swab specimens should be discouraged because they dry out and also because they expose anaerobes, if present, to ambient oxygen. Once collected, precautions should be taken to protect specimens from oxygen exposure through use of anaerobic transport containers (see Chapter 1) and to deliver them to the laboratory promptly.

Anaerobic Blood Cultures

Blood culture techniques should permit optimal recovery of obligate anaerobes as well as aerobes and facultative anaerobes. For many years, anaerobes were encountered in 9% to 20% of all positive

Table 11-3
Commonly Encountered and Medically Important Anaerobic Bacteria

Gram-Negative Anaerobic Bacilli

Bacteroides fragilis group (especially *B. fragilis* and *B. thetaiotaomicron*)*

Porphyromonas group (especially *P. asaccharlytica*)†

Prevotella group (especially *P. melaninogenica* and *P. intermedia*)‡

Prevotella oralis group (especially *P. oralis* and *P. veroralis*)

Prevotella bivia and *P. disiens*

Bacteroides ureolyticus group (*B. ureolyticus, B. gracilis,* and others)

Fusobacterium nucleatum, F. necrophorum, and "other" *Fusobacterium* species (eg, *F. naviforme, F. mortiferum, F. varium,* and *F. russii*)

Bilophila wadsworthia

Gram-Positive Cocci

Peptostreptococcus species (especially *P. magnus, P. asaccharolyticus, P. prevotii, P. anaerobius,* and *P. micros*)

Streptococcus species (especially *S. intermedius* ["microaerophilic," but not obligate anaerobes])

Gram-Positive Non–Spore-Forming Anaerobic Bacilli

Actinomyces species (especially *A. israelii, A. odontolyticus, A. naeslundii, A. meyeri,* and *A. viscosus*)

Propionibacterium acnes

Propionibacterium propionicum

Eubacterium lentum

Bifidobacterium dentium (formerly *B. eriksonii*)

Gram-Positive Spore-Forming Anaerobic Bacilli

Clostridium perfringens

C. ramosum

C. clostridioforme

C. difficile

C. septicum

C. sordellii

C. bifermentans

C. novyi

C. innocuum

C. tertium

C. sporogenes

C. botulinum

C. tetani

Includes B. fragilis, B. thetaiotaomicron, B. vulgatus, B. distasonis, B. ovatus, B. uniformis, B. caccae, and others.

†*Includes P. asaccharolytica, P. gingivalis, P. endodontalis, and others.*

‡*Includes P. melaninogenica, P. intermedia, P. corporis, and others.*

(Data from SD Allen and JA Siders, April 1993)

Table 11-4
Specimens That Should Not Be Cultured
for Anaerobic Bacteria

Throat or nasopharyngeal swabs

Gingival swabs

Sputum or bronchoscopic specimens

Gastric contents, small bowel contents, feces, rectal
swabs, colocutaneous fistulas, colostomy stomata*

Surfaces of decubitus ulcers, swab samples of encrusted
walls of abscesses, mucosal linings, and eschars

Material adjacent to skin or mucous membranes other
than the above that have not been properly
decontaminated

Voided urine

Vaginal or cervical swabs

*When indicated clinically, specimens from these sources may be
used for the diagnosis of botulism and for intestinal disease
caused by Clostridium difficile and C. perfringens.

---

blood culture sets at a number of medical centers. Recently, however, the percent of gram-positive cocci (eg, staphylococci, enterococci, streptococci), Enterobacteriaceae, and fungi has increased at Indiana University Hospitals, probably as a result of shifting antimicrobial treatments and greater proportions of tertiary care of immunocompromised patients. In addition, there has been a steady decline in blood cultures positive for *Propionibacterium acnes* at Indiana University Hospitals. Nonetheless, the numbers of patients with clinically significant anaerobic bacteremia at this institution have been relatively similar to those seen 10 years ago, in contrast to the experience at the Mayo Clinic,[22] Duke University (Reller B, personal communication, May 1991), and the University of Iowa Hospitals (Koontz F, personal communication, May 1991), where smaller percentages of anaerobes were isolated from blood cultures. Recently, Murray and colleagues[76] reviewed their experience with anaerobic bacteremia and reported also that anaerobic bacteremia is decreasing relative to bacteremia caused by nonanaerobic bacteria and fungi.

Direct Examination of Clinical Materials

Gross examination of specimens is particularly valuable in bringing to light the possible presence of anaerobes. A foul odor, purulent appearance of fluid specimens, and the presence of necrotic tissue and gas or sulfur granules are all valuable clues. For example, sulfur granules are clues to the diagnosis of actinomycosis (discussed in the latter part of this chapter).

The importance of *microscopic examination* of clinical specimens has been emphasized by several authors, and the information derived may give immediate presumptive evidence that anaerobes are present.[24,45,94] In preparing slides for Gram staining, methanol fixation is much better than traditional heat fixation. The background and cellular characteristics of the smear should be observed. The Gram reaction, the size, shape, and arrangement of bacteria, and the relative number of organisms present should be recorded. The presence of spores, their shape and position in the bacterial cell, and other distinctive morphologic features such as branching filaments, spherical bodies, pointed ends, and granular forms should be noted. Acridine orange stains are most worthwhile for detecting bacteria in blood cultures, cerebrospinal fluid, pleural fluid, joint fluid, and exudates.[60] The morphology of several anaerobes in stained preparations examined microscopically is illustrated in the photomicrographs included in Color Plates 11-1 through 11-3.

Selection and Use of Media

The media most commonly used for recovering anaerobes from specimens should include nonselective, selective, and enrichment types, as illustrated in Table 11-5. Other media may also be substituted; for example, colistin and nalidixic acid agar may be used instead of phenylethyl alcohol agar. Either paromomycin-vancomycin blood agar or kanamycin-vancomycin blood agar can be used for the selective isolation of the gram-negative non–spore-forming anaerobes. *Bacteroides* bile esculin agar is recommended in the *Wadsworth Anaerobic Bacteriology Manual* for the selection and presumptive identification of the *Bacteroides fragilis* group[94] and has also been found useful as a selective medium for *Bilophila wadsworthia*.[12] Results obtained with plating media formulations such as Schaedler, Columbia, *Brucella*, or others may not be entirely comparable to the morphology and growth characteristics of anaerobes seen on the

Table 11-5

Representative Media for Primary Isolation of Anaerobes From Clinical Specimens

MEDIUM*	MAJOR INGREDIENTS AND COMMENTS	PURPOSE
CDC anaerobe blood agar (AnBAP)	Trypticase soy agar base with 5% sheep blood; supplemented with yeast extract, hemin, vitamin K₁ and L-cystine for anaerobes requiring additional growth factors (eg, *Prevotella melaninogenica, Fusobacterium necrophorum,* and others). Additional media bases, including *Brucella,* brain–heart infusion, Schaedler, and Columbia blood agar support excellent growth of many anaerobes, but morphology and other characteristics tend to differ on these media.	Nonselective blood agar plating medium for primary isolation of essentially all types of anaerobes found in clinical materials.
Anaerobe phenylethyl-alcohol blood agar (PEA)	In addition to containing the same ingredients as the CDC anaerobe blood agar formulation above, the medium has phenylethyl alcohol (2.5 g/L). PEA inhibits the swarming of *Proteus* species and inhibits the growth of many other gram-negative facultatively anaerobic bacteria, including most Enterobacteriaceae. PEA is volatile. Plates should be tightly sealed in cellophane or plastic bags and stored at 4°C. A batch of plates that no longer inhibits the swarming of *Proteus* should be discarded, regardless of the expiration date.	PEA medium aids in selective isolation of anaerobes from infected materials containing a mixture of bacteria. It should support good growth of most gram-positive and gram-negative obligately anaerobic bacteria. Facultatively anaerobic gram-positive bacteria such as staphylococci, streptococci, *Bacillus* species, and coryneform bacteria also grow well on it.
Anaerobe kanamycin-vancomycin blood agar (KV)	Contains the same CDC anaerobe blood agar formulation as AnBAP above but, in addition, contains 100 mg/L of kanamycin and 7.5 mg/L of vancomycin. The kanamycin inhibits many (but not all) facultatively anaerobic gram-negative rods and the vancomycin inhibits gram-positive bacteria in general (including most gram-positive anaerobes and nonanaerobes). Vancomycin in this concentration can also inhibit the *Porphyromonas* species.	KV medium is useful for selective isolation of most *Bacteroides, Prevotella, Fusobacterium,* and *Veillonella* species from clinical specimens containing mixed aerobic and anerobic bacteria.
Anaerobe paromomycin-vancomycin laked blood agar (PV)	Laked PV medium is similar to the KV formulation above, except that 100 mg/L of paromomycin is substituted for the kanamycin. Also in PV, the blood is laked before it is added (by freezing and thawing the blood). Performance is similar to KV, except that the paromomycin may inhibit some additional facultative anerobes that are resistant to kanamycin such as some strains of *Klebsiella* species. Like KV agar, laked PV should inhibit growth of gram-positive organisms in general. The laked blood may aid in early recognition of pigmented *Prevotella.*	Laked PV is an excellent medium for selective primary isolation of organisms in the *Bacteroides fragilis* group, the pigmented and nonpigmented *Prevotella* species, *Fusobacterium nucleatum, F. necrophorum, F. mortiferum, Veillonella,* and other obligately anaerobic gram-negative non–spore-forming anaerobes. It is not necessary to use both KV and PV; rather, it is reasonable to select one or the other of these media based on preferences of the microbiologist.

(continued)

Table 11-5 (continued)

MEDIUM*	MAJOR INGREDIENTS AND COMMENTS	PURPOSE
Cycloserine-cefoxitin fructose agar (CCFA)	Tryticase soy or proteose peptone base containing fructose and neutral red indicator. In addition, cycloserine (500 mg/L) and cefoxitin (16 mg/L) are added to inhibit intestinal flora. *C. difficile*, at 48 hours of incubation, forms 4 mm or greater yellowish rhizoid colonies that have birefringent crystalline internal structures ("speckled opalescence"). *C. difficile* colonies show yellow-green fluorescence under long-wave ultraviolet light (their odor is reminiscent of horse manure). *C. difficile* is negative for both lipase and lecithinase activity.	CCFA is for selective isolation of *Clostridium difficile* from stool specimens or other intestinal materials. However, growth on CCFA is not specific for only *C. difficile;* therefore, identification of pure culture isolates is still required. (It is common to find breakthrough growth on the medium of unwanted Enterobacteriaceae, *Bacillus* species, staphylococci, and other clostridia.)
Enriched thioglycolate medium (THIO)	THIO is an enriched liquid medium prepared by supplementing the BBL-0135C Formula Thioglycolate Medium (without indicator) with hemin and vitamin K_1.	This is a noninhibitory broth that is especially useful for primary isolation of actinomycetes. THIO is also an excellent supplement or backup to solid plating media for isolation of slow-growing or fastidious organisms. It should support good growth of essentially all anaerobes commonly found in clinical materials.

*All the media in this table are available in prepared form from several manufacturers (see text). All but CCFA are described in detail by Dowell, Lombard, and colleagues in an excellent CDC manual (1977).[27] The publication by George and colleagues (J Clin Microbiol 1979;9:214–219)[38] is recommended for those who desire more information on CCFA. Also, publications by Bartley and Dowell (Lab Med 1991;22:335–338)[17] and Marler and associates (J Clin Microbiol 1992;30:514–516)[67] are recommended.

Centers for Disease Control (CDC) anaerobe blood agar base media formulations[27] (see Color Plates 11-1 through 11-3).

The anaerobe blood agar developed and evaluated originally by Lombard, Dowell, and others at the CDC is recommended as a nonselective medium. It contains 5% defibrinated rabbit or sheep blood added to trypticase soy agar (Becton Dickinson Microbiology Systems, Cockeysville, MD), with L-cystine, yeast extract (Difco Laboratories, Detroit, MI), vitamin K_1, and hemin.[27]

Before use, the plates are held for 4 to 16 hours in an anaerobic jar or an anaerobic glove box in an atmosphere of 85% N_2, 10% H_2, and 5% CO_2. Allen and colleagues found that the L-cystine in CDC anaerobe blood agar permits growth of thiol-dependent *Fusobacterium necrophorum* and fastidious, thiol-dependent streptococci that have been isolated from patients with endocarditis.[7] As an added benefit, this medium also supports excellent growth of the strict anaerobes *Clostridium novyi* type B and *C. haemolyticum.*[7]

The phenylethyl alcohol blood agar is prepared by supplementing the anaerobe blood agar described above with 0.25% phenylethyl alcohol. Similarly, the kanamycin-vancomycin or the paromomycin-vancomycin blood agar is prepared by adding 100 μg of kanamycin or paromomycin and 7.5 μg of vancomycin per milliliter of the blood agar medium.

The enriched thioglycolate medium (BBL-135C with hemin and vitamin K_1 supplement; Becton Dickinson Microbiology Systems, Cockeysville, MD) is recommended primarily as a back-up to the plating media.[27] This medium aids in cultivating slow-growing species of *Actinomyces*. Chopped meat glucose broth is a good alternative to enriched thioglycolate medium. Prereduced anaerobically sterilized (PRAS) media in roll tubes are recommended by the Virginia Polytechnic Institute (VPI) anaerobe laboratory for isolating anaerobes.[45] These media are available from Carr-Scarborough Microbiologicals (Stone Mountain, GA). Other special-purpose selective media for primary isolation of anaerobes have been described in detail by Sutter and colleagues in the *Wadsworth Anaerobic Bacteriology Manual*[94] and in the current literature.[4,17]

ANAEROBIC SYSTEMS FOR CULTIVATION OF ANAEROBIC BACTERIA

Comparative studies have shown that the following systems are satisfactory for the cultivation of anaerobic bacteria commonly associated with human disease if used properly:[55]

- Jar techniques
- Evacuation-replacement
- GasPak, Difco, Marion (now Becton Dickinson Microbiology Systems), or Oxoid disposable gas generator method
- Anaerobic glove box techniques

The following general principles must be followed for optimal results:

- Proper collection and transport of the clinical specimens
- Processing of specimens with minimal exposure to atmospheric oxygen
- Use of fresh or prereduced media
- Proper use of an anaerobic system with inclusion of an active catalyst to allow removal of oxygen (from jar or glove box systems)

Anaerobic Jar Techniques

Some of the different jars used for cultivating anaerobic bacteria have included the Brewer, Baird-Tatlock, GasPak, McIntosh-Fildes, Oxoid, and Torbal jars. The GasPak jar (Becton Dickinson Microbiology Systems, Cockeysville, MD), illustrated in Figure 11-2, is the system most commonly used in clinical laboratories in the United States. The Oxoid jar (Oxoid USA, Inc, Columbia, MD) (Fig. 11-3) has a metal lid, Schrader valves, and a pressure gauge. Otherwise, it is used similarly to the other jars.

The basic principle of these jars is the same, namely, removal of oxygen from the chamber by

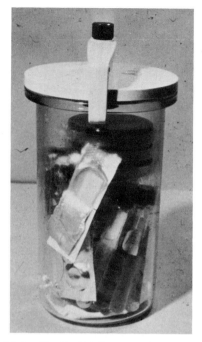

Figure 11-2. The GasPak (Becton Dickinson Microbiology Systems, Cockeysville, MD) anaerobic system. The jar contains inoculated plates, broth tubes, a GasPak hydrogen and carbon dioxide generator envelope, a disposable methylene blue indicator strip, and a catalyst basket in the lid.

reaction with hydrogen added to the system in the presence of the catalyst. Oxygen is reduced to water as follows:

$$2H_2 + O_2 \xrightarrow{\text{catalyst}} 2H_2O$$

The use of an active catalyst in each system is important. The GasPak jar uses a "cold" catalyst composed of palladium-coated alumina pellets. The palladium catalyst can be inactivated in the jar by hydrogen sulfide or other volatile metabolic products of bacteria. It is recommended that the catalyst pellets be replaced with new or rejuvenated pellets each time the jar is used.[5] The pellets can be rejuvenated by heating them in a dry heat oven at 160°C for 2 hours. After heating, the pellets are stored at room temperature in a clean, dry container or in a desiccator until the time of use.

Anaerobic conditions can be produced in jar systems with either the disposable H_2–CO_2 generator (GasPak, Oxoid, and others) or by the evacuation-replacement procedure. The evacuation-replacement procedure, in which the air in the jar is removed and replaced with a mixture of 85% N_2,

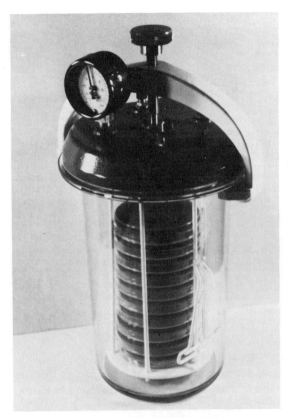

Figure 11-3. The Oxoid Anaerobic Jar (Oxoid USA, Columbia, MD) contains a 3.5-liter polycarbonate jar closed by a heavy-duty metal lid and metal clamp. The lid center has two Schrader valves and a plus/minus pressure gauge with two valves to facilitate the evacuation/replacement (E/R) technique. There is also a safety valve in the lid to prevent extra gas pressure caused by incorrect use of the E/R technique. A sachet low temperature catalyst is clipped to the undersurface of the lid. In lieu of using the E/R technique, the jar can be used with the Oxoid Generating Kit available from the manufacturer.

with a new generator. A defective gasket in the lid that allows escape of gas or inactivated catalyst pellets are the two most common causes of failure of this system.

Evacuation-Replacement Jar Procedure

Whaley and Gorman described an inexpensive device for evacuating and gassing jars.[104] This device can be used with an in-house vacuum, thereby eliminating the need for a vacuum pump when the evacuation-replacement procedure is used. Air is evacuated from the jar by drawing a vacuum of 20 to 24 inches of mercury. This procedure is repeated three times. The jar is filled with nitrogen after the first two evacuations and the final replacement is made with the 85% N_2, 10% H_2, and 5% CO_2 gas mixture.

Anaerobic conditions should always be monitored when using either of the two jar techniques by including an oxidation-reduction indicator. Methylene blue strips are available commercially for this purpose (Becton Dickinson Microbiology Systems, Cockeysville, MD). Methylene blue is blue when oxidized and clear when reduced.

Use of the Anaerobic Glove Box

An anaerobic glove box is a self-contained anaerobic system that allows the microbiologist to process specimens and perform most bacteriologic techniques for isolation and identification of anaerobic bacteria without exposure to air. The flexible vinyl plastic anaerobic chamber developed at the University of Michigan has enjoyed wide popularity[9]), and a modification of this design is available in varying sizes from Coy Laboratory Products, Inc, Ann Arbor, Michigan (Fig. 11-4).

PRAS Media

Prereduced anaerobically sterilized (PRAS) media are inoculated under a stream of oxygen-free CO_2, which minimizes exposure to air and helps to maintain a reduced oxidation-reduction potential in the media. A needle and syringe are used to inoculate PRAS media in Hungate tubes through a rubber

10% H_2, and 5% CO_2, is more economical than gas generators and allows anaerobic conditions to be established more rapidly. Any airtight container can be used, including a GasPak jar with a vented lid, a Brewer jar, an Oxoid jar, or even a modified pressure cooker.

A disposable H_2–CO_2 generator is used by opening the generator envelope and placing it into the jar to be used. After 10 mL of water is added to allow the generation of H_2 and CO_2, the lid is tightly sealed. If the lid is not warm to the touch within 40 minutes after it is sealed, or if condensation does not appear on the inner surface of the glass within 25 minutes, the jar should be opened and the generator envelope discarded and replaced

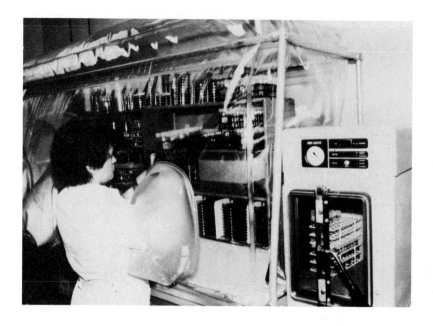

Figure 11-4. The anaerobic glove box (Coy Laboratory Products, Inc., Ann Arbor, MI). Materials are passed in and out of the large flexible plastic chamber through an automatic entry lock. Anaerobic conditions are maintained by constant recirculation of the atmosphere within the plastic chamber (85% N_2, 10% H_2, 5% CO_2) through palladium catalyst. Cultures are incubated either within a separate incubator inside the glove box or by maintaining the entire chamber at 35°C through use of heated catalyst boxes.

stopper–screw cap closure assembly.[45] PRAS media used for the performance of conventional biochemical tests and gas–liquid chromatography (GLC) are available from Carr-Scarborough Microbiologicals, Inc (Stone Mountain, GA).

Anaerobic Disposable Plastic Bags

The Bio-Bag system, originally developed by Marion Scientific (Kansas City, MO) is now available from Becton Dickinson Microbiology Systems (Cockeysville, MD) (Fig. 11-5). A second system, the Anaerobic Pouch System Catalyst-Free, is marketed by Difco Laboratories (Detroit, MI). A third anaerobic disposable bag system, the Anaerocult A, is manufactured by Merck Darmstadt (Gibbstown, NJ).

The anaerobic Bio-Bag consists of a clear-plastic bag (sold in varying sizes capable of holding one to three, 100-mm diameter Petri dishes), an H_2–CO_2 gas generator (analogous to the generator used in a GasPak jar), palladium catalyst pellets, and a resazurin indicator. The generator is activated, then the bag is heat-sealed.

The Difco Anaerobic Pouch and the Anaerocult both achieve anaerobic conditions differently, without catalyst, to remove oxygen from the atmosphere. In these disposable systems, water is added to sodium carbonate resulting in production of CO_2 and H_2. Oxygen is removed from within the

sealed plastic pouch by combining it with iron powder to produce iron oxides. In one study, the Bio-Bag was reported to be less effective than the Difco Anaerobic Pouch for recovery of anaerobes from clinical specimens, while the latter system was found comparable to the anaerobic chamber methods that were used.[28] Thus, the Anaerobic Pouch and Anaerocult systems may be practical alternatives to glove box or anaerobic jar systems for the incubation of anaerobes when only one or two plates are to be incubated.

Use of the Anaerobic Holding Jar

A modification of the Martin holding jar procedure is a convenient and inexpensive adjunct to the jar and glove box anaerobic systems that allows primary plating, inspection of cultures, and subculture of colonies at the bench with only minimal exposure to atmospheric oxygen.[7,68] The holding jar assembly is illustrated in Figure 11-6, and its use is briefly described as follows:

1. Three holding jars are used, the first to hold uninoculated media, the second for plates that are growing colonies to be subcultured, and the third to receive freshly inoculated plates.
2. Commercially prepared agar plates or agar media freshly prepared in the laboratory can be used.

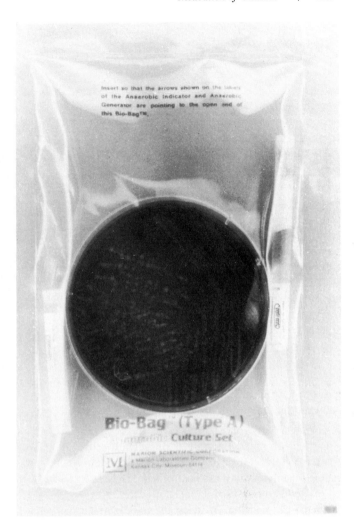

Figure 11-5. The Bio-Bag anaerobic Culture Set (Becton Dickinson Microbiology Systems, Cockeysville, MD). This culture set includes a plate of CDC-anaerobic blood agar contained within an oxygen-impermeable bag. The system contains its own gas-generating kit and cold catalyst.

3. The plates to be used on any given day should first be placed in an anaerobic glove box or an anaerobic jar for 4 to 15 hours before use to reduce the media.
4. As needed, the reduced media are placed in the first holding jar and continuously flushed with a gentle stream of nitrogen.
5. The plates of reduced media are inoculated one at a time in ambient air and immediately placed in the third holding jar, which is also flushed with nitrogen. The second holding jar is used to hold any plates removed from the GasPak jar that require subculture.
6. After the jar containing the newly inoculated plates is filled, the plates can be transferred to a conventional anaerobic system, such as a GasPak jar or into an anaerobic glove box for incubation.

Inexpensive, commercial-grade nitrogen can be used in the holding jar system. The operator opens the small needle valve on the gas manifold (see Fig. 11-6) and sets the gas-tank regulator to 4 psi for 20 to 30 seconds to rapidly purge the jar of air. Then the regulator pressure is turned down to about 0.5 to 1 psi and the flow to each jar is regulated at 50 to 100 mL/min, using the small needle valve on the manifold. This is equivalent to a flow rate of one to two bubbles per second when the rubber tubing in the jar is placed just beneath the surface of water in a beaker.

INCUBATION OF CULTURES

In most instances, 35° to 37°C is the temperature most satisfactory for primary isolation of anaerobic bacteria from clinical specimens. Plates inoculated

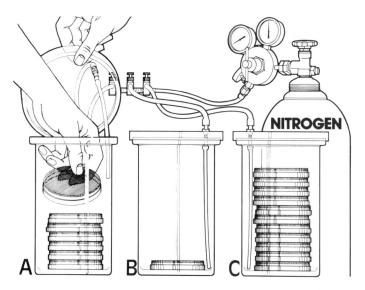

Figure 11-6. Illustration of the anaerobic holding jar system. The flow rate of nitrogen to each jar is regulated by the needle valves on the manifold (three-gang valve, available where aquarium supplies are sold). Jars A, B, and C contain uninoculated plates, plates with colonies to be subcultured, and freshly inoculated plates, respectively.

at the bench and placed in anaerobic jars should be incubated for at least 48 hours and reincubated for another 2 to 4 days to allow slow-growing organisms to form colonies; some anaerobes, such as certain species of *Actinomyces* and *Eubacterium*, grow rather slowly, and colonies may not be detected if jars are opened sooner. Also, if the jar is opened too soon, some of the slow-growing organisms may be killed because of oxygen exposure. Also, prolonged exposure of freshly inoculated plates to ambient air must be avoided. If a holding jar procedure is not used, inoculated plates must be immediately placed in an anaerobic system (anaerobic jar or anaerobic glove box) to allow for effective cultivation of these anaerobes. Unless growth is apparent visually, broth cultures should be held a minumum of 5 to 7 days before discarding them as negative.

INSPECTION AND SUBCULTURE OF COLONIES

Use of the stereoscopic dissecting microscope during examination of colonies is extremely helpful because a number of anaerobes have distinctive colonial features.[24] The dissecting microscope is also a valuable aid during the subculture of colonies to obtain pure culture isolates.

During the inspection of colonies, any action on the medium, such as hemolysis of blood agar or clearing of egg yolk agar, as well as the size and distinctive features of the colonies should be recorded. A number of characteristic colonies of an-

aerobes are illustrated in Color Plates 11-1 through and 11-3. When recording colony characteristics, the following should be noted: the age of the culture and the name of the medium, the diameter in millimeters of each colony in addition to its color, surface features (glistening, dull), density (opaque, translucent), consistency (butyrous, viscid, membranous, brittle), and other descriptive features (see Fig. 1-19).

Gram-stained smears of colonies from the anaerobic and CO_2-incubated plates should also be examined. Do not assume on the basis of colony and microscopic features only that colonies on plates that have been incubated in an anaerobic system are obligate anaerobes. Although the morphology and colony characteristics of certain anaerobes are distinctive, it is often impossible to distinguish some facultative anaerobes from obligate anaerobes without aerotolerance tests, even when the CO_2-incubated plates show no growth.

The number of different colony types on the anaerobe plates should be determined and a semiquantitative estimate of the number of each type should be recorded (light, moderate, or heavy growth). Transfer each different colony to another anaerobe blood agar plate to obtain a pure culture and an aerobic blood agar plate for aerotolerance testing. If colonies are well separated on the primary isolation plate, a tube of enrichment broth, such as enriched thioglycolate or chopped meat glucose medium, should be inoculated to provide a source of inoculum for differential tests.

After incubation, the enriched thioglycolate and chopped meat glucose subcultures are Gram stained. If the organisms appear to be in pure culture, they can be used to inoculate appropriate differential media for identification of isolates.

The enriched thioglycolate and chopped meat glucose cultures that were inoculated with the original specimen along with all primary isolation plates are examined. If no growth is evident on the primary anaerobic plates, or if the colonies isolated fail to account for all the morphologic types found in the direct Gram-stained smear of the specimen, each broth medium should be subcultured to two anaerobe blood agar plates, one for anaerobic incubation and the other incubated in a 5% to 10% CO_2 air incubator. Alternatively, a chocolate agar plate can be used for the subculture plate to be incubated in the 5% to 10% CO_2 air incubator. These subculture plates should then be examined as described earlier.

AEROTOLERANCE TESTS

Each colony type from the primary anaerobic isolation plate is subcultured to an aerobic (5% to 10% CO_2, or candle jar) and anaerobic blood agar plate for overnight incubation.

Haemophilus influenzae, which grows on anaerobe blood agar anaerobically but not on ordinary blood agar aerobically, can be mistaken for an anaerobe. This can be avoided by inoculating a chocolate agar plate (in place of the aerobic blood agar plate) for incubation in a 5% to 10% CO_2 air incubator. It may be expedient to inoculate quadrants or sixths of the chocolate agar plate for testing the aerotolerance of four to six colonies from a primary anaerobic isolation plate (Fig. 11-7).

PRELIMINARY REPORTING OF RESULTS

Organisms that are shown to be obligate anaerobes should be reported to the clinician immediately, together with the results from observing a Gram-stained preparation and characteristics of colonies. It is not justified to report the presence of an obligate anaerobe until aerotolerance studies have been completed.

Unfortunately, a period of 3 days or longer is often required for these studies to be completed. Clinicians should be made aware that this lengthy time cannot be avoided with some slow-growing anaerobes (eg, some species of *Actinomyces* and *Propionibacterium*). Fortunately, the colonial and microscopic morphology of certain anaerobic bacteria is often so distinctive that *preliminary* or *presumptive* reports of these isolates can be made before aerotolerance studies. Examples include *Clostridium perfringens*, members of the *Bacteroides fragilis* group, the pigmented *Prevotella-Porphyromonas* group, and others.

DETERMINATION OF CULTURAL AND BIOCHEMICAL CHARACTERISTICS FOR DIFFERENTIATION OF ANAEROBIC ISOLATES

Once the presence of anaerobes has been confirmed by aerotolerance tests and a description of morphologic features has been reported, the next priority is to identify the pure-culture isolates as rapidly and as accurately as possible and to report

Figure 11-7. Quadrant plating technique used for aerotolerance testing of four anaerobe isolates. The left plate has been incubated in an anaerobe jar for 18 to 24 hours, while the plate on the right was incubated in a candle jar. Isolates A and C are obligate anaerobes. Isolate B is facultatively anaerobic. Isolate D is either a microaerophile or an obligate aerobe and should be further tested for its ability to grow in ambient air compared with the environment containing increased CO_2. A candle jar is not adequate for testing *Campylobacter jejuni*; this species grows optimally in 5% CO_2, and 85% N_2.

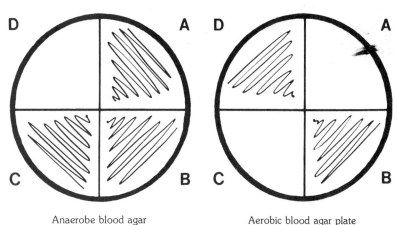

Anaerobe blood agar incubated anaerobically

Aerobic blood agar plate incubated in candle jar

the results to the clinician within a relevant time. Although probably more than 500 species of anaerobes are recognized by taxonomists, the task of identifying anaerobes for the clinical microbiologist is not nearly as formidable as it might seem because only a relatively small number are involved in anaerobic infections with any frequency (see Table 11-3).

Presumptive Identification

Nearly all clinically significant isolates are moderate obligate or aerotolerant anaerobes and with practice are not particularly difficult to isolate and identify. In addition to organisms of the *Bacteroides fragilis* group, the pigmented *Prevotella-Porphyromonas* group, *Fusobacterium nucleatum*, and the anaerobic cocci, which are quite frequently isolated, certain other, less common anaerobes nonetheless have major pathogenic potential. Consequently, it is important to be familiar with and be able to recognize *Actinomyces israelii, A. naeslundii, A. meyeri, Propionibacterium propionicum,* and *Bifidobacterium dentium,* all of which may cause serious acute suppurative and chronic inflammatory disease; *Prevotella bivia* and *Prevotella disiens,* which are commonly resistant to various penicillins and cephalosporins; *Fusobacterium necrophorum* (which may be highly virulent); *F. mortiferum* and *F. varium,* which vary in susceptibility to certain penicillins, cephalosporins, and clindamycin; *Clostridium septicum,* an organism frequently associated with carcinoma of the colon or hematopoietic malignancy when isolated from patients' blood; the "histotoxic" clostridia in addition to *C. perfringens,* which can cause gas gangrene and various wound infections; *C. difficile,* a major cause of antibiotic-associated diarrhea and colitis; and *C. tetani* and *C. botulinum* because of the diseases they cause.[4,14,16,34]

Reference laboratories commonly use large batteries of tests in characterizing anaerobe isolates referred to them for identification or confirmation. Certain of these are listed below; a full description of these tests is beyond the scope of this text.

Characterization of Anaerobic Bacteria
Relation to oxygen
Colony morphology
Gram stain reaction
Microscopic features

Motility
Growth in liquid media
Biochemical tests
Metabolic products (GLC)
Antibiotic susceptibility
Serologic tests
Toxicity, toxin neutralization, pathogenicity in animals
Polyacrylamide gel electrophoresis of soluble proteins
Cell wall long-chain fatty acids; menaquinones

In addition, new species are being recognized by use of deoxyribonucleic acid (DNA)-DNA homology studies and other sophisticated methods. The data derived from the characterization of cultures with a large number of tests provide a valuable base for compiling tables of differential characteristics such as those published by the CDC, VPI, and Wadsworth Anaerobe Laboratories.[25,45,94] In most clinical diagnostic laboratories it is not practical or economically feasible to use such a large number of differential media and biochemical determinations to identify isolates.

Fortunately, certain characteristics are especially useful in the identification of anaerobes. These characteristics form the basis of a practical approach for identifying anaerobic isolates that are commonly encountered in the clinical laboratory and additional species that are less common or are potential major pathogens. Some cardinal identifying characteristics of anaerobes follow:

Relation to oxygen
Colonial characteristics
Pigment
Hemolysis
Pitting of medium
Gram stain reaction
Morphology
Spores
Motility
Flagella
Miscellaneous
    Growth in thioglycolate broth, catalase, lecithinase, lipase; reactions on milk medium; production of indole; hydrolysis of starch, esculin, and gelatin; reduction of nitrate; fermentation of key carbohydrates (eg, glucose, mannitol, lactose, rhamnose); growth in presence of bile, penicillin, rifampin, and kanamycin; inhibition by sodium poly-

anetholsulfonate [SPS]; production of toxins; metabolic products

Use of Differential Agar Media

Several important characteristics for identifying anaerobic bacteria can be obtained with pure cultures on CDC anaerobe blood agar and in enriched thioglycolate medium.[26] These characteristics, outlined in Table 11-6, provide important clues for differentiating anaerobes in general. Additional characteristics are determined by use of differential disks, which are added to freshly inoculated anaerobe blood agar plates. A 2-unit penicillin disk, 1000-µg kanamycin disk and 15-µg rifampin disk aid in the differentiation of anaerobic, non–spore-forming, gram-negative bacilli. Colistin and vancomycin disks may also be extremely useful, as described elsewhere.[94] An SPS disk test is a practical way to separate *Peptostreptococcus anaerobius* from other anaerobic cocci. A nitrate disk test is a convenient method to demonstrate nitrate reduction during the work-up of anaerobic bacteria.

Presumpto Plates

Developed by Dowell, Lombard, and associates,[25–27] a practical approach to the identification of anaerobes that uses a series of three quadrant plates–called Presumpto 1, 2, and 3–can be recommended (Carr-Scarborough Microbiologicals, Stone Mountain, GA). This system of media plates allows the determination of 20 different characteristics (Table 11-7) of anaerobe isolates at a minimal cost.[25] The information derived from using the three quadrant plates, along with the other characteristics obtained from anaerobe blood agar and enriched thioglycolate medium plus metabolic product analysis using GLC, permits definitive identification of many clinically significant anaerobic bacteria that are encountered in the laboratory. In addition, the quadrant plates, especially the Presumpto 1 and 2 plates, can be used to supplement several of the commercial packaged kit systems, as well as traditional broth identification systems, with important tests or characteristics these nonagar systems lack.

Preparation of the media and reagents used in the Presumpto quadrant plate system, their inoc-

ulation, the method of incubation, and their use and interpretation of the various differential inhibitory and antibiotic disk tests, including a plate of color photographs illustrating the key reactions, are presented in detail elsewhere.[55]

Growth Inhibition on Anaerobe Blood Agar Using Antibiotic Disk Test

Zones of growth inhibition around the antibiotic disks are recorded as follows:

Penicillin, 2-unit disk: sensitive (S) if zone of growth inhibition is 12 mm or greater in diameter and resistant (R) if the zone is less than 12 mm.

Rifampin, 15-µg disk: sensitive (S) if zone of growth inhibition is 15 mm or larger and resistant (R) if zone is less than 15 mm.

Kanamycin, 1000-µg disk: sensitive (S) if zone of growth inhibition is 12 mm or greater and resistant (R) if zone is less than 12 mm.

SPS Disk Test

The zone of inhibition is measured. A 12-mm or greater zone of inhibition is recorded as sensitive (S).

Nitrate Disk Test

Nitrate reduction is tested for by adding 1 drop of nitrate A reagent (sulfanilic acid) and 1 drop of nitrate B reagent (1,6 Cleave's acid) to the disk.[94] A pink or red color indicates that nitrate has been reduced to nitrite. If the disk was colorless after addition of reagents A and B, zinc dust is sprinkled on the disk to confirm a negative reaction. The development of a red color after zinc dust is added confirms that nitrate is still present in the disk (a negative reaction).

Characterization of Anaerobes Using Conventional Biochemical Tests in Large Tubes

Conventional tube culture procedures are covered briefly below. For further details, refer to the laboratory manuals on anaerobic bacteriology by Hold-

Table 11-6
Differentiation of Anaerobic, Gram-Negative, Non–Spore-Forming Rods to the Genus Level

DESCRIPTION	GENUS

Nonmotile or Motile With Peritrichous Flagella; Straight or Coccobacillary Rods

A. Recently proposed to include only the highly fermentative and bile resistant species resembling *B. fragilis* (ie, *B. distasonis, B. caccae, B. ovatus, B. thetaiotaomicron, B. merdae, B. vulgatus, B. uniformis, B. eggerthii,* and *B. stercoris*). Several other species remain in this genus and are awaiting further studies to determine their correct place (ie, *B. capillosus, B. polyprogmatus, B. putredinis, B. pyogenes, B. forsythus, B. gracilis, B. pneumosintes, B. salivosus, B. tectum,* and *B. ureolyticus.*) Until the latter group is moved this genus remains heterogenous. — *Bacteroides**

B. Most often black pigmented colonies. Produces acetic, butyric, and succinic acids with minor amounts of propionic, isobutyric, and isovaleric acids. One strain produces phenylacetic acid. All are asaccharolytic and indole positive. — *Porphyromonas†*

C. Nonpigmented to pigmented colonies. Bile inhibited and saccharolytic. Usually oral flora. — *Prevotella**

D. Bile resistant, catalase positive, nitrate reduced, and urease positive. — *Bilophila†*

E. Found as a part of the human normal flora but rarely encountered in properly selected clinical specimen. — *Anaerorhabdus‡*
Fibrobacter‡
Megamomas‡
Mitsuokella‡
Tissierella‡

F. Found in animals and nature. — *Pectinatus*
Rikenella
Roseburia
Ruminobacter
Sebaldella

G. Produces butyric acid (but little or no isoacids) as the major product. Succinic acid is not produced. All species are nonmotile. — *Fusobacterium**

H. Lactic acid is the only major product. *L. buccalis,* the only species, is nonmotile. — *Leptotrichia†*

I. Acetic acid is the major acid metabolic product. Produces hydrogen sulfide; reduces sulfate. *D. pigra,* the only species, is nonmotile. — *Desulfomonas‡*

Motile, Peritrichous Flagella Not Produced

A. Curved rods with monotrichous or lophotrichous polar flagella or subpolar flagella. Butyric acid is major product of fermentation. — *Butyrivibrio†*

B. Succinic and acetic acids are major products of fermentation.
  1. Short, straight rods to coccobacilli; a single polar flagellum. Found only in bovine rumen. — *Succinimonas‡*
  2. Curved, helically twisted rods with pointed ends. Vibrating type motility by a single polar flagellum. — *Succinivibrio†*
  3. Helical, curved rods; bipolar tufts of flagella. — *Anaerobiospirillum†*

C. Helical, curved, or straight rods; single polar flagellum; carbohydrates not fermented; produce succinic acid from fumaric acid. Oxidase positive (difficult to distinguish from *Campylobacter sputorum* and *C. concisus*). — *Wolinella†*

D. Curved rods with multiple subterminal flagella. Fermentative in peptone yeast glycogen broth, supplemented with rabbit serum. Succinic and acetic acids as major fermentation products, with or without lactic acid. Oxidase-negative. — *Mobiluncus†*

E. Propionic and acetic acids as major fermentation products.
  1. Tufts of flagella on concave side of crescent-shaped cells. — *Selenomonas†*
  2. Single polar flagellum; lipolytic; curved rods. — *Anaerovibrio†*
  3. Flagella are inserted in a spiral along the cell. — *Centipeda†*

*Commonly found in clinical specimens.
†Rarely found in clinical specimens.
‡Normal flora only.
(Data from Holdeman LV, et al. Anaerobic gram-negative straight, curved, and helical rods. Family 1. Bacteroidaceae Pribram 1933, 10^AL. In: Krieg NR, Holt JG, eds. Bergey's manual of systematic bacteriology. Baltimore, Williams & Wilkins, 1984;1:602–662; Holdeman LV, et al. Bacteroides oris and Bacteroides buccae: new species from human periodontitis and other human infections. Int J Syst Bacteriol 1982;32:125–131; and Spiegel CA, Roberts M. Mobiluncus gen. nov., Mobiluncus curtisii subsp. curtisii sp. nov., Mobiluncus curtissi subsp. holmesii subsp. nov., and Mobiluncus mulieris sp. nov., curved rods from the human vagina. Int J Syst Bacteriol 1984;34:177–184.)

Table 11-7

Media and Characteristics of Cultures That Can Be Determined Using the Differential Agar Media System for Identifying Anaerobes

MEDIA	CHARACTERISTICS
Blood agar	Relation to O_2,* colonial characteristics, hemolysis, pigment, fluorescence with ultraviolet light (Wood's lamp), pitting of agar, cellular morphology, Gram stain reaction, spores, motility (wet mount); inhibition by penicillin, rifampin, and kanamycin
Enriched thioglycolate medium	Appearance of growth, rapidity of growth, gas production, odor, cellular morphology
Presumpto 1 plate	
LD agar	Indole, growth on LD medium, catalase†
LD esculin agar	Esculin hydrolysis, H_2S, catalase
LD egg yolk agar	Lipase, lecithinase, proteolysis
LD bile agar	Growth in presence of 20% bile (2% oxgall), insoluble precipitate under and immediately surrounding growth
Presumpto 2 plate	
LD glucose agar	Glucose fermentation; stimulation of growth by fermentable carbohydrate
LD starch agar	Starch hydrolysis
LD milk agar	Casein hydrolysis
LD DNA agar	Deoxyribonuclease activity
Presumpto 3 plate	
LD mannitol agar	Mannitol fermentation
LD lactose agar	Lactose fermentation
LD rhamnose agar	Rhamnose fermentation
LD gelatin	Gelatin hydrolysis

*By comparing growth on anaerobe plate with blood agar (or chocolate agar) incubated in 5% to 10% CO_2 incubator (or candle jar) or in room air.

†The catalase test can be performed by adding 3% hydrogen peroxide to the growth on LD agar, but the reactions of catalase-positive cultures are more vigorous on LD esculin agar.

eman and coworkers,[45] Moore and colleagues,[72] Sutter and associates,[94] Dowell and Hawkins,[24] and Dowell and coworkers.[27]

Instead of the differential tests in agar media described, one may use PRAS media in large test tubes for determining biochemical characteristics. These are inoculated either through a rubber diaphragm in Hungate tubes or with a special gassing device according to procedures of the *VPI Anaerobe Laboratory Manual.*[45] PRAS media can be prepared in the laboratory or can be obtained from commercial sources (Carr-Scarborough Microbiologicals, Stone Mountain, GA). If PRAS media are used for characterization of isolates, the identification tables of Holdeman and associates[45] and Moore and colleagues[72] should also be used.

The pH of PRAS peptone yeast (PY)–based carbohydrate fermentation tests is determined directly by using a pH meter; a long, thin, combination electrode is inserted into each culture tube. According to the *VPI Manual*, pH 5.5 to 6.0 is recorded as weak acid, whereas pH below 5.5 is strong acid. The pH of PY carbohydrate cultures should be compared with that of plain PY cultures (without carbohydrate). The pH of PY broth ranges between 6.2 to 6.4 when inoculated under CO_2.

Alternate Procedures

Use of conventional media in Hungate or other large tubes is relatively time-consuming, and the media are costly to prepare or purchase. Therefore, various alternative procedures have been described for characterizing isolates and identification schemas based on smaller volumes of media in containers that can be manipulated with reasonable speed at the bench.[2,5,6] In addition, descriptions of several rapid tests for preliminary grouping of isolates are given in the *Wadsworth Anaerobic Bacteriology Manual.*[94] These include the use of *Bac-*

teroides bile-esculin agar for selective isolation as well as presumptive identification of *B. fragilis* group organisms, the use of a battery of antibiotic disk tests somewhat different from those described previously, an indole spot test (the procedure differs from that used with the Presumpto 1 plate), a rapid gelatin hydrolysis test using unexposed Pan-X film in a turbid broth suspension, a rapid urease test, and others.

Glutamic Acid Decarboxylase Microtube Test

A rapid glutamic acid decarboxylase (GDC) microtube test (Carr-Scarborough Microbiologicals, Stone Mountain, GA) was investigated in detail by Banks and coworkers,[10] who established a data base for use in presumptive identification of clinically encountered anaerobic bacteria. The GDC test was found to be positive for only a relatively small number of anaerobes. Species of bile-stimulated *Bacteroides*, including the *B. fragilis* group, were likely to be positive, whereas *Prevotella* and *Porphyromonas* species were negative. Nearly all *Clostridium perfringens*, *C. barati*, and *C. sordellii* were GDC-positive, while a wide variety of other *Clostridium* species gave negative reactions.

API-20A and Minitek Packaged Microsystems

Since the early 1970s two commercial packaged micromethod kits have been widely used in clinical laboratories for identification of anaerobes: the API-20A (bioMérieux Vitek, Hazelwood, MO) and the Minitek (Becton Dickinson Microbiology Systems, Cockeysville, MD). The construction of these systems is similar to similar systems described in Chapter 2. Without the use of supplemental tests, only about 50% of 330 anaerobes tested could be identified with these systems. When supplemental tests were used along with these kits for identification of the same group of isolates, there was still only about 75% agreement between the kit results and the Mayo Laboratories Anaerobe Laboratory conventional system identification.[82] Neither the API-20A 24-hour system nor the Minitek Anaerobe II was found to be an adequate replacement for conventional test methods.[82] Both these systems lack a sufficient number of differential tests to characterize and adequately identify asaccharolytic organisms.

Commercial Packaged Kits for Aerobic Identification of Anaerobes After 4 Hours of Incubation

Several manufacturers have marketed packaged kits that test for preformed enzymes. Most of these systems utilize a battery of chromogenic substrates to rapidly test for a number of amino peptidases and glycosidases. Each system requires the preparation of a heavy cell suspension from the surface of a purity plate culture. These packaged kits enable the microbiologist to determine multiple enzymatic characteristics of a pure culture isolate after 4 hours of aerobic incubation. Except for the API-ZYM kit (bioMérieux Vitek, Hazelwood, MO),[65] all of these packaged systems provide numerical codes, computerized data bases, and identification tables to aid in identification once an isolate has been characterized using the system. In addition to the API-ZYM, the rapidly expanding list of products includes the following:

- API An-Ident (bioMérieux Vitek, Hazelwood, MO)
- IDS RapID-ANA II (Innovative Diagnostic Systems, Inc, Atlanta, GA)
- Vitek Anaerobe Identification (ANI) Card (bioMérieux Vitek, Hazelwood, MO)
- MicroScan Rapid Anaerobe Identification System (American Microscan, Sacramento, CA)
- ATB 32A Anaerobes ID (bioMérieux Vitek, Hazelwood, MO)

These kits are being used widely in diagnostic microbiology laboratories. In general, they are simple to use and less time consuming than conventional methods. Several of the systems have been evaluated in many different laboratories. Without the use of additional tests, the identification accuracies of these systems have generally been disappointing (range of 60% to 70%).[20,49,67,75]

DETERMINATION OF METABOLIC PRODUCTS BY GAS–LIQUID CHROMATOGRAPHY

Analysis of metabolic products by GLC is a practical, inexpensive procedure that is easily performed by personnel in the clinical laboratory. Metabolic products, released into broth culture media during anaerobic growth, are key characteristics of anaerobic bacteria and many facultatively anaerobic bacteria. Together with determining the relationship to oxygen, most anaerobic bacteria can be identified to the genus level based on presence or lack of spores, Gram reaction, cellular morphology, and results of GLC analysis. This technique improves the speed and accuracy of identification; cost actually decreases because of the time saved.[63,74] Gas chromatographs are relatively inexpensive, safe, simple to operate, and reliable and are commercially available from various scientific instrument manufacturing companies. Equipment and procedures for determining metabolic products by GLC are described in more detail by Holdeman and coworkers,[45] Sutter and associates,[94] and Lombard and Dowell.[63]

IDENTIFICATION OF ANAEROBES

Only 12 to 15 groups or species of anaerobic bacteria account for about 75% or more of the isolates from properly collected species (see Table 11-3). Laboratory personnel should be familiar with these species, either because they are so commonly isolated or because they may be highly pathogenic for patients (even though they are not so common).

Beyond considerations of the need to be familiar with the common and medically significant anaerobes, it has been proposed that microbiologists in clinical laboratories may wish to limit the extent of anaerobe identification, based on levels of capability.[1,7] As proposed previously, laboratories with limited capability (*Level One or Extent One*) should be able to isolate anaerobes in pure culture and to evaluate microscopic and colonial morphology. Together with results of aerotolerance testing, this information would then be reported to the clinician (as a preliminary report).

The *second level* of capability that was proposed would require, in addition to *Level One*, some identification capability.[1] Specifically, the differentiation of the *Bacteroides fragilis* group from the other Gram-negative anaerobes and identification of *Clostridium perfringens* would be performed. Like the first level of identification, isolates and direct smears from clinically relevant cases would be transported to a reference laboratory for further identification of isolates.

The *third level* of capability that was proposed

would require the presumptive identification of most of the 12 or so common anaerobe groups and species mentioned previously. This third category or extent of identification can be accomplished without the use of GLC. The common and clinically important anaerobes that can be presumptively identified, using a few simple rapid tests, include the *Bacteroides fragilis* group, the pigmented *Prevotella-Porphyromonas* groups (when pigment is formed), *Fusobacterium nucleatum*, *Peptostreptococcus anaerobius*, *P. asaccharolyticus*, *Propionibacterium acnes*, *Clostridium perfringens*, *C. ramosum*, *Actinomyces israelii*, and several less common species.

Isolates requiring GLC and further characterization to permit accurate identification include most *Clostridium* species other than *C. perfringens* or *C. ramosum*, most species of *Fusobacterium*, most genera and species of anaerobic gram-negative non–spore-forming bacilli other than the *B. fragilis* group, some of the anaerobic cocci, and most of the anaerobic non–spore-forming gram-positive rods. This is mentioned again because the *fourth level* of identification (or *definitive identification*), including the tests done in the previous levels, also includes GLC for organisms that require it. In addition to determining morphology, growth characteristics, relationships to oxygen, preliminary spot tests, use of the Presumpto system, and GLC, definitive identification (*Level Four*) includes determining whatever additional characteristics are needed (within reason) to arrive at an accurate identification to species (including those species that are not frequently isolated). A description of the activities involved in these higher level laboratories is beyond the scope of discussion here.

Anaerobic Gram-Negative Non–Spore-Forming Bacilli

The anaerobic, gram-negative, non–spore-forming bacteria are now classified in the genera as listed in Table 11-1. Key characteristics for differentiation of these bacilli are given in Table 11-6. The anaerobic gram-negative bacilli are among the normal flora of the oropharynx, lower digestive tract, vagina, cervix, urethra, and external genitalia. Only *Bacteroides*, *Prevotella*, *Porphyromonas*, and *Fusobacterium* among these genera are commonly isolated from properly selected and collected specimens (ie, those specimens without contamination with normal flora) from humans with signficant infections. Others, such as *Anaerobiospirillum succiniciproducens*, are still relatively obscure organisms that have been found infrequently in positive blood cultures, and little is known about their role in health and disease.[71,79]

Presumptive or Preliminary Group Identification of *Bacteroides, Prevotella, Porphyromonas,* and *Fusobacterium*

The presence of anaerobic gram-negative rods suggestive of *Bacteroides, Prevotella, Porphyromonas,* or *Fusobacterium* species (based on determining relationships to oxygen), together with the Gram stain results and colony observations, should be promptly reported to the clinician. Presumptive or preliminary identification of this group of gram-negative anaerobes can be made using the information included in Table 11-8.

BACTEROIDES

Bacteroides fragilis Group.   Organisms of the *B. fragilis* group are the anaerobic bacteria most often isolated from infections of humans, and these bacteria are particularly important clinically (see Table 11-3). They are a part of the indigenous microbiota of the intestinal tract of most persons but are seldom found in the mouth. *B. fragilis* is the most common species of the group found in properly collected clinical specimens, but it is not often isolated from feces during studies of the intestinal flora. In contrast, *B. ovatus* is not as frequently isolated but is common in fecal materials. *B. ovatus* can be isolated from the blood of compromised patients with polymicrobial bacteremia secondary to massive trauma or necrosis of the bowel. *B. thetaiotaomicron* is the second most common species of this group in clinical infections (see Table 11-3). For information on pathogenic properties and infections caused by the *B. fragilis* group, the reader

Table 11-8

Characteristics That Are Especially Useful for Identifying Commonly Encountered *Bacteroides, Porphyromonas, Prevotella,* and *Fusobacterium* Species

CHARACTERISTIC	SPECIES
Brick-red fluorescence (with long-wave ultraviolet light) or brown-black pigment	*Prevotella melaninogenica* group,* *Porphyromonas* species
Good growth in 20% bile; resistant to penicillin (2-IU disk) and kanamycin (1-mg disk) and inhibited by rifampin (15-μg disk)	*Bacteroides fragilis* group*
Catalase produced on LD esculin agar	*B. fragilis, B. thetaiotaomicron, B. distasonis, B. ovatus*
Lipase produced on LD egg yolk agar	*Prevotella intermedia, Fusobacterium necrophorum*
Asaccharolytic (glucose or other carbohydrates not fermented)	*Bacteroides* CDC group F₂, *Prevotella asaccharolytica, Porphyromonas gingivalis, B. capillosis* (this species is rare), *B. ureolyticus, F. gonidiaformans* (rare), *F. naviforme, F. nucleatum*
Agar pitted; urease positive	*B. ureolyticus; B. gracilis*
Gelatin hydrolyzed; milk digested	*Prevotella bivia, P. disiens, P. intermedia*
DNase-positive; enhanced growth on 20% bile	*B. thetaiotaomicron, B. uniformis, B. ovatus*
Resistant to rifampin; esculin hydrolyzed	*F. mortiferum*
Resistant to rifampin; esculin not hydrolyzed	*F. varium*
Long, thin, filamentous rods; internal speckling of colonies; propionate produced from threonine	*F. nucleatum*

*See text for listing of species included.

is referred to the excellent texts of Finegold and George[35] and Smith and Williams.[89]

Organisms of the *B. fragilis* group are non-motile, small to medium size gram-negative rods with rounded ends.[89] Cells obtained from a broth culture tend to be pleomorphic, often with vacuoles. Colonies of *B. fragilis* on CDC anaerobe blood agar are nonhemolytic, gray, entire, and semiopaque with concentric whorls or ringlike structures inside the colonies (see Color Plate 11-1). Colonies of other species of the group are similar in size and shape but differ with regard to their internal structures. A key characteristic of species of the *B. fragilis* group is that growth is enhanced by bile. In addition, they are all resistant to penicillin and kanamycin but sensitive to rifampin by the disk technique. All are saccharolytic and their carbohydrate fermentation patterns (along with indole, divided into the indole-positive and the indole-negative groups) help to differentiate between the species. The most commonly encountered species of the indole-negative group include *B. fragilis*, *B. distasonis*, and *B. vulgatus*. The most frequently isolated indole-positive species include *B. thetaiotamicron*, *B. ovatus*, and *B. uniformis*. This distinction is useful clinically because of differences in resistance to antimicrobial agents between the indole-positive and indole-negative groups (see Table 11-13).

Pigmenting Anaerobic Gram-Negative Bacilli. In 1989, Shah and Collins proposed that the genus *Bacteroides* be restricted to the *Bacteroides fragilis* group and related species, which actively ferment glucose, grow in the presence of 20% bile, and hydrolyze esculin.[84] Thus, the pigmenting anaerobic gram-negative bacilli are no longer classified in the genus *Bacteroides*. The moderately saccharolytic, pigmenting species were placed in the genus *Prevotella*[85] the asaccharolytic pigmenting species were reclassified in the genus *Porphyromonas*.[83]

Presumptive clues for the recognition of anaerobic gram-negative bacilli that belong to the genus *Porphyromonas* include the formation of tan to buff colonies that fluoresce brick-red under long-wave ultraviolet light or brown-black colonies, inhibition of growth in the presence of vancomycin (ie, failure to grow on kanamycin-vancomycin blood agar), inhibition by bile, inhibition by penicillin and rifampin but resistance to kanamycin, formation of indole, and failure to ferment glucose. Although definitive identification of *Porphyromonas* to

the species level is difficult, the determination of enzyme activities through the use of a rapid, 4-hour test system (ie, the API ZYM, ATB 32A Anaerobes ID or RapID ANA) has become a practical way to characterize and identify *Porphyromonas* to the species level.[21,99,100]

Inhibition by bile is a key characteristic of the genus *Prevotella*. In contrast to *Porphyromonas*, the pigmented species of *Prevotella* ferment glucose and other carbohydrates. The "pigmenting" *Prevotella* group may take from 2 days to 3 weeks to form pigment on CDC-anaerobe blood agar or may even fail to produce pigmented colonies. Before showing pigmentation, young colonies often exhibit a brick-red fluorescence when examined under long-wave (365 nm) ultraviolet light.

Species of the pigmented *Prevotella-Porphyromonas* group are part of the normal flora of the oropharynx, nose, and gastrointestinal and genitourinary tracts. They are the second most common group of anaerobic bacteria encountered in human infections (see Table 11-3). Details of the clinical significance, gross and microscopic characteristics, and biochemical test results for less commonly recovered miscellaneous species including *Prevotella oralis* and related species, *Bacteroides ureolyticus*, *B. gracilis*, *Bilophila* species, and other asaccharolytic, nitrate-positive species can be found in other texts.[21,46,47,55,98-100]

FUSOBACTERIUM. Production of butyric acid as the major metabolic product, separates the genus *Fusobacterium* from *Bacteroides*, *Prevotella*, *Porphyromonas*, and *Leptotrichia*. *Fusobacterium* species are normally found in the gastrointestinal, genitourinary, and upper respiratory tracts. Fusobacteria are commonly involved in serious infections in various body sites. They were described in 54 cases of bacteremia by Felner and Dowell.[31]

Fusobacterium nucleatum and members of the *Prevotella-Porphyromonas* group are the anaerobic bacilli most frequently involved in anaerobic pleuropulmonary infections (eg, aspiration pneumonia, lung abscess, necrotizing pneumonia, thoracic empyema). Fusobacteria are also fairly common pathogens in brain abscess, chronic sinusitis, metastatic osteomyelitis, septic arthritis, liver abscess, and other intraabdominal infections.[32]

Fusobacterium nucleatum is the most common species found in clinical materials. The spindle-shaped cells are long, slender filaments with tapered ends (see Color Plate 11-1*E* and *F*). Colonies on anaerobe blood agar are slightly convex with slightly irregular margins and have a characteristic internal flecking that was aptly called speckled opalescence by the late G. L. Lombard (see Color Plate 11-1). Biochemically, *F. nucleatum* is relatively inactive. *F. necrophorum* has the ability to cause serious infections (eg, liver abscess), and it is not unusual to isolate it alone (in pure culture) from soft tissue lesions.[89] The cells are pleomorphic, often with curved forms and spherical areas within cells (see Color Plate 11-1*G* and *H*). They also produce free coccoid bodies. Most strains produce lipase on LD egg yolk agar. *F. necrophorum* is pathogenic, producing liver abscesses in mice, and is susceptible to penicillin (500 units/mL).[86]

Fusobacterium mortiferum and *F. varium* are often resistant to clindamycin, penicillin G, and certain other antibiotics (Allen SD, Siders JA, unpublished data, April 1993). The cells are highly pleomorphic and coccoid to filamentous, with spherical swellings near the center or one end of unevenly stained rods. Colonies on blood agar are 1 to 2 mm in diameter and have a distinctive fried-egg appearance, with raised, opaque centers and a flat, translucent margin. *F. mortiferum* and *F. varium* are resistant to rifampin (15-μg disk), which helps separate them from other *Fusobacterium*, *Bacteroides*, *Porphyromonas*, and *Prevotella* species. Additional characteristics of these and other species are presented elsewhere.[45,47,93]

Mobiluncus and Bacterial Vaginosis

The name *Mobiluncus* was proposed for a new genus of gram-variable or gram-negative, motile, curved, non–spore-forming anaerobic rods, which occur singly or in pairs and with a "gull wing" appearance.[93] The organisms tend to stain gram-variable in young culture and gram-negative in older culture. The name *Mobiluncus* was derived from the words *mobilis* (meaning "capable of movement") and *uncus* (which means "hook").[92] The organisms are motile by means of multiple subpolar flagella. *Mobiluncus* has been found in urogenital tract specimens of women who had nonspecific bacterial vaginosis as well as in urogenital tract specimens of asymptomatic women without vaginosis and in urogenital secretions of asymptomatic heterosexual males.[43] Although the role of *Mobiluncus* species in nonspecific bacterial va-

ginosis remains controversial, the organism is one of many genera of anaerobes that colonizes the vagina in both health and disease.[91]

Identification of the Anaerobic Cocci

The anaerobic cocci, compared with the anaerobic gram-negative bacilli, are the second most common group of anaerobes encountered in human infections (see Table 11-3). Like the anaerobic gram-negative rods, they are frequently encountered in the clinical laboratory in blood cultures, in other body fluids, and in a wide variety of wound and abscess specimens. The gram-positive cocci encountered clinically that belong to the genus *Peptostreptococcus* are listed in Table 11-9, including a new species, *P. hydrogenalis*.[29,73] The former *Peptostreptococcus parvulus* is now called *Streptococcus parvulus*.[19] Other anaerobic streptococci are *Streptococcus hansenii*, *S. intermedius*, and *S. pleomorphus*. The species formerly called *Streptococcus morbillorum* is now *Gemella morbillorum*.[54] The susceptibility of anaerobic cocci (isolated at the Indiana University Medical Center) to antimicrobial agents can be found in Table 11-13.

Identification of the Anaerobic Non–Spore-Forming Gram-Positive Bacilli

Included in this group of anaerobes are members of the genera *Actinomyces*, *Bifidobacterium*, *Eubacterium*, *Propionibacterium*, and *Lactobacillus* (see Chapter 10). Important characteristics of species of non–spore-forming, gram-positive bacilli are given in Table 11-10. The microscopic morphology and colonial characteristics of *Actinomyces israelii* and *Eubacterium lentum* are shown in Color Plate 11-2.

Identification of the anaerobic, gram-positive bacilli requires the use of GLC for metabolic product analysis. Cellular morphology of many of these organisms tends to vary with the type of culture medium and growth conditions. On morphologic grounds alone, they can sometimes be confused with several other genera, including *Clostridium*, *Corynebacterium*, *Lactobacillus*, *Leptotrichia*, *Listeria*, *Nocardia*, *Peptostreptococcus*, and *Streptococcus*. Thus, GLC results and morphologic characteristics, considered together, aid in practical differentiation.

Table 11-9
Some Key Characteristics of Anaerobic Cocci Commonly Isolated from Clinical Specimens

SPECIES	GRAM REACTION	BLACK PIGMENT	INDOLE	NITRATE	COAGULASE	UREASE	INHIBITED BY SPS	ALKALINE PHOSPHATASE	FERMENTATION OF Glucose	FERMENTATION OF Lactose	FERMENTATION OF Maltose	ACID METABOLIC PRODUCTS IN PYG, 48 HOURS, 35°C
Peptococcus niger	+	+	−	−	−	−	−	NT	−	−	−	A, (P), IB, B, IV, (V), C
Peptostreptococcus												
P. asaccharolyticus	+	−	+	−	−	−	−	−	−	−	−	A, (P), B
P. hydrogenalis	+	−	+	+	−	−	−	+	+	NT	−	A, B
P. indolicus	+	−	+	+	+	−	−	+	−	−	−	A, (P), B
P. anaerobius	+	−	−	−	−	−	+	−	w/−	−	w/−	A, (IB), (B), (IV), IC
P. prevotii	+	−	−	−/+	−	−/+	−	+	+	−	−	A, (P), B
P. tetradius	+	−	−	−	−	+	−	−	+*	−	+	A, B
P. magnus	+	−	−	−	−	−	−	+	−	−	−	A
P. micros†	+	−	−	−	−	−	−	+	−	−	−	A
P. productus	+	−	−	−	−	−	−	NT	+	+	+	A
Staphylococcus saccharolyticus	+	−	−	+	−	−	−	NT	+	−	−	A
Streptococcus intermedius	+	−	−	−	−	−	−	NT	+	+	+	A, L
Gemella morbillorum	+	−	−	−	−	−	−	NT	+	−	w	A, L
Veillonella species	−	−	−	+	−	−	−	NT	−	−	−	A, P

+, positive reaction; −, negative reaction; w, weakly fermentative; −/+, occasional strains positive; w/−, most strains positive; w/−, most strains weakly fermentative but occasional strains negative; SPS, sodium polyanethol sulfonate; A, acetic acid; P, propionic acid; IB, isobutyric acid; B, butyric acid; IV, isovaleric acid; V, valeric acid; IC, isocaproic acid; C, caproic acid; L, lactic acid; parentheses, variable; NT, not tested.

*P. tetradius strains lose their ability to ferment sugars rapidly after subculturing, so it is not uncommon for these reactions to be negative.

†Most strains of P. micros produce a slight β-hemolysis on CDC anaerobe blood agar (Carr-Scarborough, Stone Mountain, GA), which helps to distinguish them from P. magnus.

Table 11-10
Differentiation of Anaerobic, Gram-Positive Rods Encountered in Human Specimens to the Genus Level

DESCRIPTION	GENUS
I. Bacterial endospores produced	*Clostridium*
II. Endospores not produced	
A. Produce major amounts of propionic and acetic acids; catalase usually produced; irregular or regular shaped rods, coccoid cells; occasional branching	*Propionibacterium*
B. Produce acetic and lactic acids (>1:1 ratio); very irregular rods with bifid forms and branching	*Bifidobacterium*
C. Produce lactic acid as sole major product	
1. Short to long and slender rods; chain formation common; irregular rods uncommon; usually grow on tomato juice agar at $pH \leq 4.5$	*Lactobacillus*
2. Irregular rods predominant; filament forms with some branching	*Actinomyces*
D. Produce (1) moderate acetic and major succinic, (2) major lactic and major succinic, or (3) a major amount of lactic acids (see C, 2 above). Irregular rods; filaments with branching	*Actinomyces*
E. roduce mixture of acid metabolic products including (1) butyric acid and others, (2) acetic and formic acids, or (3) no major acids; obligate anaerobes; pleomorphic diphtheroid cells common, or uniform	*Eubacterium*

(Adapted from Allen SD. Gram-positive, nonsporeforming anaerobic bacilli. In: Lennette EH, Balows A, Hausler WJ Jr, Shadomy EJ, eds. Manual of clinical microbiology. 4th ed. Washington, DC, American Society for Microbiology, 1985:461–472; and Jones D, Collins MD. Irregular, nonsporing gram-positive rods. In: Sneath PHA, Mair NS, Sharpe MG, Holt JG, eds. Bergey's manual of systematic bacteriology. Baltimore, Williams & Wilkins, 1986;2:1261–1434.)

At times some strains of anaerobic bacilli resemble cocci, particularly in Gram-stained preparations of young colonies on blood agar. In addition, some streptococci, such as *S. mutans, S. intermedius, S. constellatus,* and *Gemella morbillorum* and certain peptostreptococci, may appear rod shaped when cells from colonies on blood agar are examined microscopically. On the other hand, these bacteria usually form long chains of cells in enriched thioglycolate broth and other liquid media. Many gram-positive bacteria tend to become gram-negative as they age. Also, some clostridia (eg, *C. perfringens, C. ramosum,* and *C. clostridioforme*) fail to produce spores in media routinely used in the clinical laboratory, whereas other clostridia do so as they age. Thus, Gram-stained preparations of very young cultures may aid in demonstration of gram variability, and observation of smears from older cultures may aid in demonstrating spores of clostridia.

Propionibacterium Species

Propionibacterium acnes is by far the most common gram-positive, anaerobic rod encountered in clinical specimens. It is part of the normal flora of the skin, nasopharynx, oral cavity, and gastrointestinal and genitourinary tracts. It is frequently a contaminant of blood cultures and occasionally causes endocarditis, central nervous system shunt infections, and other infections.

The cells are markedly pleomorphic and occur in varying shapes and sizes, ranging from coccoid to definite rods. Cells are often unevenly stained by the Gram procedure. Like the corynebacteria, the cells reveal Chinese letters, birds-in-flight, and picket fence arrangements, presumably because of "snapping" after they divide. *P. acnes* typically grows as an obligate anaerobe; some strains, however, show sparse growth in a candle jar (but better growth anaerobically), and have been described as aerotolerant or microaerophilic. Colonies of *P. acnes* on anaerobe blood agar are 1 to 2 mm in diameter, circular, entire, convex, glistening, and opaque. Some strains produce a narrow zone of hemolysis. *P. acnes* can be recognized without the use of GLC when it produces both indole and catalase.

While its pathogenicity and morphologic characteristics resemble those of certain species of *Actinomyces*, *P. propionicum* differs from *Actinomyces* species by producing propionic acid as a major metabolic product. *P. propionicum* should still be considered as a potential etiologic agent of human actinomycosis. *P. propionicum* is morphologically indistinguishable, in tissue and in culture, from *Actinomyces israelii*. Both *P. propionicum* and *A. israelii* form pleomorphic "diphtheroidal" rods and long, branched filaments. Both species are microaerophilic to anaerobic and grow optimally under anaerobic conditions.

Eubacterium Species

Eubacterium species are not nearly as common as *P. acnes*. When isolated from wounds and abscesses, they are often mixed with other bacteria. Their pathogenic significance in clinical specimens is often uncertain; like *P. acnes*, they may cause endocarditis and other infections. *E. lentum* is the species isolated most often. It shows little biochemical activity.

A report by Hill and colleagues[42] focused attention on one of the more recently described species, *E. nodatum*, which shares morphologic similarity with *Actinomyces* species. This species has been isolated from a wide variety of clinical sources, similar to sites that are expected to contain species of *Actinomyces*. In contrast to *A. israelii* and other actinomycetes, *E. nodatum* does not ferment carbohydrates and produces only acetic and butyric acids.

Actinomyces Species

The bacteria that can cause actinomycosis in humans include *Actinomyces israelii*, *A. naeslundii*, *A. odontolyticus*, *A. viscosus*, *A. meyeri*, *A. pyogenes* (formerly *Corynebacterium pyogenes*), *Propionibacterium propionicum*, and *Bifidobacterium dentium*. These bacteria are part of the normal flora of the mouth,

and many of them can be found in the genitourinary tract. *A. israelii* is the most common species in clinical infections. Actinomycosis (with lesions in tissue) is rare.

In Gram-stained smears prepared from lesions, one may observe characteristic *sulfur granules*, which are granular microcolonies of the organism surrounded by purulent exudate. The cells of *A. israelii* are gram-positive rods and are extremely variable in length. The cells may be short diphtheroid rods, club shaped, branched, or unbranched filaments (see Color Plate 11-2).

Rough colonies composed of branched rods or filaments usually develop slowly on blood agar. Young colonies (2 to 3 days old), when viewed with the dissecting microscope, appear as thin radiating filaments known as *spider colonies*. When the colonies get to be about 7 to 14 days old, they are often raised, heaped-up, white, opaque, and glistening; have irregular or lobate margins; and are called *molar tooth colonies* (see Color Plate 13-2). Smooth strains (about one third of *A. israelii*) produce colonies more rapidly than rough strains. Smooth strains may produce 1- to 2-mm, circular, slightly raised white, opaque, smooth, glistening colonies after only 2 to 3 days of incubation. *A. naeslundii* may also produce smooth or rough colonies. Colonies of *A. viscosus* are most often 0.5 to 2 mm in diameter, entire, convex, grayish, and translucent. *A. odontolyticus* colonies may develop a red color on blood agar after 7 to 14 days of anaerobic incubation or after the plates have been left out in room air at ambient temperature for several days. Detailed descriptions of these gram-positive anaerobic bacteria are provided in other textbooks.[3,52,87]

Bifidobacterium dentium is part of the normal microflora of the mouth and gastrointestinal tract and has been found in polymicrobial infections of the lower respiratory tract. The morphology of *B. dentium* is somewhat similar to that of *Actinomyces*, but it differs in not producing branched filaments in thioglycolate medium. Gram-stained smears prepared from solid media or broth cultures show gram-positive diphtheroidal forms that are much more variable in size and shape than *P. acnes*. Cells vary from coccoid to long, often curved forms, with characteristic swollen ends, or bifid forms, regularly produced by *B. dentium*. Other *Bifidobacterium* species are not known to be pathogenic for humans.[3]

Identification of *Clostridium* Species

The anaerobic gram-positive, spore-forming bacilli, by definition, are members of the genus *Clostridium*. In the clinical laboratory the problem
sometimes arises of determining whether an isolate
is an aerotolerant *Clostridium* or a facultatively anaerobic *Bacillus*. Aerotolerant clostridia rarely form
spores when grown aerobically and are catalase-
negative; species of the genus *Bacillus* rarely form
spores when grown anaerobically, and they produce catalase.[89]

Although the clostridia are considered gram-
positive, many are gram-negative by the time
smears of growing cultures are prepared. For example, *C. ramosum* and *C. clostridioforme* are usually
gram-negative. The demonstration of spores is frequently difficult with some species, for example,
C. perfringens, *C. ramosum*, and *C. clostridioforme*.
Demonstration of spore production is not necessary for identifying these three species. They have
several other distinctive properties. To demonstrate spores, Gram-stained preparations are usually sufficient; special spore stains generally offer
no particular advantage. In our experience, the best
way to demonstrate production of spores is to inoculate a cooked-meat agar slant and incubate it anaerobically for 5 to 7 days at 30°C. The cells from
the growth on the slant are then observed in a
Gram-stained preparation. In addition, a heat-
shock or alcohol spore selection technique may be
used.[4,56] Identifying characteristics for most of the
clostridia encountered in human infections are
given in Tables 11-11 and 11-12.

Clostridium perfringens

Some of the key reactions for identifying *C. perfringens* are illustrated in Color Plate 11-3. The
double zone of hemolysis on blood agar, production of lecithinase on egg-yolk agar, and stormy
fermentation of milk (or proteolysis of milk agar)
are characteristic of this species. The cells of *C.
perfringens* usually have blunt ends, and they are
often described as boxcar shaped. Cells examined
during early growth in broth culture tend to be
short and coccoid, while older cultures contain
longer cells that may be almost filamentous. Colonies are usually flat, somewhat rhizoid, and raised
centrally, often referred to as Chinese hat colonies.

Some colonies tend to spread, but they do not
swarm. *C. perfringens* is nonmotile.

Clostridium perfringens is by far the most commonly isolated species of *Clostridium* from human
sources, yet the clostridia account for only 10% to
13% of the anaerobic bacteria isolated from clinical
specimens. *C. perfringens* and other clostridia are
often found among the normal flora of the gastrointestinal tract. They also transiently inhabit the
skin. Many clostridia isolated from clinical specimens, even blood cultures, are accidental contaminants and may have no clinical significance. In
other circumstances, the presence of certain
clostridia in a lesion can have dire consequences to
the host. Communication between the microbiologist and the attending physician is usually necessary to assess the significance of a given isolate. *C.
perfringens* is also encountered in myonecrosis (gas
gangrene[4,16,89]), gangrenous cholecystitis, septicemia, and intravascular hemolysis after abortion
and anaerobic pleuropulmonary infections; it is
a major cause of food poisoning in the United
States[4,37] and a major worldwide cause of necrotizing
enterocolitis, involving children and adults.[4,44,89] Details of these conditions can be found elsewhere.[55]

Miscellaneous Clostridia
in Other Clinical Settings

CLOSTRIDIUM RAMOSUM.   Clostridium ramosum
is particularly common in posttraumatic intraabdominal infections and is especially important
clinically because of its resistance to penicillin G,
clindamycin, and other antibiotics. Cells are usually extremely pleomorphic, may appear gram-
negative, and sometimes produce short chains or
long filaments. Spores are usually not demonstrated on blood agar, and colonies are usually
nonhemolytic, slightly irregular or circular, low
convex, and translucent. Isolates of *C. ramosum* are
characteristically resistant to a 15-μg rifampin disk
but inhibited by the 2-IU penicillin disk and the
1-mg kanamycin disk. *C. ramosum* shows enhanced
growth on bile agar, hydrolyzes esculin, and is
negative for indol, catalase, lipase, and lecithinase.
It is among the few clostridia that ferment mannitol. Acetic, lactic, and succinic acids are the major
metabolic products.

CLOSTRIDIUM SEPTICUM.   C. septicum is usually
isolated from serious, often fatal infections. *C. sep-*

Table 11-11
Characteristics That Are Especially Useful for Identifying Some *Clostridium* Species

CHARACTERISTIC	SPECIES
Aerotolerant	*C. histolyticum, C. tertium, C. carnis*
Nonmotile	*C. innocuum, C. perfringens, C. ramosum*
Terminal spores	*C. barati, C. cadaveris, C. innocuum, C. ramosum, C. tertium, C. tetani*
Lecithinase produced on egg-yolk agar	*C. bifermentans, C. limosum, C. novyi, C. perfringens, C. sordellii, C. subterminale, C. barati, C. haemolyticum*
Lipase produced on egg-yolk agar	*C. botulinum, C. novyi* type A, *C. sporogenes*
Asaccharolytic and proteolytic (ie, gelatin-positive)	*C. histolyticum, C. limosum, C. subterminale, C. tetani, C. malenominatum* (weak to negative gelatin)
Urease-positive	*C. sordellii (C. bifermentans,* which it resembles, is urease-negative)
Do not hydrolyze gelatin	*C. butyricum, C. clostridioforme, C. malenominatum, C. paraputrificum, C. barati, C. ramosum*
Mannitol fermented	*C. difficile, C. innocuum, C. ramosum, C. sphenoides, C. symbiosum, C. tertium*
Rhamnose fermented	*C. clostridioforme, C. ramosum, C. sporogenes*
Saccharolytic and proteolytic	*C. bifermentans, C. botulinum, C. cadaveris, C. difficile, C. haemolyticum, C. novyi, C. perfringens, C. putrificum, C. septicum, C. sordellii, C. sporogenes*
Asaccharolytic and nonproteolytic	*C. barati, C. beijerinckii, C. butyricum, C. clostridioforme, C. glycolicum, C. innocuum, C. paraputrificum, C. ramosum, C. tertium*

ticum bacteremia, for unknown reasons, is often associated with underlying malignancy, particularly carcinoma of the colon, carcinoma of the breast, and hematologic malignancies (eg, leukemia, lymphoma).[57,58] The cells tend to be pleomorphic, sometimes producing long, thin filaments. Chain formation is common, as are intensely staining citron (lemon-shaped) forms. Spores are oval and subterminal and distend the organism. After 48 hours of incubation on blood agar, colonies are 2 to 5 mm in diameter, surrounded by a 1- to 4-mm zone of complete hemolysis; they are flat, slightly raised, gray, glistening,

(*text continues on page 276*)

Table 11-12
Some Key Characteristics of *Clostridium* Species Associated With Disease in Humans

SPECIES*	AERO-TOLERANT	DOUBLE ZONE HEMOLYSIS	TERMINAL SPORES	MOTILITY	VOLATILE METABOLIC PRODUCTS (GLC) IN PYG 48 HOURS, 35°C	OTHER
C. bifermentans	–	–	–	+	A, (P), (IB), (B), (IV), IC	Urease-negative; indole-positive
C. botulinum†	–	–	–	+	A, (P), (IB), B, IV, (V), (IC)	Lipase-positive
C. butyricum	–	–	–	+	A, B	Very saccharolytic
C. difficile	–	–	–	+	A, IB, B, IV, IC	
C. innocuum	–	–	+	–	A, B	Lactose- and maltose-negative
C. limosum	–	–	–	+	A	Asaccharolytic; gelatin-positive
C. novyi type A	–	–	–	+	A, P, B	Rarely encountered in clinical species

SPECIES*	AERO-TOLERANT	DOUBLE ZONE HEMOLYSIS	TERMINAL SPORES	MOTILITY	VOLATILE METABOLIC PRODUCTS (GLC) IN PYG 48 HOURS, 35°C	OTHER
C. perfringens	–	+	–	–	A, (P), B	Spores seldom observed
C. ramosum	–	–	+	–	A	Spores seldom observed; frequently gram-negative
C. septicum	–	–	–	+	A, B	Saccharolytic but sucrose-negative
C. sordellii	–	–	–	+	A, (P), (IB), (IV), IC	Urease-positive; indole-positive
C. sporogenes†	–	–	–	+	A, P, IB, B, IV, V, IC	Lipase-positive
C. subterminale	–	–	–	+	A, (P), IB, B, IV	Asaccharolytic; gelatin-positive
C. tetani	–	–	+	+	A, (P), B	May appear gram-negative
C. tertium	+	–	+	+	A, B	No spores under aerobic conditions

+, positive reaction for 90%–100% of strains tested; –, negative reaction for 90%–100% of strains tested; V, variable reaction; parentheses, variable; A, acetic acid; P, propionic acid; IB, isobutyric acid; IV, isovaleric acid; V, valeric acid; IC, isocaproic acid.

*For additional information on definitive identification of these species and other clostridia that may be encountered in clinical specimens, see references 4, 24, 45, and 94.

† Toxin neutralization tests required for definitive identification.

and semitranslucent and have markedly irregular to rhizoid margins, often surrounded by a zone of swarming. Extremely motile strains may swarm across a wide area of the plate. Stiff blood agar, which contains 4% to 6% instead of the usual 1.5% agar, is sometimes used in plating media to minimize swarming. Some key characteristics of *C. septicum* are that it hydrolyzes gelatin; does not produce indole, lipase, or lecithinase; and ferments lactose but not mannitol, rhamnose, or sucrose. Acetic and butyric acids are the major metabolic products.

Clostridium difficile-Associated Intestinal Disease

In the late 1970s, *C. difficile* was implicated as the major causative agent of antibiotic-associated diarrhea and pseudomembranous colitis.[13,15,30] Antimicrobial agents implicated in *C. difficile*-associated gastrointestinal illness have included numerous aminoglycosides, penicillins, cephalosporins, second- and third-generation β-lactam compounds, clindamycin, erythromycin, lincomycin, metronidazole, rifampin, trimethoprim-sulfamethoxazole, and amphotericin B.[13,39,97] Antibiotic-associated diarrhea manifests most often as a mild diarrhea in hospitalized patients receiving antibiotics. In other patients, the intestinal symptoms may be more severe and the diarrhea may persist. These patients may have antibiotic-associated colitis or life-threatening pseudomembranous colitis.[13,70]

The severity of illness, as well as pathologic findings, are highly variable, depending on whether the patient has pseudomembranous colitis, antibiotic-associated colitis, or antibiotic-associated diarrhea without anatomic evidence of colitis or is simply colonized with *C. difficile* (or is an asymptomatic carrier). The pathologic findings in pseudomembranous colitis and antibiotic-associated colitis have been reviewed elsewhere.[80] Factors that may be involved in *C. difficile*-associated disease include (1) toxin A, which is an enterotoxin capable of producing fluid accumulation in rabbit ligated ileal loop assays; (2) toxin B, which is a potent cytotoxin capable of producing cytopathogenic effects in several tissue culture cell lines; and (3) a "motility-altering factor" that stimulates smooth muscle contractions of intestine and is distinct from toxins A and B.[11,53,61,96] Toxin A is

also cytotoxic in certain cell lines but is not as cytotoxic as toxin B in the cell lines used for over a decade for toxin B testing.[64] Reviews of *C. difficile* and its toxins are available in other sources.[13,15,41,64]

Clostridium difficile is ubiquitous and has been isolated from soil, water, intestinal contents of various animals, the vagina and urethra of humans, and the feces of many healthy infants (but from the stools of only about 3% of healthy adult volun-

COLLECTION AND TRANSPORT OF SPECIMENS CONTAINING *CLOSTRIDIUM DIFFICILE*. Ordinarily, passed liquid or semisolid, unformed fecal specimens (about 5 g, or 5 mL if liquid) are the preferred specimens for laboratory diagnosis. Swab specimens, because of the small volume obtained, are inadequate. Formed stool specimens are inappropriate unless an epidemiologic study of stool carriage is being conducted. Other suitable specimens include biopsy material or lumen contents obtained by colonoscopy and involved bowel (surgical removal; autopsy). Leakproof plastic containers should be used for transport of specimens. Optimally, specimens should not remain at room temperature longer than 2 hours before either being processed or refrigerated. Specimens transported to a reference laboratory for a toxin assay, should be shipped on ice. Specimens to be processed for the *C. difficile* latex agglutination test should not be frozen, because the antigen detected is unstable on freezing.

LABORATORY DIAGNOSIS OF *CLOSTRIDIUM DIFFICILE*. Diagnostic testing in cases of suspected *C. difficile*-associated disease can be accomplished in the laboratory by demonstrating the cytotoxin, by recovering the organism from stool specimens, by tissue culture assay (the Toxi-titer microtiter plate, Bartels Immunodiagnostics, Bellevue, WA, is an available commercial product), by performing a latex agglutination test to detect *C. difficile* common protein antigen (Culturette Brand CDT LA Test, Becton Dickinson Microbiology Systems, Cockeysville, MD), by using an enzyme-linked immunosorbent assay (ELISA) to detect toxin A (premier Toxin A EIA, Meridian Diagnostics, Cincinnati, OH) or toxin A and B (Cambridge Biotech Corp), or by a combination of methods.

Clostridium difficile can be isolated by the use of a spore selection technique (ie, heat shock or alcohol spore selection procedures)[4,67] and by use of selective plating media such as phenylethyl alcohol blood agar (Carr-Scarborough Microbiologicals, Stone Mountain, GA) or cycloserine-cefoxitin, egg yolk, fructose agar (CCFA) plus nonselective CDC-anaerobe blood agar.[4,38,56,67] The alcohol or heat-treated sample is inoculated onto CDC anaerobe blood agar after the treatment. After 48 hours of incubation anaerobically, colonies of *C. difficile* are nonhemolytic, 2 to 4 mm in diameter, grayish-translucent, slightly raised, flat, and spreading, with rhizoid margins. As seen through a dissecting microscope, the colonies appear iridescent, speckled, or opalescent.

In addition to the spore selection procedure, a CCFA plate can be inoculated with untreated stool. The appearance of *C. difficile* colonies on CCFA medium after 48 hours of incubation is described in Table 11-5. Marler and colleagues[67] and Bartley and Dowell[17] have evaluated selective media formulations for the primary isolation of *C. difficile.*

Identification of *C. difficile* is described in several manuals.[4,24,45,94] In addition to the colony characteristics already described, there is a distinctive odor. The gram-positive to gram-variable rods have subterminal spores. Metabolic product analysis reveals acetic, propionic, isobutyric, butyric, isovaleric, valeric, and isocaproic acids (see Table 11-12). Esculin and gelatin are hydrolyzed. The cultures are negative for indole, nitrate, and urease. Most strains ferment glucose, mannitol, and mannose.

Botulism (*Clostridium botulinum*)

Botulism is a life-threatening neuroparalytic disease caused by heat-labile protein toxins of *C. botulinum.*[40,88] Botulinal toxin acts primarily by binding to synaptic vesicles of cholinergic nerves, preventing the release of acetylcholine at the peripheral nerve endings. Patients develop acute, flaccid, descending paralysis.[23]

Four different categories of botulism are recognized by the CDC. Classic *food-borne botulism*, typically seen in adults, results from the ingestion of preformed toxin in contaminated food. The second category, *wound botulism*, is the rarest form; it results from production of botulinal toxin in vivo after *C. botulinum* has multiplied in an infected wound. The third category, *infant botulism,*[9] is the most common; it results from in vivo multiplica-

tion of *C. botulinum* with production of the neurotoxin within the infant gut. The fourth category, *classification undetermined*, is for cases of botulism in persons who are older than 1 year of age in whom no food or wound source of *C. botulinum* can be implicated.[23]

The diagnosis of classic food-borne botulism is confirmed in reference laboratories such as the CDC by demonstrating botulinal toxin in serum, feces, gastric contents, or vomitus. Also, the organism may be isolated from the patient's feces.[23]

When infant botulism is suspected, serum (2 to 3 mL) and as much stool as possible (ideally 25 to 50 g) should be collected in a leakproof plastic container and refrigerated or placed on ice for shipment.

Tetanus (*Clostridium tetani*)

Tetanus is an infectious disease, caused by *C. tetani*, that largely involves unimmunized persons in the United States—mostly of the rural South.[4] It is a dramatic illness characterized by spastic contractions of voluntary muscles and hyperreflexia, caused by a protoplasmic, heat-labile protein toxin (tetanospasmin) elaborated by *C. tetani.*[23,33] Patients with tetanus have spastic muscle contractions, difficulty opening the jaw (called lockjaw, "trismus"), a characteristic smile called "risus sardonicus," and contractions of back muscles resulting in backward arching. The spores of *C. tetani*, like those of *C. botulinum*, are widely distributed in the soil, as well as in aquatic environments. Tetanus usually results from spore contamination of puncture wounds, lacerations, or even crush injuries.[23] The antecedent wound is often minor or trivial. Fecal contamination of the umbilical cord has been the source of *C. tetani* in some cases of neonatal tetanus.

Direct Gram-stained smears and anaerobic cultures of the wound site are often negative, failing to reveal the organism. *C. tetani* forms round, terminal spores, produces spreading or swarming growth on anaerobe blood agar, produces major amounts of acetate and butyrate, with only a minor amount of propionate, is lipase and lecithinase-negative on egg yolk agar, and is asaccharolytic. For more information on *C. tetani*, the books by Finegold and George[33] and Smith and Williams[89]

(*text continues on page 280*)

Table 11-13
Percentage of Anaerobes Susceptible to Concentrations of Antimicrobial Agents at Minimal Inhibitory Concentration Breakpoints Indicating Susceptibility*

BACTERIA (NO. STRAINS TESTED)	AMPICILLIN/SULBACTAM (16/8)	CEFOPERAZONE (32)	CEFOTAXIME (32)	CEFOTETAN (32)	CEFOXITIN (32)	CEFTRIAXONE (32)	CHLORAMPHENICOL (16)	CLINDAMYCIN (4)	IMIPENEM (8)	METRONIDAZOLE (16)	PENICILLIN G (4)	PIPERACILLIN (64)	TICARCILLIN/CLAVULANATE (64/2)
Bacteroides fragilis (236)	99	40	61	95	84	79	100	91	99	100	3	91	100
Bacteroides ovatus (84)	99	32	50	20	93	76	100	76	100	100	1	86	100
Bacteroides thetaiotaomicron (47)	98	40	60	30	94	79	100	79	98	100	0	94	100
Bacteroides vulgatus (64)	98	39	45	73	81	55	100	63	100	100	17	72	100
Bacteroides distasonis (28)	93	64	82	25	82	79	100	68	100	100	36	93	100
Prevotella melaninogenica "group" (21)	100	95	100	95	100	100	100	100	100	100	76	100	100
Prevotella oralis "group" (34)	100	100	97	100	100	97	100	100	100	100	53	100	100
Fusobacterium nucleatum (67)	99	99	100	100	99	100	100	100	100	100	87	97	100
Actinomyces species (22)	100	100	100	91	91	100	100	91	100	25	95	100	100
Eubacterium lentum (32)	100	31	28	81	97	66	100	94	100	97	100	100	100

278

BACTERIA (NO. STRAINS TESTED)	AMPICILLIN/SULBACTAM (16/8)	CEFOPERAZONE (32)	CEFOTAXIME (32)	CEFOTETAN (32)	CEFOXITIN (32)	CEFTRIAXONE (32)	CHLORAMPHENICOL (16)	CLINDAMYCIN (4)	IMIPENEM (8)	METRONIDAZOLE (16)	PENICILLIN G (4)	PIPERACILLIN (64)	TICARCILLIN/CLAVULANATE (64/2)
Propionibacterium acnes (245)	100	100	100	100	100	100	100	99	100	5	100	100	100
Lactobacillus species (50)	100	92	92	58	62	72	100	94	98	38	94	100	96
Clostridium perfringens (42)	100	100	100	100	100	100	100	98	100	98	100	100	100
Clostridium ramosum (35)	100	100	100	94	89	100	100	60	100	91	94	100	100
Clostridium difficile (25)	100	84	20	100	0	100	100	56	88	96	100	100	100
Clostridium clostridioforme (39)	97	90	85	100	100	90	100	92	100	100	95	97	100
Peptostreptococcus species (350)	100	96	99	100	100	100	99	87	100	96	97	99	100
Streptococcus intermedius (27)	100	100	100	96	100	100	96	85	100	7	100	100	100
Veillonella species (63)	100	92	100	100	100	100	100	98	100	100	83	94	97

Data given are from the Indiana University Medical Center Anaerobe Laboratory, December 1988 through April 1990.

*Breakpoints listed are given in µg/mL and are from the NCCLS document M100-S4, vol 12, no. 20 (Performance Standards for Antimicrobial Susceptibility Testing, Fourth Informational Supplement, December 1992).[77,78]

and the review articles by Dowell[23] and Hatheway[41] are recommended.

ANTIMICROBIAL SUSCEPTIBILITY TESTING OF ANAEROBIC BACTERIA

Successful management of diseases involving anaerobic bacteria requires selection and treatment with appropriate antimicrobial agents, often in conjunction with removal of bacteria by drainage of abscesses, elimination of foreign bodies, debridement of necrotic tissue, and other surgical measures. It was once believed that most anaerobes had predictable antimicrobial susceptibility patterns and that accurate identification of isolates was all that was necessary for one to predict the susceptibility of individual isolates to various antibiotics. This is an oversimplification. Although some antimicrobial agents are active against almost all anaerobic bacteria (including ampicillin/sulbactam, chloramphenicol, imipenem, and ticarcillin/clavulanate), several other antimicrobial agents that might be selected for use in treatment are not nearly as predictable in their activities against selected genera and species of anaerobes.[103] It is this variability in the susceptibility patterns of clinically significant anaerobes that indicates in vitro susceptibility testing of individual isolates should be performed to aid clinicians with the management of serious infections and those that require prolonged therapy, such as brain abscess, endocarditis, lung abscess, infections involving joints, infections involving prosthetic devices, vascular grafts, recurrent or refractory bacteremia, and osteomyelitis or when patients fail to respond to empiric therapy.[35,36,77] Another indication for testing is the setting in which there has not been a clear-cut clinical precedent on which to base treatment decisions.

Organisms to be considered for antimicrobial susceptibility testing, because of their virulence, or because they are commonly resistant to certain antimicrobial agents, include species of the *Bacteroides fragilis* group; species of the pigmented *Prevotella-Porphyromonas* group; *B. gracilis;* the *Prevotella oralis* group; *Fusobacterium mortiferum, F. varium,* and *F. necrophorum; Clostridium perfringens, C. ramosum, C. clostridioforme;* and nonintestinal isolates (eg, from blood cultures) of *C. difficile.* The antimicrobial susceptibility profiles of clinically

important anaerobic bacteria, based on studies conducted at the Indiana University Medical Center Anaerobic laboratory, are presented in Table 11-13.

The agar dilution and broth dilution methods for antimicrobial susceptibility testing discussed in Chapter 12 also apply in principle to the anaerobes. The broth disk elution and disk agar diffusion techniques should not, however, be used for anaerobe testing despite their convenience. Most anaerobes other than some *B. fragilis* group and *Clostridium* species grow too slowly for the disk diffusion procedure to work; the Bauer-Kirby interpretive charts were not designed for anaerobes, and interpretive charts based on standardized media and methods for disk-diffusion testing of anaerobes are lacking; also, there has been poor correlation between zone size measurements and the results from minimal inhibitory concentration dilution tests.

Guidelines have been published by the National Committee for Clinical Laboratory Standards (NCCLS; most recently M11-A2, 1990) describing their recommended methods for antimicrobial susceptibility testing of anaerobes.[57,77] NCCLS document M100-S4[78] describes minimal inhibitory concentration breakpoints indicating susceptibility, designates control strains (*B. fragilis,* ATCC 25285; *B. thetaiotaomicron,* ATCC 29741; *C. perfringens,* ATCC 13124; and *E. lentum,* ATCC 43055), and provides acceptable ranges of minimal inhibitory concentrations for control strains for the reference agar dilution method and for the broth microdilution method.

REFERENCES

1. Allen SD. Identification of anaerobic bacteria: how far to go. Clin Microbiol Newsl 1979;1(6):3–5.
2. Allen SD. Systems for rapid identification of anaerobic bacteria. In: Tilton RC, ed. Rapid methods and automation in microbiology. Washington, DC, American Society for Microbiology, 1982: 214–217.
3. Allen SD. Gram-positive, nonsporeforming anaerobic bacilli. In: Lennette EH, Balows A, Hausler WJ Jr, Shadomy EJ, eds. Manual of clinical microbiology. 4th ed. Washington, DC, American Society for Microbiology, 1985:461–472.
4. Allen SD, Baron EJ. *Clostridium.* In: Balows A, Hausler WJ Jr, Herrmann K Jr, et al, eds. Manual of clinical microbiology. 5th ed. Washington,

DC, American Society for Microbiology, 1991.

5. Allen SD, Siders JA, Marler LM. Isolation and examination of anaerobic bacteria. In: Lennette EH, Balows A, Hausler WJ Jr, Shadomy EJ, eds. Manual of clinical microbiology. 4th ed. Washington, DC, American Society for Microbiology, 1985:413–443.

6. Allen SD, Siders J, Marler L, O'Bryan N. Rapid identification of anaerobes. In: Sanna A, Morace G, eds. New horizons in microbiology. New York, Elsevier Science Publishers, 1984:233–240.

7. Allen SD, Lombard GL, Armfield AY, et al. Development and evaluation of an improved anaerobic holding jar procedure. Abstract C142. Presented before the annual meeting of the American Society of Microbiology, 1977:59.

8. Aranki AS, Syed A, Kenney EB, Freter R. Isolation of anaerobic bacteria from human gingiva and mouse cecum by means of a simplified glove box procedure. Appl Microbiol 1969;17:568–576.

9. Arnon SS. Infant botulism. In: Finegold SM, George WL, eds. Anaerobic infections in humans. New York, Academic Press, 1989:601–609.

10. Banks R, Allen SD, Siders JA, et al. Characterization of anaerobic bacteria by using a commercially available rapid tube test for glutamic acid decarboxylase. J Clin Microbiol 1989;27:361–363.

11. Banno Y, Kobayashi T, Kono H, Watanabe K, et al. Biochemical characterization and biologic actions of two toxins (D-1 and D-2) from *Clostridium difficile*. Rev Infect Dis 1984;6:S11–S20.

12. Baron EJ, Summanen P, Downes J, et al. *Bilophila wadsworthia* gen. nov., sp. nov., a unique gram-negative anaerobic rod recovered from appendicitis specimens and human faeces. J Gen Microbiol 1989;135:3405–3411.

13. Bartlett JG. Antibiotic-associated colitis. Dis Month 1984;30:1–54.

14. Bartlett JG. Anaerobic bacteria: general concepts. In: Mandell GL, Douglas RG Jr, Bennett JE, eds. Principles and practices of infectious diseases. 3rd ed. New York, Churchill Livingstone, 1990: 1828–1842.

15. Bartlett JG. *Clostridium difficile*: clinical considerations. Rev Infect Dis 1990;12(Suppl 1):S243–S251.

16. Bartlett JG. Gas gangrene (other *Clostridium*-associated diseases). In: Mandell GL, Douglas RG Jr, Bennett JE, eds. Principles and practice of infectious diseases. 3rd ed. New York, Churchill Livingstone, 1990:1850–1860.

17. Bartley SL, Dowell VR Jr. Comparison of media for the isolation of *Clostridium difficile* from fecal specimens. Lab Med 1991;22:335–338.

18. Brock TD, Madigan MT. Biology of microorganisms. 6th ed. Englewood Cliffs, NJ, Prentice-Hall, 1991.

19. Cato EP. Transfer of *Peptostreptococcus parvulus* (Weinberg, Nativelle, and Prevot 1937) Smith 1957 to the genus *Streptococcus: Streptococcus parvulus* (Weinberg, Nativelle and Prevot 1937) comb. nov., nom. rev., emend. Int J Syst Bacteriol 1983;33:82–84.

20. Celig DM, Schreckenberger PA. Clinical evaluation of the RapID-ANA II panel for identification of anaerobic bacteria. J Clin Microbiol 1991;29: 457–462.

21. Dellinger CA, Moore LVH. Use of the RapID-ANA system to screen for enzyme activities that differ among species of bile-inhibited *Bacteroides*. J Clin Microbiol 1986;23:289–293.

22. Dorsher CW, Wilson WR, Rosenblatt JE. Anaerobic bacteremia and cardiovascular infections. In: Finegold SM, George WL, eds. Anaerobic infections in humans. San Diego, Academic Press, 1989:289–310.

23. Dowell VR Jr. Botulism and tetanus: selected epidemiologic and microbiologic aspects. Rev Infect Dis 1984;6:S202–S207.

24. Dowell VR Jr, Hawkins TM. Laboratory methods in anaerobic bacteriology. (CDC laboratory manual.) DHEW Publication No. (CDC) 78-8272. Atlanta, Centers for Disease Control, 1977

25. Dowell VR Jr, Lombard GL. Differential agar media for identification of anaerobic bacteria. In: Tilton RC, ed. Rapid methods and automation in microbiology. Washington, DC, American Society for Microbiology, 1982:258–262.

26. Dowell VR Jr, Lombard GL. Presumptive identification of anaerobic non–spore-forming gram-negative bacilli. Atlanta, Centers for Disease Control, 1977.

27. Dowell VR Jr, Lombard GL, Thompson FS, Armfield AY. Media for isolation, characterization, and identification of obligately anaerobic bacteria. (CDC laboratory manual.) Atlanta, Centers for Disease Control, 1977.

28. Downes J, Mangels JI, Holden J, et al. Evaluation of two single-plate incubation systems and the anaerobic chamber for the cultivation of anaerobic bacteria. J Clin Microbiol 1990;28:246–248.

29. Ezaki T, Yamamoto N, Ninomiya K, et al. Transfer of *Peptococcus indolicus, Peptococcus asaccharolyticus, Peptococcus prevotii* and *Peptococcus magnus* to the genus *Peptostreptococcus* and proposal of *Peptostreptococcus tetradius* sp. nov. Int J Syst Bacteriol 1983;33:683–698.

30. Fekety R. Recent advances in management of bacterial diarrhea. Rev Infect Dis 1983;5:246–257.

31. Felner JM, Dowell VR Jr. *Bacteroides* bacteremia. Am J Med 1971:787–796.

32. Finegold SM. General aspects of anaerobic infection. In: Finegold SM, George WL (eds). Anaer-

obic infections in humans, pp 137–153. San Diego, Academic Press, 1989.

33. Finegold SM. Therapy of anaerobic infections. In: Finegold SM, George WL, eds. Anaerobic infections in humans. New York, Academic Press, 1989:793–818.

34. Finegold SM. Anaerobes: problems and controverises in bacteriology, infections, and susceptibility testing. Rev Infect Dis 1990;12:S223–S230.

35. Finegold SM, George WL, eds. Anaerobic infections in humans. San Diego, CA, Academic Press, 1989.

36. Finegold SM. The National Committee for Clinical Laboratory Standards Working Group on Anaerobic Susceptibility Testing: susceptibility testing of anaerobic bacteria. J Clin Micriboil 1988;26:1253–1256.

37. Foodborne disease outbreaks, annual summary, 1982. In: CDC surveillance summaries. Atlanta, Centers for Disease Control, 1986;35:7SS–16SS.

38. George WL, Sutter VL, Citron D, Finegold SM. Selective and differential medium for isolation of *Clostridium difficile.* J Clin Microbiol 1979;9:214–219.

39. Gerding DN, Olsen, MM, PeTerson LR, Teasley DG. *Clostridium difficile*–associated diarrhea and colitis in adults: a prospective case-controlled epidemiologic study. Arch Intern Med 1986;146:95–100.

40. Hatheway CL. Botulism. In: Balows A, Hausler WJ Jr, Ohashi M, et al, eds. Laboratory diagnosis of infectious diseases: principles and practice. New York, Springer, 1988;1:111–133.

41. Hatheway CL. Toxigenic clostridia. Clin Microbiol Rev 1990;3:66–98.

42. Hill GB, Ayers OM, Kohan AP. Characterization and sites of infection of *Eubacterium nodatum, Eubacterium timidum, Eubacterium brachy*, and other asaccharolytic eubacteria. J Clin Microbiol 1987;25:1540–1545.

43. Hiller SL, Eschenbach DA. Bacterial vaginosis: role of *Mobiluncus* species. Infect Dis Newsl 1984;5:65–68.

44. Hobbs BC. *Clostridium welchii* as a food-poisoning organism. J Appl Bacteriol 1965;28:74–83.

45. Holdeman LV, Cato EP, Moore WEC, eds. Anaerobe laboratory manual. 4th ed. Blacksburg, Virginia Polytechnic Institute and State University, 1977.

46. Holdeman LV, Cato EP, Moore WEC. Taxonomy of anaerobes: present state of the art. Rev Infect Dis 1984;6:S3–S10.

47. Holdeman LV, Kelley RW, Moore WEC. Anaerobic gram-negative straight, curved, and helical rods. Family 1. Bacteroidaceae Pribram 1933, 10^AL. In: Krieg NR, Holt JG, eds. Bergey's manual of systematic bacteriology. Baltimore, Williams & Wilkins, 1984:602–662.

48. Holdeman LV, Moore WEC, Churn PJ, Johnson JL. *Bacteroides oris* and *Bacteroides buccae*: new species from human periodontitis and other human infections. Int J Syst Bacteriol 1982;32:125–131.

49. Hussain Z, Lannigan R, Schieven BC, et al. Comparison of RapID-ANA and Minitek with a conventional method for biochemical identification of anaerobes. Diagn Microbiol Infect Dis 1987;6:69–72.

50. Jarkowski TL, Wolf PL. Unusual gas *Bacillus* infections including necrotic enteritis. JAMA 1962;181:845–850.

51. Johnson CC, Reinhardt JF, Edelstein MAC, Mulligan ME, et al. *Bacteroides gracilis*, an important anaerobic bacterial pathogen. J Clin Microbiol 1985;22:799–802.

52. Jones D, Collins MD. Irregular, nonsporing gram-positive rods. In: Sneath PHA, Mair NS, Sharpe MG, Holt JG, eds. Bergey's manual of systematic bacteriology. Baltimore, Williams & Wilkins, 1986:1261–1434.

53. Justus PG, Martin JL, Gooldberg DA, et al. Myoelectric effects of *Clostridium difficile*: myoelectric-altering factors distinct from its cytotoxin and enterotoxin in rabbits. Gastroenterology 1982;83:836–843.

54. Kilper-Balz R, Wenzig P, Schleifer KH. Molecular relationship and classification of some viridans streptococci as *Streptococcus oralis* and emended description of *Streptococcus oralis* (Bridge and Sneath, 1982). Int J Syste Bacteriol 1984;35:482–488.

55. Koneman EW, Allen SD, Dowell VR Jr, et al. Color atlas and textbook of diagnostic microbiology. 4th ed. Philadelphia, JB Lippincott, 1991.

56. Koransky JR, Allen SD, Dowell VR Jr. Use of ethanol for selective isolation of spore-forming microorganisms. Appl Environ Microbiol 1978;35:762–765.

57. Koransky JR, Stargel MD, Dowell VR Jr. *Clostridium septicum* bacteremia: the clinical significance. Am J Med 1979;66:63–66.

58. Kornbluth AA, Danzig JB, Bernstein LH. *Clostridium septicum* infection and associated malignancy. Medicine 1989;68:30–37.

59. Krieg NR, Hold JG, eds. Bergey's manual of systematic bacteriology, vol 1. Baltimore, Williams & Wilkins, 1984.

60. Kronvall G, Mylore E. Differential staining of bacteria in clinical specimens using acridine orange buffered at low pH. Acta Pathol Scand [B] 1977;85:249–254.

61. Laughon BE, Viscidi RP, Gdouin SL, Yolken RH, Bartlett JG. Enzyme immunoassay for de-

tection of *Clostridium difficile* toxins A and B in fecal specimens. J Infect Dis 1984;149:781–788.

62. Loesche WJ. Oxygen sensitivity of various anaerobic bacteria. Appl Microbiol 1969;8:723–727.

63. Lombard GL, Dowell VR Jr. Gas liquid chromatography: analysis of acid products of bacteria. Atlanta, Centers for Disease Control, 1982.

64. Lyerly DM, Krivan HC, Wilkins TD. *Clostridium difficile*: its disease and toxins. Clin Microbiol Rev 1988;1:1–18.

65. Marler LM, Allen SD, Siders JA. Rapid enzymatic characterization of clinically encountered anaerobic bacteria with the API ZYM system. Eur J Clin Microbiol 1984;3:294–300.

67. Marler LM, Siders JA, Wolters LC, et al. Evaluation of the new RapID ANA II system for the identification of clinical anaerobe isolates. J Clin Microbiol 1991;29:874–878.

68. Martin WJ. Practical method for isolation of anaerobic bacteria in the clinical laboratory. Appl Microbiol 1971;22:1168–1171.

69. Mayrand D. Identification of clinical isolates of selected species of *Bacterioides*: production of phenylacetic acid. Can J Microbiol 1979;25:927–928.

70. McFarland LV, Stamm WE. Review of *Clostridium difficile*–associated diseases. Am J Infect Control 1986;14:99–109.

71. McNeil MM, Martone WJ, Dowell VR Jr. Bacteremia with *Anaerobiospirillum succiniciproducens*. Rev Infect Dis 1987;9:737–742.

72. Moore LVH, Cato EP, Moore WEC, eds. Anaerobe laboratory manual update: supplement to the VPI anaerobe laboratory manual. 4th ed. 1977. Blacksburg, Virginia Polytechnic Institute and State University, 1987.

73. Moore LVH, Johnson JL, Moore WEC. Genus *Peptostreptococcus* Kluyver and van Niel 1936, 401[AL]. In: Sneath PHA, Mair NS, Sharpe ME, Holt JG, eds. Bergey's manual of systematic bacteriology. Baltimore, Williams & Wilkins, 1986; 2:1083–1092.

74. Moore WEC. Chromatography for the clinical laboratory: All you wanted to know (and possibly more). API Species 1980;4:21–28.

75. Murray PR, Weber CJ, Niles AC. Comparative evaluation of three identification systems for anaerobes. J Clin Microbiol 1985;22:52–55.

76. Murray PR, Traynor P, Hopson D. Critical assessment of blood culture techniques: analysis of recovery of obligate and facultative anaerobes, strict aerobic bacteria and fungi in aerobic and anaerobic blood culture bottles. J Clin Microbiol 1992;30:1462–1468.

77. National Committee for Clinical Laboratory Standards. Methods for antimicrobial susceptibility testing of anaerobic bacteria. 2nd ed. Approved standard, NCCLS publication M11-A2. Villanova, PA, NCCLS, 1990.

78. National Committee for Clinical Laboratory Standards: Performance standards for antimicrobial susceptibility testing. Third information supplement. NCCLS Document M100-S3. Villanova, PA, NCCLS, 1991

79. Park CH, Hixon DL, Endlich JF, O'Connell P. *Anaerobiospirillum succiniproducens*: two case reports. Am J Clin Pathol 1986;85:73–76.

80. Price AB. Histopathology of clostridial gut diseases in man. In: Borriello SP, ed. Clostridia in gastrointestinal disease. Boca Raton, FL, CRC Press, 1985:177–193.

81. Rolfe RD, Hentges DJ, Barrett JT, Campbell BJ. Oxygen tolerance of human intestinal anaerobes. Am J Clin Nutr 1977;30:1762–1769.

82. Rosenblatt JE. Anaerobic identification systems. Clin Lab Med 1985;5:59–65.

83. Shah HN, Collins DM. Proposal for re-classification of *Bacteroides asaccharolyticus*, *Bacteroides gingivalis*, and *Bacteroides endodontalis* in a new genus, *Porphyromonas*. Int J Syst Bacteriol 1988;38:128–131.

84. Shah HN, Collins DM. Proposal to restrict the genus *Bacteroides* (Castellani and Chalmers) to *Bacteroides fragilis* and closely related species. Int J Syst Bacteriol 1989;39:85–87.

85. Shah HN, Collins DM. *Prevotella*, a new genus to include *Bacteroides melaninogenicus* and related species formerly classified in the genus *Bacteroides*. Int J Syst Bacteriol 1990;40:205–208.

86. Shinjo T, Hiraiwa K, Miyazato S. Recognition of biovar C of *Fusobacterium necrophorum* (Flugge) Moore and Holdeman as *Fusobacterium pseudonecrophorum* sp. nov., nom. rev. (ex Prevot 1940). Int J Syst Bacteriol 1990;40:71–73.

87. Slack JM, Genercser MA. *Actinomyces*, filamentous bacteria biology and pathogenicity. Minneapolis, Burgess Publishing, 1975.

88. Smith LDS. Botulism: the organism, its toxins, the disease. Springfield, IL, Charles C Thomas, 1977.

89. Smith LDS, Williams BL. The pathogenic anaerobic bacteria. 3rd ed. Springfield, IL, Charles C Thomas, 1984.

90. Sneath PHA, Mair NS, Sharpe ME, Holt JG, eds. Bergey's manual of systematic bacteriology, vol 2. Baltimore, Williams & Wilkins, 1986.

91. Spiegel CA. Bacterial vaginosis. Clin Microbiol Rev 1991;4:485–502.

92. Spiegel CA, Eschenbach DA, Amsel R, et al. Curved anaerobic bacteria in bacterial (nonspecific) vaginosis and their response to antimicrobial therapy. J Infect Dis 1983;148:817–822.

93. Spiegel CA, Roberts M. *Mobiluncus* gen. nov., *Mobiluncus cutisii* subsp. *curtisii* sp. nov., *Mobiluncus curtisii* subsp. *holmesii* subsp. nov., and *Mobiluncus mulieris* sp. nov., curved rods from the human vagina. Int J Syst Bacteriol 1984;34:177–184.

94. Sutter VL, Citron DM, Edelstein MAC, Finegold SM. Wadsworth anaerobic bacteriology manual. 4th ed. Belmont, CA, Star Publishing, 1985.

95. Tally FP, Goldin BR, Jacobus NV, Gorbach SL. Superoxide dismutase in anaerobic bacteria of clinical significance. Infect Immunol 1977;16:20–25.

96. Taylor NS, Thorne GM, Bartlett JG. Comparison of two toxins produced by *C. difficile*. Infect Immun 1981;34:1036–1043.

97. Trnka YM, Lamont JT. *C. difficile* colitis. Adv Intern Med 1984;29:85–106.

98. Van Winkelhoff AJ, Clement M, de Graaf J. Rapid characterization of oral and non-oral pigmented *Bacteroides* species with the ATB Anaerobes ID system. J Clin Microbiol 1988;26:1063–1065.

99. Van Winkelhoff AJ, Van Steenbergen TJM, de Graaff J. Enzymatic characterization of oral and nonoral pigmented *Bacteroides* species. Antonie van Leeuwenhoek 1986;52:163–171.

100. Van Winkelhoff AJ, Van Steenbergen TJM, Kippuw N, et al. Further characterization of *Bacteroides endodontalis*, an asaccharolytic black-pigmented *Bacteroides* species from the oral cavity. J Clin Microbiol 1985;22:75–79.

101. Walden WC, Hentges DJ. Differential effects of oxygen and oxidation-reduction potential on the multiplication of three species of anaerobic intestinal bacteria. Appl Microbiol 1975;30:781–785.

102. Walker PD. Pig-bel. In: Borriello SP, ed. Clostridia in gastrointestinal disease. Boca Raton, FL, CRC Press, 1985:94–115.

103. Wexler HM. Susceptibility testing of anaerobic bacteria: myth, magic, or method? Clin Microbiol Rev 1991;4:470–484.

104. Whaley DN, Gorman GW. An inexpensive device for evacuating and gassing systems with in-house vacuum. J Clin Microbiol 1977;5:668–669.

Antimicrobial Susceptibility Testing

Initial optimism following Alexander Fleming's 1928 discovery of penicillin[25] that antibiotics would put an end to bacterial infection has given way to reluctant acceptance that chemotherapeutic resources must be managed wisely to control disease.

A few bacteria, such as *Streptococcus pyogenes* (group A β-hemolytic streptococci), have maintained their predictable susceptibility to penicillin. This persistent susceptibility is, unfortunately, the exception rather than the rule. The ingenuity of the chemists in the pharmaceutical industry is reflected in the large number of antibiotics available to physicians (Table 12-1).

BACTERIAL RESISTANCE TO ANTIMICROBIAL AGENTS

The mechanisms of bacterial resistance are complex, varied, and not completely understood. Interested readers should consult Lorian's *Antibiotics in Clinical Medicine*.[41] or an excellent discussion in Mandell's *Principles and Practice of Infectious Diseases*.[42] A comprehensive review is provided by Jacoby and Archer,[32] who have tabulated the major resistance mechanisms of the most important human pathogens.

LABORATORY GUIDANCE OF ANTIMICROBIAL THERAPY

A chemotherapeutic drug is a chemical compound that is used in the treatment of a disease. The compound may come from natural sources or may have been synthesized by a chemist in the labora-

tory. The disease may be of any type, including infectious and neoplastic processes. An antibiotic is an antimicrobial agent that is derived from a microorganism; an antimicrobial agent is a drug that acts primarily against infectious organisms.

Microbiologists can be of great assistance to clinicians in guiding effectual antibiotic therapy. They can evaluate the in vitro interactions between an isolated microbe and antimicrobial agents that would be appropriate for treatment of an infection in vivo. Their work in the laboratory can provide data to help the clinician decide whether the selected doses of an antibiotic are adequate.

In this chapter, the evaluation of antimicrobial agents that are active against aerobic and facultatively anaerobic bacteria is discussed. Testing of anaerobic bacteria, mycobacteria, and fungi are discussed in Chapters 11, 13, and 16.

Antimicrobial test procedures are summarized in Table 12-2, which includes a brief description of each test and a list of specimens that the laboratory must have in hand. The tests may be divided conveniently into two groups: tests that *predict* the effectiveness of therapy and those that *monitor* the effectiveness of therapy.

Several types of antimicrobial susceptibility (or

Table 12-1
Classification of Antibiotics

CLASS	GROUP	EXAMPLES
β-Lactam	Penicillins	Penicillin G, ampicillin, amoxicillin
	Penicillinase-resistant penicillins	Methicillin, nafcillin, oxacillin, cloxacillin, dicloxacillin
	Broad-spectrum penicillins	Carbenicillin, piperacillin, mezlocillin, ticarcillin
	First-generation cephalosporins	Cephalothin, cefazolin
	Second-generation cephalosporins	Cefoxitin, cefotetan, cefuroxime
	Third-generation cephalosporins	Cefotaxime, ceftazidime, ceftizoxime, ceftriaxone
	Monobactams	Aztreonam
	Carbapenem	Imipenem
β-Lactam/β-lactamase inhibitors	Penicillins	Ampicillin/sulbactam, amoxicillin/clavulanic acid, ticarcillin/clavulanic acid
Aminoglycosides		Gentamicin, tobramycin, netilmycin, amikacin, streptomycin, kanamycin
Macrolides		Erythromycin, clindamycin
Glycopeptides		Vancomycin, teicoplanin
Quinolones		Norfloxacin, ciprofloxacin, ofloxacin

Table 12-2
Guidance of Antimicrobial Therapy

PROCEDURE	DEFINITION	SPECIMENS	INDICATIONS
Minimum inhibitory concentration (broth or agar)	Lowest concentration of antibiotic that inhibits visible growth	Microbial isolate	Antimicrobial susceptibility of isolates if etiologic role established and susceptibility not predictable
Disk diffusion	Diameter of inhibition of growth around paper disk impregnated with antibiotic	Microbial isolate	Simplified method to approximate MIC with interpretative correlates
Minimum bactericidal concentration	Lowest concentration of antibiotic that kills 99.9% of the inoculum	Microbial isolate	Streptococcal endocarditis; potentially for osteomyelitis; potentially tolerant isolates if unresponsive to therapy
Antimicrobial levels	Concentration (μg/mL) of antibiotic in serum	Peak serum Trough serum	Unpredictability of peak levels or potential for toxicity
Serum bactericidal titers	Dilution of serum that kills 99.9% of the inoculum	Peak serum Trough serum Microbial isolate	Bacterial endocarditis; osteomyelitis; gram-negative sepsis in immunosuppressed patients
Synergy tests	Synergistic activity of multiple antibiotics	Microbial isolate	Research procedure for development of therapeutic regimens; rarely, confirmation of synergy against individual isolates

sensitivity) tests have been devised. The two reference tests are the macroscopic broth dilution and agar dilution procedures. Both are designed to quantitate the lowest concentration of an antibiotic that inhibits visible in vitro growth of the microbe—the minimal inhibitory concentration (MIC). The test used most frequently to guide antibiotic therapy is the disk diffusion procedure (Bauer-Kirby test), in which clinical interpretations are derived from correlations with the reference tests. In recent years, an increasing number of laboratories have routinely used a miniaturized broth test (microdilution broth test) or an automated commercial system.

Antibiotic susceptibility tests are intended to be a *guide* for the clinician, not a guarantee that an antimicrobial agent will be effective in therapy. A goal of microbiologists has been, and should continue to be, the provision of standardized in vitro tests that can be reproduced from day to day and from laboratory to laboratory. Without reproducibility there is no scientific basis for therapy. In striving for standardization, however, it is possible that the variability of each infection and each patient is not addressed. The factors that determine the outcome of an infectious process are complex and, in many instances, are incompletely addressed by in vitro tests.[68]

TESTS FOR DETERMINING INHIBITORY ACTIVITY OF ANTIBIOTICS

Indications

Tests of inhibitory activity of antibiotics are designed for bacteria that grow well after overnight incubation in air and have unpredictable susceptibilities. Fastidious bacteria, which grow more slowly or require nutritional or atmospheric supplements, should be tested with a dilution test only if careful use of control bacterial strains demonstrates the absence of inhibitory effects on the interactions. The disk diffusion test may be modified for such organisms if the procedure has been validated by comparison to reference tests and to clinical experience.[47]

Microbiologists should resist pressure from clinicians to extend the procedures beyond their established limits. Many mistakes were made by participants in the proficiency testing surveys of the College of American Pathologists in the determination of the susceptibility of *Listeria monocytogenes* to penicillin and ampicillin because the published guidelines were not designed for this bacterium.[33] Further studies made it possible to establish valid guidelines for *Listeria* species, and results of the surveys have improved. The recent demonstration that a commercial broth microdilution test did not detect resistance to penicillin among certain strains of *Streptococcus pneumoniae* emphasizes that caution is required even if dilution tests are employed and the conventional bacterial controls are included.[60]

The list of bacteria that have consistently predictable susceptibilities is, unfortunately, becoming shorter. The prevalence of β-lactamase–producing strains of *Haemophilus influenzae* and *Neisseria gonorrhoeae* is sufficiently high that susceptibility to penicillin analogues can no longer be assumed.[16] Although pneumococci that are relatively resistant to penicillin (MIC of 0.12 to 1 μg/mL) or have high-level resistance (MIC of greater than 1 μg/mL) are still uncommon in the United States, the possibility must be considered in serious infections,[31] and pneumococcal strains should be tested for resistance. With extremely rare exceptions, isolates of *Neisseria meningitidis* and *Streptococcus pyogenes* remain susceptible to penicillin.

Choice of Test

In most situations either a disk diffusion or a microdilution broth test is adequate to guide clinical therapy. Advantages of dilution tests are that they provide more quantitative information and may be applied to a wider range of isolates than the diffusion test. There is, however, definite potential for misinterpretation of a quantitative result if physicians do not understand how to use the information and the laboratory fails to provide sufficient guidance in interpretation. The disk diffusion test has a long and successful track record; it is still the most common test for antimicrobial susceptibility offered in hospital laboratories. The choice of which method to use depends on local needs and resources.

Selection of Antimicrobial Agents

The final selection of antibiotics for the hospital formulary should be decided in consultation with members of the medical staff. A list of antimicrobial agents that has been suggested by the National Committee for Clinical Laboratory Stan-

dards (NCCLS) is detailed in Table 12-3.* Many antibiotics are grouped by class because the spectrum of activity is similar. The recent recommendations of the NCCLS address selective testing and selective reporting, recognizing that the issues are complex and vary from institution to institution. Washington has provided a guide to the antimicrobial groupings[69] (Table 12-4). It is not necessary to test each antibiotic in the list. Patterns of antibiotic usage and bacterial resistance in each community should be known and considered when selecting antibiotics for testing. Distinctions may be made between antibiotics that are tested routinely and those for which results are reported routinely to physicians.

Standardization

The major improvement in laboratory guidance of susceptibility testing over the past several decades has come from the development of standardized procedures that have been widely adopted. It is extremely important to adhere to the recommended protocols if reproducible results are to be achieved. The NCCLS publishes standards for these and other tests on a continuing basis. (Copies of the *Performance Standards for Antimicrobial Disk Susceptibility Tests*[45] and the *Methods for Dilution Antimicrobial Susceptibility Tests for Bacteria that Grow Aerobically*[46] may be obtained on request by writing the NCCLS at 771 East Lancaster Avenue, Villanova, PA 19085.) It is important that revised procedures and current recommendations be promptly promulgated in all clinical laboratories. An institutional membership in the NCCLS ensures the timely receipt of all new and revised recommendations. Washington has summarized the resources and

(text continues on page 292)

---

*Permission to reprint portions of Tables 12-3, 12-6, 12-7, and 12-8 from M2–A4 and Tables 12-5 and 12-9 from M7–A2 has been granted by the National Committee for Clinical Laboratory Standards. NCCLS is not responsible for errors or inaccuracies. The data in the tables are valid only if the methods in M2–A4 and M7–A2, are followed. These documents and current supplements may be obtained from National Committee for Clinical Laboratory Standards, 771 E. Lancaster Avenue, Villanova, PA 19085. Because these tables show only a portion of the data and are to be used as educational aids only, they have been labeled "Sample." The reader is encouraged to obtain the complete tables from NCCLS.

Table 12-3
Suggested Groupings of Antimicrobial Agents That Should Be Considered for Routine
Testing and Reporting by Clinical Microbiology Laboratories

	ENTEROBACTERIACEAE	PSEUDOMONAS AERUGINOSA AND OTHER NONENTEROBACTERIACEAE[a]	STAPHYLOCOCCI	ENTEROCOCCI[b]	STREPTOCOCCI (NOT ENTEROCOCCI)[b]	HAEMOPHILUS
Group A Primary Test and Report	Ampicillin[c]	Mezlocillin Ticarcillin	Penicillin G	Penicillin G[d] or ampicillin	Penicillin G	Ampicillin[e]
	Cefazolin[c,f] Cephalothin[c,f]	Gentamicin	Oxacillin or methicillin			Trimethoprim- sulfamethoxazole[g]
	Gentamicin[c]					
Group B Primary Test Report Selectively	Mezlocillin or piperacillin Ticarcillin	Azlocillin or piperacillin / Ticarcillin–clavulanic acid[p]	Amoxicillin– clavulanic acid[h] **or** ampicillin-sulbactam[h]	Vancomycin[i]	Cephalothin[f]	Amoxicillin– clavulanic acid[g] **or** ampicillin-sulbactam
	Amoxicillin-clavulanic acid **or** Ampicillin- sulbactam Ticarcillin–clavulanic acid	Cefoperazone Ceftazidime[k] Aztreonam	Vancomycin			Cefaclor[g] Cefixime[g]
	Cefmetazole Cefoperazone Cefotetan Cefoxitin		Clindamycin[i] Erythromycin[i]		Vancomycin	**Cefuroxime**
	Cefamandole or cefonicid or cefuroxime	Imipenem				Cefotaxime[m] or Ceftazidime[m] or Ceftizoxime[m] or Ceftriaxone[m]
	Cefotaxime[k] or ceftizoxime or ceftriaxone[k]	Trimethoprim[p]- sulfamethoxazole	Trimethoprim- sulfamethoxazole		Chloramphenicol[f]	Chloramphenicol[m]
	Imipenem	Amikacin				
	Amikacin	Tobramycin			Clindamycin	Chloramphenicol[m]
	Ciprofloxacin[c]	Ciprofloxin			Erythromycin	**Tetracycline**[g]
	Trimethoprim- sulfamethoxazole[c]					

(continued)

Table 12-3 (continued)

	ENTEROBACTERIACEAE	PSEUDOMONAS AERUGINOSA AND OTHER NONENTEROBACTERIACEAE[a]	STAPHYLOCOCCI	ENTEROCOCCI[b]	STREPTOCOCCI (NOT ENTEROCOCCI)	HAEMOPHILUS
Group C[c] Supplemental Report Selectively	**Ceftazidime Aztreonam**	Cefotaxime or Ceftriaxone	**Cefotaxime[h] or ceftriaxone[h]**		**Cefotaxime or ceftriaxone**	Cefamandole Cefonicid
	Kanamycin	Netilmicin	Imipenem[h]		**Tetracycline**	**Imipenem[o]**
	Netilmicin	Chloramphenicol[p]	**Gentamicin**		Ofloxacin	**Aztreonam**
	Tobramycin		**Ciprofloxacin or ofloxacin**			**Ciprofloxacin[g] or ofloxacin[g]**
	Tetracycline[c]		Chloramphenicol[l]			Rifampin
	Chloramphenicol[l]		**Tetracycline[q]**			
Group D Supplemental For Urine Only	**Carbenicillin**	**Carbenicillin**	Norfloxacin	Ciprofloxacin Norfloxacin	Norfloxacin	
	Cinoxacin Norfloxacin **or ofloxacin**	Ceftizoxime	Nitrofurantoin	Nitrofurantoin	Nitrofurantoin	
	Nitrofurantoin	Tetracycline[p,q]	Sulfisoxazole	Tetracycline		
	Sulfisoxazole	Norfloxacin **or ofloxacin**	Trimethoprim			
	Trimethoprim	Sulfisoxazole				

SAMPLE

NOTE 1: Selection of the most appropriate antimicrobial agents to test is a decision best made by each clinical laboratory in consultation with the infectious disease practitioners, the pharmacy, and the pharmacy or infection control committees of the medical staff. The lists comprise agents of proven efficacy for that organism group that show acceptable in vitro test performance. **Considerations in the assignment of agents to groups A, B, C, and D included clinical efficacy, prevalence of resistance, minimizing emergence of resistance, cost, and current consensus recommendations for first choice and alternative drugs, in addition to the specific comments in footnotes i and n.** Tests on selected agents may be useful for infection control purposes.

NOTE 2: The boxes in the table designate clusters of comparable agents that need not be duplicated in testing because interpretive results usually will be similar and clinical efficacy comparable. In addition, an "or" designates a related group of agents that show a nearly identical spectrum of activity and interpretive results and for which cross-resistance and susceptibility is nearly complete. Therefore, usually only one of the agents within each selection box (cluster or related group) needs to be selected for testing. Agents reported must be tested **(unless reporting based on testing another agent provides a more accurate result, eg, susceptibility to cefazolin or cephalothin based on oxacillin testing)** and usually should match those included in the hospital formulary, or else the report should include footnotes indicating the agents that usually show comparable interpretive results. **Lastly, unexpected results should be considered for reporting (eg, resistance of Enterobacteriaceae to third-generation cephalosporins or imipenem).**

NOTE 3: Information in boldface type is considered tentative for 1 year.

a Non-Enterobacteriaceae other than Pseudomonas aeruginosa and Acinetobacter should be tested by the dilution method (see M7-A2).

b Antimicrobial agents not listed in this column such as the cephalosporins, clindamycin, and the aminoglycosides should not be tested or reported against the enterococci because the reporting of their results can be dangerously misleading (except for high-level aminoglycoside screening for resistance; see text 2.5.3.3 in M7-A2).

c May be appropriate for inclusion in a panel for testing of urinary tract isolates along with the agents in group D.

d **Penicillin G susceptibility may be used to predict the susceptibility to ampicillin, amoxicillin, acylampicillins, ampicillin-sulbactam, and amoxicillin–clavulanic acid to which non–β-lactamase-producing enterococci are also "moderately susceptible." However, combination therapy of penicillin G or ampicillin, plus an aminoglycoside, is usually indicated for serious enterococcal infections such as endocarditis. For blood and cerebrospinal fluid isolates a β-lactamase test is also recommended.**

e The results of ampicillin susceptibility tests may be used to predict the activity of amoxicillin. Most clinical isolates of Haemophilus influenzae that are resistant to ampicillin and amoxicillin produce a TEM-type β-lactamase. As a result, in most cases, a β-lactamase test alone can be used to predict the activity of these two agents.

f **Cephalothin should be tested to represent cephalothin, cefaclor (except against Haemophilus), cephapirin, cephradine, cephalexin, cefadroxil, and loracarbef. Cefazolin can be tested additionally against Enterobacteriaceae because strains resistant to cephalothin and other first-generation cephalosporins may be susceptible to cefazolin.**

g The results of tests with agents that are administered only by the oral route should be reported only with isolates of Haemophilus species from localized, non–life-threatening infections (eg, uncomplicated cases of otitis media and sinusitis, and selected bronchopulmonary infections).

h **Staphylococci exhibiting resistance to methicillin, oxacillin, or nafcillin should be reported as also resistant to cephalosporins, carbapenems, and β-lactamase inhibitor combinations despite apparent in vitro susceptibility of some strains to the latter agents. This is because infections with methicillin-resistant staphylococci have not responded favorably to therapy with β-lactam antibiotics.**

i **Group B represents agents that may warrant primary testing but that should be reported only selectively, such as when the organism is resistant to agents of the same family in group A.** Other indications for reporting the result might include selected specimen sources (eg, third-generation cephalosporin for isolates of enteric bacteria and H. influenzae from cerebrospinal fluid, or trimethoprim-sulfamethoxazole for urinary tract isolates), **stated allergy or intolerance or failure to respond to an agent in group A, polymicrobial infections, infections involving multiple sites with different microorganisms, or reports to infection control for epidemiologic aid.**

j Vancomycin is often used for serious enterococcal infections in patients with significant penicillin allergy. It should be reported selectively (or footnoted) as being indicated only in such patients. **Combination therapy with vancomycin plus an aminoglycoside is usually indicated for serious enterococcal infections such as endocarditis.**

k **Should be reported on isolates from cerebrospinal fluid along with agents in group A.**

l Not routinely tested against organisms isolated from the urinary tract.

m The result of testing with one of the extended spectrum cephalosporins and chloramphenicol should be reported routinely with all isolates of Haemophilus influenzae recovered from patients with serious, life-threatening infections (eg, meningitis, bacteremia, epiglottitis, facial cellulitis).

n Group C represents alternative or supplemental antimicrobial agents that may require testing in those institutions harboring endemic or epidemic strains resistant to one or more of the primary drugs (especially in the same family, eg, β-lactams or aminoglycosides), or for treatment of unusual organisms (eg, chloramphenicol for some **Pseudomonas species), or reporting to infection control as an epidemiologic aid.**

o **Haemophilus is usually susceptible to imipenem, and routine testing may not be necessary.**

p **May be indicated for primary testing of some Pseudomonas species other than P. aeruginosa, X. maltophila (moxalactam may also be tested) and Acinetobacter species (ampicillin-sulbactam may be tested for strains resistant to other agents).**

q Doxycycline or minocycline may be tested in place of or in addition to tetracycline for some isolates of S. aureus and nonfermentative, gram–negative bacilli (eg. Acinetobacter species) but should not be used to predict tetracycline susceptibility.

Table 12-4
Grouping of Recommended Antibiotics for Testing and Reporting

GROUP	CATEGORY	TYPE OF ANTIMICROBIAL AGENT
A	Primary test and report	Include in routine panel and report routinely
B	Primary test; report selectively	Second-line or back-up antibiotics for group A, because of greater expense or toxicity, appropriateness for a specific site, or clinical failure with a group A antibiotic. Results may be needed but on a selective basis.
C	Supplemental testing; selective reporting	Testing in institutions with specific bacterial resistance problems, or in patients who are allergic to other antibiotics, or in unusual infections
D	Supplemental	Testing of lower urinary tract infections only

(Adapted from Washington JA. Functions and activities of the area committee on microbiology of the National Committee for Clinical Laboratory Standards. Clin Microbiol Rev 1991;4:150–155.)

processes of this national consensus organization that affect clinical microbiologists.[69]

The following discussion is of some of the important facets of susceptibility testing that have been standardized.

Growth Medium

Mueller-Hinton broth and agar have been selected for testing aerobic and facultatively anaerobic bacterial isolates. These formulations most closely approximate the criteria for a reproducible medium. They contain dehydrated beef infusion, acid digest of casein, and cornstarch. Most pathogens grow satisfactorily, and the media have minimal inhibitory effect on sulfonamides, trimethoprim, and tetracycline.[4] Large quantities of thymidine are present in some lots of media. Some organisms can use the thymidine to bypass the mechanism of action of trimethoprim and grow, even though they are innately resistant to the antibiotic. Enterococci are particularly affected; isolated colonies may appear within the established zone of inhibition around disks that contain trimethoprim.

pH

The pH of the medium should be between 7.2 and 7.4 at room temperature. The pH of broth media may be tested directly with a pH electrode, and agar media may be tested by macerating enough agar so that the tip of the electrode can be submerged, by allowing a portion of agar to solidify around the electrode, or by using a properly calibrated surface electrode.

Serum

Antibiotics differ greatly in the degree to which they bind to proteins. In the bloodstream, free antibiotic is in equilibrium with serum protein-bound antibiotic. Free and protein-bound antibiotic can be measured, but it is not clear what the more useful result is. In the laboratory, different values can be obtained for highly protein-bound antibiotics if serum is added to the medium. The NCCLS method does not include added serum because of the difficulty in standardization of the product and uncertainty about how to interpret the results. Perl and colleagues[54] studied the effect of serum on 11 broad-spectrum antibiotics used to treat nosocomial gram-negative bacillary infections. The results were identical with 9 of the 11 antibiotics. Only in the case of ceftriaxone (over 95% protein bound) and cefoperazone (90% protein bound) were there substantial differences when serum was incorporated into the reference procedure.

Cation Concentration

The concentration of the divalent cations Ca^{2+} and Mg^{2+} affects the susceptibility results when certain combinations of bacterial species and antibiotic are tested.[56] When the organisms are grown in media deficient in cations, cell-wall permeability to the aminoglycoside antibiotics and other compounds is increased. The organisms, therefore, are more sensitive to the action of the aminoglycosides, producing falsely low MIC results or large inhibitory zone sizes. Mueller-Hinton broth has very low concentrations of divalent cations and should be supplemented to physiologic concentrations to conform with NCCLS standards (12.5 g/L Mg^{2+} and 25 g/L Ca^{2+}). Some batches of Mueller-Hinton agar may actually have an abnormally high concentration of these cations, so that small inhibitory zones are produced when *Pseudomonas aeruginosa* is tested against aminoglycosides. Such lots, which can be identified by testing with reference strains of known reactivity, should be discarded.

Detection of resistance of certain strains of staphylococci to semisynthetic penicillins is improved by including 2% NaCl in the broth media or 4% NaCl in the agar media.[9,65] The NaCl should be added only to tubes, wells, or plates that contain methicillin or oxacillin.

Atmosphere

Agar or broth is incubated in an ambient air incubator. A CO_2 incubator should not be used for routine tests. The carbonic acid formed on the surface of the agar or in the broth can cause a decrease in pH, which can affect the antibacterial activity of certain antibiotics, as previously discussed. In laboratories with a small workload and where only a CO_2 incubator is available, it is acceptable to place the susceptibility plates or tubes in a sealed jar to prevent access of the CO_2 from the incubator.

Temperature

Plates and tubes should be incubated routinely at 35°C. At higher temperatures, the detection of oxacillin-resistant staphylococci is compromised. If oxacillin resistance is suspected and not manifested at 35°C, the plates or tubes may be incubated at 30°C.

Inoculum

The inoculum is usually prepared from a broth culture that has been incubated for 4 to 6 hours, when growth is considered to be in the logarithmic phase. Several similar-appearing colonies should be sampled to minimize variation in the bacterial population. The density of the suspension is adjusted to about 10^8 colony-forming units per milliliter by comparing its turbidity to a McFarland 0.5 $BaSO_4$ standard. The standard is prepared by adding 0.5 mL of 0.048 M $BaCl_2$ (1.175% w/v $BaCl_2 \cdot H_2O$) to 99.5 mL of 0.36 N H_2SO_4. Aliquots of 4 to 6 mL of the barium sulfate turbidity standard are distributed to screw-capped tubes of the same size, sealed tightly, and stored in the dark at room temperature. Nephelometers may be used to determine turbidity. Commonly, the degree of cloudiness in the broth is compared with the standard, visualizing the two against a white background on which black lines have been drawn (Composite 12-1C). Further adjustments to the inoculum depend on the type of test employed. Alternatively, commercially available devices for preparing a standardized inoculum have worked well[5] (Composite 12-2).

If time does not permit incubation for 4 to 6 hours, young colonies may be removed from the surface of an agar plate that has been incubated overnight and diluted to the proper density. This method is recommended when staphylococci are tested for resistance to methicillin and when testing isolates of *Streptococcus pneumoniae* and *Haemophilus influenzae*.

It is useful to document the number of organisms in the inoculum periodically by inoculating serial dilutions of the suspension onto agar plates.

Antibiotics

Reference antibiotic powders for use in dilution tests should be obtained from the manufacturer or from the US Pharmacopeia in Rockville, Maryland. These reference powders are documented with an assay of antimicrobial activity. For example, the label may indicate that the powder contains 1075 g of active chemical in each 1000 g of powder. The amount of powder weighed must be adjusted for the activity of each lot. Vials should not be obtained from the hospital pharmacy because they may contain fillers and are not assayed for biologic activity. The antibiotics should be stored in a desiccator as indicated for each agent. Many antibiotics, especially those of the β-lactam class, are more stable at temperatures below −20°C. Suspensions of antibiotic should be stored at −20°C or less, preferably at −70°C; they should not be refrozen after dispensing. Imipenem, which is particularly affected by freezing and thawing, should be reconstituted each time a batch of plates or tubes is prepared. A frost-free freezer should not be used because repeated cycles of freezing and thawing occur.

Antimicrobial-impregnated disks should be

stored at $-20°C$ or lower in an anhydrous condition. Under guidelines established by the US Food and Drug Administration, manufacturers of antibiotic disks must carefully control the concentration of antibiotics in the disks to within 60% to 120% of the stated content; the actual variation is usually considerably less. A small working supply may be maintained at refrigerator temperatures in a desiccator. Disks should always be allowed to warm to room temperature before opening the desiccator, so that condensation of moisture from the air does not partially rehydrate the disks.

Quality Control

Rigorous quality control is important for antimicrobial susceptibility testing because of the large numbers of variables that may affect the results. Some of the physical and chemical characteristics of the media, such as pH and depth of agar, may be monitored, but the final control is provided by a series of reference bacterial strains, including *Escherichia coli* (ATCC 25922), *Pseudomonas aeruginosa* (ATCC 27853), *Staphylococcus aureus* (ATCC 29213 for dilution tests; ATCC 25923 for disk tests), *Streptococcus faecalis* (ATCC 29212), *Haemophilus influenzae* (ATCC 49247), and *Neisseria gonorrhoeae* (ATCC 49226), for which expected results have been established. These reference strains are available from the American Type Culture Collection in Washington, DC, or from various commercial sources. The ideal control strains have susceptibility end points in the mid range of antimicrobial concentrations tested and have minimal tendencies to change susceptibility patterns over time.

These reference strains must be stored in a condition that minimizes the possibility of mutation. They may be stored frozen (below $-20°C$ or preferably below $-60°C$) after suspension in a stabilizer, such as defibrinated whole blood, 50% fetal calf serum in bacteriologic broth, or 10% glycerol in broth. Alternatively, the strains may be lyophilized. For short-term storage, the bacteria may be grown on soybean-casein digest agar and stored at $2°$ to $8°C$. Fresh slants should be prepared every 2 weeks, and a new stock culture should be obtained when aberrant results are noted. A fresh subculture should be prepared each day that the control strain is used.

Interpretation of Results

A clinician who receives the results of a dilution susceptibility test knows the concentrations of a group of drugs that inhibited growth of the pathogen under carefully defined conditions in the laboratory. To make a rational selection of the most appropriate antibiotic for a patient, the physician needs at least three other pieces of information: (1) the pharmacokinetics of the antimicrobial agent, including the peak level that can be expected at the site of infection and the rapidity with which that level will decrease, that is, the half-life; (2) how the isolated bacterium compares with other isolates of the same species; and (3) any available clinical data on the in vivo response of similar isolates in similar situations.

Without complete knowledge of these factors, it is easy to misinterpret the raw data. For instance, a β-lactam antibiotic such as ampicillin, with an MIC of 2 μg/mL for an isolate of *E. coli*, might be considered less effective than an aminoglycoside antibiotic, such as gentamicin, with an MIC of 0.5 μg/mL. In fact, the achievable levels of drug in serum are far greater for ampicillin than for gentamicin and the risk of toxicity is much lower in the absence of a history of allergic reactions to the drug. The appropriate choice of therapy would, therefore, be ampicillin, and not the antibiotic with the lowest MIC.

Four categories of antibiotic susceptibility are recognized by the NCCLS for dilution tests (Table 12-5). *Susceptible* implies that the organism should respond to usual doses of the antimicrobial agent administered by an appropriate route, including orally. *Moderately susceptible* implies that the isolate may be inhibited by concentrations of drug that are achieved when the maximum parenteral doses are given; the antibiotic may be selected, but consideration should be given to other choices that may provide more optimal therapy. An additional choice for the middle category is *intermediate*, a designation for results that are considered equivocal or indeterminant, because of potential toxicity, inadequate data, or other reasons. *Resistant* indicates that the bacterium is not inhibited by achievable concentrations of drug and, therefore, the drug should not be selected for therapy, except in certain body fluids where high concentrations of the antibiotic may accumulate. The number of "major and very major errors"—those that trans-

Table 12-5
MIC Interpretive Standards (μg/mL) of Three Categories of Susceptibility for Organisms Other Than
Haemophilus and *Neisseria gonorrhoeae*

ANTIMICROBIAL AGENT	SUSCEPTIBLE[a]	MODERATELY SUSCEPTIBLE[b]	INTERMEDIATE[c]	RESISTANT
β-Lactams—Penicillins				
Ampicillin[d]				
When testing Enterobacteriaceae	≥8	16	—	≤32
When testing staphylococci[e] and *Brahamella catarrhalis*[f]	≥0.25	—	—	≤0.5
When testing *Listeria monocytogenes*	≥2	—	—	≤4
When testing enterococci[g]	—	≥8	—	≤16
When testing streptococci (not enterococci) and other gram-positives[g]	≥0.12	0.25–2	—	≤4
Azlocillin when testing *Pseudomonas*[k]	≥6.4	—	—	≤128
Carbenicillin				
When testing *Pseudomonas*	≥128	256	—	≤512
When testing other gram-negative organisms	≥16	32	—	≤64
Methicillin				
When testing staphylococci[i]	≥8	—	—	≤16
Others				
Chloramphenicol	≥8	—	16	≤32
Clindamycin[h]	≥0.5	—	1–2	≤4
Nitrofurantoin[r]	≥32	—	64	≤128
Rifampin	≥1	—	2	≤4
Sulfonamides[r]	≥256	—	—	≤512
Trimethoprim[r]	≥8	—	—	≤16
Trimethoprim/sulfamethoxazole[s]	≥2/38	—	—	≤4/76

[a] ***Policies regarding generation of cumulative antibiograms should be developed in concert with the infectious disease service, infection control, and the pharmacy and therapeutics committee.***

[b] ***The interpretive category "moderately susceptible" should be reported. MICs for these isolates approach attainable serum levels, and response rates may be lower than for susceptible isolates. The "moderately susceptible" category implies clinical applicability in body sites where the drugs are physiologically concentrated (eg, quinolones in urine), when high dosage of drug can be used (eg, β-lactams), or when combination drug therapy is required for a bactericidal effect in serious infections (eg, penicillin, ampicillin, teicoplanin, or vancomycin plus an aminoglycoside with enterococci).***

[c] ***The category "intermediate" should be reported. It represents a "buffer zone" that should prevent small uncontrolled technical factors from causing major discrepancies in interpretation, especially for drugs with narrow pharmacotoxicity margins.***

See current NCCLS tables for complete information.

pose susceptible and resistant—should be kept to the absolute minimum.

If the laboratory performs a disk diffusion test, the standardized method and interpretations suggested by the NCCLS should be reported (Table 12-6). Occasionally, a physician may derive useful information from the closeness of the actual zone size to the MIC breakpoints, but this information is rarely reported.

A laboratory that performs dilution susceptibility tests may report the interpretative correlate alone, that is, susceptible, moderately susceptible, intermediate, or resistant, or may report the MIC value along with the interpretative correlate. If the MIC value is included in the report, the physicians must be educated as to its purpose. A convenient mechanism is to publish the data on achievable antibiotic levels and the relation of MIC to interpretative correlate in a form that is easily accessible to physicians.

Selection of Antibiotics to be Reported

Only antibiotics appropriate for the infection should be included in a report. Drugs that are active only in the urinary tract should not be reported if the isolate comes from another site. Antibiotics that do not penetrate into a site, such as cefazolin or cephalothin in the meninges, should not be reported for organisms isolated from that site. Use of chloramphenicol for uncomplicated urinary tract infections is inappropriate; its use should not be encouraged by including the susceptibility results in a laboratory report. There are, unfortunately, few of these absolute prohibitions. Most of the decisions should be made in consultation with members of the medical staff and pharmacy. All accredited hospitals have pharmacy and therapeutics committees (or the equivalent) that provide a useful forum for coordinated effort.

Disk Diffusion Susceptibility Test

Figure 12-1 illustrates the basic principle of the disk diffusion method of antimicrobial susceptibility testing.[4] As soon as the antibiotic-impregnated disk comes in contact with the moist agar surface, water is absorbed into the filter paper and

the antibiotic diffuses into the surrounding medium. The rate of extraction of the antibiotic out of the disk is greater than its outward diffusion into the medium, so that the concentration immediately adjacent to the disk may exceed that in the disk itself. As the distance from the disk increases, however, there is a logarithmic reduction in the antibiotic concentration. If the plate has been previously inoculated with a bacterial suspension, simultaneous growth of bacteria occurs on the surface of the agar. When a critical cell mass of bacteria is reached, the inhibitory activity of the antibiotic is overcome and bacterial growth occurs. The time (critical time) required to reach the critical cell mass (4 to 10 hours for commonly tested bacteria) is characteristic of each species but is influenced by the composition of the medium and temperature of incubation. The lateral extent of antimicrobial diffusion before the critical time is reached is affected by the depth of the agar because diffusion occurs in three dimensions. The points at which the critical cell mass is reached appear as a sharply marginated circle of bacterial growth, with the middle of the disk forming the center of the circle if the test has been performed properly (Fig. 12-2). The concentration of diffused antibiotic at this interface of growing and inhibited bacteria is known as the critical concentration and approximates the MIC obtained in dilution tests. Although direct calculation of the inhibitory concentration is not done in practice, the MIC can actually be calculated with reasonable accuracy if the characteristics of antimicrobial diffusion and bacterial growth are known.[4]

Development of a Standardized Disk Diffusion Procedure

A World Health Organization committee was formed in 1961 to lay the groundwork to develop standardized antimicrobial test procedures.[70] The test that has become standard in the United States is based on the work of Bauer, Kirby, and coworkers.[6,7,45] The procedure for the disk diffusion test as recommended by the NCCLS is illustrated in Composite 12-1.

If the test is properly performed, the edges of the inhibitory zones should be clear and easy to measure. The following are situations, however, in which the technologist must learn to interpret unclear results correctly:

Table 12-6

Zone Diameter Interpretive Standards and Equivalent Minimum Inhibitory Concentration (MIC) Breakpoints for Organisms Other Than *Haemophilus* and *Neisseria gonorrhoeae*

ANTIMICROBIAL AGENT	DISK CONTENT	RESIST-ANT	ZONE DIAMETER, NEAREST WHOLE MM			EQUIVALENT MIC BREAKPOINTS[d] (μg/mL)	
			Inter-mediate[a]	Moderately Susceptible[b]	Sus-ceptible[c]	Resistant	Sus-ceptible
β-Lactams—Penicillins							
Ampicillin[e]							
When testing gram-negative enteric organisms	10 μg	≤13	—	14–16	≥17	≥32	≤8
When testing staphylococci[f]	10 μg	≤28	—	—	≥29	β-lactamase[f]	≤0.25
When testing enterococci[g]	10 μg	≤16	—	≤17[g]	—	≥16	—
When testing streptococci (not enterococci)[g]	10 μg	≤21	—	22–29	≥30	≥4	≤0.12
When testing *Listeria monocytogenes*	10 μg	≤19	—		≥20	≥4	≤2
Azlocillin when testing *Pseudomonas*[f,h]	75 μg	≤17	—		≥18	≥128	≤64
Carbenicillin[f]							
When testing *Pseudomonas*	100 μg	≤13	—	14–16	≥17	≥512	≤128
When testing other gram-negative organisms	100 μg		—	20–22	≥23	≥64	≤16
Methicillin when testing staphylococci[i]	5 μg	≤9	10–13	—	≥14	≥16	≤8
Others							
Chloramphenicol	30 μg	≤12	13–17	—	≥18	≥32	≤8
Clindamycin[s]	2 μg	≤14	15–20	—	≥21	≥4	≤0.5
Nitrofurantoin[r]	300 μg	≤14	15–16	—	≥17	≥128	≤32
Rifampin	5 μg	≤16	17–19	—	≥20	≥4	≤1
Sulfonamides[r,t]	250 or 300 μg	≤12	—	13–16	≥17	≥350	≤100
Trimethoprim[r,t]	5 μg	≤10	—	11–15	≥16	≥16	≤4
Trimethoprim/sulfamethoxazole[t]	1.25/23.75 μg	≤10	—	11–15	≥16	≥8/152	≤2/38

[a] **The category "Intermediate" should be reported. It indicates a "buffer zone" that should prevent small uncontrolled technical factors from causing major discrepancies in interpretation, especially for drugs with narrow pharmacotoxicity margins.**

[b] **The interpretive category "moderately susceptible" should be reported. MICs for these isolates approach attainable serum levels and response rates may be lower than for susceptible isolates. The "moderately susceptible" category implies clinical applicability in body sites where the drugs are physiologically concentrated (eg, quinolones in urine), when high dosage of drug can be used (eg, β-lactams), or when combination drug therapy is required for a bactericidal effect in serious infections (eg, penicillin, ampicillin, teicoplanin, or vancomycin plus an aminoglycoside with enterococci).**

[c] **Policies regarding generation of cumulative antibiograms should be developed in concert with the infectious disease service, infection control, and the pharmacy and therapeutics committee.**

See current NCCLS tables for complete information.

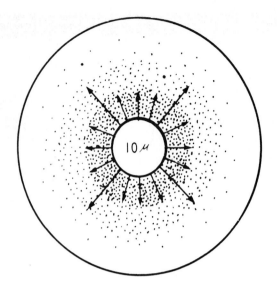

Figure 12-1. The principle of antibiotic diffusion in agar. The concentration of antibiotic decreases as the distance from the disk increases.

1. Motile organisms such as *Proteus mirabilis* or *P. vulgaris* may swarm when growing on agar surfaces, resulting in a thin veil that may penetrate into the zones of inhibition around antibiotic susceptibility disks (Fig. 12-3). This zone of swarming should be ignored; the outer margin, which is usually clearly outlined, should be measured. Similarly, with sulfonamide disks, growth may not be completely inhibited at the outer margin, resulting in a faint veil where 80% or

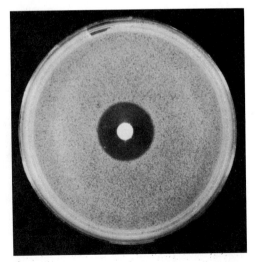

Figure 12-2. Disk antibiotic susceptibility plate showing the same principle as in Figure 12-1. At the area where the concentration of antibiotic is insufficient to prevent bacterial growth, a distinct margin can be seen.

more of the organisms are inhibited. Again, the outer margin of heavy growth inhibition should be used as the point of measurement.

2. The phenomenon shown in Figure 12-4 must be interpreted differently from that shown in Figure 12-3. Distinct colonies are present within the zone of inhibition. This does not represent swarming. Instead, these colonies are either mutants that are more resistant to the antibiotic than the major portion of the bacterial strain being tested or the culture is not pure and the separate colonies are of a different species. Isolation, identification, and susceptibility testing of the resistant colonies may be required to resolve this problem. If it is determined that the separate colonies represent a variant of a mutant strain, the bacterial species being tested must be considered resistant, even though a wide zone of inhibition may be present for the remainder of the growth.

3. Figure 12-5 demonstrates the difficulty in measuring one zone diameter when there is overlapping with adjacent antibiotic zones, or when the zone extends beyond the margin of the Petri dish. Oval or elliptical zones may occur, and it is difficult to determine whether to measure the short or long diameters. Unless the zones are very wide and the organism being tested is obviously susceptible, the test must be repeated with more careful placement of the antibiotic disks so that overlapping will not occur.

4. Figure 12-6 illustrates a poorly prepared plate. The lines of streaking are irregular, leaving spaces between adjacent colonies. The margins of the zones are indistinct, making it difficult to pick the exact points at which to make the measurements. Readings should not be attempted on a poorly inoculated plate such as this, and the test should be repeated.

Interpretation of Results

The zone size that is observed in a disk diffusion test has no meaning in and of itself. The interpretative standards provided by the NCCLS are derived from a correlation between zone sizes and MICs of those species that can be tested by the disk diffusion method. A prototype of a regression curve providing such a correlation is illustrated in Figure 12-7. A large number of strains have been tested against a single antibiotic both by the disk diffusion

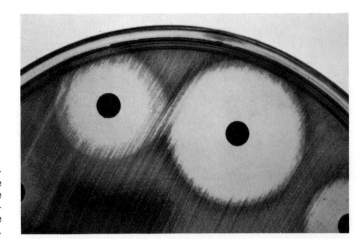

Figure 12-3. Photograph of an antibiotic susceptibility plate using a species of *Proteus* as the test organism. Note the swarming into the zone of inhibition at the peripheral margins. The second outer zone of growth inhibition should be used when measuring the width of the zone.

technique and by a dilution method. Each triangle represents the results of both tests for a single strain. A regression line has been drawn through the many individual points. Once the regression line is established, an approximate MIC result can be inferred from any zone diameter. In this example, a zone size of 18 mm corresponds to an MIC of 6.25 μg/mL—the susceptible breakpoint of the broth dilution test.

Thus, an antimicrobial agent that produces a zone diameter greater than 18 mm would theoretically have an MIC less than 6.25 μg/mL, and

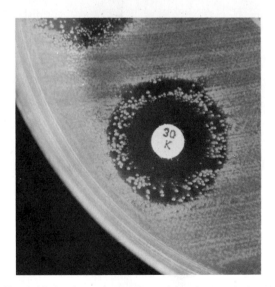

Figure 12-4. An antibiotic susceptibility plate in which colonies resistant to kanamycin are growing within the zone of inhibition. Biochemical tests must be performed to determine if the resistant strain is a mutant of the organisms being tested or represents a second species growing in mixed culture.

the organism would be considered susceptible; one producing a zone size less than 18 mm would, conversely, be considered resistant. In actual practice, regression curves are not that clearly defined, and a 2- to 4-mm zone may be established where it is not possible to determine whether the organism is susceptible or resistant (see Table 12-6). Isolates that produce an inhibitory zone in this range are characterized as intermediate in susceptibility. In studies conducted late in the 1950s, Bauer, Perry, and Kirby first demonstrated that bacterial strains tested against a given antibiotic tend to fall either into the resistant or the susceptible categories; only a small percentage (5% or less) fall into the intermediate range.[8] Thus, if a high percentage of intermediate reports is issued by a certain laboratory, a reexamination of the procedure is indicated.

The interpretative guidelines for the disk diffusion test (see Table 12-6) permit the user to make approximations of the MIC for each of the antibiotics listed (last two columns) with zone diameters as determined by the disk diffusion technique. These correlates are not intended to match the breakpoints for susceptibility and resistance established for the dilution tests, but they do give the user an appreciation of the meaning of the report. For example, a microorganism showing an 11-mm zone of inhibition against ampicillin would be considered resistant at a level of greater than 32 μg/mL.

If the infection is in the lower urinary tract, however, very high concentrations of ampicillin are achieved, and the organism might be treatable even in the presence of an apparently resistant result. It may be necessary to perform a dilution test to obtain a more precise result.

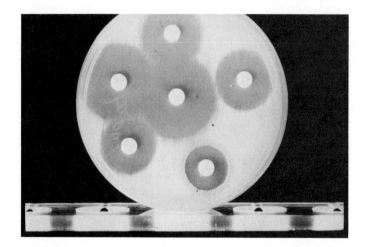

Figure 12-5. A poorly prepared antibiotic susceptibility plate showing objectionable overlapping of the zones of growth inhibition from adjacent disks.

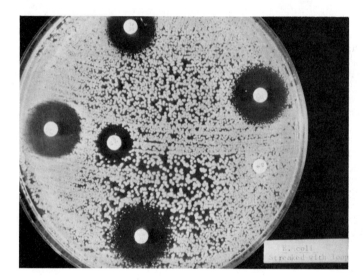

Figure 12-6. A poorly streaked antimicrobial susceptibility plate showing uneven growth. The zone margins are indistinct, compromising accurate measurement.

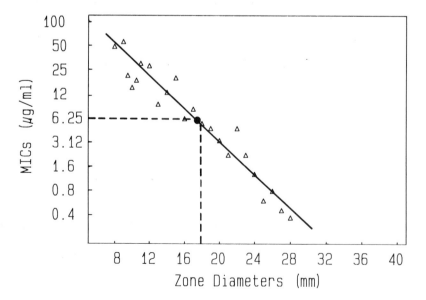

Figure 12-7. Prototype regression curve comparing MICs in micrograms per milliliter with zone size in millimeters. Each triangle represents the MIC (vertical axis) and inhibitory zone (horizontal axis) of a single isolate. A zone diameter of 18 mm corresponds with the MIC breakpoint of 6.25 μg/mL.

Quality Control

Control cultures of *Staphylococcus aureus* (ATCC 25923), *Escherichia coli* (ATCC 25922), and *Pseudomonas aeruginosa* (ATCC 27853) should be kept in stock. A β-lactamase–producing *E. coli* (ATCC 35218) can be used to control results of disks that contain combinations of β-lactam antibiotics and a β-lactamase inhibitor. *Haemophilus influenzae* (ATCC 49247) or *Neisseria gonorrhoeae* (ATCC 29226) must be used if these organisms are tested. Control cultures can be maintained on soybean-casein digest agar at 4° to 8°C and subcultured weekly; alternately, lyophilized samples are available from several commercial suppliers. These cultures can be used as long as the zone diameter measurements remain within acceptable limits.

Quality control should be performed each time a new lot of disks or agar is used. In the interim, controls should be tested each day the procedure is performed unless stringent criteria for weekly testing are met. The NCCLS has established limits on zone sizes that are acceptable for the quality control strains (Table 12-7); these limits provide a means by which to measure the accuracy of testing. Similarly, the precision can be assessed by examining the range of values in a series of tests (Table 12-8). If the largest minus smallest zone diameter in a group of five consecutive test results falls within the limits listed in Table 12-8, the probability of a major interpretive error is less than 1%. Corrective action must be taken if the results are out of control (Table 12-9; see also Table 12-7).

The results of quality control testing may give

Table 12-7
Control Limits for Monitoring Antimicrobial Disk Susceptibility Tests: Zone Diameter (mm) Limits for Individual Tests on Mueller-Hinton Medium Without Blood or Other Supplements

ANTIMICROBIAL AGENT	DISK CONTENT	E. coli (ATCC 25922)	S. aureus (ATCC 25923)	P. aeruginosa (ATCC 27853)	E. coli (ATCC 35218)
Amikacin	30 μg	19–26	20–26	18–26	—
Amoxicillin/clavulanic acid	20/10 μg	19–25	28–36	—	18–22
Ampicillin	10 μg	16–22	27–35	—	—
Ampicillin/sulbactam	10/10 μg	20–24	29–37	—	13–19
Azithromycin	**15 μg**	—	**21–**	—	—
Azlocillin	75 μg	—	—	24–30	—
Aztreonam	30 μg	28–36	—	23–29	—
Carbenicillin	100 μg	23–29	—	18–24	—
Cefaclor	30 μg	23–	27–31	—	—
Cefamandole	30 μg	26–32	26–34	—	—
Cefazolin	30 μg	23–29	29–35	—	—
Ticarcillin/clavulanic acid	75/10 μg	25–29	—	20–28	21–25
Tobramycin	10 μg	18–26	19–29	19–25	—
Trimethoprim	5 μg	21–28	19–26	—	—
Trimethoprim/sulfamethoxazole	1.25/23.75 μg	24–32	24–32	—	—
Vancomycin	30 μg	—	15–19	—	—

NOTE 1: To determine whether the Mueller-Hinton medium has sufficiently low levels of thymidine and thymine, an E. faecalis (ATCC 29212 or 33186) may be tested with trimethoprim/sulfamethoxazole disks. An inhibition zone of ≥20 mm that is essentially free of fine colonies indicates a sufficiently low level of thymine and thymidine.

NOTE 2: Information in boldface type is considered tentative for 1 year.

See current NCCLS table for complete information.

Table 12-8
Maximum Zone Diameter Range That Should Be Observed in a Series of Five Consecutive Control Test Results

ANTIMICROBIAL AGENT	DISK CONTENT	E. coli (ATCC 25922)	S. aureus (ATCC 25923)	P. aeruginosa (ATCC 27853)	E. coli (ATCC 35218)
Amikacin	30 µg	6	6	6	—
Amoxicillin/ clavulanic acid	20/10 µg	7	9	—	4
Ampicillin	10 µg	6	8	—	—
Ampicillin/sulbactam	10/10 µg	4	9	—	7
Azithromycin	**15 µg**	—	4	—	—
Azlocillin	75 µg	—	—	8	—
Aztreonam	30 µg	10	—	10	—
Carbenicillin	100 µg	10	—	8	—
Cefaclor	30 µg	4	4	—	—
Cefamandole	30 µg	8	8	—	—
Cefazolin	30 µg	—	8	—	—
Tobramycin	10 µg	6	6	6	—
Trimethoprim	5 µg	10	10	—	—
Trimethoprim/sulfa- methoxazole	1.25/23.75 µg	10	10	—	—
Vancomycin	30 µg	—	6	—	—

NOTE 1: *Zone diameter range is defined as the largest minus the smallest zone diameter in a group of five consecutive control tests results.*

NOTE 2: *Maximum zone diameter ranges have been calculated using formulae for determining control charts for ranges (ASTM Manual on Quality Control of Materials, Special Technical Publication 15-C, American Society for Testing and Materials, Philadelphia, PA, 1951). Performance within these limits indicates that test precision is sufficient to ensure that the probability of major interpretative error (RS S) is less than 1%.*

NOTE 3: *Information in boldface type is considered tentative for 1 year.*

See current NCCLS table for complete information.

---

clues as to the nature of the problem. Certain errors are particularly common. Some of the possible problems and explanations are summarized in Table 12-10.

Limitations

The Bauer-Kirby test, as modified by the NCCLS, has been accepted as the standard technique for performing disk diffusion susceptibility tests, giving useful information in most instances. There are, however, a few distinct limitations. The test should be applied only to bacterial species that have been thoroughly evaluated. Bacteria that grow slowly, need special nutrients, or require CO_2 or anaerobic conditions for growth should not be tested, unless the validity of the procedure has been documented.[33]

Microdilution Broth Susceptibility Test

Concurrent with the development of a usable disk diffusion test, other investigators have attempted to simplify the broth dilution test. The microtube dilution procedure is similar in principle to the macrotube method, except that the susceptibility of microorganisms to antibiotics is determined in a series of microtube wells that are molded into a plastic plate. Each plate may contain 80, 96, or more wells, depending on the number and concentration of antibiotics that are to be included in the susceptibility test panel.

The advantages of the microtube method are that small volumes of reagents are used and that large numbers of bacteria can be tested simply and inexpensively against a panel of antibiotics. The

Table 12-9
Acceptable Quality Control Ranges of MICs (µg/mL) for Reference Strains

ANTIMICROBIAL AGENT	S. aureus ATCC 29213	E. faecalis ATCC 29212	E. coli ATCC 25922	P. aeruginosa ATCC 27853	E. coli ATCC 35218
Amikacin	1–4 [a]	64–256	0.5–4	**0.5–8**	—
Amoxicillin/clavulanic acid	—	—	2/1–8/4	—	4/2–16/8
Ampicillin	0.25–1	0.5–2	2–8	—	—
Ampicillin/sulbactam	—	—	1/0.5–4/2	—	4/2–16/8
Azithromycin	**0.25–1**	**—**		**—**	**—**
Azlocillin	2–8	1–4	8–32	2–8	—
Aztreonam	—	—	0.06–0.25	2–8	—
Tobramycin	0.12–1	8	0.25–1	**0.12–2**	—
Vancomycin	0.5–2	1	—	—	—
Nalidixic acid	—		1–4	—	—
Nitrofurantoin	8–32	4–16	4–16	—	—
Norfloxacin	0.5–2	2–8	0.03–0.12	1–4	—
Sulfisoxazole[b]	32–128	32-128	8–32	—	—
Trimethoprim[b]	1–4	≤1	0.5–2	>64	—
Trimethoprim/sulfa-methoxazole (1/19)[b]	≤0.5/9.5	≤0.5/9.5	≤0.5/9.5	3/152–32/608	—

NOTE 1: *These MICs obtained in several reference laboratories by broth microdilution. If four or fewer concentrations are tested, quality control may be more difficult.*
NOTE 2: *Information in boldface is considered tentative for 1 year.*
[a]All results represent a bimodal distribution of MICs; results at the extremes of the acceptable range should be suspect. Verify control validity with data from other control strains.
[b]Highly medium dependent, especially with enterococci.

intensive labor involved in preparing the multiwell plates has been a major impediment to their routine use.

Manufacturers have eased the burben by preparing plates that contain lyophilized antibiotic solutions—the laboratory equivalent of instant coffee. Rehydration of the wells adds another step to the procedure, but the extended shelf-life of the freeze-dried plates is valuable, especially for laboratories in which small numbers of tests are performed. Both the frozen and lyophilized broth dilution systems have performed well in comparison to the reference methods.[11,27,28,55,58] As might be expected, the interlaboratory reproducibility of the commercial systems that use standardized batches of very large volume has been greater than that for homemade plates, even when the plates were prepared for investigational use.[27]

The procedure for the microdilution broth test as recommended by the NCCLS is summarized in Table 12-11. The interpretative guidelines suggested by the NCCLS, which should be reported along with or in place of the actual MIC values, are listed in Table 12-5. Separate guidelines for interpreting *Haemophilus* species have been published by the NCCLS. The guidelines for quality control are similar to those for the disk diffusion test (see Tables 12-8 and 12-10). Some of the sources of error with dilution tests are summarized in Table 12-10.

End points are usually easily defined (Fig. 12-8). Examination of the microplates is facilitated by use of a viewing mirror (Fig. 12-9). Occasionally, growth may be inhibited in a well that is adjacent to wells with uninhibited growth (skipped well). If a single well is skipped and the interpretation of the result is not affected, the skipped well may be ignored. If multiple wells are skipped, if the skipped

Table 12-10
Trouble-Shooting Quality Control (QC) Problems in Susceptibility Tests

OBSERVATION	DIAGNOSIS	CORRECTIVE ACTION
MICs too large or zone sizes too small (Isolates too resistant)	1. Inoculum too high 2. Deterioration of antibiotic 3. Change in QC strain 4. Agar too deep 5. Incorrect reading of results	1. Check and adjust inoculum if necessary 2. Check potency of disks or powder; try new lot 3. Test new stock of QC strain 4. Check depth of agar 5. Repeat with multiple observers
MICs too small or zone sizes too large (Isolates too susceptible)	1. Inoculum too low 2. Antibiotic too potent 3. Change in QC strain 4. Agar too thin 5. Incorrect reading of results	1. Check and adjust inoculum if necessary 2. Check potency of disks or powder; try new lot 3. Test new stock of QC strain 4. Check depth of agar 5. Repeat with multiple observers
Results for *Pseudomonas* and aminoglycosides out of control	Cation content incorrect	Use cation-supplemented broth or try different lot of agar
Results for *Pseudomonas* and carbenicillin out of control	Mutation of QC strain	Test new stock of QC strain
Aminoglycosides and macrolides too resistant; tetracycline too susceptible	Medium too acid	Check pH of media
Aminoglycosides and macrolides too susceptible; tetracycline too resistant	Medium too alkaline	Check pH of media
Trimethoprim MICs too large or zone sizes too small; results difficult to read	Excess thymidine in medium	Test medium with *Streptococcus faecalis* (ATCC 29212 or 33186); add thymidine phosphorylase or lysed horse blood

well occurs at a dilution that is critical for determining susceptibility of the isolate, or if multiple isolates demonstrate the phenomenon, the problem should be investigated and the test repeated.

SPECIAL ISSUES IN SUSCEPTIBILITY TESTING

β-Lactamases

β-Lactamases are heterogeneous bacterial enzymes that cleave the β-lactam ring of penicillins and cephalosporins to inactivate the antibiotic.

β-Lactamases are found in a wide variety of gram-positive and gram-negative bacterial species;

at present, the enzymes produced by *Staphylococcus* species, *Haemophilus* species, *Moraxella (Branhamella) catarrhalis*, and *Neisseria gonorrhoeae* are clinically most important. The significance of the enzymes produced by many enteric bacteria is less clear, and these bacteria should not be tested for β-lactamase.

The presence of β-lactamases may be detected quickly, providing an early clue that an isolate will not respond to the β-lactam antibiotics in question. The chromogenic cephalosporin test, employing Nitrocefin, is the most sensitive.[2] Filter-paper disks impregnated with Nitrocefin are commercially available. A loopful of a colony is smeared on the disk and placed in a closed Petri dish to prevent rapid desiccation. Organisms that contain β-lacta-

Table 12-11
Performance of Microdilution Broth Susceptibility Tests

Introduction

The microdilution test is an adaptation of the reference macroscopic test. Large numbers of isolates can be tested against multiple drugs easily, so the procedure is well adapted to routine use. This test generates more quantitative information, which may be useful in certain circumstances, than does the disk diffusion test.

Principle

The principle of the microdilution test is the same as that of the macroscopic test. Bacterial isolates are exposed to serial dilutions of each antimicrobial agent, after which the concentration of drug that inhibits growth is determined by visual inspection.

Media and Reagents

Nutrient broth (soybean-casein digest broth is recommended)
0.5 McFarland standard for adjusting inoculum
White background with black lines for comparison of turbidity of inoculum with 0.5 McFarland standard
Frozen or lyophilized microtiter plates containing antibiotics in cation-supplemented Mueller-Hinton broth
Multiprong inoculators—either wire loops or disposable plastic pins
Viewing mirror and template for visualization of end points. A photometric or fluorometric analysis of end points may be done if demonstrated to be equivalent to visual inspection.

Procedure

Preparation of Inoculum

At least five similar appearing colonies are selected, as described in the disk diffusion test (see Composite 12-1). The turbidity of an actively growing broth culture is adjusted to the density of a 0.5 McFarland standard. A direct method, in which bacteria from a plate that has been incubated overnight are adjusted directly, has also produced satisfactory results. The extent to which the inoculum must be diluted further will depend on the system, because replicate inoculating devices deliver various volumes of fluid. Each well should contain approximately 5×10^5 CFU/mL.

Inoculation of Plates

Inoculate the bacterial suspension into each well of the microplate within 15 minutes of adjusting the density of the inoculum. One well should contain bacteria without antibiotic (growth control), and one well should contain broth only (sterility control). If the volume of the inoculum exceeds 10% of the volume of the well, the dilution effect on the antimicrobial agent must be calculated. To prevent drying, seal the plates in a plastic bag, with plastic tape, or with a tight-fitting plastic cover. A portion of a nutrient agar plate, such as blood agar, should be inoculated to detect contamination (see Composite 12-2).

Incubation

Incubate the plates at 35°C for 16 to 20 hours in a forced air incubator. Do not place more than four plates in a stack, so that a uniform temperature of incubation is maintained.

Interpretation

The MIC is the lowest concentration of antibiotic that inhibits growth of the isolate. It may be determined by viewing the wells with the unaided eye, comparing the growth in the wells that contain antibiotics to that in the growth control well. A viewing mirror, with which the bottom of the microtubes may be visualized, facilitates observation (see Fig. 12-9). A template on which the contents of each well are detailed is useful. The end points may also be determined in a semiautomated fashion.

Refer to the guidelines for interpretation of MIC results as susceptible, moderately susceptible, intermediate, or resistant (see Table 12-5).

Examine the purity plate and repeat the test if contamination is present.

Quality Control

Quality control should be performed with each new lot of plates. During use, controls may be performed daily or at weekly intervals if strict criteria have been fulfilled.

The organisms used for the dilution test are *Straphylococcus aureus* (ATCC 29213), *Enterococcus faecalis* (ATCC 29212), *Escherichia coli* (ATCC 25922), *Pseudomonas aeruginosa* (ATCC 27583), *Neisseria gonorrhoeae* (ATCC 49226), and *Haemophilus influenzae* (ATCC 49247). Note that the *S. aureus* strain differs from that used in the disk diffusion test. *E. coli* (ATCC 35218) may be used to control combinations that include clavulanic acid, a β-lactamase inhibitor.

Bibliography

National Committee for Clinical Laboratory Standards. Methods for dilution antimicrobial susceptibility tests for bacteria that grow aerobically (approved standard M7-A2). Villanova, PA, National Committee for Clinical Laboratory Standards, 1985.

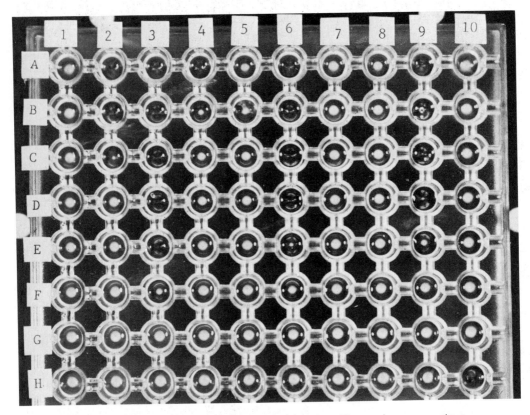

Figure 12-8. Microtube broth dilution antibiotic susceptibility plate. The numbers across the top indicate the different antibiotics being tested within each vertical column; the letters along the left border reflect the concentration of antibiotics contained within each well. The appearance of a button of bacterial growth in any well indicates resistance to that concentration of antibiotic.

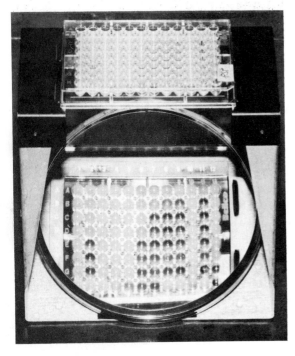

Figure 12-9. Viewing mirror for visualization of bacterial growth in broth microdilution test.

mase change the color of the disk from yellow to red. The reaction usually occurs within 30 seconds, but tests are read finally after 15 minutes.

Iodometric and acidometric tests are less expensive to perform but are less sensitive than the Nitrocefin assay.

Staphylococcus Species

The β-lactamases of staphylococci are induced by exposure to penicillins. They are responsible for most of the resistance to penicillin G and related compounds but are not active against the cephalosporins or the penicillinase-resistant penicillins, such as methicillin and nafcillin, unless produced in large amounts. Detection of these enzymes is particularly difficult with the microbroth dilution test, because the bacteria in the relatively small inoculum used in this test may be killed before the enzyme is induced.

If the MIC of a staphylococcal strain to penicillin is greater than 0.25 μg/mL, the presence of a β-lactamase can be inferred. Isolates with penicillin MICs less than 0.03 μg/mL are considered nonproducers and susceptible. Isolates for which the MIC falls between these limits (0.06 or 0.12 μg/mL) should be tested for the presence of β-lactamase before the results are reported. Use of bacterial growth from a well that contains a penicillin-class drug or from the edge of a zone of inhibition around a disk that contains a penicillin compound may induce activity and enhance detection of the enzyme. The results from the testing of penicillin can be extrapolated to ampicillin.

Haemophilus Species

As many as 20% to 40% of type B *Haemophilus influenzae* isolates from serious infections produce β-lactamases.[16] Detection of the enzymes should be performed on any isolate that is considered a pathogen. A few strains have demonstrated resistance to ampicillin by other mechanisms, so a non–enzyme-producing strain should also be tested against ampicillin by a diffusion or dilution susceptibility test.[8]

Neisseria gonorrhoeae

Penicillinase-producing gonococci were detected initially in the Far East but are now widely distrib-

uted. All isolates should be tested for β-lactamase. As with *Haemophilus* species, some strains that are resistant to penicillin by nonenzymatic means have now been identified,[57] so that a susceptibility test should also be performed if the treatment fails.

Moraxella (Branhamella) catarrhalis

Moraxella (Branhamella) catarrhalis has been recognized in recent years as an important cause of upper respiratory tract infection and of nosocomial lower respiratory tract infection. There is little reason to perform any test routinely other than β-lactamase on *Moraxella (Branhamella) catarrhalis* because the susceptibility of the organism to other antibiotics is predictable.[18] Doern and colleagues found that the Nitrocefin tube or disk test was the most effective means of detecting β-lactamase.[17] The subject has been reviewed by Doern and Jones.[15]

Enterococcus Species

Isolates of enterococci that produce β-lactamase have been identified.[43,52,53] This high-level resistance to penicillin can be detected by the Nitrocefin test. The β-lactamase, which resembles that of staphylococci, is carried on a plasmid.[44] Strains that express high-level aminoglycoside resistance and produce β-lactamase have been described.[51] The infection produced by this strain was successfully treated with vancomycin.

Oxacillin- and Vancomycin-Resistant *Staphylococcus* Species

The resistance of *S. aureus* and *S. epidermidis* to penicillinase-resistant penicillins is particularly difficult to detect in the laboratory. These species are heteroresistant; that is, only a small fraction of the bacteria in a culture express resistance, a characteristic that is chromosomally mediated. The resistant cells grow more slowly than the susceptible bacteria, unless incubated at reduced temperature. The relatively low inoculum used in the microdilution broth test may compromise detection of the small fraction of resistant cells. Variations in the ability of different lots of Mueller-Hinton agar to detect heteroresistance have been reported.[30]

It is probable that no single procedure detects staphylococcal resistance to oxacillin with absolute reliability. It is also likely that false estimates of resistance can be generated by some manipulations, such as prolonged incubation of susceptibility tests.[9] If there is a possibility of resistance to oxacillin in a clinically significant isolate of *Staphylococcus*, a variety of tests for detection of resistance should be performed. If resistance to oxacillin remains in question, other effective antibiotics, such as vancomycin alone or combined with rifampin, should be used.[3]

The following guidelines may be offered to maximize detection of methicillin-resistant staphylococci:

1. For *S. aureus*, oxacillin is more likely to detect cross-resistance among penicillinase-resistant penicillins than other compounds. Cloxacillin and dicloxacillin should not be used. Nafcillin should not be used if the media contain blood.[46] Coudron and colleagues[9] have suggested that methicillin may detect resistance in *S. epidermidis* better than oxacillin.
2. Addition of 2% NaCl to broth and 4% NaCl to agar that contains penicillinase-resistant penicillins enhances detection of resistance.[9,65]

3. The inoculum should be prepared by the alternate direct method, using colonies from a fresh overnight plate (see Tables 12-7 and 12-12).
4. The cultures should be incubated at temperatures below 37°C to facilitate growth of the resistant bacteria. A temperature of 35°C is a reasonable compromise for routine use. Incubation at 30°C may be used if resistance is highly suspected.
5. If the disk diffusion procedure is used, the edge of the apparent zone of inhibition should be examined closely. The border is sharp and clear when oxacillin-susceptible organisms are tested. Growth of oxacillin-resistant organisms "feathers" or "trails" off as the disk is approached, so that the inner edge of growth may be difficult to define (Fig. 12-10).

Resistance to cephalosporins among staphylococci is difficult to detect. There is clinical evidence that isolates of *S. aureus* that are resistant to oxacillin do not respond in vivo to cephalosporin therapy; the same phenomenon has also been suggested for *S. epidermidis*.[46] If resistance to nafcillin, oxacillin, or methicillin is demonstrated, the bacte-

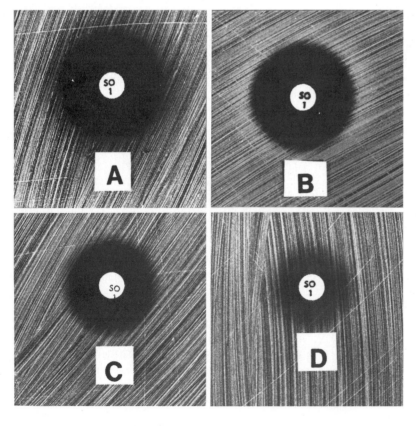

Figure 12-10. The effect of salt on the expression of methicillin resistance to staphylococci is shown. A susceptible strain was tested against a 1-μg oxacillin disk on Mueller-Hinton agar that had no supplemental salt (*A*) or that contained 4% NaCl (*B*). The zone of bacterial inhibition was unaffected by addition of the salt. A methicillin-resistant strain was also tested against oxacillin on Mueller-Hinton agar without (*C*), and with (*D*) the addition of 4% NaCl. Without NaCl, a clear zone of inhibition was produced (*C*), and the isolate would be considered susceptible. In the presence of NaCl, there was a gradually decreasing growth or "feathering" right up to the disk; this organism should be considered resistant to oxacillin and other penicillinase-resistant penicillins.

rial strain should be reported as resistant to other β-lactam antibiotics, including all cephalosporins, such as cefazolin or cephalothin, and the carbapenem antibiotic imipenem.

A strain of *S. haemolyticus* that developed resistance to vancomycin during treatment of a patient with recurrent episodes of peritonitis has been described.[59] Fortunately, no isolates of *S. aureus* have yet displayed resistance to vancomycin.

Haemophilus Species

Haemophilus organisms require hemin (factor X) or nicotinamide adenine dinucleotide (NAD) (factor V) for growth. The validity of adding supplements both to dilution and also to diffusion susceptibility media has been established. A new supplement for *Haemophilus* has been suggested by Jorgensen and colleagues.[35] The NCCLS has adopted the *Haemophilus* test medium, which may contain cation supplements if appropriate. Proper preparation of the inoculum is important for testing *Haemophilus* species. The alternate direct method of standardizing the bacterial suspension from an overnight culture should be used (see Table 12-11).

A new approach to susceptibility testing, called the E test, has been applied to *Haemophilus influenzae*. The E test consists of a plastic strip impregnated with graduated concentrations of antibiotics.[34] To perform the test a technologist must streak an agar plate with a bacterial suspension, as for a disk diffusion test, after which strips containing the antibiotics of interest are laid on the surface of the agar. After overnight incubation, the point at which the elliptical zone of growth inhibition intersects a quantitative scale on the strip determines the MIC. Jorgensen and colleagues found a good correlation of the E test and standardized microdilution tests.[34]

Antimicrobial susceptibility testing of *H. influenzae* has been reviewed by Doern and Jones.[15]

Streptococcus pneumoniae

For many years, penicillin was the standard treatment for pneumococcal infections and susceptibility testing was not indicated. The emergence of strains that are resistant to multiple antibiotics, including penicillin, has breached even this bastion of antimicrobial therapy. Strains that have MICs between 0.12 and 1 µg/mL are considered relatively resistant to penicillin; those with MICs greater than 1 µg/mL are designated as resistant. In one study, nearly 7% of patients in Denver who had pneumococcal bacteremia or meningitis were infected by relatively resistant strains.[31] Although the frequency of resistance has not been so high in all communities, testing of isolates from serious infections should be performed routinely. Pneumococcal resistance to penicillin has been reviewed by Klugman.[38]

Five percent sheep blood may be added to agar media and 2% to 5% lysed horse blood may be added to broth media for growth of *S. pneumoniae*. Quality control of these tests should include known resistant pneumococcal strains in addition to standard control organisms, because one commercial system has been shown to be insensitive to the detection of these relatively resistant strains.[60] If the commercial system that is used in a laboratory does not detect resistance reliably, the disk screening test described below should be employed. Incubation in CO_2 is acceptable if necessary for growth of the strain.

In most laboratories, the simplest screening test for resistance is a variation of the disk diffusion test. Although penicillin disks have been used in some studies, the procedure recommended by the NCCLS for detection of resistance to penicillin incorporates a 1-g disk of oxacillin. Strains that have a zone diameter of 19 mm or less should be reported as provisionally resistant to penicillin; confirmation by a dilution susceptibility test should be arranged. Swenson and colleagues[64] found that oxacillin was a better predictor of penicillin susceptibility than was methicillin, and nafcillin disks should not be used on agar-containing media.[45] The disk diffusion test does not differentiate strains that are relatively resistant (MIC of 0.12 to 1 µg/mL) from strains that are resistant (MIC greater than 1 µg/mL). A strain of *S. pneumoniae* that is presumptively resistant to penicillin should be tested in a reliable quantitative susceptibility test. Although some strains of relatively resistant pneumococci have responded to penicillin therapy,[49,67] meningitis may not be treated successfully because concentrations of antibiotic are lower.[50] Strains that have an MIC greater than 1 µg/mL are unlikely to respond to penicillin therapy. Unfortunately, many of these overtly resistant strains are resistant to multiple antibiotics.

The newly developed E test may be applied to *S. pneumoniae* as well as to *Haemophilus* species.[34]

Neisseria gonorrhoeae

For many years the gonococcus was uniformly susceptible to penicillin and the therapeutic approach to gonococcal infection was relatively straight forward. In the mid 1970s strains of *N. gonorrhoeae* that produced β-lactamase appeared[23] and spread rapidly.[61] A second mechanism of resistance appeared a few years later when Dougherty and colleagues[19] described resistant strains that lacked β-lactamase but contained altered penicillin-binding proteins. These strains have produced epidemic as well as sporadic infection.[24]

A second weapon in the antigonococcal armamentarium was removed when a plasmid that mediated high-level resistance to tetracycline appeared in *N. gonorrhoeae*.[39]

The tests recommended by the NCCLS for detection of chromosomally mediated resistance in *N. gonorrhoeae* are agar dilution and agar diffusion. The subject has been reviewed by Doern and Jones.[15]

All isolates of *N. gonorrhoeae* should be tested for β-lactamase production, preferably using the Nitrocefin method. An agar dilution or disk diffusion test should be performed on β-lactamase negative isolates if the frequency of intrinsic resistance to penicillin or the prevalence of tetracycline resistance in the population is high. Any isolates from treatment failures should be tested locally or referred to a reference laboratory.

Enterococcus Species

The mainstay of antimicrobial therapy of serious enterococcal infections has been the use of combinations of β-lactam and aminoglycoside antibiotics. The underpinnings of this approach have been seriously undermined in recent years. The subject has been reviewed by Herman and Gerding.[29]

Aminoglycoside Antibiotics

Two mechanisms of resistance to aminoglycosides are available to enterococci. The primary mechanism is production of inactivating enzymes, but strains of *E. faecalis* with ribosomal resistance to streptomycin have been described.[21] *E. faecium* is more resistant to both aminoglycosides and penicillin than is the more common *E. faecalis*.[66]

Detection of high-level resistance of enterococci to aminoglycosides is important because these strains are not inhibited synergistically by combination therapy with β-lactam antibiotics. Resistance of *E. faecium* to kanamycin, amikacin, netilmicin, and tobramycin can be assumed. Resistance of *E. faecium* to gentamicin and streptomycin and of *E. faecalis* to all of the aminoglycosides can be predicted by in vitro testing with large concentrations of antibiotic in a dilution test or by disks with a high antibiotic content.[22,62] Concentrations of 500 or 2000 μg/mL of gentamicin are most commonly used. Problems with detection of this resistance by commercial susceptibility systems are being addressed by the manufacturers.

β-Lactam Antibiotics

Many strains of enterococci are intrinsically resistant to β-lactam antibiotics because they possess binding proteins with low affinity for these drugs. In particular, the cephalosporins are uniformly ineffective against enterococci and should not be tested. In general, ampicillin is more effective than penicillin in vitro. The recent emergence of enterococcal strains that produce β-lactamase has been discussed previously.

Vancomycin

The last therapeutic resort for enterococci was vancomycin until Leclercq and colleagues described strains of *E. faecium* that contained a plasmid-mediating resistance to the glycopeptide antibiotics vancomycin and teicoplanin.[40] Vancomycin-resistant isolates of *E. faecalis* have also been described.[48] Fortunately such strains have been rare. Resistance to glycopeptides appears to be transferred by dissemination of a gene rather than a plasmid.[20] Vancomycin-resistant enterococci from serious infections should be referred to a reference laboratory for confirmation.

Rapid and Automated Susceptibility Testing

To perform and report laboratory tests more rapidly has been the goal of microbiologists for many years. Theoretically, identification of bacterial isolates and same-day determination of their antimicrobial susceptibility can better guide clinical use of antibiotics, shorten the length of hospitalization, and improve patient care. It is not easy to demonstrate an influence of rapid reporting on the use of antibiotics. It is much more difficult to demonstrate an effect on the outcome of the infectious process or the length of hospitalization.[14]

Advances in rapid antimicrobial susceptibility testing fall into two categories: (1) adaptations of standard manual methods and (2) use of semiautomated instruments, often equipped with computers for analysis of results. The microbiology laboratory and blood bank are the least automated of the clinical laboratories. Even the most advanced instruments for microbiologic analysis have not yet achieved the degree of automation that is available in clinical chemistry or hematology.

Adaptations of Standard Methods

Direct susceptibility testing of clinical specimens is not generally recommended because the inoculum is not standardized and mixed bacterial species are often present. Direct susceptibility testing of broth from positive blood culture bottles has correlated well with standard tests from isolated colonies. The tests have been performed both with unadjusted broth from the bottles[10] and after adjustment of the density of the culture by comparison to a 0.5 McFarland standard.[37] In addition, urine from patients with urinary tract infections may be tested directly if a single bacterial strain is present.[13] Some degree of mechanization has been achieved with the standard tests. Interpretation of the end points in microbroth dilution susceptibility tests by using commercially available microplate readers has compared well with visual inspection.[12] These instruments can be programmed to enter results directly into a computer and to provide interpretative correlates of susceptibility. An alternative system, which also performed well in comparison to traditional methods, incorporates a fluorescent dye into the microwells or bacterial inoculum; fluorescence that has been liberated by bacterial enzymatic alteration of the fluorescent substrates is measured.[63]

Commercial Systems

Multiple semiautomated systems for performance of antimicrobial susceptibility tests are commercially available. The largest market share belongs to two products, Vitek (bioMérieux Vitek, Hazelwood, MO) and MicroScan (MicroScan, Baxter Healthcare Corporation, West Sacramento, CA). A detailed description is beyond the scope of this text; manufacturers should be consulted for more information.

Certain combinations of drug and bacterial species present difficulties for the instruments, and the laboratory must make other arrangements for testing these combinations. Resistance of *Staphylococcus aureus* to oxacillin and the difficulty in detecting resistance of pneumococci to penicillin have been mentioned.[60] Problems in recognition of aminoglycoside-resistant enterococci have been encountered with several systems,[26] but the companies have worked diligently to correct them.

Quality control of the automated results has been difficult and largely unsatisfactory. For most drug–organism combinations, the standard control strains produce results that are at the extremes of the parameter measured and cannot be quantitated precisely.[36]

Serum Antimicrobial Levels

Indications

The concentration of antibiotic (in micrograms per milliliter) should be determined if it is assumed that adequate levels cannot be achieved or if the toxic level is close to the optimum therapeutic level. The overwhelmingly prevalent indication for serum drug assays is the administration of aminoglycoside antibiotics. Many isolates of *Pseudomonas aeruginosa* have MICs to gentamicin of 4 to 8 μg/mL. These concentrations may not be achieved in all patients, even if recommended doses are administered. Gentamicin toxicity is a concern if concentrations exceed 10 μg/mL.

The other major indication for measurement of antimicrobial levels is to document that oral antibiotics are being absorbed from the gastrointestinal tract, particularly when the patient has a serious infection that requires prolonged therapy or has lost a large segment of bowel. A description of the methods for assaying antibiotic levels is beyond the scope of this text.

REFERENCES

1. Anhalt JP. Assays for antimicrobial agents in body fluids. In: Balows A, Hausler WJ Jr, Herrmann KL, et al, eds. Manual of clinical microbiology. Washington, DC, American Society for Microbiology, 1991:1192–1198.

2. Anhalt JP, Washington JA II, eds. Laboratory procedures in clinical microbiology. New York, Springer-Verlag, 1985:281–313.

3. Archer GL. *Staphylococcus epidermidis*: the organism, its disease, and treatment. Curr Clin Topics Infect Dis 1984;5:25–48.

4. Barry AL. Procedure for testing antimicrobial agents in agar medium: theoretical considerations. In: Lorian V, ed. Antibiotics in laboratory medicine. Baltimore, Williams & Wilkins, 1986:1–26.

5. Barry AL, Badal RE, Hawkinson RW. Influence of inoculum growth phase on microdilution susceptibility tests. J Clin Microbiol 1983;18:645–651.

6. Bauer AW, Kirby WMM, Sherris JC, et al. Antibiotic susceptibility testing by a standardized single disk method. Am J Clin Pathol 1966;45:493–496.

7. Bauer AW, Perry DM, Kirby WMM. Single-disk antibiotic-sensitivity testing of staphylococci. Arch Intern Med 1959;104:208–216.

8. Bell SM, Plowman D. Mechanisms of ampicillin resistance in *Haemophilus influenzae* from respiratory tract. Lancet 1980;1:279–280.

9. Coudron PE, Jones DL, Dalton HP, et al. Evaluation of laboratory tests for detection of methicillin-resistant *Staphylococcus aureus* and *Staphylococcus epidermidis*. J Clin Microbiol 1986;24:764–769.

10. Coyle MB, McGonagle LA, Plorde JJ, et al. Rapid antimicrobial susceptibility testing of isolates from blood cultures by direct inoculation and early reading of disk diffusion tests. J Clin Microbiol 1984; 20:473–477.

11. D'Amato RF, Isenberg HD, McKinley GA, et al. Collaborative evaluation of the UniScept qualitative antimicrobial susceptibility test. J Clin Microbiol 1985;21:293–297.

12. DeGirolami PC, Eichelberger KA, Salfity LC, et al. Evaluation of the AutoSCAN-3, a device for

13. Dennstedt FE, Stager CE, Davis JR. Rapid method for identification and susceptibility testing of *Escherichia coli* bacteriuria. J Clin Microbiol 1983;18: 150–153.

14. Doern GV. Clinical impact of rapid susceptibility testing. Diagn Microbiol Infect Dis 1985;3: 59S–64S.

15. Doern GV, Jones RN. Antimicrobial susceptibility testing of *Haemophilus influenzae, Branhamella catarrhalis*, and *Neisseria gonorrhoeae*. Antimicrob Agents Chemother 1988;32:1747–1753.

16. Doern GV, Jorgensen JH, Thornsberry C, et al. Prevalence of antimicrobial resistance among clinical isolates of *Haemophilus influenzae*: a collaborative study. Diagn Microbiol Infect Dis 1986;4: 95–107.

17. Doern GV, Tubert TA. Detection of beta-lactamase activity among clinical isolates of *Branhamella catarrhalis* with six different beta-lactamase assays. J Clin Microbiol 1987;25:1380–1383.

18. Doern GV, Tubert TA. In vitro activities of 39 antimicrobial agents for *Branhamella catarrhalis* and comparison of results with different quantitative susceptibility test methods. Antimicrob Agents Chemother 1988;32:259–261.

19. Dougherty TJ, Koller AE, Tomasz A. Penicillin-binding proteins of penicillin-susceptible and intrinsically resistant *Neisseria gonorrhoeae*. Antimicrob Agents Chemother 1988;18:730–737.

20. Dutka-Malen S, LeClercq R, Coutant V, et al. Phenotypic and genotypic heterogeneity of glycopeptide resistance determinants in gram-positive bacteria. Antimicrob Agents Chemother 1990; 34:1875–1879.

21. Eliopoulos GM, Farber BF, Murray BE, et al. Ribosomal resistance of clinical enterococcal to streptomycin isolates. Antimicrob Agents Chemother 1984;25:398–399.

22. Eliopoulos GM, Wennersten C, Reiszner E, et al. High-level resistance to gentamicin in clinical isolates of *Streptococcus (Enterococcus) faecium*. Antimicrob Agents Chemother 1988;32:1528–1532.

23. Elwell LP, Roberts M, Mayer LW, et al. Plasmid-mediated beta-lactamase production in *Neisseria gonorrhoeae*. Antimicrob Agents Chemother 1977; 11:528–533.

24. Faruki H, Kohmescher RN, McKinney WP, et al. A community-based outbreak of infection with penicillin-resistant *Neisseria gonorrhoeae* not producing penicillinase (chromosomally mediated resistance). N Engl J Med 1985;313:607–611.

25. Fleming A. On the antibacterial action of cultures of a penicillium with special reference to their use

in isolation of *B. influenzae*. Br J Exp Pathol 1929; 110:226–236.

26. Fuller SA, Low DE, Simor AE. Evaluation of a commercial microtiter system (MicroScan) using both frozen and freeze-dried panels for detection of high-level aminoglycoside resistance in *Enterococcus* spp. J Clin Microbiol 1990;28:1051–1053.

27. Gavan TL, Jones RN, Barry AL. Evaluation of the Sensititre System for quantitative antimicrobial drug susceptibility testing: a collaborative study. Antimicrob Agents Chemother 1980;17:464–469.

28. Gerlach EH, Jones RN, Barry AL. Collaborative evaluation of the Microbial Profile System for quantitative antimicrobial susceptibility testing. J Clin Microbiol 1983;17:436–444.

29. Herman DJ, Gerding DN. Antimicrobial resistance among enterococci. Antimicrob Agents Chemother 1991;35:1–4.

30. Hindler JA, Inderlied CB. Effect of the source of Mueller-Hinton agar and resistance frequency on the detection of methicillin-resistant *Staphylococcus aureus*. J Clin Microbiol 1985;21:205–210.

31. Istre GR, Humphreys JT, Albrecht KD, et al. Chloramphenicol and penicillin resistance in pneumococci isolated from blood and cerebrospinal fluid: a prevalence study in metropolitan Denver. J Clin Microbiol 1983;17:472–475.

32. Jacoby GA, Archer GL. New mechanisms of bacterial resistance to antimicrobial agents. N Engl J Med 1991;324:601–612.

33. Jones RN, Edson DC. Antibiotic susceptibility testing accuracy: review of the College of American Pathologists Microbiology Survey, 1972–1983. Arch Pathol Lab Med 1985;109:595–601.

34. Jorgensen JH, Howell AW, Maher LA. Quantitative antimicrobial susceptibility testing of *Haemophilus influenzae* and *Streptococcus pneumoniae* by using the E-test. J Clin Microbiol 1991;29:109–114.

35. Jorgensen JH, Redding JS, Maher LA, et al. Improved medium for antimicrobial susceptibility testing of *Haemophilus influenzae*. J Clin Microbiol 1987;25:2105–2113.

36. Kellogg JA. Inability to adequately control antimicrobial agents on AutoMicrobic System Gram-Positive and Gram-Negative Susceptibility Cards. J Clin Microbiol 1985;21:454–456.

37. Kiehn TE, Capitolo C, Armstrong D. Comparison of direct and standard microtiter broth dilution susceptibility testing of blood culture isolates. J Clin Microbiol 1982;16:96–98.

38. Klugman KP. Pneumococcal resistance to antibiotics. Clin Microbiol Rev 1990;3:171–196.

39. Knapp JS, Zenilman JM, Biddle JW, et al. Frequency and distribution in the United States of strains of *Neisseria gonorrhoeae* with plasmid-medi-

40. Leclercq R, Derlot E, Duval J, et al. Plasmid-mediated resistance to vancomycin and teicoplanin in *Enterococcus faecium*. N Engl J Med 1988;319: 157–161.

41. Lorian V, ed. Antibiotics in clinical medicine. 2nd ed. Baltimore, Williams & Wilkins, 1986.

42. Mayer KH, Opal SM, Medeiros AA. Mechanisms of antibiotic resistance. In: Mandell GL, Douglas RG Jr, Bennett JE, eds. Principles and practice of infectious diseases. New York, Churchill Livingstone, 1990.

43. Murray BE, Church DA, Wanger A, et al. Comparison of two β-lactamase-producing strains of *Streptococcus faecalis*. Antimicrob Agents Chemother 1986;30:861–864.

44. Murray BE, Mederski-Samoraj B, Foster SK, et al. In vitro studies of plasmid-mediated penicillinase from *Streptococcus faecalis* suggest a staphylococcal orgin. J Clin Invest 1986;77:289–293.

45. National Committee for Clinical Laboratory Standards. Performance standards for antimicrobial disk susceptibility tests (approved standard, M2-A4). Villanova, PA, National Committee for Clinical Laboratory Standards, 1984.

46. National Committee for Clinical Laboratory Standards. Methods for dilution antimicrobial susceptibility tests for bacteria that grow aerobically (approved standard, M7-A2). Villanova, PA, National Committee for Clinical Laboratory Standards, 1985.

47. Neumann MA, Sahm DF, Thornsberry C, et al. New developments in antimicrobial agent susceptibility testing: a practical guide. Cumitech 1991; 6A:1–26.

48. Nicas TI, Cole CT, Preston DA, et al. Activity of glycopeptides against vancomycin-resistant gram-positive bacteria. Antimicrob Agents Chemother 1989;33:1477–1481.

49. Pallares R, Gudiol F, Linares J, et al. Risk factors and response to antibiotic therapy in adults with bacteremic pneumonia caused by penicillin-resistant pneumococci. N Engl J Med 1987;317: 18–22.

50. Paredes A, Taber LH, Yow MD, et al. Prolonged pneumococcal meningitis due to an organism with increased resistance to penicillin. Pediatrics 1976; 58:378–381.

51. Patterson JE, Colodny SM, Zervos MJ. Serious infection due to β-lactamase–producing *Streptococcus faecalis* with high-level resistance to gentamicin. J Infect Dis 1988;158:1144–1145.

52. Patterson JE, Masecar BL, Zervos MJ. Characterization and comparison of two penicillinase-pro-

ducing strains of *Streptococcus (Enterococcus) faecalis.* Antimicrob Agents Chemother 1988;32:122–124.

53. Patterson JE, Zervos MJ. Susceptibility and bactericidal activity studies of four β-lactamase–producing enterococci. Antimicrob Agents Chemother 1989;33:251–253.

54. Perl TM, Pfaller MA, Houston A, et al. Effect of serum on the in vitro activities of 11 broad-spectrum antibiotics. Antimicrob Agents Chemother 1990;32:2234–2239.

55. Peterson EM, Evans KD, Shigei JT, et al. Evaluation of four antimicrobic susceptibility testing systems for gram-negative bacilli. Am J Clin Pathol 1986;86:619–623.

56. Reller LB, Schoenknecht FD, Kenny MA, et al. Antibiotic susceptibility testing of *Pseudomonas aeruginosa*: selection of a control strain and criteria for magnesium and calcium content in media. J Infect Dis 1974;130:454–462.

57. Rice RJ, Biddle JW, Jeanlouis YA, et al. Chromosomally mediated resistance in *Neisseria gonorrhoeae* in the United States: results of surveillance and reporting, 1983–1984. J Infect Dis 1986;153:340–345.

58. Schieven BC, Hussain Z, Lannigan R. Comparison of American MicroScan dry and frozen microdilution trays. J Clin Microbiol 1985;22:495–496.

59. Schwalbe RS, Stapleton JT, Gilligan PH. Emergence of vancomycin resistance in coagulase-negative staphylococci. N Engl J Med 1987;316:927–931.

60. Shanholtzer CJ, Peterson LR. False susceptible penicillin G MIC's for *Streptococcus pneumoniae* with a commercial microdilution system. Am J Clin Pathol 1986;85:626–629.

61. Siegel MS, Thornsberry C, Biddle JW, et al. Penicillinase-producing *Neisseria gonorrhoeae*: results of surveillance in the United States. J Infect Dis 1978;137:170–175.

62. Spiegel CA. Laboratory detection of high-level aminoglycoside-aminocyclitol resistance in *Enterococcus* spp. J Clin Microbiol 1988;26:2270–2274.

63. Staneck JL, Allen SD, Harris EE, et al. Automated reading of MIC microdilution trays containing fluorogenic enzyme substrates with the Sensititre Autoreader. J Clin Microbiol 1985;22:187–191.

64. Swenson JM, Hill BC, Thornsberry C. Screening pneumococci for penicillin resistance. J Clin Microbiol 1986;24:749–752.

65. Thornsberry C, McDougal LK. Successful use of broth microdilution in susceptibility tests for methicillin-resistant (heteroresistant) staphylococci. J Clin Microbiol 1983;18:1084–1091.

66. Tompsett R, McDermott W. Recent advances in streptomycin therapy. Am J Med 1949;7:371–381.

67. Ward J. Antibiotic-resistant *Streptococcus pneumoniae*: clinical and epidemiologic aspects. Rev Infect Dis 1981;3:254–266.

68. Washington JA II. Discrepancies between in vitro activity of and in vivo response to antimicrobial agents. Diagn Microbiol Infect Dis 1983;1:25–31.

69. Washington JA. Functions and activities of the area committee on microbiology of the National Committee for Clinical Laboratory Standards. Clin Microbiol Rev 1991;4:150–155.

70. World Health Organization. Standardization of methods for conducting microbic sensitivity tests. WHO Tech Rep Ser 1961;210.

Chapter 12
Composites

Disk Diffusion Susceptibility (Kirby-Bauer) Test

A

Using a Dacron-tipped swab or a bacteriologic loop, touch the tops of four or five bacterial colonies of the same morphology.

B

Transfer the bacteria to a tube containing 4 to 5 mL of an appropriate broth and incubate the broth at 35°C.

C

Match the density of the bacterial suspension to the 0.5 McFarland density standard, using a calibrated nephelometer or visual inspection. Here, the density of painted lines is viewed through the standard (S) suspension and the test suspension. The lines are more difficult to visualize through the test suspension, so it must be diluted to match the standard.

D

Within 15 minutes of adjusting the bacterial suspension, insert a cotton-tipped swab into the suspension, rotate the swab firmly against the wall of the tube to express excess fluid, and streak the surface of a dried Mueller-Hinton agar plate.

E

Swab the surface of the plate three times, rotating the plate 60 degrees each time.

F

Allow 3 to 5 minutes, but no more than 15 minutes, for the inoculum to dry. Using a manual or multichannel dispenser, place antibiotic impregnated disks on the surface of the agar.

G

Tamp the disks down firmly onto the surface of the agar. Do not move the disks once they have touched the agar surface.

H

After overnight incubation, use a ruler, calipers (*shown here*), or template to measure the diameters of zones of inhibition. Reflected light should be used, not transmitted light. The diameters can be measured from the surface of the plate or through the bottom of the plate.

A

B

C

D

E

F

G

H

Standardized Direct Inoculation of Microdilution Susceptibility Test, Using the Prompt System (Baxter Healthcare Corporation, West Sacramento, CA)

A
Holding the wand *perpendicular* to the agar plate, touch the tops of three isolated colonies that are at least as wide as the wand.

B
Without bending or twisting the wand, pull firmly to break the connection between the handle and the protective collar. Remove the protective collar from the wand.

C
Place the inoculation wand into an inoculation bottle and press down firmly with a twisting motion to ensure a tight seal. Shake the bottle vigorously 8 to 10 times to release the bacteria from the wand.

D
Within 4 hours, pour the contents of the inoculation bottle into an inoculation tray. Here a plastic, disposable system is pictured. The plastic inoculating pins (P) are affixed to the top of the panel, which is placed into the well after the inoculum has been poured. The final step is to place the pins into the microdilution tray to inoculate the susceptibility test.

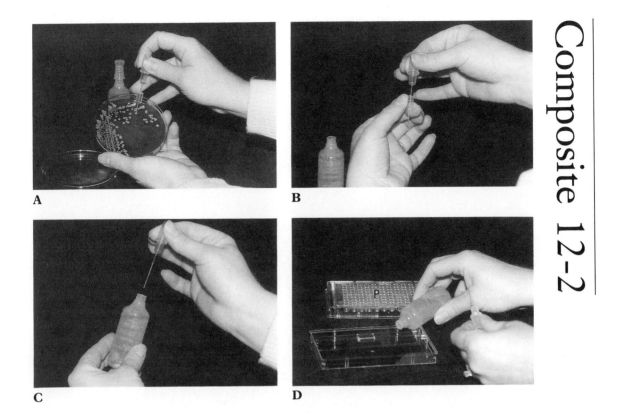

A

B

C

D

13

Mycobacteria

The mycobacteria have certain distinguishing characteristics by which they can be recognized:

1. Most strains are slow growing, often requiring several weeks before visible colonies are observed in culture media.
2. The slightly curved or straight bacilli, measuring 0.2 to 0.6 μm by 1 to 10 μm, either do not stain with the Gram method or stain faintly gram-positive.
3. Because of the high concentration of waxy materials in their cell walls, mycobacteria are acid-fast; that is, they resist decolorization with acidified alcohol and strong mineral acids once stained with carbolfuchsin.
4. They are obligate aerobes and require increased

concentrations of CO_2 during incubation to grow.

The recovery of *Mycobacterium tuberculosis* from clinical specimens is almost always associated with infection, and tuberculosis is known to be a highly communicable disease. Reinfection or adult-type tuberculosis is a slowly progressive inflammatory process in the lungs, characterized by intense chronic granulomatous inflammation, usually with the formation of many Langhans-type giant cells, necrosis, and caseation, with the propensity of the process to break into bronchi. Large numbers of tubercle bacilli are spread to fresh foci within the lung when a cavity ruptures and may be coughed up in profusion if the cavity breaks into a bronchus, potentially infecting others in close contact. Coughing, weight loss, low-grade fever, dyspnea, and chest pain are the usual clinical signs and symptoms of chronic progressive pulmonary tuberculosis.

Yet, over the past decade, classic tuberculosis and mycobacterial infections caused by species other than *M. tuberculosis*, have undergone profound changes. The progressive annual decline in incidence and prevalence of tuberculosis in the United States in every decade since the turn of the century gave way to significant increases in the 1980s. In 1988, 22,436 cases of tuberculosis were reported to the Centers for Disease Control (CDC; 9.1 per 1 million population), 14,678 more than expected. This upsurge was caused primarily by an increase of infections caused by organisms other than *M. tuberculosis*, primarily by the *M. avium-intracellulare* complex of organisms.

The disease manifestations of tuberculosis have become altered, particularly in patients with the acquired immunodeficiency syndrome (AIDS). The course of *M. tuberculosis* infections in these patients often does not follow the classic slowly progressive course; instead, a rapidly spreading miliary type of tuberculosis has become common. Disease progression is often rapid, no longer measured in months and years as with the classic disease but in time frames of a few weeks. Disseminated disease, particularly in infections with *M. avium-intracellulare*, may be observed in several unusual organ systems, including the bowel, deep visceral organs, and the central nervous system with massive organism concentrations never before witnessed. Cases of septicemia, once only rarely encountered, can almost be expected in patients with these heavy infections.

To accommodate to these changes in the clinical manifestations of mycobacterial infections, clinical microbiology laboratories have implemented new technologies directed toward the more rapid recovery and identification of mycobacteria. Included are the use of radiometric instruments (BACTEC 460 + BACTEC 12B vials, Becton Dickinson Microbiology Systems, Cockeysville, MD), both to shorten the time of recovery of mycobacteria from clinical specimens by as much as 2 to 3 weeks and for rapid antimycobacterial susceptibility testing; determining the inhibitory properties of *p*-nitro-acetylamino-hydroxypropiophenone (NAP) against *M. tuberculosis;* the introduction of isotopic and nonisotopic nucleic acid probes (commercially available are probes for the culture confirmation of *M. tuberculosis* complex, *M. avium* and *M. intracellulare, M. kansasii,* and *M. gordonae*) and the potential use of polymerase chain reaction for the direct detection of mycobacteria.

New techniques have also been introduced for the more rapid recovery of mycobacteria from virtually all specimen types, including such previously unlikely sources as blood and stool. Decontamination and concentration procedures have been revised to recover mycobacteria from stools, and lysis centrifugation techniques have enhanced recovery from peripheral blood and bone marrow samples. Bronchoalveolar lavage and fine-needle biopsies have allowed the more rapid diagnosis of pulmonary and disseminated diseases, respectively, minimizing the need for more invasive surgical procedures.

SPECIMEN COLLECTION AND PROCESSING

Respiratory Samples

Sputum samples collected by expectoration or by ultrasonic nebulization are best obtained shortly after the patient awakens in the morning, since mycobacteria are then in the highest concentration in the respiratory secretions. Twenty-four-hour collections are now discouraged because the sample containing the highest concentration of mycobacteria will be proportionally diluted by subsequent low-yield samples and the chances for bacterial and fungal contamination during the prolonged collection process are significantly increased.[17,22]

The irregular and intermittent release of mycobacteria into the bronchial lumen from mucosal ulcers or loculated cavities often results in a variable pattern of recovery from respiratory secretions. Cultures obtained from patients with pulmonary and renal tuberculosis in particular may be positive on one day but negative on the next; thus, a minimum of three to five early-morning sputum and urine specimens should be collected in successive 24-hour periods to maximize the chance of recovery of mycobacteria. All specimens should be transported promptly to the laboratory and refrigerated if processing is delayed.

Recovery of Mycobacteria from the Blood

The use of the lysis centrifugation blood culture system (Isolator, Wampole Laboratories, Cranbury, NJ) has increased the yield and shortened the time of recovery of mycobacteria from blood cultures.[8,25] The lysis centrifuge tube contains an anticoagulant and a lysing agent to effect rupture of both erythrocytes and neutrophils that are present in the broth. Thus, intracellular mycobacteria are released into the broth milieu, further enriched by the lysis of the red blood cells. Each tube holds 5 mL of blood, and cell lysis can be enhanced by gently inverting the tube several times immediately after adding the sample. After centrifugation of the tube at 3000 g for 20 to 30 minutes, the eluate is discarded and 1.6 mL of sediment is divided into 0.2-mL aliquots for transfer to appropriate culture media. In many laboratories, it is common practice to transfer one such aliquot to a BACTEC 12B blood culture vial.

The BACTEC (Becton Dickinson Microbiology Systems, Cockeysville, MD) is a semiautomated blood culture system that is based on the detection of radioactive $^{14}CO_2$ released in the blood culture vial from ^{14}C palmitic acid included in the broth medium (ie, Middlebrook). For those laboratories in which the BACTEC system is being

used, a new 13A bottle has been designed specifically for the recovery of mycobacteria from blood.

Stool Specimens

In certain patients with AIDS, the concentration of mycobacteria, particularly *M. avium-intracellulare*, may be sufficiently high in the lower intestinal tract to be recovered in culture. Kiehn and colleagues[19] have outlined a procedure for the processing of stool specimens for mycobacterial culture. Stool specimens are collected in a clean (not necessarily sterile) container with a tightly fitting lid, as for routine bacterial cultures. A direct smear is first prepared from a small quantity of the specimen and stained for acid-fast bacilli, using either the Ziehl-Neelsen or Kinyoun carbolfuchsin techniques or the rhodamine-auramine fluorescence method. If the smears are negative for acid-fast bacteria, the specimen is not further processed. If acid-fast bacilli are seen in the smear, 1 g of feces is suspended in 5 mL of Middlebrook 7H9 broth or equivalent and subjected to the same sodium hydroxide digestion/decontamination as for sputum specimens. Culture contamination with intestinal bacteria was not a problem after the digestion procedure.

Miscellaneous "Sterile" Specimens

Specimens submitted for acid-fast culture that are normally sterile, such as cerebrospinal fluid, synovial fluid, and other body fluids, need not be decontaminated before culture. Processing can commence with centrifugation, and a small aliquot of the sediment can be transferred to appropriate culture media. Low-volume fluid samples can be added directly to about 10 mL of Middlebrook 7H9 or 7H11 broth and incubated directly. Urine samples can usually be processed without decontamination and centrifuged and a portion of the sediment used for culture. After centrifugation, a portion of the sediment is cultured. Tissue and needle biopsy material should be placed in a small quantity of Middlebrook 7H9 or 7H11 broth as a holding medium. Depending on the size and nature of the material obtained, the specimen should be ground in a small amount of broth with a mortar and pestle and aliquots of the suspension transferred to appropriate culture media.

The use of swabs for the culture of mycobacteria is discouraged; if a swab is received, the tip should be placed directly on the surface of the culture medium or into a tube containing about 5 mL of Middlebrook 7H9 broth and incubated for 4 to 8 weeks. Mycobacteria, if present, may be found forming colonies in the fibers of the swab at the junction with the culture media.

SPECIMEN PREPARATION

Specimens likely to contain a mixed bacterial flora, notably sputum, are treated with a decontaminating agent to reduce undesirable bacterial overgrowth and to liquefy mucus. After treatment with the decontaminating agent for a carefully controlled period of time, the acid or alkali used is neutralized and the mixture is centrifuged at high speed to concentrate the mycobacteria.

Digestion/Decontamination Agents

Several chemical solutions are used for the decontamination of clinical specimens. Sodium hydroxide alone or in combination with other agents is used in most laboratories. This reagent is effective but may also kill or seriously injure mycobacteria. Thus, the concentration of sodium hydroxide in the final mixture should not exceed 2%, and the time of exposure should be rigidly limited to no more than 15 minutes. Mild decontaminating agents, such as trisodium phosphate alone or combined with benzalkonium chloride (Zephiran; Winthrop Laboratories, New York, NY) is popular in some laboratories. Specimens containing large numbers of M. tuberculosis can withstand the action of these agents as long as overnight, and careful timing is not required.[21,22] Trisodium phosphate–treated specimens must be neutralized if agar base medium is used; egg-based medium inherently contain neutralizers, and the addition of buffer solutions is not required. Table 13-1 lists additional agents for decontaminating and concentrating specimens, along with comments about their use. Each clinical mycobacteriologist should select the agents to employ on the basis of the number and types of specimens received and the time and technical staff available to process the specimens. Dithiothreitol is also an effective mycolytic agent when used with 2% sodium hydroxide. Cetylpyridinium chloride has also been recommended for the decontamination of specimens, particularly those mailed from remote sites of collection.[47,50]

The decontamination/digestion process can be facilitated by adding a mucolytic agent such as N-acetyl-L-cysteine (NALC) to the digestion mixture. This agent has the property of splitting mucoprotein disulfide linkages, thereby liquefying mucin and releasing trapped mycobacterial cells, which in turn can be more readily concentrated in the sediment by high-speed centrifugation. Shah and Dye[43] have found the sulfhydryl reducing agent dithiothreitol, a white solid that is soluble in water and alcohol, to be superior to NALC for the recovery of mycobacteria from sputum samples. Aqueous dithiothreitol is stable in atmospheric storage and possesses little odor.

Centrifugation

Centrifugation of the digestion mixture is necessary to ensure the best recovery of mycobacteria. Generally, if the organism is to be maximally concentrated during centrifugation, the specific gravity of the suspending fluid should be kept as low as possible and the centrifugal force applied to the specimen should be as high as practical. Improved recovery of mycobacteria by culture occurred as the relative centrifugal force (RCF) was increased from 1260 to 3000 g.[37] When the RCF was increased to 3800 g, a twofold increase in the correlation of positive smears to positive cultures from 40% to 82% was realized, or more than a threefold increase from the correlation when the RCF was only 1260 g. Therefore, it is recommended that centrifugation with the relative centrifugal force of 3000 g be used. As pointed out by Sommers and Good,[50] with the centrifugation forces produced at RCFs of 3000 g or greater, glass or plastic centrifuge tubes may collapse and must be placed in sealed cups. Additionally, considerable heat is generated at high-speed centrifugation and refrigerated centrifuges may be required when RCFs exceed 3000 g.

Table 13-1
Commonly Used Agents for Decontamination and Concentration of Specimens

AGENT	COMMENTS
N-acetyl-L-cysteine plus 2% NaOH	Mild decontamination solution with mucolytic agent NALC to free mycobacteria entrapped in mucus. Limit exposure to NaOH to 15 minutes.
Dithiothreitol plus 2% NaOH*	Very effective mucolytic agent used with 2% NaOH. Trade name of dithiothreitol is Sputolysin. Reagent is more expensive than NALC. Limit exposure to NaOH to 15 minutes.
Trisodium phosphate, 13%, plus benzalkonium chloride (Zephiran)	Preferred by laboratories that cannot carefully control time of exposure to decontamination solution. Zephiran should be neutralized with lecithin not inoculated to egg-based culture medium.
NaOH, 4%	Traditional decontamination and concentration solution. Time of exposure must be carefully controlled to no more than 15 minutes. NaOH, 4%, effects mucolytic action to promote concentration by centrifugation.
Trisodium phosphate, 13%	Can be used for decontamination of specimens when exposure time can be completely controlled. It is not as effective as TSP-Zephiran mixture.
Oxalic acid, 5%	Most useful in the processing of specimens that contain *Pseudomonas aeruginosa* as a contaminant.
Cetylpyridium chloride, 1%, plus 2% NaCL	Effective as a decontamination solution for sputum specimens mailed from outpatient clinics. Tubercle bacilli have survived 8-day transit without significant loss.

*See Shah and Dye.[43]
†See Smithwick et al.[47]

Safety Precautions

The emergence of multidrug-resistant mycobacteria strains, both of *M. tuberculosis* and mycobacteria other than *M. tuberculosis* (MOTT), and the high concentrations of organisms achieved in some patients significantly increases the chances for human-to-human transmission. Therefore, laboratory personnel must carry out several safety practices when handling potentially positive specimens. An approved class I or IIA biologic safety hood, preferably located in a separate room with a slightly negative pressure and an outside exhaust, should be used when transferring sputum and other clinical specimens from collection containers to centrifuge tubes, when dissecting surgical tissues for sectioning, when preparing smears for acid-fast staining, when inoculating cultures, and when transferring isolated mycobacterial colonies for further studies. Personnel are advised to wear gloves and a gown when handling specimens suspected of harboring mycobacteria; cap, mask, and shoe covers are optional depending on local laboratory policies. Every attempt must be made to prevent drying and aerosolization of specimens during handling. The use of either 50- or 250-mL centrifuge cups with aerosol-free tops that can be adapted to hold 50-mL centrifuge tubes is strongly recommended to prevent aerosolization of specimens from broken tubes. Precautions should be taken to prevent the spontaneous rupture of fluid surface tension membranes when inoculating broth cultures or liquid specimens. All working surfaces, particularly dissecting boards used for the processing of surgical specimens, should be thoroughly cleaned and decontaminated after the processing of all specimens.

CULTURE OF MYCOBACTERIA SPECIMENS

Culture media containing whole eggs, potato flour, glycerol, and salts, solidified by heating to 85° to 90°C for 30 to 45 minutes, has served as the classic formula for the laboratory recovery of *M. tuberculosis*. The process of solidifying protein-containing medium by heat is known as inspissation. Certain aniline dyes, such as malachite green or crystal violet, may be added to the inspissated medium to control the overgrowth of contaminating bacteria. The concentration of dye must be carefully adjusted; if too high, the growth of mycobacteria may also be inhibited along with the contaminating bacteria. Malachite green is the dye most commonly incorporated in nonselective culture media, in concentrations ranging between 0.0025 and 0.052 g/dL.

Löwenstein-Jensen medium is most commonly used in most clinical diagnostic laboratories; it is less inhibitory to the growth of mycobacteria than is Petragnani medium, which is used primarily to recover mycobacteria from specimens heavily contaminated with bacteria. Conversely, the American Thoracic Society medium, which contains only 0.02 g/dL of malachite green, is less inhibitory to the growth of mycobacteria and is recommended for use in usually sterile specimens such as cerebrospinal fluid, pleural fluid, and tissue biopsy samples.

During the 1950s, Cohen and Middlebrook developed a series of synthetic culture media prepared from defined salts and organic chemicals; some contained agar, but all were found to require the addition of albumin for optimal growth of mycobacteria. Middlebrook 7H9 is the designation for a popular liquid medium; both Middlebrook 7H10 and 7H11 agar media are widely used for both the isolation of mycobacteria and for susceptibility testing. The antimycobacterial agents should be incorporated into the medium just before it solidifies to reduce the loss of activity known to occur with some drugs during the long heating period needed to prepare the inspissated egg-based media. Middlebrook 7H11 agar differs from 7H10

agar only in also containing 0.1% casein hydrolysate, an additive found to improve the rate and amount of growth of mycobacteria resistant to isoniazid.[5]

Culture media can also be made selective by the addition of one or more antibacterial agents. The selective medium described by Gruft,[12] which consists of Löwenstein-Jensen medium with penicillin, nalidixic acid, and ribonucleic acid (RNA), is used in some laboratories. Middlebrook 7H10 medium containing malachite green, cycloheximide, lincomycin, and nalidixic acid is also commonly used (see Table 13-2). Selective Middlebrook 7H11 is a modification of an oleic acid agar medium first described by Mitchison and coworkers.[30] Mitchison's medium contains carbenicillin, polymyxin, trimethoprim lactate, and amphotericin B. McClatchy and associates[27] suggested reducing the concentration of carbenicillin from 100 to 50 g/mL and using Middlebrook 7H11 medium instead of oleic acid agar. They called this modification Selective 7H11, or S7H11. The use of S7H11 medium with Löwenstein-Jensen and Middlebrook 7H11 has shown that recovery of mycobacteria is definitely improved, particularly when the S7H11 medium is used with the NALC-1% sodium hydroxide decontamination procedure.[27] One advantage of these selective media is that sputum and other normally contaminated specimens can be inoculated directly to the medium without the use of a decontaminating agent, thus reducing the chance for killing mycobacteria in the process.

Although essentially all culture media yield more growth and larger colonies of mycobacteria when incubated in 5% to 10% CO_2, the Middlebrook media absolutely require capneic incubation in 5% to 10% CO_2 for proper performance. Exposure of Middlebrook 7H10 and 7H11 media to strong light, or storage of the media at 4°C for more than 4 weeks, may result in deterioration and release of formaldehyde, a chemical inhibitory to mycobacteria.[29]

STAINING OF ACID-FAST BACILLI

The lipid-rich cell walls of mycobacteria have the unique capability of binding fuchsin dye so that it is not de-stained by acid alcohol. This acid-fast staining reaction of mycobacteria, along with their

Table 13-2
Selective Mycobacterial Isolation Media

MEDIUM	COMPONENTS	INHIBITORY AGENTS
Gruft modification of Löwenstein-Jensen	Coagulated whole eggs, defined salts, glycerol, potato flour, RNA–5 mg/dL	Malachite green, 0.025 g/dL Penicillin, 50 IU/mL Nalidixic acid, 35 μg/mL
Löwenstein-Jensen	Coagulated whole eggs, defined salts, glycerol, potato flour	Malachite green, 0.025 g/dL Cycloheximide, 400 μg/mL Lincomycin, 2 μg/mL Nalidixic acid, 35 μg/mL
Middlebrook 7H10	Defined salts, vitamins, cofactors, oleic acid, albumin, catalase, glycerol, glucose	Malachite green, 0.0025 g/dL Cycloheximide, 260 μg/mL Lincomycin, 2 μg/mL Nalidixic acid, 20 μg/mL
Selective 7H11 (Mitchison's medium)	Defined salts, vitamins, cofactors, oleic acid, albumin, catalase, glycerol, glucose, casein hydrolysate	Carbenicillin, 50 μg/mL Amphotericin B, 10 μg/mL Polymyxin B, 200 IU/mL Trimethoprim lactate, 20 μg/mL

characteristic size and shape, is a valuable aid in the early detection of infection and in the monitoring of therapy for mycobacterial disease. After therapy with antimycobacterial drugs is started, cultures become negative before the smears do, suggesting that the organisms are not capable of replicating but are capable of binding the stain. With continued treatment, more organisms are killed and fewer shed, so that assessing the number of organisms in the sputum during treatment can provide an early objective measure of response. Two types of acid-fast stains are commonly used:

Carbolfuchsin stains: a mixture of fuchsin with phenol (carbolic acid)
 Ziehl-Neelsen (hot stain)
 Kinyoun (cold stain)
Fluorochrome stain: auramine O, with or without a second fluorochrome, rhodamine

Both stains in these techniques are reported to bind to mycolic acid in the mycobacterial cell wall. The reagents and procedures for these acid-fast stains are included in Table 13-3. Smears stained fluorochrome dyes can be screened using a microscope fitted with an appropriate ultraviolet light source, filters and a $25 \times$ objective. This lower magnification objective increases the field of view and considerably reduces the time needed to scan a smear compared with carbolfuchsin-stained smears, which must be examined under oil immersion. The $40 \times$ objective can then be used to confirm any suspicious forms.

Mycobacteria stained with either the Ziehl-Neelsen or the Kinyoun's procedure, using methylene blue as a counterstain, appear as bright red-staining rods against a blue background. The size, shape, and specific nature of staining (eg, beaded, banded) are features that may be used by experienced workers to support the species identifications of certain species of mycobacteria. Fluorochrome-stained bacteria are bright yellow (auramine) or orange-red (rhodamine) against a dark background. False-positives may be due to fluorescence of nonspecific tissue or cellular debris that can be mistaken for bacilli. Fluorochrome-stained smears can be restained with one of the carbolfuchsin reagents to confirm any suspicious forms observed. Dead mycobacterial cells also stain with rhodamine and auramine, leading to a smear-positive/culture-negative situation about 10% of the time. This feature is also important to remember when using acid-fast smears to assess treatment efficacy—the

Table 13-3
Acid-Fast Staining Procedure

ZIEHL-NEELSEN PROCEDURE	KINYOUN'S COLD PROCEDURE	AURAMINE FLUOROCHROME PROCEDURE
Carbolfuchsin: dissolve 3 g of basic fuchsin in 10 mL of 90%–95% ethanol. Add 90 mL of 5% aqueous solution of phenol.	**Carbolfuchsin:** dissolve 4 g of basic fuchsin in 20 mL of 90%–95% ethanol and then add 100 mL of a 9% aqueous solution of phenol (9 g of phenol dissolved in 100 mL of distilled water).	**Phenolic auramine:** dissolve 0.1 g of auramine 0 in 10 mL of 90%–95% ethanol and then add to a solution of 3 g of phenol in 87 mL of distilled water. Store the stain in a brown bottle.
Acid-alcohol: Add 3 mL of concentrated HCL *slowly* to 97 mL of 90%–95% ethanol, in this order. Solution may get hot!	**Acid-alcohol:** add 3 mL of concentrated HCL *slowly* to 97 mL of 90%–95% ethanol, in this order. Solution may get hot!	**Acid-alcohol:** add 0.5 mL of concentrated HCL to 100 mL of 70% alcohol.
Methylene blue counterstain: dissolve 0.3 g of methylene blue chloride in 100 mL of distilled water.	**Methylene blue counterstain:** dissolve 0.3 g of methylene blue chloride in 100 mL of distilled water.	**Potassium permanganate:** dissolve 0.5 g potassium permanganate in 100 mL of distilled water.
Procedure	**Procedure**	**Procedure**
Cover a heat-fixed, dried smear with a small rectangle (2×3 cm) of filter paper.	Cover a heat-fixed, dried smear with a small rectangle, 2×3 cm) of filter paper.	Cover a heat-fixed, dried smear with carbol auramine and allow to stain for 15 minutes. Do not heat or cover with filter paper.
Apply 5 to 7 drops of carbolfuchsin stain to thoroughly moistened filter paper	Apply 5 to 7 drops of carbolfuchsin to thoroughly moisten filter paper. Allow to stand for 5 minutes. Add more stain if paper dries. Do not steam!	Rinse with water and drain.
Heat the stain-covered slide to steaming but do not allow to dry. Heating may be done by gas burner or over an electric staining rack.	Remove paper with forceps, rinse slide with water, and drain.	Decolorize with acid-alcohol (2 minutes).
Remove paper with forceps, rinse slide with water, and drain.	Decolorize with acid-alcohol until no more stain appears in the washing (2 minutes).	Rinse with water and drain.
Decolorize with acid-alcohol until no more stain appears in the washing (2 minutes)	Counterstain with methylene blue (1 to 2 minutes).	Flood smear with potassium permanganate for 2 and not more than 4 minutes.
Counterstain with methylene blue (1 to 2 minutes).	Rinse, drain, and air dry (1 to 2 minutes).	Rinse with tap water. Drain
Rinse, drain, and air dry (1 to 2 minutes).	Examine with 100× oil immersion objective. Mycobacteria are stained red and the background light blue.	Examine with 25× objective using a mercury vapor burner and BG-12 filter or a strong blue light. Mycobacteria are stained yellowish orange against a dark background.
Examine with 100× oil immersion objective. Mycobacteria are stained red and the background light blue.		

presence of acid-fast bacilli in fluorochrome-stained smears does not necessarily indicate treatment failure, and carbolfuchsin stains should also be performed.

The recommendations of the American Thoracic Society for reporting mycobacteria seen on acid-fast stained smears are given in Table 13-4. These recommendations are followed by many laboratories to provide consistency of observations between technologists in a given laboratory and uniformity of reporting from one laboratory to another.

Table 13-4
Method for Reporting Numbers of Acid-Fast Bacilli Observed in Stained Smears*

NUMBER OF BACILLI OBSERVED	CDC METHOD REPORT	
0	Negative	(−)
1–2/300 fields	Number seen†	(±)
1–9/100 fields	Average no./100 fields	(1+)
1–9/10 fields	Average no./10 fields	(2+)
1–9/field	Average no./field	(3+)
Greater than 9/field	Greater than 9/field	(4+)

*Examination at × 800 to × 1000 is assumed. Magnifications less than × 800 should be clearly stated. If a microscopist uses consistent procedure for smear examination, relative comparisons of multiple specimens should be easy for the clinician regardless of magnification used. To equate numbers of bacilli observed at less than × 800 with those seen under oil immersion, adjust counts as follows: for magnifications about × 650, divide count by 2; near × 450, divide by 4; near × 250, divide by 10; eg, if 8 bacilli per 10 fields were seen at × 450, the count at × 1000 would be equivalent to about 2/10 fields (8÷4).

†Counts less than 3/3000 fields at × 800 to × 1000 are not considered positive; another specimen (or repeat smear of same specimen) should be processed if available.

(American Thoracic Society. Diagnostic standards and classification of tuberculosis and other mycobacterial diseases. Am Rev Respir Dis 1981;123:343–358)

INCUBATION

Different species of mycobacteria show striking dependence on the temperature of incubation for optimal growth. Species having a predilection for infecting skin, such as *M. marinum, M. ulcerans,* and *M. haemophilum,* grow best at the temperature of the skin (30° to 32°C) and very poorly or not at all at 37°C. *M. tuberculosis* grows best at 37°C and poorly or not at all at 30°C or at 42° to 45°C (the body temperature of birds). *M. xenopi,* a species not commonly found as a cause of infection in humans, grows best at 42°C and has been implicated as an environmental contaminant in the hot water system of a large hospital.[11]

Mycobacteria grow best in an atmosphere of 3% to 11% CO_2. Use of CO_2 is mandatory if Middlebrook 7H11 medium is used. If lack of incubator space to maintain cultures is a problem, however, cultures can be removed from the CO_2 atmosphere after 7 to 10 days of incubation since organisms growing in log phase are less CO_2 dependent. For reasons that are not well understood, mycobacteria do not grow well in candle extinction jars. The CO_2 concentration in incubators should be monitored daily and the temperature and CO_2 levels recorded.

PHENOTYPIC CHARACTERISTICS FOR THE IDENTIFICATION OF MYCOBACTERIA

Several phenotypic characteristics are used to identify the clinically important mycobacteria. Detailed identification tables are included in many textbooks and monographs. Following is a brief summary of these characteristics and specific applications in the identification of key mycobacteria.

Temperature of Incubation

Each *Mycobacterium* species has an optimum temperature and range of time for recovery in culture media. The time of recovery varies depending on the types of media used—the average time of recovery of mycobacteria on egg-based media is around 21 days (as short as 3 to 5 days and as long as 60 days depending on the species). Times of recovery are generally shorter by several days when using Middlebrook 7H10 or 7H11 agar if the technique of microscopic observation for microcolonies is employed; and, as mentioned earlier, the use of BACTEC vials, both for the inoculation of blood cultures and other body fluids, can shorten the times of detection considerably.[6, 20, 38]

Pigment Production

Strains of mycobacteria that produce pigmented colonies in the dark are known as scotochromogens (*M. scrofulaceum* and *M. gordonae* most common); those that product pigmented colonies only after exposure to light are called photochromogens (*M. kansasii* and *M. marinum* most common). Several species, including *M. tuberculosis,* do not produce pigment. Although previously classified as a non–pigment producer, *M. avium-intracellulare* (particularly those patients that are recovered from patients with AIDS) has the capability of producing a yellow pigment. Nevertheless, pigment production remains a helpful clue in making presumptive identifications.

Biochemical Characteristics

The determination of several biochemical characteristics is essential for making phenotypic separations of the various *Mycobacterium* species. Only a brief summary of the principles, reagent requirements, procedures, and interpretation of results for these tests are included here.

Niacin Accumulation

All mycobacteria produce niacin; in particular, *M. tuberculosis*, *M. simiae*, and rare strains of *M. africanum*, *M. bovis*, *M. marinum*, and *M. chelonei* lack the enzyme necessary to further convert the niacin to niacin ribonucleotide. Thus, for these species, niacin accumulates in the culture medium and can be detected by the addition of appropriate reagents. Reagent-impregnated filter paper strips are commercially available that facilitate the performance of this test. The development of a yellow color in the test medium incubated with a reagent strip is indicative of niacin accumulation and a positive test.

Nitrate Reduction

Only a few species of mycobacteria, notably *M. tuberculosis*, produce nitroreductase, which catalyzes the reduction of nitrate to nitrite. The development of a red color on addition of sulfanilic acid and *n*-naphthylethylenediamine to an extract of the unknown culture is indicative of the presence of nitrite and a positive test. In addition to supporting the identification of *M. tuberculosis*, the nitrate reduction test is also a key test in the identification of *M. kansasii* and, in particular, *M. szulgai*.

Catalase Activity

Most of the mycobacteria produce catalase, but not all species are capable of producing a positive reaction after heating the culture at 68°C for 20 minutes (heat-stable catalase). Most strains of *M. tuberculosis*, and other members of the *M. tuberculosis* complex, do not produce heat-stable catalase, except for certain isoniazid-resistant strains, when the results of this test are of particular value. Catalase activity can be semiquantitatively assessed by measuring the height achieved by the column of bubbles produced by adding hydrogen peroxide to a colony of the *Mycobacterium* species to be identified growing on the surface of a nonslanted tube of Löwenstein-Jensen agar. A column of bubbles in excess of 45 mm high is considered a positive test.

Growth Inhibition by Thiophene 2-Carboxylic Acid Hydrazide

Thiophene-2-carboxylic acid hydrazine (T_2H) selectively inhibits the growth of *M. tuberculosis*, making this an important differential test from most other species, including the phenotypically closely related *M. bovis*, which can grow in a medium containing this compound.

Tween 80 Hydrolysis

Tween 80 is the trade name of a detergent that can be useful in identifying those mycobacteria that possess a lipase that splits the compound into oleic acid and polyoxyethylated sorbitol. This test is helpful in identifying *M. kansasii*, which can produce a positive result as soon as 3 to 6 hours. A positive reaction is indicated by a change in the color of the substrate from straw yellow to pink after 3 days after inoculation and incubation of a positive strain.

Arylsulfatase Activity

Arylsulfatase is an enzyme that splits the tripotassium salt of phenolphthalein disulfate, which is incorporated in the test substrate, into free phenolphthalein. The development of a red color in the test medium, indicating a release of free phenolphthalein, indicates a positive result. This test is particularly helpful in identifying members of the rapidly growing *M. fortuitum-chelonei* complex.

Pyrazinamidase

Pyrazinamidase is an enzyme that deaminates pyrazinamide to form pyrazinoic acid, resulting in the production of a red band in the culture medium.[54] The test is useful in distinguishing *M. kansasii* (positive) from *M. marinum* (negative) and weakly niacin-positive *M. bovis* (negative) from *M. tuberculosis* (positive; see Table 13-5).

Growth on MacConkey Agar

Modified MacConkey agar from which crystal violet has been removed supports the growth of the *M.*

fortuitum-chelonei complex; most other *Mycobacterium* species cannot grow on this medium.

Urease Activity

Urease activity of mycobacteria can be determined by inoculating the organism to be tested into distilled water containing a urea-based concentrate and observing for a red color change after up to 3 days of incubation at 35°C. The test is helpful to differentiate *M. scrofulaceum* (positive) from *M. gordonae* (negative) and *M. gastri* (positive) from other members of the group III nonchromogenic mycobacteria.

Growth in 5% Sodium Chloride

The ability to grow on an egg-based culture medium containing 5% sodium chloride when incubated at 28°C is shared by *M. flavescens*, *M. triviale*, and the rapidly growing mycobacteria, with the exception of *M. chelonei* subspecies *chelonei* (see Table 13-5).

Iron Uptake

Of all the mycobacteria (except for *M. smegmatis*), *M. fortuitum* uniquely has the ability to take up soluble iron from inorganic iron-containing reagent added to the surface of a culture actively growing on the surface of a Löwenstein-Jensen slant. The development of a rusty brown pigment in the colonies after up to 21 days of incubation is a positive test result.

CLASSIFICATION OF MYCOBACTERIA

In the late 1950s, as species of mycobacteria other than *M. tuberculosis* were being encountered with increasing frequency in medical practices, Runyon proposed the following grouping of these "atypical" organisms based on growth rate and pigment production:

Mycobacteria Other Than *Mycobacterium tuberculosis* and *Mycobacterium bovis*

Group I: photochromogens
Group II: scotochromogens
Group III: nonphotochromogens
Group IV: rapid growers

Advances in knowledge of the genetics, cell structure, and aberrant phenotypic properties of old and newly discovered strains of the mycobacteria have advanced our knowledge beyond the neat packaging of species under the classic Runyon system. Woods and Washington[57] have suggested the following clinically oriented classification of mycobacteria based on their potential for causing human infections, refined from an earlier published proposal by Wolinski:[56]

Species Potentially Pathogenic in Humans

M. avium-intracellulare
M. kansasii
M. fortuitum-chelonei complex
M. scrofulaceum
M. xenopi
M. szulgai (rarely recovered in clinical laboratories)
M. malmoense (rarely recovered in clinical laboratories)
M. simiae (rarely recovered in clinical laboratories)
M. marinum
M. ulcerans (rarely recovered in clinical laboratories)
M. haemophilum (rarely recovered in clinical laboratories)

Saprophytic Mycobacteria Rarely Causing Disease in Humans

M. gordonae
M. asiaticum
M. terrae-triviale complex
M. gastri
M. nonchromogenicum
M. paratuberculosis

Other species are considered to be of little clinical importance when recovered from clinical specimens. This clinical orientation, however, is of limited usefulness to laboratory mycobacteriologists, and the Runyon system still may serve as a helpful initial clue to the presumptive identification of mycobacteria. Observation of whether an mycobacteria colony grows rapidly or is pigmented from inception or only after exposure to light (or is nonpigmented) still affords valuable information early in the study of an unknown isolate.

Review of *Mycobacterium* Species: Laboratory Aspects and Clinical Correlations

Only a brief review of the key laboratory features by which the more commonly encountered *Mycobac-*

terium species can be identified in the laboratory and their clinical implications is presented here. The reader is advised to consult the other microbiology and infectious disease texts if more detailed information is desired.

Mycobacterium tuberculosis

Mycobacterium tuberculosis, as the most common cause of mycobacterial disease in humans, is often the major focus for making definitive identifications in most microbiology laboratories. A few relatively simple tests identify most isolates of *M. tuberculosis*:

▸ Formation of nonpigmented, rough, buff colonies after 14 to 28 days of incubation at 37°C on Löwenstein-Jensen and Middlebrook media
▸ Accumulation of niacin (*M. simiae*, certain strains of *M. bovis*, and occasional strains of *M. marinum* and *M. chelonei* may also be niacin-positive; therefore, this is not an absolute characteristic).
▸ Reduction of nitrates to nitrites
▸ Lack of catalase activity
▸ Selective inhibition of growth in culture media containing NAP (particularly useful in those laboratories in which a BACTEC System is employed)

Most cases of classic tuberculosis have been of the reinfection or adult-type in patients who have had a previous exposure, presenting as a slowly progressive inflammatory process in the lungs leading to fibrosis, scarring, loss of lung function, cavitation, and caseation necrosis. Human-to-human transmission occurs when an infected cavity of an infected person, teeming with high concentrations of acid-fast bacilli, breaks into bronchi and bacterial cells become airborne in droplets that are spread by means of coughing and sneezing. Cough, weight loss, low-grade fever, dyspnea, and chest pain are the usual clinical signs and symptoms of chronic progressive pulmonary tuberculosis. Occurring less commonly were cases of primary or miliary tuberculosis, which are characterized by rapid spread of acute infection from the lungs to other organs in the body, usually occurring in patients with chronic debilitating diseases or in immunosuppressed patients. This form of disease is being reported in patients with AIDS. The disease is often rapidly progressive, is accompanied by septicemia, and is less likely to progress

to fibrosis, caseation, and cavitary formation. Miliary dissemination can involve virtually any organ in the body.

Mycobacterium bovis

Mycobacterium bovis is one of the mycobacteria that is now included within the *M. tuberculosis* complex. Phenotypic characteristics by which *M. bovis* can be differentiated from classic strains of *M. tuberculosis* include the following:

▸ Most strains negative for niacin
▸ No reduction of nitrates to nitrites
▸ No production of pyrazinamidase
▸ Selective inhibition of growth by thiophene-2-carboxylic acid hydrazide (T_2H). *M. bovis* will not grow in medium containing T_2H.

The classic human strains have a very slow growth rate, producing "dysgonic"-appearing colonies on Löwenstein-Jensen medium. It may be necessary to prolong the period of incubation beyond the conventional 4 weeks to recover certain strains. Typical colonies on Löwenstein-Jensen medium are buff colored, low, and small and may appear either smooth or rough on egg-based medium. On Middlebrook 7H11 agar, colonies are very thin ("water droplet–like"), often show little or no stranding, closely simulating the dysgonic forms of *M. avium-intracellulare*.

Mycobacterium bovis typically infects cattle but may also infect other animals, including dogs, cats, swine, rabbits, possibly certain birds of prey, and humans. The human disease closely resembles that caused by *M. tuberculosis* and is treated similarly.

Mycobacterium kansasii

Mycobacterium kansasii is a photochromogen classified within Runyon group 1. Although infections occur throughout the United States, most cases have been reported from the southern states (Texas, Louisiana, Florida), Midwest (Illinois), and California. Typical strains of *M. kansasii* grow at about the same rate or slightly more rapidly than *M. tuberculosis* at 37°C. The distinctive feature is the dependence on light exposure for the production of a visible yellow pigment (photochromogenicity, see Color Plate 13-1*A*). The colonies are typically intermediate between fully rough and fully smooth (certain strains are totally one or the other). The bacterial cells in acid-fast smear preparations are characteristically long and broad and distinctly cross-banded or barred, presumably from utilization of the fatty material of the medium.

The group of phenotypic properties, in addition to photochromogenicity, by which the identification of *M. kansasii* can be confirmed include the following:

- Rapid hydrolysis of Tween 80, within 3 days
- Strong reduction of nitrate to nitrite
- Rapid catalase reaction, including 68°C test
- Strong pyrazinamidase activity

Chronic pulmonary disease simulating classic tuberculosis is the most common manifestation, usually involving the upper lobes. Cavitation with scarring is evident in most cases, and disease is slowly progressive.[41] Extrapulmonary or disseminated infections are less common, although cases of scrofula-like lymphadenitis, sporotrichosis-like cutaneous infections, osteomyelitis, soft tissue infections, and tenosynovitis have been reported. Disseminated disease may be seen in the presence of severe immunosuppression and has been reported in patients with AIDS.[15,53] Most strains of *M. kansasii* are susceptible to rifampin but slightly resistant to isoniazid, ethambutol, and streptomycin.

Mycobacterium marinum

Mycobacterium marinum, when recovered from clinical specimens, grows optimally at 30° to 32°C and grows poorly, if at all, at 37°C. Subcultures may grow at 37°C. Colonies appear in 8 to 14 days; those grown in the dark may appear nonpigmented. When exposed to light, a deep yellow pigment develops in the colony (photochromogen). Colonies vary between wrinkled and rough, to smooth and hemispheric, particularly if grown on Middlebrook 7H10 and 7H11 agar. Microscopically the cells are relatively long rods with frequent cross-barring. Following are additional characteristics by which an identification can be made:

- Positive niacin accumulation by some strains
- No reduction of nitrates to nitrites
- Hydrolysis of Tween 80
- Positive urease test
- Production of pyrazinamidase
- No production of heat-stable catalase

Typical infections involve the skin, usually resulting when traumatized skin comes in contact with inadequately chlorinated fresh water or salt water (swimming pools, tropical fish aquariums, water cooling towers). Some patients present with sporotrichosis-like lesions, with central spread along the lymphatics emanating from an ulcerated area at the primary site of inoculation. More typically, the lesions present as tender, red or blue-red subcutaneous nodules, usually involving the elbow, knee, toe, or finger ("swimming pool granuloma"). Such lesions may be mistaken for rheumatoid nodules.[2] Treatment is usually directed to resecting the primary lesions if possible (curettage, electrodesiccation, excision). Most strains are susceptible to rifampin and ethambutol but resistant to isoniazid and streptomycin.

Mycobacterium scrofulaceum

The species name *scrofulaceum* (derived from the Latin *scrofula* meaning "brood sow") was used in 1956 by Prissick and Masson in reference to the most common form of disease by this organism, cervical lymphadenitis in children.[36] Colonies of *M. scrofulaceum* grow slowly (4 to 6 weeks) at various temperatures (25°, 31°, and 37°C). They are typically smooth, buttery, and globoid, with pigmentation ranging from light yellow to deep orange. Pigment production is not dependent on light exposure; thus, the organism is included in the scotochromogen group II of Runyon (see Color Plate 13-1*B*).

Key biochemical test reactions include the following:

- Failure to hydrolyze Tween 80
- No reduction of nitrates to nitrites
- Positive 68°C catalase test
- Production of urease

Lymphadenitis is the classic presenting symptom, occurring most commonly in children between ages 18 months and 4 years of age. The lymphadenitis is unilateral, involving nodes high in the neck adjacent to the mandible. Colonization of the organism in the mouth and throat is presumed to be the site of origin. The high incidence of disease among young children is believed to be related to disruption of the gums during tooth eruptions, during an age when the immune system is still relatively immature. Only a few cases of progressive pulmonary disease and dissemination to other organs, primarily in patients with serious debilitating illness, have been reported. Treatment of serious infections should involve use of at least three drugs: isoniazid, streptomycin, and rifampin or cycloserine.[41]

Mycobacterium xenopi

Mycobacterium xenopi (*Xenopus* is a genus of frog) was first isolated from an African toad.[55] Previously considered to be nonpathogenic, *M. xenopi* has been incriminated in several infections. Hot and cold water taps, including water storage tanks and hot water generators of hospitals, are potential sources for nosocomial infections.[46,56]

Mycobacterium xenopi colonies are slow growing, small, and erect and produce characteristic yellow pigment (occasional strains are nonpigmented). Growth is more rapid at 42°C than at 37°C; growth is absent at 25°C. Colonies tend to be rough, and an aerial mycelium may be evident. Examination of young microscopic colonies on Middlebrook 7H10 agar reveals a distinctive "bird's nest" appearance with sticklike projections. Branching and filamentous extensions appear in older colonies, particularly those grown on cornmeal-glycerol agar. Microscopically, acid-fast stained smears reveal long, filamentous rods that are tapered at both ends, tending to arrange in palisades. The characteristics leading to a species identification are listed below:

- Optimum growth at 42°C
- Yellow scotochromogenic pigment
- No niacin accumulation
- Nitrate reduction–negative
- Heat-stable catalase production
- Arylsulfatase-positive
- Pyrazinamidase-positive

Most human cases of *M. xenopi* infections have been pulmonary, resembling those seen in patients with *M. tuberculosis*, *M. kansasii*, or *M. avium-intracellulare* infections. Multinodular densities, often showing cavitation and fibrosis, are often seen radiologically. Infections usually occur in patients with preexistent lung disease or predisposing conditions (alcoholism, malignancy, diabetes mellitus).

Mycobacterium gordonae

Of the group of *Mycobacterium* species "rarely causing human infections," as designated in the outline presented earlier, perhaps *M. gordonae* is recovered in clinical laboratories with most frequency. It is found particularly in aqueous environments, leading to the alternate designation of *M. aquae* or the "tap water bacillus."[55] *M. gordonae* is a scotochromogen, readily recognized by the smooth, deeply yellow-orange pigmented colonies that develop after 7 days of incubation at 37°C (see Color Plate 13-1*D*). The organism hydrolyzes Tween 80 and produces heat-stable catalase.

Several isolated reports of infections in the literature are cited by Woods and Washington[57] and include cases of meningitis secondary to ventriculoatrial shunts, hepatoperitoneal disease, endocarditis in a prosthetic aortic valve, cutaneous lesions of the hand, and possible cases of pulmonary involvement. *M. gordonae* is resistant to isoniazid, streptomycin, and *p*-aminosalicylic acid but susceptible to rifampin and ethambutol.

Mycobacterium avium-intracellulare

The *M. avium-intracellulare* complex of organisms is characterized on primary isolation media by slowly growing, thin, transparent, homogeneous, smooth colonies, sometimes with "asteroid" margins. A small proportion of *M. intracellulare* colonies may be partially or completely rough; for *M. avium*, the proportion of rough colonies may often be greater. Many of these strains also show yellow pigmentation, conflicting with the inclusion of this organism in the Runyon nonpigmented group III mycobacteria (see Color Plate 13-1*E* and *F*). Microscopic examination of acid-fast smears reveals cells that are typically short and coccobacillary. Early in culture and under certain conditions, long, thin bacilli may be seen. Staining is usually uniform without beading or banding.

Phenotypically, *M. avium-intracellulare* complex strains are best characterized by a battery of negative reactions. The organism does produce heat-stable catalase and has the ability to grow on T_2H; otherwise, the biochemical reactions are inert.

The greatest upsurge in *M. avium-intracellulare* complex infections during the past decade has been in patients with AIDS, to the point that in some settings, this organism is more frequently recovered than *M. tuberculosis*. From our experience, the following features of *M. avium-intracellulare* complex infections in patients with AIDS seem evident. The organism load in biopsy or autopsy tissue sections is often extremely heavy, with intracellular bacterial aggregates often seen within large foamy macrophages, simulating the lepra cells seen in *M. leprae* infections. Involvement of the gastrointestinal tract is also often heavy. In some instances, large foamy macrophages simulating the cells seen in Whipple's disease seem to predominate the areas of inflammation. Lesions in other organs, notably the lungs, liver, spleen, and lymph nodes, may also show a massive invasion with acid-fast bacilli. In some cases, little inflammation may be seen at the time of death. Necrotizing inflammation rather than granuloma formation and caseation necrosis is more characteristic of the histologic appearance of these lesions. Most strains are resistant to antituberculous drugs.

Mycobacterium fortuitum-chelonae Complex

An unknown isolate can be suspected of belonging to the *M. fortuitum-chelonei* complex if growth of an acid-fast organism is observed after 2 to 4 days of incubation. The young colonies of both species appear smooth and hemispheric, usually with a butyrous or waxy consistency. Colonies are typically nonchromogenic but may appear off-white or faintly cream colored (see Color Plate 13-1*G* and *H*). *M. fortuitum* produces branching, filamentous extensions on from 1- to 2-day-old colonies on cornmeal-glycerol or Middlebrook 7H11 agar. Some strains produce rougher colonies with short aerial hyphae, which are best observed under a stereomicroscope. *M. chelonae* lacks these filamentous extensions.

Microscopically, in acid-fast stained preparations, the bacterial cells are generally pleomorphic, ranging from long filamentous forms to short, thick rods. Branching is absent or rudimentary at best; at times the cells may appear beaded or swollen, with nonstaining ovoid bodies present at one end.

Silcox and coworkers[45] have identified the following characteristics for an isolate to belong to the *M. fortuitum-chelonae* complex:

- Acid-fastness
- Lack of pigment production
- Growth in less than 7 days at its optimum temperature
- Evidence of arylsulfatase activity at 3 days
- Grow at 28°C on special MacConkey agar (devoid of crystal violet)

Additional tests can be performed to separate *M. fortuitum* from *M. chelonae*:[52]

- *M. chelonae* does not reduce nitrates (*M. fortuitum* is positive).
- *M. chelonae* is incapable of assimilating iron from ferric ammonium citrate, a property uniquely possessed by *M. fortuitum*.
- *M. fortuitum* is susceptible to ciprofloxacin and pipemidic acid but resistant to polymyxin B; *M. chelonae* has the opposite reactions.

A wide variety of infections have been associated with *M. fortuitum* and *M. chelonae*, with involvement of the lungs, skin, bone, central nervous system, and prosthetic heart valves and also accompanied by disseminated disease.[13,42,45] Skin infections are particularly common, often evolving into draining subcutaneous abscesses.[13]

The rapidly growing mycobacteria vary in their in vitro susceptibilities.[43] Amikacin is predictably active; other aminoglycosides, cefoxitin, doxycycline, and erythromycin have also been selectively active. Newer agents that have shown in vitro activity against some strains include imipenem-cilastatin, amoxicillin-clavulanate, and ciprofloxacin.

The presentation of other *Mycobacterium* species is beyond the scope of this book. Human infections are only rarely encountered and are limited to isolated case presentations in the medical literature. Following are selected citations for those readers who require further information: *M. simiae*,[14,20,40] *M. szulgai*,[26,55] *M. paratuberculosis*,[3,4,9,28] *M. malmoense*,[1] and *M. haemotilium*.[10,32] *M. paratuberculosis* is of interest because of its possible association with Crohn's disease; *M. szulgai* does not fit in the classic Runyon classification of mycobacteria because it is a scotochromogen when incubated at 35°C but a photochromogen when held at room temperature (see Color Plate 3-1*C*). A more detailed summary of these and other MOTT bacilli can be found elsewhere.[21]

SUSCEPTIBILITY TESTING OF MYCOBACTERIA

A discussion of antimycobacterial susceptibility testing is beyond the scope of this book, only a brief outline is included here. More information can be found elsewhere.[21] The agar method for performing antimycobacterial susceptibility tests is commonly employed. In this method, plates are inoculated either from digested and concentrated smear-positive sputum (direct test) or from a pure culture of mycobacteria isolated from a clinical specimen (indirect test). The first-line drugs to which clinical isolates are tested include isoniazid, rifampin, ethambutol, streptomycin, and pyrazinamide. The second-line drugs are *p*-aminosalicylic acid, cycloserine, ethionamide, kanamycin, amikacin, viomycin, and capreomycin.[48,49,51] The first-line drugs, except ethambutol, are considered bactericidal; the remaining drugs included in the secondary list are to be used only when resistance to the primary drug develops.

The agar plate method is rapidly being superseded by the use of radiometric methods, primarily the BACTEC 460 instrument fitted with a "TB hood." The test is based on the radiometric detection of carbon 14 released from Middlebrook 7H12 liquid medium containing ^{14}C palmitic acid by the metabolizing bacteria. In either of above-cited methods, at least 99% of the mycobacterial strain being tested must be killed for a drug to be considered susceptible. Several published studies confirm that the level of agreement between standard and radiometric susceptibility test methods exceed 90%, at least for susceptible organisms.[23,39,44]

The emergence of drug-resistant *M. tuberculosis* has become a major problem in the United States, with an overall incidence in 1980 of 8%.[35] A Public Health Service study of primary drug resistance for *M. tuberculosis* showed marked variation in ethnic groups, ranging from 15% to 19% in Hispanics and Asians in Texas and Los Angeles to 3% of those in Detroit.[16] Primary drug resistance for *M. tuberculosis* is defined as resistance to an antimycobacterial drug in an organism isolated from a patient who has not previously received antituberculous therapy.

With the advent of AIDS and the increase in other immunosuppressed or debilitated patients undergoing prolonged therapeutic regimens, rapidly progressive and disseminated forms of tuberculosis are being reported with increasing frequency. Therefore, in contrast to the past when a 3- to 6-week delay in receiving definitive culture and susceptibility results could be tolerated because of the chronic nature of the illness, such time delays are no longer acceptable. Research efforts and clinical trial studies are focused on finding new methods for the rapid assessment of mycobacteria recovered in culture.

The BACTEC 460 instrument can also be used in the detection of mycobacteria from sputum, blood, and other clinical specimens. Its effectiveness has been demonstrated in a number of field trial and clinical correlation studies.[6,8,31,38] In a multicenter collaborative study, the recovery of *M. tuberculosis* from clinical specimens known to be smear-positive can be accomplished by the BACTEC system in 14 days compared with 21 days by the standard culture method.[38]

The BACTEC instrument can also be used to differentiate *M. tuberculosis* and *M. bovis* from nontuberculous mycobacteria using blood culture vials containing NAP. *M. tuberculosis* and *M. bovis* cannot grow in NAP-containing culture media and therefore will not produce a positive growth index after several days of incubation.

Practical applications of nucleic acid probes, coupled with the rapid radiometric detection methods discussed previously and the newly emerging polymerase chain reaction technology, portend to revolutionize the direct and culture detection of mycobacteria in clinical specimens. The probe technology is based on the ability of complementary nucleic acid strands to bond and form stable, double-stranded complexes under appropriate test conditions. Organism identification is possible if the ribosomal RNA released from the test bacterium through the action of a lysing agent, heat, and sonication is hybridized with the complementary single-stranded iodine-125–labeled DNA probe to form a stable DNA–RNA complex.[33,39]

Several studies have authenticated the accuracy, specificity, and sensitivity of these probes in the culture confirmation of clinical *Mycobacterium* species isolates.[7,18,31] Beyond culture confirmation, the detection of mycobacteria directly in clinical specimens through the use of polymerase chain reaction methodology is on the horizon. Clinical studies to determine the applicability of this technology in patient care settings are just beginning to emerge.

REFERENCES

1. Albers WM, Chandler KW, Solomon DA, Goldman AL. Pulmonary disease caused by *Mycobacterium malmoense*. Am Rev Respir Dis 1987;135: 1375–1378.

2. Aubrey M, Fam AG. A case of clinically unsuspected *Mycobacterium marinum* infection. Arthritis Rheum 1987;30:1317–1318.

3. Chiodini RJ. Crohn's disease and the mycobacterioses: a review and comparison of two disease entities. Clin Microbiol Rev 1989;2:90–117.

4. Chiodini RJ, Van Kruiningen HJ, Merkal RS, et al. Characteristics of an unclassified *Mycobacterium* species isolated from patients with Crohn's disease. J Clin Microbiol 1984;20:966–971.

5. Cohn ML, et al. The 7H11 medium for the culture of mycobacteria. Am Rev Respir Dis 1976;98: 295–296.

6. Damato JJ, Collins MT, Rothlauf MV, et al. Detection of mycobacteria by radiometric and standard plate procedures. J Clin Microbiol 1983;17: 1066–1073.

7. Drake TA, Hindler JA, Berlin OGW, Bruckner DA. Rapid identification of *Mycobacterium avium* complex in culture using DNA probes. J Clin Microbiol 1987;25:1442–1445.

8. Gill VJ, Park CH, Stock F, et al. Use of lysis-centrifugation (Isolator) and radiometric (BACTEC) blood culture systems for the detection of mycobacteria. J Clin Microbiol 1985;22:543–546.

9. Gitnick G, Collins J, Beaman B, et al. Preliminary report on isolation of mycobacteria from patients with Crohn's disease. Dig Dis Sci 1989;34: 925–932.

10. Gouby A, Branger B, Oules R, Ramuz M. Two cases of *Mycobacterium haemophilum* infections in a renal dialysis unit. J Med Microbiol 1988;25: 299–300.

11. Gross W, Hawkins J, Murphy B. *Mycobacterium xenopi* in clinical specimens. I. Water as a source of contamination. (Abstract) Am Rev Respir Dis 1976;113:78.

12. Gruft H. Isolation of acid-fast bacilli from contaminated specimens. Health Lab Sci 1971;8:79–82.

13. Hanson PJV, Thomas JM, Collins JV. *Mycobacterium chelonae* and abscess formation in soft tissue. Tubercle 1987;68:297–299.

14. Heap BJ. *Mycobacterium simiae* as a cause of intra-abdominal disease: a case report. Tubercle 1989; 70:217–221.

15. Jacobson MA, Isenberg WM. *M. kansasii* diffuse pulmonary infection in a patient with acquired immune deficiency syndrome. Am J Clin Pathol 1989;91:236–238.

16. Kapanoff DE, Kilburn JO, Glassroth JL, et al. A continuing survey of tuberculous primary resistance in the United States: March 1975–November 1977. A United States Public Health Service Cooperative Study. Am Rev Respir Dis 1978;118: 835–842.

17. Kestle DG, Kubica GP. Sputum collection for cultivation of mycobacteria: an early morning specimen or the 24 to 72 hour pool? Am J Clin Pathol 1967;48:347–351.

18. Kiehn TE, Edwards FF. Rapid identification using a specific DNA probe of *Mycobacterium avium* complex from patients with acquired immunodeficiency syndrome. J Clin Microbiol 1987;25: 1551–1552.

19. Kiehn TE, Edwards FF, Brannon P, et al. Infections caused by *Mycobacterium avium* complex in immunocompromised patients: diagnosis by blood culture and fecal examination, antimicrobial susceptibility tests and morphological and seroagglutination characteristics. J Clin Microbiol 1985; 21:168–173.

20. Kirihara JM, Hillier SL, Coyle MB. Improved detection times for *Mycobacterium avium* complex and *Mycobacterium tuberculosis* with the BACTEC radiometric system. J Clin Microbiol 1985;22: 841–845.

21. Koneman EW, Allen SD, Janda WM, Schreckenberger PC, and Winn WC Jr. Color atlas and textbook of diagnostic microbiology, ed 4. Philadelphia, JB Lippincott, 1992.

22. Krasnow I. Sputum digestion. I. The mortality rate of tubercle bacilli in various digestion systems. Am J Clin Pathol 1969;45:352–355.

23. Laszlo A, Siddiqui SH. Evaluation of a rapid radiometric differentiation test for the *Mycobacterium tuberculosis* complex by selective inhibition with p-nitro-acetylamino-hydroxy-propiophenone. J Clin Microbiol 1984;19:694–698.

24. Levy-Frebault V, Pangon B, Bure A, et al. *Mycobacterium simiae* and *Mycobacterium avium-intracellulare* mixed infection in acquired immune deficiency syndrome. J Clin Microbiol 1987;25: 154–157.

25. Macher AM, Kovacs JA, Gill V, et al. Bacteremia due to *Mycobacterium intracellulare* in the acquired immune deficiency syndorme. Ann Intern Med 1983;99:782–785.

26. Maloney JM, Clark RG, Stephans DS, et al. Infections caused by *Mycobacterium szulgai* in humans. Rev Infect Dis 1987;9:1120–1126.

27. McClatchy JK, Waggoner RF, Kanes W, et al. Isolation of mycobacteria from clinical specimens by use of selective 7H11 medium. Am J Clin Pathol 1976;65:412–415.

28. McFadden JJ, Butcher PD, Chiodini R, Hermon-Taylor J. Crohn's disease-isolated mycobacteria are identical to *Mycobacterium paratuberculosis*, as determined by DNA probes that distinguish between mycobacterial species. J Clin Microbiol 1987;25:796–801.

29. Millner R, Stottmeier KD, Kubica GP. Formaldehyde: a photothermal activated toxic substance

produced in Middlebrook 7H10 medium. Am Rev Respir Dis 1969;99:603–607.

30. Mitchison DA, et al. A selective oleic acid albumin agar medium for tubercle bacilli. J Med Microbiol 1972;5:165–175.

31. Morgan MA, Horstmeier CD, DeYoung DR. Comparison of a radiometric method (BACTEC) and conventional culture media for recovery of mycobacteria from smear negative specimens. J Clin Microbiol 1983;18:384–388.

32. Moulsdale MT, Harper JM, Thatcher GN. Infection by *Mycobacterium haemophilum*, a metabolically fastidious acid-fast bacillus. Tubercle 1983; 64:29–36.

33. Musial CE, Tice LS, Stockman L, Roberts GD. Identification of mycobacteria from culture by using the Gen-Probe rapid diagnostic system for *Mycobacterium avium* complex and *Mycobacterium tuberculosis* complex. J Clin Microbiol 1988;26: 2120–2123.

34. Prantera C, Bothamley G, Levenstein S, et al. Crohn's disease and mycobacteria: two cases of Crohn's disease with high antimycobacterial antibody levels cured by dapsone therapy. Biomed Pharmacother 1989;43:295–299.

35. Primary resistance to antituberculous drugs, United States. MMWR 1980;29:345.

36. Prissick FH, Mason AM. Cervical lymphadenitis in children caused by chromogenic mycobacteria. Can Med Assoc J 1956;75:798–803.

37. Ratman SM, Marsh SB. Effect of relative centrifugal force and centrifugation time on sedimentation of mycobactgeria in clinical specimens. J Clin Microbiol 1986;23:582–585.

38. Roberts GD, Goodman NL, Heifets L, et al. Evaluation of the radiometric method for recovery of mycobacteria and drug susceptibility testing of *Mycobacterium tuberculosis* from acid-fast smear positive specimens. J Clin Microbiol 1983;18: 689–696.

39. Roberts GD, Koneman EW, Kim YK. *Mycobacterium*. In: Balows A, ed. Manual of clinical microbiology. 5th ed. Washington, DC, American Society for Microbiology, 1991.

40. Rose HD, Dorff GJ, Lauwasser M, et al. Pulmonary and disseminated *Mycobacterium simiae* infection in humans. Am Rev Respir Dis 1982;126: 1110–1113.

41. Sanders WE Jr, Horowitz EA. Other mycobacteria species. In: Mandell GL, Douglas RG Jr, Bennett JE, eds. Principles and practice of infectious diseases. 3rd ed. New York, Churchill Livingstone, 1990.

42. Schlossberg D, Aaron T. Aortitis caused by *Mycobacterium fortuitum*. Arch Intern Med 1991; 151:1010–1011.

43. Shah RR, Dye WE. The use of dithiolthreitol to replace N-acetyl-L-cysteine for routine sputum digestion-decontamination for the culture of mycobacteria. Am Rev Respir Dis 1966;94:454.

44. Siddiqui SH, Libonati JP, Middlebrook G. Evaluation of a rapid radiometric method for drug susceptibility testing of *Mycobacterium tuberculosis*. J Clin Microbiol 1981;13:908–912.

45. Silcox VA, Good RA, Floyd MM. Identification of clinically significant *Mycobacterium-fortuitum* complex isolates. J Clin Microbiol 1981;14:686–691.

46. Simor WE, Salit IE, Vellend H. Role of *Mycobacterium xenopi* in human disease. Am Rev Respir Dis 1984;129:435–438.

47. Smithwick RW, et al. Use of cetylpyridium chloride and sodium chloride for the decontamination of sputum specimens that are transported to the laboratory for the isolation of *Mycobacterium tuberculosis*. J Clin Microbiol 1975;1:411–413.

48. Snider DE Jr, Cohn DL, Davidson PT, et al. Standard therapy for tuberculosis. Chest 1985;87 (Suppl):S117–S124.

49. Snyder DE, Good RC, Kilburn JO, et al. Rapid drug-susceptibility testing of *Mycobacterium tuberculosis*. Am Rev Respir Dis 1981;123:402–406.

50. Sommers HM, Good RC. *Mycobacterium*. In: Lennette EH, ed. Manual of clinical microbiology. 4th ed. Washington, DC, American Society for Microbiology, 1985.

51. Stead WW, Dutt AK. Chemotherapy for tuberculosis today. Am Rev Respir Dis 1982;125 (Suppl 3):94–101.

52. Steele LC, Wallace RJ Jr. Ability of ciprofloxicin but not pipemidic acid to differentiate all three biovariants of *Mycobacterium fortuitum* from *Mycobacterium chelonae*. J Clin Microbiol 1987;25: 456–457.

53. Valainis GT, Cardona LM, Greer DL. The spectrum of *Mycobacterium kansasii* disease associated with HIV-1 infected patients. J Acquir Immune Defic Syndr 1991;4:516–520.

54. Wayne LG. Simple pyrazinamidase and urease tests for routine identification of mycobacteria. Am Rev Respir Dis 1974;109:147–151.

55. Wayne LG, Kubica GP. Genus *Mycobacterium*. In: Sneath PHA, Mair NS, Sharpe ME, Holt JG, eds. Bergey's manual of systematic bacteriology. Baltimore, Williams & Wilkins, 1986;2:1436–1457.

56. Wolinski E. Nontuberculous mycobacteria and associated diseases. Am Rev Respir Dis 1979;119: 107–159.

57. Woods GL, Washington JA II. Mycobacteria other than *Mycobacterium tuberculosis*: review of microbiologic and clinical aspects. Rev Infect Dis 1987;9:275–294.

14

Spirochetal Infections

TAXONOMY

The order Spirochaetales contains the spirochetes most commonly pathogenic for humans. They are all helically shaped motile bacteria that measure 0.1 to 3 μm in diameter by 5 to 120 μm in length.[9] The flagella of most spirochetes are encased within the multilayered outer membrane that is referred to as an outer sheath. The genus *Spirillum* has external flagella. In contrast to other bacteria, the spirochetes propel themselves by rotation through a liquid environment and are able to maintain their motility even in high viscosity liquids.

The classification of the pathogenic spirochetes is detailed in Table 14-1. The pathogens are con-centrated in three genera: *Treponema*, *Borrelia*, and *Leptospira*. In this chapter the discussion concerns the most important human diseases caused by spirochetes: syphilis (*Treponema pallidum*) and Lyme disease (*Borrelia burgdorferi*).

TREPONEMA

The four major pathogens in the genus *Treponema* are genetically related, infect only humans, and have not been cultivated for more than one passage in vitro. Despite these similarities, they produce very different diseases.

Table 14-1
Classification of Spirochetes

ORGANISM	GEOGRAPHIC LOCATION	DISEASE
Order Spirochaetales		
Family Spirochaetaceae		
Genus III. *Treponema*		
T. pallidum subspecies *pallidum*	Worldwide	Venereal syphilis
T. pallidum subspecies *pertenue*	Tropical Asia, Africa, South and Central America	Yaws
T. pallidum subspecies *endemicum*	Africa, SE Asia, Middle East, Yugoslavia	Endemic, nonvenereal syphilis
T. carateum	Central and South America	Pinta
T. pallidum–like oral spirochetes	Worldwide	Necrotizing gingivitis
Genus IV. *Borrelia*		
Borrelia species	Worldwide	Tick-borne relapsing fever
B. recurrentis	South America, Europe, Africa, Asia	Louse-borne relapsing fever
B. burgdorferi	North America, Europe, Australia	Lyme disease
Family Leptospiraceae		
Genus I. *Leptospira*		
L. interrogans	Worldwide	Leptospirosis

(Adapted from Krieg NR, Holt IR, eds. Bergey's manual of systematic bacteriology. Baltimore, Williams & Wilkins, 1984:38–64)

Treponema pallidum Subspecies *pallidum*

Treponema pallidum subspecies *pallidum* (hereafter called *T. pallidum*) is the dominant pathogen among the spirochetes. It shares 100% genetic homology with *T. pallidum* subspecies *pertenue*, which causes a nonvenereal cutaneous disease.[48] *T. pallidum*, the cause of venereal syphilis, has been infamous for 500 years. It was known as the "Great Pox," whereas variola virus produced the small pox. Each country chose to associate the disease with its neighbor. To the English, syphilis was the "French disease." The French considered it the "Italian pox."

The clinical presentation of venereal syphilis is varied and complex. Sir William Osler, one of the founders of modern medicine, referred to the disease as "the great imitator" and admonished students that if they knew syphilis, they would know medicine. The clinical disease has been somewhat arbitrarily divided into a series of stages.[72]

Incubation Period

The treponemes are introduced into the body through a mucous membrane or a cut or abrasion on the skin. It has been estimated epidemiologically that as many as 50% of sexual contacts of infectious persons escape infection. Experimental studies in human volunteers have documented, however, that the ID_{50} (the number of organisms needed to infect 50% of volunteers) for *T. pallidum* is as few as 57 organisms.[47] Shortly after inoculation the spirochetes are disseminated throughout the body, where they may eventually cause disease. The incubation period varies from 3 to 90 days, with a mean of 3 weeks.

Primary Syphilis

The primary phase encompasses the development of the primary lesion at the site of inoculation. The inflammatory reaction creates an ulcerated lesion called a chancre. The chancre has a clean, smooth base, and the edge is raised and firm. The ulcer is usually painless, although slightly tender. There is scant exudate unless the chancre is secondarily infected. There is usually a single primary chancre, but multiple primary ulcers may occur in patients with the acquired immunodeficiency syndrome. The base contains spirochetes that can be visualized after scraping of the lesion.

The chancre occurs at the inoculation site, most commonly on the genitalia. Occasionally, syphilis may occur without a visible ulcer.[61] The regional lymph nodes are enlarged but painless and firm. The chancre heals in 3 to 6 weeks (range of 1 to 12 weeks).

Secondary Syphilis

This phase of dissemination is the most florid part of the disease and the period when organisms are most numerous. The secondary phase begins 2 to 8 weeks after the appearance of the chancre and lasts for a few days to months. The most dramatic presentation is a widespread rash, which may be macular, maculopapular, or pustular but not vesicular. The rash in syphilis characteristically involves the palms of the hands and soles of the feet. In moist intertriginous areas, broad, moist, gray-white plaques called condylomata lata are teeming with infectious spirochetes. Similarly, infectious lesions, called mucous patches, are found on mucous membranes. There may be loss of hair or thinning of the eyebrows.

Systemic symptoms include generalized lymphadenopathy, fever, and malaise. Virtually any organ may be involved in secondary syphilis. Keratitis, hepatitis, and osteitis may be found. Infection of the central nervous system may occur at any stage of syphilis but is most common in the secondary phase. Meningismus and headache are common. Aseptic meningitis may develop, but spirochetes can be cultured from the cerebrospinal fluid without any evidence of inflammation and without clinical disease.[44]

The borderline between the primary and secondary phases is not cleanly drawn. On occasion the primary chancre may still be present when the secondary rash appears.

Latent Syphilis

After the secondary phase, the disease becomes subclinical, although not necessarily dormant. The latent phase has been arbitrarily divided into an initial 4-year period, referred to as the early latent phase, and a subsequent late latent period. During early latency, relapses may occur and the patient is infectious. Ninety percent of the relapses occur within the first year. The late latent period is of indefinite duration, and late complications may never appear. During the latent stage of syphilis the presence of the disease can be detected only serologically.

Late Syphilis

Late complications of syphilis include central nervous system disease, cardiovascular abnormalities, and tumors, called gummas, in any organ.

Late neurovascular syphilis may be symptomatic or asymptomatic.[31] Asymptomatic disease is characterized by cerebrospinal fluid abnormalities in the absence of symptoms. Pleocytosis, elevated protein levels, or depressed glucose levels are usually found in the cerebrospinal fluid. A positive serologic test for syphilis in the cerebrospinal fluid defines the disease. Symptomatic disease is either meningovascular or parenchymatous, but there is considerable overlap in the categories. Meningovascular syphilis resembles the aseptic meningitis of the secondary stage. Any cranial nerve may be affected by the inflammation, leading to deafness or visual impairment. Parenchymatous disease may involve the neurons of either the cerebrum or the spinal cord. Cerebral involvement is manifested as a wide variety of neuropsychiatric disturbances, including physical changes such as paralysis and psychiatric problems such as delusions of grandeur ("general paresis of the insane"). The posterior columns (sensory tracts) of the spinal cord are preferentially affected, causing severe pain and inability to perceive sensual impulses from the extremities. The disease, called tabes dorsalis, includes a peculiar "slapping" gait and deformed knees (Charcot's joints), which are caused by the lack of the feedback loop that tells the body to go easy on the joints.

The interval between primary disease and neurologic complication is 5 to 10 years for meningovascular syphilis, 15 to 20 years for general paresis, and 25 to 30 years for tabes dorsalis.

CARDIOVASCULAR SYPHILIS. The cardiovascular lesion in tertiary (late) syphilis, syphilitic aortitis, occurs in about 10% of untreated patients. It is caused by inflammation in the small vessels that feed the aorta (syphilitic endarteritis) and affects primarily the ascending aorta. Two complications may result: an aortic aneurysm and dilatation of the aortic ring causing insufficiency and regurgitation of blood through the aortic valve. Aortic aneurysms may grow to such a size that they erode through the sternum and are visualized under the skin of the chest.

LATE BENIGN SYPHILIS. This phase is characterized by the formation of nonspecific granulomatous lesions called gummas. This lesion is the most common complication in late syphilis and occurs in about 15% of untreated patients. The formation of the granuloma indicates a fully active cellular immune response. In the earliest stages of syphilis, patients may be reinfected. By the late stage, the patient is immune to reinfection. The gumma, however, may destroy surrounding tissue as it enlarges.[55] Clinically, gummas are destructive mass lesions in virtually any organ and may be mistaken initially for carcinomas.

CONGENITAL SYPHILIS. The greatest tragedy of syphilis is the intrauterine infection of the fetus.[73] Transplacental infection is most likely to occur during the primary or secondary stages of syphilis. The spirochetes may infect the fetus at any time during pregnancy, but the likelihood of clinical disease increases with the duration of pregnancy. Many of the infected fetuses die. In some areas of the country, congenital syphilis is the most common cause of nonimmune hydrops, a disease of the placenta that causes fetal death.[73] Of those who survive, half have no symptoms and the other half have the lesions of secondary syphilis without detectable primary lesions because they do not have a single primary portal of entry. Hepatosplenomegaly, meningitis, thrombocytopenia, anemia, and bone lesions characterize the infection. Intrauterine infection of bone may result in visible abnormalities of bone and teeth, such as deformed tibias (saber shins) or teeth (mulberry molars). To prevent this tragedy, prenatal screening has been recommended.[75]

Epidemiology

Syphilis can be transmitted by only a few routes: sexual contact,[56] direct introduction into the vascular system by shared needles or transfusions,[11] direct cutaneous contact with infectious lesions, or transplacental transfer of spirochetes[73] (Table 14-2).

Despite successful antitreponemal therapy and knowledge of the epidemiology for decades, the problem of syphilis remains and the incidence of infection is increasing. The treatment of choice for syphilis remains penicillin. Alternate therapeutic choices for penicillin-allergic patients have limitations, but a third-generation cephalosporin, ceftriaxone, has been promising in clinical trials.[30]

Table 14-2
Transmission of Spirochetes

ORGANISM	TRANSMISSION
Treponema pallidum pallidum	Venereal; blood transfusion (human only)
Treponemia pallidum pertenue	Direct skin contact (human only)
Treponema carateum	Direct skin contact (human only)
Treponema pallidum endemicum	Direct mucosal contact (human only); contaminated eating or drinking vessels
Borrelia recurrentis	Human host, human louse vector *(Pediculus humanus humanus)*
Borrelia species	Rodents, primates, human host; tick vector *(Ornithodoros, Rhipicephalus)*
Borrelia burgdorferi	Rodent, deer host; tick vector *(Ixodes, Amblyomma)*
Leptospira interrogans	Rat hosts; contaminated water

Laboratory Diagnosis of Treponemal Infection

The following discussion is applicable to the diagnosis of *T. pallidum*, and serologic cross-reactions make many of the techniques applicable to other treponemal species as well. The laboratory diagnosis may be accomplished by culture, by direct detection of spirochetes in lesions, and by serologic analysis. Diagnosis by culture is a research laboratory procedure because experimental animals must be inoculated. Direct detection is limited to the early stages when numerous spirochetes are present.

Direct Detection of Spirochetes

If a primary chancre or an infectious secondary lesion is present, an attempt should be made to visualize the spirochetes directly. Darkfield microscopy is the traditional technique for visualizing the motile spirochetes. A presumptive diagnosis of syphilis can be made if organisms with typical morphology and motility are observed in a lesion that is characteristic of syphilis (Fig. 14-1). *T. pallidum* must be differentiated from artifacts and nonpathogenic spirochetes in genital lesions. The mouth contains many spirochetes. It has been esti-

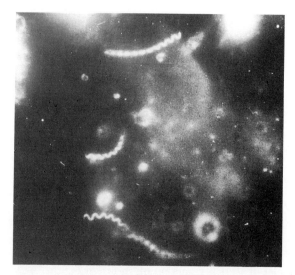

Figure 14-1. Positive darkfield examination for *Treponema pallidum*. The tightly coiled spiral nature of the organisms is evident. The background consists of debris and occasional red blood cells, indicating an adequate specimen (× 1000). (Courtesy of Centers for Disease Control and Prevention, Atlanta, GA)

Table 14-3
Characteristics of Serologic Tests for Syphilis

TEST	TYPE	POSITIVE AT INFECTIOUS STAGE (%)		
		Primary	Secondary	Late
VDRL	Non-treponemal	70	99	1
RPR	Non-treponemal	80	99	0
FTA-ABS	Treponemal	85	100	98
TPHA	Treponemal	65	100	95
TPI	Treponemal	50	97	95

(Adapted from Tramont EC. Treponema pallidum [syphilis]. In: Mandell GL, Douglas RG, Bennett JE, eds. Principles and practice of infectious diseases. 3rd ed. New York, Churchill Livingstone, 1990)

mated that more than 10,000 spirochetes must be present on the slide to produce a positive darkfield examination.[47] If the examination is negative, therefore, it should be repeated or the patient should be treated and observed for serologic evidence of syphilis. Darkfield examination requires considerable experience and should be reserved for facilities that can maintain proficiency.

Serologic Tests

The serologic tests for syphilis can be divided into two groups: nontreponemal tests and treponemal tests. The two groups have distinctive characteristics that make them useful for different purposes. They are complementary, not mutually exclusive. The nontreponemal tests are most useful as screening tests. The treponemal tests should be reserved as confirmatory tests when a nontreponemal test is positive or when clinical suspicion of syphilis is high despite a nonreactive nontreponemal test. The general characteristics of these tests are summarized in Table 14-3.

The procedures for performance of these tests have been standardized and published in great detail by the US Public Health Service.[42] When these tests are performed in the laboratory, it is imperative that the manual or manufacturer's directions be consulted and followed exactly. The *Manual of*

Tests for Syphilis even contains a classic typographic error: in Chapter 3 readers are instructed in the "Collection Procedure for Venus [sic] Blood."

NONTREPONEMAL TESTS. The nontreponemal tests take advantage of antibodies to a tissue lipid, called cardiolipin, that are produced as a byproduct of treponemal infection. The association was recognized early in this century when a variety of complement fixation tests were developed. The procedures are all flocculation tests. They use a form of cardiolipin that is complexed with cholesterol and lecithin. The most commonly used procedures are the Venereal Disease Research Laboratory (VDRL) and the rapid plasma reagin (RPR) tests. Other tests that have been used are the reagin screen test (RST), the unheated serum reagin (USR) test, and the toluidine red unheated serum test (TRUST).[41]

The nontreponemal tests have a sensitivity of 70% to 99%, depending on the stage of disease. The tests may not be positive in primary syphilis, so they should be repeated after 1 week, 1 month, and 3 months if a negative result is obtained in a patient suspected of having syphilis. The sensitivity of these tests approaches 100% during the secondary phase of the disease. Plasma and cord blood should not be used because borderline reactions may be obtained.[41]

The nontreponemal tests are affected by antitreponemal therapy. As a result they are useful for following the progression of disease and response to therapy. The results of any positive test should be titered to an end-point dilution. In addition, serum from patients with large amounts of antibody may produce a prozone phenomenon. When a prozone occurs, the relative concentrations of antibody and antigen are not in balance and precipitation or flocculation does not occur. The false-positive results caused by the prozone phenomenon continue to be a clinical problem.[5] The prozone results are often marked by a "rough" appearance to the flocculated antigen. Any serum that produces this rough appearance should be titered. In addition, sera should be diluted and retested if a patient with negative tests is strongly suspected of having syphilis on clinical grounds.

If the titer of the antibody does not fall progressively with treatment, the possibility of a treatment failure should be considered. There should be at least a fourfold decrease in antibody titer after 3 months of antitreponemal therapy. Patients who are treated in the late stages of syphilis or who are reinfected may develop titers that decline very slowly or remain stable. Some of these "chronic persisters" may maintain positive nontreponemal tests for life.[20]

The nontreponemal tests cannot be used to diagnose late syphilis, especially if treated, because the titer of antibody will eventually decline to undetectable levels.

The VDRL test has become the standard nontreponemal test. Preparation of the antigen must be done with great precision and attention to detail. It is the only serologic test that is universally accepted for the diagnosis of neurosyphilis. Examples of VDRL reactions are shown in Figure 14-2.

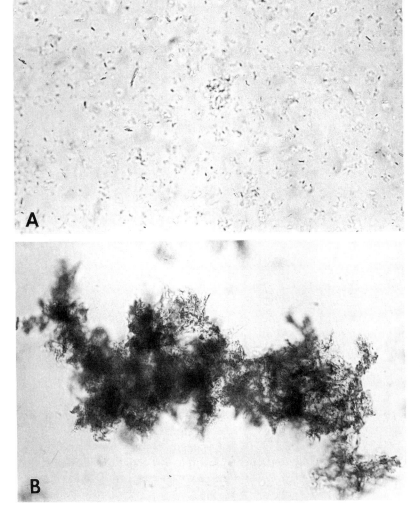

Figure 14-2. VDRL test. The reactions in this test are evaluated microscopically. (*A*) Nonreactive serum. The particles of VDRL antigen are uniform and freely dispersed without clumping. (*B*) Reactive serum. The VDRL antigen particles are strongly agglutinated by this syphilitic serum. The individual particles have aggregated into sheaves and large clumps (×100). (Preparation by Burton Wilcke, PhD, and Mary Celotti)

The RPR test is an adaptation of the flocculation principle to a card format. The visibility of the flocculation is enhanced by incorporation of charcoal particles. The uses of the RPR test are similar to those of the VDRL test except that the RPR test cannot be used to test cerebrospinal fluid. The simplicity of the RPR test has led most laboratories to adopt it as the primary screening test (Fig. 14-3).

The specificity of the nontreponemal tests averages 98% with a range from 93% to 99%. The lack of specificity is mostly a problem when the tests are used for screening populations with a low prevalence of syphilis, in whom positive reactions are likely to be false-positive. The false-positive reactions occur in patients who have other treponemal infections and also in patients with diseases that elicit anticardiolipin antibodies. These biologic false-positives may be transient, usually from viral infections, or may be persistent, usually related to immunologically mediated diseases. Biologic false-positive reactions have been reported in drug addicts, a population at increased risk of developing syphilis.[38] A positive reaction in a nontreponemal test should be confirmed, therefore, with a more specific treponemal test. Pedersen and colleagues have evaluated an enzyme immunoassay that incorporates the VDRL antigen.[50] They found that the specificity of the nontreponemal test was improved when it was adapted to the enzyme immunoassay format. Harris and colleagues have developed an enzyme immunoassay that distinguishes between antibodies to syphilitic cardiolipin and cardiolipin antigens in patients with connective tissue diseases.[25] These new approaches have not yet supplanted the traditional methods, but they represent the tests of the future.

TREPONEMAL TESTS. The treponemal tests incorporate specific treponemal antigens into the system. The traditional gold standard was the *T. pallidum* immobilization (TPI) test, in which the motility of live, virulent treponemes was inhibited by the presence of specific antibody. This expensive and cumbersome test has been replaced by the fluorescent treponemal antibody absorption test (FTA-ABS). Subsequently, another test specific for treponemal antigens, the microhemagglutination test for *T. pallidum* (MHA-TP) was developed. The specificity of the FTA-ABS test is increased by absorption of the test sera with a nonpathogenic spirochete, the Reiter strain of *T. phagadenis*. The FTA-ABS test has a higher rate of positivity in early syphilis than do the nontreponemal tests (see Table 14-3). The positivity rate approaches 100% in the secondary stage and remains so for life. It is not affected by antitreponemal therapy. The FTA-ABS test is, therefore, a good test for screening late syphilis, but it cannot be used to follow treatment. The degree of positivity in the FTA-ABS test has no biologic meaning, so the intensity of fluores-

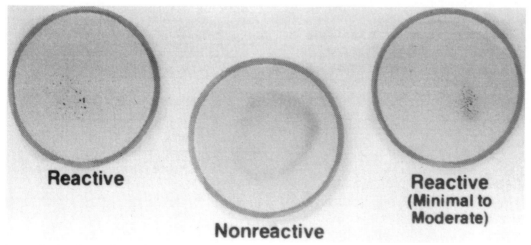

Figure 14-3. RPR card test. The reactions in this test are read with the naked eye, using incandescent light illumination. This control card contains reactive, weakly reactive, and nonreactive sera. The modified VDRL antigen is made visible by complexing with charcoal particles. The charcoal-antigen particles are evenly dispersed and finely distributed in the nonreactive serum and are grossly clumped. The serum with minimal to moderate activity produces small aggregates and clumps of charcoal-VDRL antigen particles.

cence is not reported and positive sera are not titered. The specificity of the FTA-ABS test is high, but problems can arise when it is used as a screening test in a low prevalence population. The biologic false-positive reactions of the nontreponemal tests do not occur with few exceptions. Sera from some patients, especially those with systemic lupus erythematosus or other connective tissue diseases, may produce an unusual beaded staining reaction.[40] It has been estimated that 1% of the normal population will have a positive FTA-ABS test.[42] Cross-reactions occur with other pathogenic treponemes.

The microhemagglutination test uses antigens specific to *T. pallidum*. The test is considerably less complicated than the FTA-ABS and does not require a fluorescence microscope. It is similar in performance to the fluorescent procedure but is less sensitive in early syphilis. The FTA-ABS test should be available to test sera that give equivocal reactions.[71]

Presentation of the methods used to perform these tests is beyond the scope of this text, but a full description is available elsewhere.[39]

BORRELIA

Borrelia are helical bacteria that measure 0.2 to 0.5 μm in diameter and 3 to 20 μm in length with 3 to 10 loose coils and 15 to 29 periplasmic flagella. Those species that have been cultivated in vitro are microaerophilic. The bacteria are gram-negative and stain well with Giemsa's stain. The human pathogens are transmitted by insect vectors (see Table 14-2). Louse-borne relapsing fever is caused by *B. recurrentis*, tick-borne relapsing fever by a variety of species, and Lyme disease by *B. burgdorferi*.

Lyme Disease

In 1977, Steere and colleagues at Yale University reported that an epidemic of arthritis had been occurring in residents of several surrounding Connecticut communities at least since 1972.[69] The alarm had been sounded by two vigilant mothers. In 1975, a mother from Old Lyme, Connecticut, informed the state health department of 12 cases of childhood arthritis in her small community of 5000 people. A second woman came to the Rheumatol-

ogy Division at Yale University with a story of acute arthritis in herself, her husband, two children, and several neighbors. The disease in all the children had been diagnosed as juvenile rheumatoid arthritis, a clinical diagnosis that depends on exclusion of known causes of arthritis. The investigators at Yale believed that they were dealing with a new disease, which they named Lyme arthritis.

Steere and colleagues recognized that the arthritis was almost always preceded by a distinctive rash, an erythematous papule that developed into a rapidly expanding annular lesion. Many of the physicians who examined the skin lesions believed that an insect bite had started the process, but an arthropod (in that case a tick) was recognized in only one patient. The nature of the primary lesion and the occurrence of cases in the summer and early fall suggested an arthropod vector. In the initial paper the authors noted the resemblance of the rash to a lesion called erythema chronicum migrans, described in Europe, especially Scandinavia.

In 1982, only 5 years after the original description of Lyme arthritis, Burgdorfer and colleagues determined the etiology by isolating a spirochete from the implicated tick vector, demonstrating that the spirochetes produced cutaneous lesions in rabbits and that the serum of patients with Lyme arthritis contained antibodies to the spirochete.[8] The next year Steere and associates clinched the issue by isolating a spirochete from blood, skin lesions, or cerebrospinal fluid of infected patients as well as from ticks.[66] Shortly thereafter spirochetes were isolated from the lesions of erythema chronicum migrans and Bannwarth syndrome in Europe.[1,53] The newly isolated spirochete is related to other *Borrelia* species[59] but shares almost no homology with species of *Treponema* and *Leptospira*.[33] It has been named *B. burgdorferi*,[36] in honor of Burgdorfer, who first isolated the organism.[8,36] *B. burgdorferi* is the longest and narrowest of the borreliae. It contains several outer membrane proteins and a 41-kd flagellar protein that may be important for pathogenesis and diagnosis.

Epidemiology

Lyme disease is now the most common arthropod-borne infection in the United States. From 1982 to 1989 there was an 18-fold increase in cases reported to the Centers for Disease Control. From

1986 to 1989 the number of cases doubled each year, but the increase now appears to have reached a plateau.[10] Cases have been reported in almost every state, but they are concentrated in the Northeast, the North Central region, and the Pacific Northwest. In 1989 to 1990 there were 6468 cases reported from New York, but smaller states such as New Jersey, Connecticut, and Wisconsin experienced more than 1000 cases each. The infection is recognized around the entire northern hemisphere, including the former Soviet republics.[16]

In the United States the distribution of Lyme disease matches the distribution of ticks of the genus *Ixodes*. In the East[68] and North Central[21] regions, the vector is usually *I. dammini*, whereas *I. pacificus* carries the spirochetes in the Northwest.[58,68] The frequency of tick infection in some areas is as high as 75%.[2] The life cycle of ixodid ticks involves three distinct stages and a life span of 2 years.[63] Ticks feed in late summer as larvae and the next year as nymphs (early spring) and adults (late summer). The larval and nymphal stages are so small that many patients do not recall having been bitten, although from experimental data the ticks must remain attached for at least 24 hours to transmit the spirochetes effectively.[52] The cycle in nature is maintained by a number of small rodents, notably the white-footed mouse (*Peromyscus leucopus*), which maintains an asymptomatic spirochetemia.[43] White-tailed deer are important for the survival of the tick but do not appear to be involved in transmission of the infection.

Clinical Disease

The clinical manifestations of *B. burgdorferi* infection are protean.[63] This spirochete has been referred to as the "latest great imitator,"[62] following in the tracks of its relative *T. pallidum*. As in syphilis the manifestations of Lyme disease may be catalogued into three stages.

The first stage begins when the tick bite elicits the classic lesion, erythema chronicum migrans. The expanding erythematous skin lesion presents in multiple locations and in varying extents.[4] In New Jersey, 93% of the patients developed erythema chronicum migrans and about half had systemic symptoms, including lymphadenopathy.[7] At this stage the spirochete is most easily cultivated and it may be visualized in as many as 40% of biopsy specimens by silver impregnation staining.[4]

The second stage of Lyme disease is a result of dissemination of the spirochete throughout the body.[64] The most common lesions are acute arthritis[70] and meningitis.[49] Bowen and colleagues documented arthritis in 26% of their patients, meningitis in 10%, and cranial nerve palsies in 8%.[7] The meningitis may appear purulent.[6] Secondary cutaneous lesions, infection of the eye, hepatitis, and myocardial damage may occur.

The third and chronic phase of the disease is characterized by chronic skin lesions, chronic neurologic symptoms, and chronic arthritis.[70] The recurrent episodes of arthritis diminish in frequency and severity each year, but some patients develop chronic synovitis and permanent disability.

The initial therapy of Lyme disease was penicillin or tetracycline, which are effective in many cases.[65,67] Treatment failures with both antibiotics have been described.[13,17] A clinical trial of ceftriaxone in late Lyme disease has documented a greater efficacy of that antibiotic than penicillin.[14] Ceftriaxone and erythromycin were most effective against *B. burgdorferi* in vitro, but ceftriaxone and tetracycline were most effective in an animal model.[35]

Laboratory Diagnosis

Lyme disease may be diagnosed by culture of the spirochete, by demonstration of the spirochetes in tissue, or by documentation of a serologic response. The erythema chronicum migrans lesion is specific, and Lyme disease may be most confidently diagnosed if this lesion is present. Culture is difficult and the yields are low except when the characteristic skin lesions are tested. Direct detection of spirochetes suffers from very low sensitivity. The diagnostic method of choice by default is serologic analysis. Immunofluorescence and enzyme immunoassays have been used most commonly. Indirect immunofluorescence,[46] quantitative fluorescence immunoassay,[51] and a fluoroimmunoassay[28] have been recommended, but many investigators have found the enzyme immunoassay to be more satisfactory.[12,57] Specific IgM titers may remain elevated throughout the course of illness, so the presence of IgM cannot be used to establish acute infection. Antibody may be absent early but is usually present after several weeks.[63]

Most assays use sonicated whole spirochetes. Investigators have suggested that using a flagellar antigen[23,24] or purified outer membrane proteins as the antigen improves the specificity of the reactions. These assays are not yet commercially available.

Cross-reactions with a variety of infectious agents have been found in sera from patients suspected of having Lyme disease. Sera of patients with other borrelial infections,[45] treponemal infections,[3,32,45,54] human immunodeficiency virus infection,[54] Epstein-Barr virus infection,[3] and rickettsial infection[3] may react in assays for *B. burgdorferi*. Reports on cross-reaction with *Leptospira* antisera are conflicting.[45,54] Although cross-reactions develop with specific treponemal antigens, the VDRL test is not positive in patients with Lyme disease.[63]

Kaeli and colleagues described four patients from an area endemic for Lyme disease who had confusing multisystemic disease that was initially attributed to *B. burgdorferi*.[37] All four patients had antibodies to the spirochete, and three of the four had positive Western blot tests; further study revealed that the cause in all four cases was subacute bacterial endocarditis.

Interlaboratory and intralaboratory variation in an immunofluorescence test was acceptable under highly controlled conditions, but in the real world the degree of variation among laboratories has been a matter of great concern.[29,74] Both false-negative and false-positive reactions occur. The procedures and the reagents, most importantly the antigens, have not been standardized. Physicians and laboratory workers alike should question suppliers of reagents or reference laboratories carefully about the test.

Immunoblots have served as reference tests for human immunodeficiency virus and might serve the same function in Lyme disease.[22] It is not yet clear, however, that immunoblots are a gold standard.[15,37] Dattwyler and colleagues have reported[17] patients who had vigorous T-cell proliferative responses when exposed to *B. burgdorferi* antigen but lacked antibody by immunofluorescence and by Western blot analysis.[15] They concluded that the patients had Lyme disease without a serologic response, but Steere warns that normal persons may have a similar blastogenic response.[63] DNA hybridization probes have been used to identify *B. burgdorferi* and *B. hermsii*, but the technique has not been applied clinically.[60]

LEPTOSPIRA

Leptospira are motile, obligately aerobic helical rods that measure 0.1 μm in diameter and 6 to 12 μm in length. They are gram-negative and are only faintly stained by aniline dyes. Darkfield microscopy must be used to visualize unstained *Leptospira* organisms (Fig. 14-4). Two species of *Leptospira* are recognized: *L. interrogans*, which contains all of the human pathogens, and the saprophytic species, *L. biflexa*. *L. interrogans* contains many individual serotypes that cause human disease. Antigenically related serovars are collected into serogroups for classification purposes. The type strain is *L. interrogans* serovar *icterohaemorrhagiae*,[34] and the clinical disease is leptospirosis. Several thorough reviews, although old, still reflect the state of knowledge in many areas.[18,19,26,27]

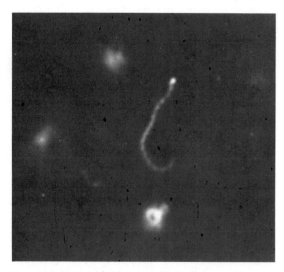

Figure 14-4. Darkfield examination of *Leptospira interrogans* culture. The spiral coils, which are not clearly demonstrated, appear as alternating bright and dark areas. The very bright upper end of the organism may represent the hooked end that many *Leptospira* organisms possess. It is easy for inexperienced observers to confuse cell debris and artifacts with *Leptospira* organisms in clinical specimens (× 1000). (Courtesy of David Miller, DVM, MS)

REFERENCES

1. Ackerman R, Kabatzki J, Boisten HP, et al. Spirochaten-Atiologie der Erythema-chronicum-migrans-Krankenheit. Dtsch Med Wochenschr 1984;109:92–97.

2. Anderson JF. Epizootiology of *Borrelia* in *Ixodes* tick vectors and reservoir hosts. Rev Infect Dis 1989;11:1451–1459.

3. Berardi VP, WEeks KE, Steere AC. Serodiagnosis of early Lyme disease: analysis of IgM and IgG antibody responses by using an antibody-capture enzyme immunoassay. J Infect Dis 1988;158:754–760.

4. Berger BW. Erythema chronicum migrans of Lyme disease. Arch Dermatol 1984;120:1014ave–1021.

5. Berkowitz K, Baxi L, Fox HE. False-negative syphilis screening: the prozone phenomenon, nonimmune hydrops, and diagnosis of syphilis during pregnancy. Am J Obstet Gynecol 1990;163:975–977.

6. Bourke SJ, Baird AG, Bone FJ, et al. Lyme disease with acute purulent meningitis. Br Med J 1988;297:460.

7. Bowen GS, Griffin M, Hayne C, et al. Clinical manifestations and descriptive epidemiology of Lyme disease in New Jersey, 1978 to 1982. JAMA 1984;251:2236–2240.

8. Burgdorfer W, Barbour AG, Hayes SF, et al. Lyme disease: a tick-borne spirochetosis. Science 1982;216:1314–1319.

9. Canale-Parola E. Spirochetales. In: Krieg NR, Holt JR, eds. Bergey's manual of systematic microbiology. Baltimore, Williams & Wilkins, 1984.

10. Centers for Disease Control: Lyme disease surveillance—United States, 1989–1990. MMWR 1991;40:417–421.

11. Chambers RW, Foley HT, Schmidt PJ. Transmission of syphilis by fresh blood components. Transfusion 1969;9:32–34.

12. Craft JE, Grodzicki RL, Steere AC. Antibody response in Lyme disease: evaluation of diagnostic tests. J Infect Dis 1984;149:789–795.

13. Dattwyler RJ, Halperin JJ. Failure of tetracycline therapy in early Lyme disease. Arthritis Rheum 1987;30:448–450.

14. Dattwyler RJ, Halperin JJ, Volkman DJ, et al. Treatment of late Lyme borreliosis: randomised comparison of ceftriaxone and penicillin. Lancet 1988;1:1191–1194.

15. Dattwyler RJ, Volkman DJ, Luft BJ, et al. Seronegative Lyme disease: dissociation of specific T- and B-lymphocyte responses to *Borrelia burgdorferi*. N Engl J Med 1988;319:1441–1446.

16. Dekonenko EJ, Steere AC, Berardi VP, et al. Lyme borreliosis in the Soviet Union: a cooperative US–USSR report. J Infect Dis 1988;158:748–753.

17. Diringer MN, Halperin JJ, Dattwyler RJ. Lyme meningoencephalitis: report of a severe, penicillin-resistant case. Arthritis Rheum 1987;30:705–708.

18. Edwards GA, Domm BM. Human leptospirosis. Medicine 1960;39:117.

19. Feigin RD, Anderson DC. Human leptospirosis. CRC Crit Rev Clin Lab Sci 1975;5:413–467.

20. Fiumara NJ. Serologic responses to treatment of 128 patients with late latent syphilis. Sex Transm Dis 1979;6:243–246.

21. Godsey MS JR, Amundson TE, Burgess EC, et al. Lyme disease ecology in Wisconsin: distribution and host preferences of *Ixodes dammini* and prevalence of antibody to *Borrelia burgdorferi* in small mammals. Am J Trop Med Hyg 1987;37:180–187.

22. Grodzicki RL, Steere AC. Comparison of immunoblotting with indirect enzyme-linked immunosorbent assay using different antigen preparations for diagnosing early Lyme disease. J Infect Dis 1988;157:790–797.

23. Hansen K, Asbrink E. Serodiagnosis of erythema migrans and acrodermatitis chronica atrophicans by the *Borrelia burgdorferi* flagellum enzyme-linked immunosorbent assay. J Clin Microbiol 1989;27:545–551.

24. Hansen K, Hindersson P, Pedersen NS. Measurement of antibodies to the *Borrelia burgdorferi* flagellum improves serodiagnosis in Lyme disease. J Clin Microbiol 1988;26:338–346.

25. Harris EN, Gharavi AE, Wasley GD, et al. Use of an enzyme-linked immunosorbent assay and of inhibition studies to distinguish between antibodies to cardiolipin from patients with syphilis or autoimmune disorders. J Infect Dis 1988;157:23–31.

26. Heath CW Jr, Alexander AD, Galton MM. Leptospirosis in the United States: analysis of 483 cases in man, 1949–1961. N Engl J Med 1965;273:857–864.

27. Heath CW Jr, Alexander AD, Galton MM. Leptospirosis in the United States (concluded): analysis of 483 cases in man, 1949–1961. N Engl J Med 1965;273:915–922.

28. Hechemy KE, Harris HL, Wethers JA, et al. Fluoroimmunoassay studies with solubilized antigens from *Borrelia burgdorferi*. J Clin Microbiol 1989;27:1854–1858.

29. Hedberg CW, Osterholm MT, MacDonald KL, et al. An interlaboratory study of antibody to *Borrelia burgdorferi*. J Infect Dis 1987;155:1325–1327.

30. Hook EW, Roddy RE, Handsfield HH. Ceftriaxone therapy for incubating and early syphilis. J Infect Dis 1988;158:881–884.

31. Hooshmand H, Escobar MR, Kopf SW. Neurosyphilis: a study of 241 patients. JAMA 1972;219:726–729.

32. Hunter EF, Russell H, Farshy CE, et al. Evaluation of sera from patients with Lyme disease in the fluorescent treponemal antibody-absorption test for syphilis. Sex Transm Dis 1986;13:232–236.

33. Hyde FW, Johnson RC. Genetic relationship of Lyme disease spirochetes to *Borrelia*, *Treponema*, and *Leptospira* spp. J Clin Microbiol 1984;20: 151–154.

34. Johnson RC, Faine S. *Leptospira* Noguchi 1917. In: Krieg NR, Holt JR, eds. Bergey's manual of systematic bacteriology. Baltimore, Williams & Wilkins, 1984:62–67.

35. Johnson RC, Kodner C, Russell M. In vitro and in vivo susceptibility of the Lyme disease spirochete, *Borrelia burgdorferi*, to four antimicrobial agents. Antimicrob Agents Chemother 1987;31:164–167.

36. Johnson RC, Schmid GP, Hyde FW, et al. *Borrelia burgdorferi* sp. nov.: etiologic agent of Lyme disease. Int J Syst Bacteriol 1984;34:496–497.

37. Kaeli AT, Volkman DJ, Gorevic PD, et al. Positive Lyme serology in subacute bacterial endocarditis: a study of four patients. JAMA 1990;264:2916–2918.

38. Kaufman RE, Weiss S, Moore JD, et al. Biological false positive serological tests for syphilis among drug addicts. Br J Vener Dis 1974;50:350–353.

39. Koneman EW, Allen SD, Janda WM, Schreckenberger PC, Winn WC Jr. Color atlas and textbook of diagnostic microbiology. 4th ed. Philadelphia, JB Lippincott, 1992.

40. Kraus SJ, Haserick JR, Lantz MA. Fluorescent treponemal antibody-absorption test reactions in lupus erythematosus: atypical beading pattern and probable false-positive reactions. N Engl J Med 282:1970;1287–1290.

41. Larsen SA. Syphilis. Clin Lab Med 1989;9: 545–557.

42. Larsen SA, Hunter EF, Kraus SJ. Manual of tests for syphilis. Washington, DC, American Public Health Association, 1990.

43. Levine JF, Wilson ML, Spielman A. Mice as reservoirs of the Lyme disease spirochete. Am J Trop Med Hyg 1985;34:355–360.

44. Lukehart SA, Hook EW, Baker-Zander SA, et al. Invasion of the central nervous system by *Treponema pallidum*: implications for diagnosis and treatment. Ann Intern Med 1988;109:855–862.

45. Magnarelli LA, Anderson JF, Johnson RC. Cross-reactivity in serological tests for Lyme disease and other spirochetal infections. J Infect Dis 1987; 156:183–188.

46. Magnarelli LA, Meegan JM, Anderson JF, et al. Comparison of an indirect fluorescent-antibody test with an enzyme-linked immunosorbent assay for serological studies of Lyme disease. J Clin Microbiol 1984;20:181–184.

47. Magnuson HJ, Thomas EW, Olansky S, et al. Inoculation syphilis in human volunteers. Medicine 1956;35:33–82.

48. Miao RM, Fieldsteel AH. Genetic relationship between *Treponema pallidum* and *Treponema pertenue*: two noncultivable human pathogens. J Bacteriol 1980;141:427–429.

49. Pachner AR, Steere AC. The triad of neurologic manifestations of Lyme disease: meningitis, cranial neuritis, and radiculoneuritis. Neurology 1985; 35:47–53.

50. Pedersen NS, Orum O, Mouritsen S. Enzyme-linked immunosorbent assay for detection of antibodies to the venereal disease research laboratory (VDRL) antigen in syphilis. J Clin Microbiol 1987;25:1711–1716

51. Pennell DR, Wand PJ, Schell RF. Evaluation of a quantitative fluorescence immunoassay (FIAX) for detection of serum antibody to *Borrelia burgdorferi*. J Clin Microbiol 1987;25:2218–2220.

52. Piesman J, Mather TN, Sinsky RJ, et al. Duration of tick attachment and *Borrelia burgdorferi* transmission. J Clin Microbiol 1987;25:557–558.

53. Preac-Mursic V, Wilske B, Schierz G, et al. Repeated isolation of spirochetes from the cerebrospinal fluid of a patient with meningoradiculitis Bannwarth. Eur J Clin Microbiol 1984;3:564–565.

54. Raoult D, Hechemy KE, Baranton G. Cross-reaction with *Borrelia burgdorferi* antigen of sera from patients with human immunodeficiency virus infection, syphilis, and leptospirosis. J Clin Microbiol 1989;27:2152–2155.

55. Rodriguez S, Teich DL, Weinman MD, et al. Gummatous syphilis: a reminder. J Infect Dis 1988;157:606–607.

56. Rolfs RT, Goldberg M, Sharrar RG. Risk factors for syphilis: cocaine use and prostitution. Am J Public Health 1990;80:853–857.

57. Russell H, Sampson JS, Schmid GP, et al. Enzyme-linked immunosorbent assay and indirect immunofluorescence assay for Lyme disease. J Infect Dis 1984;149:465–470.

58. Schmid GP, Horsley R, Steere AC, et al. Surveillance of Lyme disease in the United States, 1982. J Infect Dis 1985;151:1144–1149.

59. Schmid GP, Steigerwalt AG, Johnson SE, et al. DNA characterization of the spirochete that causes Lyme disease. J Clin Microbiol 1984;20:155–158.

60. Schwan TG, Simpson WJ, Schrumpf ME, et al. Identification of *Borrelia burgdorferi* and *B. hermsii* using DNA hybridization probes. J Clin Microbiol 1989;27:1734–1738.

61. Sperling LC, Hicks K, James WD. Occult primary syphilis: the nonerosive chancre. J Am Acad Dermatol 1990;23:514–515.

62. Stechenberg BW. Lyme disease: the latest great imitator. Pediatr Infect Dis J 1988;7:402–409.

63. Steere AC. Lyme disease. N Engl J Med 1989; 321:586–596.

64. Steere AC, Bartenhagen NH, Craft JE, et al. The early clinical manifestations of Lyme disease. Ann Intern Med 1983;99:76–82.

65. Steere AC, Green J, Schoen RT, et al. Successful parenteral penicillin therapy of established Lyme arthritis. N Engl J Med 1985;312:869–874.

66. Steere AC, Grodzicki RL, Kornblatt AN, et al. The spirochetal etiology of Lyme disease. N Engl J Med 1983;308:733–740.

67. Steere AC, Hutchinson GJ, Rahn DW, et al. Treatment of the early manifestations of Lyme disease. Ann Intern Med 1983;99:22–26.

68. Steere AC, Malawista SE. Cases of Lyme disease in the United States: locations correlated with distribution of *Ixodes dammini*. Ann Intern Med 1979; 91:730.

69. Steere AC, Malawistaates: locations correlated with distribution of *Ixodes dammini*. Ann Intern Med 1979;91:730.

69. Steere AC, Malawista SE, Snydman DR, et al. Lyme arthritis: an epidemic of oligoarticular ar-thritis in children and adults in three Connecticut communities. Arthritis Rheum 1977;20:7–17.

70. Steere AC, Schoen RT, Taylor E. The clinical evolution of Lyme arthritis. Ann Intern Med 1987;107:725–731.

71. Su SJ, Huang S, Chung CY, et al. Evaluation of the equivocal test results of *Treponema pallidum* haem-agglutination assay. J Clin Pathol 1990;43: 166–167.

72. Tramont EC. *Treponema pallidum* (syphilis). In: Mandell GL, Douglas RG Jr, Bennett JE, eds. Principles and practice of infectious diseases. New York, Churchill Livingstone, 1990:1794–1812.

73. Wendel GD. Gestational and congenital syphilis. Clin Perinatol 1988;15:287–303.

74. Wilkinson HW, Russell H, Sampson JS. Caveats on using nonstandardized serologic tests for Lyme disease. J Clin Microbiol 1985;21:291–292.

75. Zenker PN, Rolfs RT. Treatment of syphilis, 1989. Rev Infect Dis 1990;12(Suppl 6):590–609.

15

Mycoplasmas and Ureaplasmas

Mycoplasmas and ureaplasmas are organisms that differ from other bacteria in that they lack a rigid cell wall. Individual cells are bound only by a trilaminar unit membrane. The cultivation of mycoplasmas and ureaplasmas requires an enriched medium containing precursors for nucleic acid, protein, and lipid biosynthesis. Precursors for nucleic acids and proteins are provided principally by the enriched basal peptone medium and yeast extract, while lipids are provided by the inclusion of serum. These organisms are much smaller than most bacteria, measuring 0.2 to 0.3 μm; hence, they are able to pass through bacteriologic filters.

The lack of a typical bacterial cell wall containing peptidoglycans renders these organisms insensitive to cell wall–active antimicrobial agents, such as penicillins and cephalosporins.[5,33] Because of this, the recovery of these organism from clinical specimens may have significant therapeutic implications.

Mycoplasmas and ureaplasmas have been recovered from humans, animals, birds, insects, and plants, while some species have a free-living existence in soil and water. New species in both animals and plants are being continually identified and reported in the taxonomic literature. The human mycoplasmas belong to the genus *Mycoplasma* and the genus *Ureaplasma*, which contains those mycoplasmas that are able to hydrolyze urea. Several species in the genus *Mycoplasma* and only one species in the genus *Ureaplasma*, *U. urealyticum*, are found in human clinical specimens. With the exception of *M. pneumoniae*, the role of other mycoplasmas, specifically *M. hominis* and *U. urealyticum*, in human disease is controversial. *M. pneumoniae* is the well-recognized cause of primary atypical pneumonia, while *M. hominis* and *U. urealyticum* are associated primarily with genital tract colonization and disease in adults and respiratory tract colonization and disease in neonates.[12,13,16,37]

TAXONOMY OF MYCOPLASMAS AND UREAPLASMAS

Mycoplasmas and ureaplasmas are classified in the class Mollicutes. Analysis of ribosomal ribonucleic acid sequences have revealed that the Mollicutes are most closely related to the *Bacillus-Lactobacillus-Streptococcus* subdivision of the eubacteria, with the closest bacterial relatives being members of the clostridia, lactobacilli, and the genus *Erysipelothrix*. The genus *Mycoplasma* and the genus *Ureaplasma* belong to the order Mycoplasmatales and the family Mycoplasmataceae, which require sterols such as cholesterol for cultivation. The genus *Mycoplasma* contains over 90 species; they inhabit a wide variety of plants and animals, including mammals, insects, birds, and reptiles, and may exist as commensals, parasites, and pathogens.[4,21,22,34,40,41] Only six *Mycoplasma* species are found in humans. *M. hominis*, *M. genitalium*, and *M. fermentans* are isolated primarily from the human genital tract, while *M. pneumoniae*, *M. salivarium*, and *M. orale* may be recovered from the human respiratory tract. *M. salivarium* is found in the gingival crevices and may play a role in certain types of periodontal disease. *M. orale* is considered part of the normal upper respiratory tract flora and is nonpathogenic.

As with other bacteria, the human mycoplasmas recovered from clinical material differ in certain phenotypic characteristics that are exploited for their isolation and identification (Table 15-1). *M. pneumoniae* ferments glucose with the production of acidic end products, while *M. hominis* utilizes arginine, with the formation of basic end products.

Cultivation of these organisms is dependent on the use of special agar and broth media that are enriched with factors required for mycoplasmal growth in addition to specific growth substrates such as glucose and arginine. *M. pneumoniae* strains are antigenically homogeneous, with only one recognized serovar.

The genus *Ureaplasma* is composed of organisms within the family Mycoplasmataceae that are specifically able to hydrolyze urea. The genus contains three species: *U. urealyticum*, *U. diversum*, and *U. gallorale*.[2,25] *U. urealyticum* is recovered from the human respiratory and genital tracts.[37] As with the *Mycoplasma* species described earlier, the role of *U. urealyticum* as a primary pathogen in human disease is an area of debate and ongoing study.

CLINICAL SIGNIFICANCE OF THE HUMAN MYCOPLASMATACEAE

Mycoplasma pneumoniae

Mycoplasma pneumoniae causes a pneumonic process called primary atypical pneumonia.[12] This organism is one of the most common causes of respiratory tract illnesses, with over 12 million infections occurring annually. Like other organisms causing respiratory tract disease, *M. pneumoniae* is transmitted by airborne transfer of droplets containing the organisms. Although it is highly transmissible, only 3% to 10% of infected persons develop symptoms consistent with bronchopneumonia, with the remainder being either asymptomatic or having a milder, bronchitis-like illness.[32] Infections may occur year-round, but the incidence of overt disease is highest in late fall and winter. Infection occurs in young children and in older adults, but most clinical disease is seen in children older than 5 years of age, in teenagers, and in young adults.

In susceptible hosts after exposure, the organism attaches to epithelial cells in the respiratory tract and multiplies. The organisms do not penetrate the epithelial cells of the respiratory tract but remain localized. Organisms may be recovered on culture during the incubation period and for several weeks during and after clinical illness, even in the presence of specific antibodies.[3] The clinical presentation of mycoplasmal pneumonia is usually

Table 15-1
Characteristics for the Identification of Human *Mycoplasma* Species

SITE OF ISOLATION AND SPECIES	UTILIZATION OF			OPTIMAL pH	TIME TO RECOVERY	GROWTH IN			SEROVARS
	Glucose	Arginine	Urea			Air	CO_2	Anaerobic	
Respiratory tract									
Mycoplasma pneumoniae	+	−	−	6.5–7.5	4–21 days	4+	4+	1+	1
Mycoplasma salivarium	−	+	−	6.0–7.0	2–5 days	2+	NA	4+	1
Mycoplasma orale	−	+	−	7.0	4–10 days	2+	NA	4+	1
Genital tract									
Mycoplasma hominis	−	+	−	5.5–8.0	1–5 days	4+	4+	4+	Unknown
Ureaplasma urealyticum	−	−	+	5.5–6.5	1–4 days	4+	4+	4+	14
Mycoplasma fermentans	+	+	−	7.0	4–21 days	2+	NA	4+	1
Respiratory/genital tracts									
Mycoplasma genitalium	+	−	−	7.0	Slow	2+	3–4+	1+	Unknown
Acholeplasma laidlawii	+	−	−	6.0–8.0	1–5 days	4+	4+	4+	1

+, positive; −, negative; NA, not available; 1+ to 4+, relative degree and rapidity of growth under optimal incubation conditions.

insidious rather than abrupt, with the gradual onset of constitutional and pneumonic symptoms.[12] Most patients will develop fever (up to 103°F) over a few days, with chills, malaise, sore throat, nasal congestion, and a nonproductive cough appearing early in the course of disease. As lower respiratory tract symptoms develop, the sputum generally becomes more mucoid or mucopurulent. Some patients may also complain of earaches. With the onset of pneumonic symptoms, patients may feel like they have a bad cold or the flu yet will continue to function—hence the application of the term *walking pneumonia* to this disease. On physical examination of the chest, localized rhonchi and rales are usually detected. Findings on chest roentgenograms are consistent with a diffuse bronchopneumonia, generally involving multiple lobes of the lung without consolidation. These radiographic findings usually appear more extensive than the physical examination of the patient would suggest.

Mycoplasma pneumoniae pneumonia is generally self-limited, with resolution of most constitutional symptoms in 3 to 10 days without antimicrobial therapy.[32] Abnormalities on chest roentgenograms generally resolve more slowly and may take from 10 days to 6 weeks for complete resolution. Although antimicrobial therapy with tetracycline or erythromycin significantly reduces the duration of signs and symptoms and hastens resolution of abnormalities seen on chest films, the organism is generally not eradicated from the respiratory tract by therapy.[12] Complications due to *M. pneumoniae* infection are rare.

Mycoplasma hominis and *Ureaplasma urealyticum*

Both *M. hominis* and *U. urealyticum* may be isolated from the genital tracts of asymptomatic men and women.[29] They are more frequently recovered from the lower genital tract of women, with vaginal isolation rates of 35% to 80%, depending on the population studied. Rates of genital tract colonization in both men and women are related to sexual activity, and persons with multiple sexual partners are more likely to be colonized. Thus the epidemiology of organism acquisition suggests that mycoplasmas are indeed sexually transmitted.

Over the past several years, both *U. urealyticum* and *M. hominis* have been implicated in a variety of clinical conditions primarily related to lower genital tract colonization and infection, upper genital tract infections in women, and, rarely, upper genital tract infection and prostatitis in men.[16,20,33] Both organisms have been postulated to play roles in early and late endometritis, chorioamnionitis, and premature rupture of membranes.[14–16,19] The presence of these organisms in the lower and upper female genital tract has also been associated statistically with prematurity, low-birthweight infants, and infertility.[13,19,20] In a study conducted by Kass and coworkers,[23] women who were colonized with *U. urealyticum* in the genital tract and who demonstrated a fourfold or greater antibody response to the organism had low-birthweight infants at a rate of 30%, while colonized women who did not show this antibody response had low-birthweight infants at a rate of 7.3%.

Urinary tract infections caused by mycoplasmas have also been reported, and, again, most work in this area has been in pregnant women.[18] Determining the significance of mycoplasmas in clean-catch urine specimens from women is difficult, owing to the likely contamination of the specimen from organisms colonizing the vagina and the distal urethra. In men, *M. hominis* is relatively uncommon as a cause of clinical disease, and most research on mycoplasmas has concentrated on the association of *U. urealyticum* with nongonococcal, nonchlamydial urethritis. Although several studies have been done, the role of *U. urealyticum* in this clinical entity is still unclear.[1,29,30]

Among infants born to mothers who are colonized with genital mycoplasmas, colonization of the neonate also appears to occur frequently.[47] In several survey studies, 18% to 45% of neonates delivered of colonized mothers were also colonized with *M. hominis*, with positive cultures being obtained from the throat, the genital tract, or the urine.[14,16] Colonization may persist in these infants for prolonged periods of time with no ill effects. Several other studies have indicated that *U. urealyticum* may, on the other hand, be associated with chronic lung diseases in the premature in-

fant.[8,36,46] The appearance of this syndrome in the neonate has also been supported by animal models and reflects both the nature of these bacteria as opportunistic agents and the immunocompromised status of the premature infant.

Several reports and studies have also shown that both *U. urealyticum* and *M. hominis* may be frequently recovered from the central nervous system as a cause of silent or clinically symptomatic meningitis in the newborn period.[45] Many cases of *M. hominis* central nervous system infections in the neonate have been described; most of these occurred in premature infants in whom prolonged rupture of membranes had been documented.[17,28,31,39]

"AIDS-Associated *Mycoplasma*"

At this time, the role of a virus-like infectious agent in the acquired immunodeficiency syndrome (AIDS), if any, is unknown. This agent, known as the AIDS-associated mycoplasma, has been detected in brain, liver, lymph node, and splenic tissues of patients with AIDS in the absence of human immunodeficiency virus (HIV) and other viral, bacterial, parasitic, and fungal agents that cause opportunistic infections in these patients.[26] It has also been isolated from patients without AIDS but with an acute fatal disease and can cause immunosuppression in nonhuman primates. Immunohistochemical methods using monoclonal antibodies directed against the organism have detected the mycoplasmal antigens in thymus, liver, spleen, and brain tissue of patients with AIDS and in placental tissues delivered by pregnant women with AIDS.[27] Histopathology of the infected tissues showed a range of responses; in some tissues no histologic changes were observed, while in others fulminant necrosis with inflammation was noted. The significance of this organism is unknown at this time, and it may represent yet another opportunistic agent in patients with HIV-1 infection. Its recovery from patients without AIDS but with fatal immunosuppressive illness and its ability to induce immune suppression in monkeys has suggested to some workers that this organism may be immunosuppressive on its own. It may act as a cofactor that is able to facilitate disease progression in patients who are already immunocompromised by HIV-1 infection or by other infections or therapeutic interventions.

CULTURE OF THE HUMAN MYCOPLASMAS FROM CLINICAL SPECIMENS

General Considerations

Human mycoplasmas can be divided into three groups on the basis of the utilization of three substrates: glucose, arginine, and urea (see Table 15-1). Depending on the species of *Mycoplasma* that is being sought, an enriched peptone basal medium containing yeast extract and serum is supplemented with one of these three substrates and a *p*H indicator (usually phenol red) is added. *M. pneumoniae* metabolizes glucose to produce lactic acid, resulting in a shift to an acidic *p*H. *M. hominis* metabolizes arginine with the production of ammonia and a shift in *p*H from neutral to alkaline. Similarly, *U. urealyticum* produces urease enzymes that hydrolyze urea to ammonia, again resulting in an alkaline *p*H shift. *M. fermentans* produces acid from glucose and also metabolizes arginine.

Specimens for the isolation of mycoplasmas, particularly the more rapidly growing genital mycoplasmas, are routinely inoculated onto both solid agar media and into some type of selective/differential broth enrichment media. Most broth media formulations used for isolation of mycoplasmas are diphasic, with medium containing agar in the butt of a tube overlaid with broth of similar composition but without added agar. Media for isolation of mycoplasmas also contain antibiotics (eg, ampicillin, penicillin, polymyxin B, and amphotericin) to inhibit contaminant bacteria and fungi. Thallium acetate used to be commonly included as an antibacterial agent in media as well, but this compound is inhibitory for *U. urealyticum* and *M. genitalium* and is also highly poisonous for humans.[10]

Human mycoplasmas differ in their optimal *p*H for growth and in the atmospheric conditions that are required for successful recovery from clinical specimens (see Table 15-1). Media for the isolation of *M. pneumoniae* is buffered at an initial *p*H of about 7.8, while the growth medium for *M. hominis* is buffered at an initial neutral *p*H (7.0). *U. urealyticum* grows optimally in an environment with a slightly acid *p*H, so primary isolation media for this species is buffered at about *p*H 6.0. The optimal temperature for mycoplasmal growth is 35° to 37°C. *M. pneumoniae* and *M. hominis* grow well in air or in an atmosphere of 95% nitrogen and 5% carbon dioxide. *U. urealyticum* tends to be capnophilic, with optimal growth occurring in an atmosphere of 10% to 20% carbon dioxide and 80% to 90% nitrogen. Agar media inoculated directly with specimens or subcultures from broths onto agar medium should be incubated under the appropriate conditions described earlier; broth media can be incubated under aerobic conditions in all cases.

Broth media are generally inoculated with 0.1 to 0.2 mL of the specimen contained in a transport fluid. Agar plates are inoculated with a similar amount, and the inoculum is spread over the surface of the agar with a sterile bent glass rod. Agar plates are sealed with cellophane tape to prevent the agar from drying out. Media for isolation of *M. pneumoniae* should be incubated for up to 4 weeks before a final culture report is made. Cultures for genital mycoplasmas should be incubated for 7 to 8 days; most positive broth cultures will be detected after 5 days of incubation. Diphasic media are compared with co-incubated tubes of the same media inoculated with sterile transport medium and with tubes inoculated with control *Mycoplasma* strains to detect subtle differences in color, turbidity, or both. Cultures should be inspected daily for subtle changes since the organisms die rapidly once growth occurs and the substrates are exhausted. If a potentially positive culture is detected visually in diphasic medium, the broth is subcultured onto a solid agar medium, such as SP-4 agar or A7 differential agar.

Identification of the mycoplasmas requires the recognition of typical colonies on solid media directly inoculated with the specimen or with a loopful of broth medium from a presumptively positive diphasic broth medium.[11] Colonies on agar media can be directly examined under $30\times$ to $100\times$ magnification with peripherally incident light to ascertain morphology and growth characteristics. Supravital dyes, such as Dienes' stain, can be used to further characterize colonies and to differentiate them from artifacts.[44] Various identification tests may be performed directly on solid medium, such as the hemadsorption test for presumptive identification of *M. pneumoniae*, or substrates such as arginine or urea, plus a phenol red indicator, may be incorporated in the agar to provide a direct assessment of substrate utilization and, therefore, a presumptive identification.

Specimen Collection

Mycoplasma pneumoniae may be recovered from both upper and lower respiratory tract specimens, including throat swabs, nasopharyngeal swabs, throat washings, and sputum, tracheal and trans-tracheal aspirate, bronchoscopy, bronchoalveolar lavage, and lung tissue specimens. The organism may be recovered from these specimens throughout the course of the illness and for some time after symptomatic recovery. Because of the fastidious nature of these bacteria, culture media should be inoculated as soon after collection as possible. Culture media dispensed into small vials may be used for transport of swab specimens, while other specimens (eg, sputum, tissue, washings) may be transported to the laboratory in sterile screw-capped containers. Before inoculation of growth media, respiratory tract specimens should be homogenized by repeated drawing through a needle and syringe; sputolysin or other chemical treatments for sputum liquefaction are toxic to mycoplasmas.

Genital mycoplasmas may be isolated from a variety of specimens. These include urethral, vaginal, and cervical swab specimens, prostatic secretions, semen, urine, blood, miscellaneous body fluids (cerebrospinal fluid, amniotic fluid, respiratory tract secretions, synovial fluid, pericardial fluid), and tissue (eg, endometrial washings and biopsies, placental or amniotic tissues, fetal or abortus tissues, fallopian tube biopsy specimens, uterine biopsy specimens, wound biopsy specimens, rectal tissues). Swab specimens should be obtained using rayon, calcium alginate, or cotton swabs with either plastic or aluminum shafts. Swabs with wooden shafts should not be used since the wood itself may be toxic to ureaplasmas. If other genital tract pathogens are being sought simultaneously, rayon swabs on plastic shafts are probably preferable because they are nontoxic to the other genital tract pathogens as well. Contact of the swab surfaces with antiseptic solutions, creams, jellies, or lubricants should be avoided. Swab specimens should not be allowed to dry and should be placed immediately into a transport or culture medium after collection. Other body fluids and tissue biopsy specimens should be submitted in sterile containers. Saline should not be used to moisten tissue specimens because it may cause lysis of the organisms. In the laboratory, tissue specimens should be minced in sterile transport medium to produce a 10% (w/v) suspension and serially diluted 10- and 100-fold. This is necessary to prevent inhibition of mycoplasmal growth by organic materials such as hemoglobin, toxic phospholipids, antibodies, or complement that may be present in the tissue specimen. These dilutions are then used to inoculate growth media.

Transport Media

A variety of transport media may be used for genital *Mycoplasma* cultures. These include trypticase-soy broth with 0.5% bovine serum albumin, 2-sucrose-phosphate (2SP) broth with 10% heat-inactivated fetal calf serum (as is used for chlamydial cultures), or various types of *Mycoplasma* growth media. Antibiotics are generally added to decrease contamination by other bacterial and fungal organisms. These transport media are further described elsewhere.[24]

Blood for recovery of mycoplasmas should be inoculated directly into *Mycoplasma* culture media. The blood should be diluted 1 to 10 with growth medium, so culture of a substantial blood volume may require multiple vials of culture media. Sodium polyanthol sulfonate (SPS), the anticomplementary and antiphagocytic additive that is present in most routine blood culture media, is toxic to mycoplasmas. Mycoplasmas have been recovered from radiometric blood culture media, but the SPS will inhibit or delay organism recovery depending on the SPS content of the broth.[40]

Media for Culture of Mycoplasmas

Several types of media have been described in the literature for the cultivation of *M. pneumoniae* and the genital mycoplasmas. As mentioned, most broth media are diphasic; that is, the tubes contain an agar phase that is overlaid with broth medium of similar composition. One medium recommended by the Centers for Disease Control for isolation of *M. pneumoniae* is called methylene blue-glucose diphasic medium.[44] This medium contains PPLO broth and agar, yeast extract, and serum supplements along with glucose, methylene blue, and phenol red. The methylene blue in the medium inhibits the growth of other human mycoplasmas that may be found in the respiratory tract, making the medium selective for *M. pneumoniae*. During growth of *M. pneumoniae*, the medium becomes more acidic and the phenol red turns from salmon colored to yellow. At the same time, the organisms reduce the methylene blue and turn it from blue to colorless. Therefore, the color of the broth phase changes from purple to green or yellow-green, while the agar phase turns from purple to yellow or yellow orange. This medium is used in conjunction with *Mycoplasma* glucose agar medium. Colonies recovered either directly on this medium or from subcultures of positive broths are then subjected to inspection and identification procedures. Other media recommended for the isolation of *M. pneumoniae* from clinical specimens are SP-4 diphasic broth and SP-4 agar.[43]

Isolation and Identification of *Mycoplasma pneumoniae*

In general, the growth of *M. pneumoniae* from clinical specimens is detected by the ability of these organisms to produce acid from glucose. Methylene blue-glucose diphasic medium is inoculated with 0.2 mL of the specimen in transport fluid. Tubes of media are simultaneously inoculated with sterile transport medium and with a positive control culture and are incubated along with the specimens. Broth cultures are incubated at 35°C with the caps tightened. Media are inspected daily for color changes in the medium and for turbidity for 4 weeks. The development of gross turbidity and an acid or alkaline shift of the indicator within 1 to 5 days is generally due to bacterial contamination. A slight, gradual shift in the *p*H indicator over an 8- to 15-day period without gross turbidity suggests a true positive culture.

As soon as color changes in the medium are apparent, the broth must be subcultured to appropriate agar medium; as more acid accumulates in the medium, mycoplasmas rapidly become nonviable. At the earliest indication of growth, the broth is subcultured to agar medium (such as SP-4 agar) and incubated in air for 5 to 7 days. Inspection of the agar surface under the low power of the microscope will reveal small colonies of the organisms. In the absence of obvious color change in diphasic media, blind subculture to agar media should be performed after 1 and 3 weeks of incubation. A general scheme for the isolation of *M. pneumoniae* is shown in Figure 15-1.

M. pneumoniae may be identified by a variety of procedures, some of which are more involved than others. Tests that are easily adaptable to the clinical laboratory include the hemadsorption test and the tetrazolium reduction test. In the hemadsorption procedure, colonies growing on the surface of the agar are flooded with a 0.2% to 0.4% suspension of washed guinea pig erythrocytes. After incubation, the surface of the plate is gently washed with sterile saline and examined under $50\times$ to $100\times$ magnification. Colonies of *M. pneumoniae* adsorb the erythrocytes to their surface and appear as round colonies studded with red blood cells. The tetrazolium reduction test exploits the unique ability of *M. pneumoniae* to reduce the colorless compound triphenyl tetrazolium to the red compound formozan. To perform the test, the agar surface bearing the suspected colonies is flooded with a solution of 2-(*p*-iodophenyl)-3-nitrophenyl-5-phenyl tetrazolium chloride (0.21%) and incubated at 35°C for an hour. Colonies of *M. pneumoniae* will appear reddish after an hour and may appear purple to black after 3 to 4 hours. Other mycoplasmas are negative with this test. Specific serologic methods may also be used for culture confirmation of *M. pneumoniae*.[9,11] The more rapid of these is the epifluorescence procedure. Agar medium containing colonies is flooded with *M. pneumoniae*–specific antibodies conjugated to fluorescein isothiocyanate, washed to remove unbound conjugate, and subsequently examined with a microscope equipped for epifluorescence procedures. Colonies of *M. pneumoniae* will fluoresce.

Isolation and Identification of Genital Mycoplasmas

Mycoplasmas that may be recovered from the genital tract include *M. hominis*, *M. genitalium*, *M. fermentans*, and *U. urealyticum*. Although *M. hominis* and *U. urealyticum* are easily cultivated and usually grow within 1 to 5 days, *M. genitalium* and *M. fermentans* grow much more slowly and are more difficult to detect in culture. Genital mycoplasmas other than *M. hominis* and *U. urealyticum* are generally not sought in genital tract specimens. Appropriate specimens received in transport media are inoculated onto both broth and agar media. In general, about 0.2 mL of the specimen should be streaked onto agar media and placed in broth me-

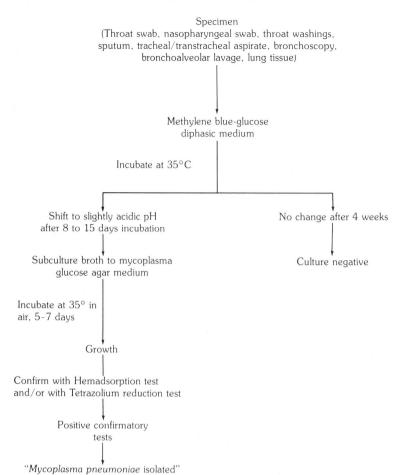

Specimen
(Throat swab, nasopharyngeal swab, throat washings, sputum, tracheal/transtracheal aspirate, bronchoscopy, bronchoalveolar lavage, lung tissue)

Methylene blue-glucose
diphasic medium

Incubate at 35°C

Shift to slightly acidic pH
after 8 to 15 days incubation

No change after 4 weeks

Subculture broth to mycoplasma
glucose agar medium

Culture negative

Incubate at 35° in
air, 5-7 days

Growth

Confirm with Hemadsorption test
and/or with Tetrazolium reduction test

Positive confirmatory
tests

"*Mycoplasma pneumoniae* isolated"

Figure 15-1. Protocol for isolation of *Mycoplasma pneumoniae* from respiratory tract specimens.

dia. Broths may be incubated aerobically at 35°C, while plates should be incubated in a CO_2 incubator or a candle jar. Both organisms may also be recovered under anaerobic conditions. Plated media should be inspected daily under $40\times$ magnification using oblique light to observe the "fried egg" colonies of *M. hominis* or the small, dense colonies of *U. urealyticum*. With broth cultures, any broths showing the slightest alkaline color change or turbidity should be subcultured to the appropriate plated media. In M broth, *M. hominis* produces a slight turbidity in addition to a change in color. In U broth, *U. urealyticum* will tend to produce a slight color change early in incubation with no distinct or obvious turbidity. Most isolates of *M. hominis* and *U. urealyticum* will grow within 5 to 7 days. If growth is not detected on primary plates or broth subcultures after this time, the culture can be reported as negative for genital mycoplasmas.

The general scheme for isolation of genital mycoplasmas is shown in Figure 15-2.

Identification of genital mycoplasmas is generally easy and straightforward. *M. hominis* colonies grow in 1 to 5 days, have the typical "fried egg" colonial morphology, and are usually 50 to 300 μm in diameter. Colonies may be stained with the Dienes stain to aid visualization. Further identification procedures are not necessary since rapidly growing, arginine-positive organisms exhibiting the typical colony morphology are invariably *M. hominis*. The small colonies of *U. urealyticum* may be difficult to distinguish from various artifacts, such as mammalian cells and cellular debris or materials present in serum. Because of these problems, suspect *U. urealyticum* colonies must be confirmed. This is done by exploiting the ability of *U. urealyticum* to hydrolyze urea. If the U agar medium contains urea and phenol red, the

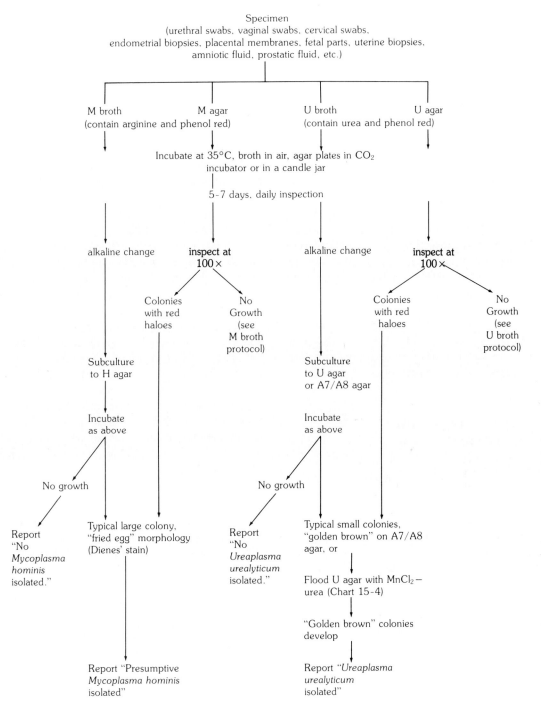

Figure 15-2. Protocol for isolation of *Mycoplasma hominis* and *Ureaplasma urealyticum* from genital specimens.

suspect *Ureaplasma* colonies will be surrounded by a red halo.

M. hominis may also be occasionally recovered from blood cultures, particularly in women with postpartum fever. Most strains are inhibited by SPS, and growth in SPS-containing medium may be inhibited or delayed. Smaron and coworkers isolated *M. hominis* from blood cultures using the radiometric BACTEC system.[40] Organisms were detected in both aerobic and anaerobic blood culture vials after 3 to 7 days of incubation. Blood bottles did not appear grossly positive, and growth indices on the instrument increased slowly over time. In addition, Gram stains from positive bottles failed to reveal any organisms, but organisms were visible when examined with the acridine orange stain. If *M. hominis* bacteremia is suspected, blood should optimally be inoculated at the patient's bedside into SPS-free media. Incubation of the cultures should be prolonged, and blind subcultures to appropriate agar and broth *Mycoplasma* isolation medium, in addition to colistin–nalidixic acid agar, should be made at frequent intervals.

SEROLOGY AND NEW TECHNOLOGIES FOR DIAGNOSIS OF *MYCOPLASMA PNEUMONIAE* INFECTION

Because of the slow growth of *M. pneumoniae*, non–growth dependent, direct specimen nucleic acid probe methods have been developed for the diagnosis of mycoplasmal respiratory tract infections. A brief discussion of DNA probe methodology can be found in Chapter 19, and a more extensive discussion can be found in the *Color Atlas and Textbook of Diagnostic Microbiology*.[24] Serologic tests are also used for the diagnosis of *M. pneumoniae*.[11] The most widely used serologic test for diagnosis of *M. pneumoniae* infection is the complement fixation (CF) test. As with other serologic tests, a fourfold rise in CF titers between acute and convalescent serum specimens is diagnostic of recent or current infection with *M. pneumoniae*. The acute specimen should be collected as soon after disease onset as possible, with the convalescent specimen being collected 3 weeks later. Single CF titers of 128 or greater collected in the convalescent period are highly suggestive of recent infection. CF titers begin to rise 7 to 10 days after infection with

the organism and reach peak titers after 4 to 6 weeks.[2,12,32] Significant CF titers may persist beyond this time. A nonspecific serologic test that is often used to support the diagnosis of *M. pneumoniae* infection is the production of cold agglutinins. These agglutinins react in the cold with human erythrocyte I antigens. Cold hemagglutinins appear about 7 days after infection and reach peak levels after 4 to 5 weeks.[32] After this, titers decline rapidly, becoming undetectable after about 5 months. As with the CF and other serologic tests, a fourfold rise in cold agglutinin titers in the presence of a compatible clinical illness is suggestive of *M. pneumoniae* infection.

Enzyme immunoassays (EIAs) for the detection of *M. pneumoniae*–specific antibodies have also been developed. In general, these assays have proven to be more sensitive than the CF test; in one study, 3 of 65 sera that had CF titers of 16 had much higher titers in the EIA.[7] EIA methods have also been described for the detection of serum antibodies against *M. hominis*, but these assays are not widely available.[6] Easily performed methods for detecting antibody responses to genital mycoplasmas may be valuable in sorting out colonization versus infection with these bacteria and may help to target individuals, such as pregnant women, who may be at risk for more serious *Mycoplasma*-associated disease.

ANTIMICROBIAL SUSCEPTIBILITY AND TREATMENT OF *MYCOPLASMA* INFECTIONS

Atypical pneumonia caused by *M. pneumoniae* is generally treated with tetracycline or erythromycin.[12] Although the organism may still be present in the upper respiratory tract during and after treatment, clinical manifestations of infection generally improve and infiltrates on the chest roentgenogram usually disappear during therapy. Because of the difficulty in culturing the organism, its slow growth rate, and the lack of a readily available method, antimicrobial susceptibility testing of *M. pneumoniae* is neither necessary or appropriate. The genital mycoplasmas are more variable in their antimicrobial susceptibility patterns, and resistance to both tetracycline and erythromycin is fairly common. Because of variability in antimicrobial susceptibility, methods for susceptibility testing on mycoplasmas have been devised but are not widely available because they require special media and may incur considerable expense for routine clinical microbiology laboratories. Therefore, susceptibility testing on mycoplasmas is usually performed only in larger institutions with special research interests in the therapy of genital *Mycoplasma* infections.

REFERENCES

1. Alfa MJ, Robertson JA. The co-existence of genital mycoplasmas and *Neisseria gonorrhoeae* isolated from the male urethra. Sex Transm Dis 1984;11: 131–136.

2. Barile MF. DNA homologies and serologic relationships among ureaplasmas from various hosts. Pediatr Infect Dis 1986;5:S296–S299.

3. Bartlett JG, Ryan KJ, Smith TF, et al. Cumitech 7A: Laboratory diagnosis of lower respiratory tract infections. Washington, DC, American Society for Microbiology, 1987.

4. Bradbury JM, Jordan FTW, Shimizu T, et al. *Mycoplasma anseris* sp. nov. found in geese. Int J Syst Bacteriol 1988;38:74–76.

5. Braun P, Klein JO, Kass EH. Susceptibility of genital mycoplasmas to antimicrobial agents. Appl Microbiol 1970;19:62–70.

6. Brown MB, et al. Measurement of antibody to *Mycoplasma hominis* by an enzyme-linked immunosorbent assay and detection of class-specific responses in women with postpartum fever. Am J Obstet Gynecol 1987;156:701–708.

7. Busolo F, Tonin E, Meloni GA. Enzyme-linked immunosorbent assay for serodiagnosis of *Mycoplasma pneumoniae* infections. 1983;18:432–435.

8. Cassell GH, Waites KB, Crouse DT, et al. Association of *Ureaplasma urealyticum* of the lower respiratory tract with chronic lung disease and death in very-low-birth-weight infants. Lancet 1988; 2:240–244.

9. Clyde WA. *Mycoplasma* species identification based upon growth inhibition by specific antisera. J Immunol 1964;92:958–965.

10. Clyde WA. Letter to the editors. Clin Microbiol Newsl 1985;7:164–165.

11. Clyde WA, Kenny GE, Schachter J. Cumitech 19: Laboratory diagnosis of chlamydial and mycoplasmal infections. Washington, DC, American Society for Microbiology, 1984.

12. Couch RB. *Mycoplasma pneumoniae* (primary atypical pneumonia). In: Mandell GL, Douglas RG, Bennett JE, eds. Principles and practice of infectious diseases. 3rd ed. New York, Churchill-Livingstone, 1990:1446–1458.

13. Cunningham CK. The role of genital mycoplasmas in neonatal disease. Clin Microbiol Newsl 1990;12:147–149.

14. Dinsmoor MJ, Ramamurthy RS, Gibbs RS. Transmission of genital mycoplasmas from mother to neonate in women with prolonged membrane rupture. Pediatr Infect Dis J 1989;8:843–847.

15. Driscoll SG. Chorioamnitonitis: perinatal morbidity and mortality. Pediatr Infect Dis 1986;5: S273–S275.

16. Embree J. *Mycoplasma hominis* in maternal and fetal infections. Ann NY Acad Sci 1988;549:56–64.

17. Gewitz M, Dinwiddie R, Rees L, et al. *Mycoplasma hominis*: a cause of neonatal meningitis. Arch Dis Child 1979;54:231–239.

18. Gilbert GL, Garland SM, Fairley KF, et al. Bacteriuria due to ureaplasmas and other fastidious organisms during pregnancy: prevalence and significance. Pediatr Infect Dis 1986;5:S239–S243.

19. Gravat MG, Eschenbach DA. Possible role of *Ureaplasma urealyticum* in preterm premature rupture of the fetal membranes. Pediatr Infect Dis 1986;5:S253–S257.

20. Harrison HR. Cervical colonization with *Ureaplasma urealyticum* and pregnancy outcome: prospective studies. Pediatr Infect Dis 1986;5:S266–S269.

21. Hill AC. *Mycoplasma testudinis*, a new species isolated from a tortoise. Int J Syst Bacteriol 1985;35: 489–492.

22. Kanamoto Y, Kotani H, Ogata M. Isolation of *Mycoplasma* and *Ureaplasma* species from raccoon dogs (*Nyctereutes procyonoides viverrinus*). J Gen Microbiol 1983;129:2447–2450.

23. Kass EH, Lin J-S, McCormack WM. Low birth weight and maternal colonization with genital mycoplasmas. Pediatr Infect Dis 1986;5:S279–S281.

24. Koneman EW, Allen SD, Janda WM, Schreckenberger PC, Winn WC Jr. Color atlas and textbook of diagnostic microbiology. 4th ed. Philadelphia, JB Lippincott, 1992

25. Koshimizu K, Harasawa R, Pan I-J, et al. *Ureaplasma gallorale* sp. nov. from the oropharynx of chickens. Int J Syst Bacteriol 1987;37:333–338.

26. Lo SC, Shih JW-K, Newton PB, et al. Virus-like infectious agent (VLIA) is a novel pathogenic mycoplasma: *Mycoplasma incognitus*. Am J Trop Med Hyg 1989;51:586–600.

27. Lo SC, Dawson MS, Wong DM, et al. Identification of *Mycoplasma incognitus* infection in patients with AIDS: an immunohistochemical, in situ hybridization and ultrastructural study. Am J Trop Med Hyg 1989;41:601–616.

28. Mardh P-A. *Mycoplasma hominis* infection of the

central nervous system in newborn infants. Sex Transm Dis 1983;10(Suppl):331–334.

29. McCormack WM. *Ureaplasma urealyticum*: ecologic niche and epidemiologic considerations. Pediatr Infect Dis 1986;5:S232–S233.

30. McCormack WM, Lee Y-H, Zinner SH. Sexual experience and urethral colonization with genital mycoplasmas: a study in normal men. Ann Intern Med 1973;78:696–698.

31. McDonald JC, Moore DL. *Mycoplasma hominis* meningitis in a premature infant. Pediatr Infect Dis J 1988;7:795–798.

32. Murray HW, Masur H, Senterfit LB. The protean manifestations of *Mycoplasma pneumoniae* infection in adults. Am J Med 1975;58:229–242.

33. Peeters, et al. Role of mycoplasmas in chronic prostatitis. Yale J Med Biol 1983;56:551.

34. Robertson JA, Coppola JE, Heisler OR. Standardized method for determining antimicrobial susceptibility of strains of *Ureaplasma urealyticum* and their response to tetracycline, erythromycin, and rosaramicin. Antimicrob Agents Chemother 1981;20:53–58.

35. Rose DL, Kocka JP, Somerson NL, et al. *Mycoplasma lactucae* sp. nov., a sterol-requiring mollicute from a plant surface. Int J Syst Bacteriol 1990;40:138–142.

36. Rudd PT, Waites KB, Duffy LB, et al. *Ureaplasma urealyticum* and its possible role in pneumonia during the neonatal period and infancy. Pediatr Infect Dis 1986;5:S288–S291.

37. Shepard MC. *Ureaplasma urealyticum*: overview with emphasis on fetal and maternal infections. Ann NY Acad Sci 1988;549:48–55.

38. Shepard MC, Lunceford CD, Ford DK, et al. *Ureaplasma urealyticum* gen. nov., sp. nov.: proposed nomenclature for the human (T-strain) mycoplasmas. Int J Syst Bacteriol 1974;24:160–171.

39. Siber GR, Alpert S, Smith AL, et al. Neonatal central nervous system infection due to *Mycoplasma hominis*. J Pediatr 1977;90:625–627.

40. Smaron MF, Boonlayangoor S, Zierdt CH. Detection of *Mycoplasma hominis* septicemia by radiometric blood culture. J Clin Microbiol 1985;21:298–301.

41. Tully JG, Rose DL, Hackett KJ, et al. *Mycoplasma ellychniae* sp. nov., a sterol-requiring mollicute from the firefly beetle *Ellychnia corrusca*. Int J Syst Bacteriol 1989;39:284–289.

42. Tully JG, Rose DL, McCoy RE, et al. *Mycoplasma melaleucae* sp. nov., a sterol-requiring mollicute from flowers of several tropical plants. Int J Syst Bacteriol 1990;40:143–147.

43. Tully JG, Rose DL, Whitcomb RF, et al. Enhanced isolation of *Mycoplasma pneumoniae* from throat washings with a newly modified culture medium. J Infect Dis 1979;139:478–482.

44. Velleca WM, Bird BR, Forrester FT. Course 8228C: laboratory diagnosis of *Mycoplasma* infections. Atlanta, Centers for Disease Control, 1980.

45. Waites KB, Rudd PT, Crouse DT, et al. Chronic *Ureaplasma urealyticum* and *Mycoplasma hominis* infections of the central nervous system in preterm infants. Lancet 1988;1:17–21.

46. Wang EEL, Drayha H, Watts J, et al. Role of *Ureaplasma urealyticum* and other pathogens in the development of chronic lung disease of prematurity. Pediatr Infect Dis J 1988;7:547–551.

47. Wientzen RL. Genital mycoplasmas and the pediatrician. Pediatr Infect Dis J 1990;9:232–235.

16

Mycology

In the presence of certain clinical signs and symptoms, to be reviewed below, counsel to the primary care physician is to "think fungus." Failure to appreciate the possibility of a mycotic infection when examining a patient may not necessarily reflect a lack of knowledge or experience. In particular, patients who are immunosuppressed may present with nonspecific, vague signs and symptoms that often are not consistent with how fungal diseases have been recognized in the past. Physicians must always suspect the possibility of fungal infections in patients with the acquired immunodeficiency syndrome (AIDS), particularly those living in an endemic region of the country.[58] Histoplasmosis and coccidioidomycosis, in particular, may appear in patients with AIDS many months or even years after they have left an endemic area.[48] An atypical presenting sign or symptom of a fungal infection may, in fact, be the initial clue to the diagnosis of AIDS. Patients with leukemia and other hematologic malignancies are also at high risk for developing systemic fungal infections, particularly during the febrile and neutropenic stages of chemotherapy or following bone marrow transplantation. Fungal infections may often be rapidly progressive and reach organ systems rarely involved in past infections. A variety of unusual fungal species, either heretofore not recognized or considered strictly as contaminants, have emerged as pathogens, and many of these are refractory to the commonly used antifungal agents.

SIGNS AND SYMPTOMS OF FUNGAL INFECTION

With the exception of candidiasis, the dermatophytes, and select agents of mycetoma and chromomycosis, most fungal infections begin in the lungs, after inhalation of aerosolized spores or hyphal fragments. Trauma, intravenous drug use, and a variety of invasive medical procedures, including the increasing use of vascular access devices, may provide a direct route of entry for pathogenic fungi into the tissues or bloodstream.[36] The primary pulmonary infection may resolve spontaneously or progress.[68] Spread throughout the body may occur by way of phagocytic cells that carry intracellular yeast forms or from vascular invasion by hyphae, resulting in thrombosis, hemorrhagic necrosis, and the release of infective mycotic emboli.

It is important that the physician elicit any relevant historical information from the patient, such as past or recent travel into areas known to be endemic for fungal infection or high-risk occupational or vocational activities (eg, road construction, archeological digs, spelunking) that entail overexposure to soil, dust, bird excreta, or other materials that have a high probability of fungal contamination. For example, outbreaks of blastomycosis have been reported among fishermen and campers along riverbanks in endemic areas in Wisconsin and other locales.[38,39]

The patient's complaints may be vague and nonspecific. Low-grade fever, night sweats, weight loss, lassitude, easy fatigability, cough, and chest pain are common presenting symptoms. Deep-seated or disseminated fungal diseases may mimic other infections such as tuberculosis, brucellosis, syphilis, sarcoidosis, or disseminated carcinomatosis. Careful examination of the skin and mucous membranes should always be performed, since systemic fungal infections may often present as mucocutaneous lesions. Rippon[56] describes ulcerating lesions in the intestine, larynx, pharynx, genitals, and tongue as complications of chronic disseminated histoplasmosis; up to 50% of patients with blastomycosis have verrucous or pustular lesions of the skin, which may be the presenting symptom, or ulcerating granulomas of mucous membranes, reported in such sites as the larynx,[18] the esophagus,[46] the tongue,[64] and the mouth.[52]

Laboratory tests may reveal nonspecific inflammatory responses. The erythrocyte sedimentation rate may be increased, the levels of serum enzymes or IgA may be high, and low-grade neutrophilia or monocytosis may be present. Radiographic findings may be helpful; often the finding of pulmonary infiltrates or of inflammatory processes in other organs is nonspecific. In some patients with severely compromised resistance, general symptoms or laboratory and radiographic abnormalities may be lacking. Fine-needle biopsies play an important role in the rapid diagnosis of fungal infections, particularly those involving subcutaneous tissues.[42]

Involvement of Specific Organ Systems

Fungal infections are often suspected because of manifestations that may be confined to one or two organ systems. These specific signs and symptoms are reviewed briefly here.

Pulmonary Disease

A cough that may or may not produce sputum, chest pain that is frequently pleuritic, dyspnea, tachypnea, and, less commonly, hemoptysis are the more common presenting symptoms of pulmonary fungal infections. In the acute phase of infection, a transient influenza-like syndrome or pneumonia that localizes in one lobe or spreads to other lobes may develop. Rales or rhonchi and a pleural friction rub may be detected on auscultation. Roentgenography of the chest may reveal small pulmonary infiltrates and hilar adenopathy or more diffuse and confluent opacities, depending on the severity of exposure and the immunologic status of the patient.

Cutaneous Disease

Certain fungi involve only the stratum corneum and rarely invade the deeper tissues. Superficial scaling lesions of the thorax or back that vary in size, shape, and color suggest tinea versicolor. The superficial dermatophytic fungi of the genera *Microsporum*, *Trichophyton*, and *Epidermophyton* most commonly cause itching, scaling lesions known as tinea or ringworm; specific anatomic designations include tinea pedis, tinea cruris, tinea corporis, tinea capitis, and so on, depending on the primary sites of involvement. Tinea capitis may appear as alopecia with scaling, as black dot ringworm (typical for *T. tonsurans*), and as a thickened, crusting, hyperkeratotic, exophytic fungoid affectation known as favus (typical for *T. violaceum* and *T. schoenleinii*). Tinea corporis classically presents as circular, ringworm lesions. Varying degrees of inflammation may accompany each of these conditions.

Scaling or crusting lesions confined to the moist intertriginous areas of skin (between the fingers and toes and under the breasts of females) suggest yeast infections with *Candida* species. A condition known as chronic mucocutaneous candidosis is less commonly encountered and occurs in patients with immune T-cell defects.[37] *Candida* species should also be considered as well as dermatophytic fungi as a cause of nail infections. Nonhealing pustules, ulcers, or draining sinuses may be the initial presenting signs of a disseminated mycotic infection. A primary subcutaneous pustular infection at the site of inoculation with proximal spread and evolution of secondary skin ulcers along the course of the lymphatics is characteristic of infections with *Sporothrix schenckii*. Deep involvement of the skin and development of draining sinus tracts (mycetoma) are caused by fungal agents such as *Pseudallescheria boydii* (*Scedosporium* species) and *Exophiala jeanselmei*; similar lesions are caused by the actinomycotic bacteria, *Actinomyces* species, and *Nocardia* species. Purpuric lesions and subcutaneous cysts may be caused by several phaeohyphomycotic fungi, with *Alternaria*, *Curvularia*, *Cladosporium*, and *Aureobasidium* being most frequently reported.[56]

Central Nervous System Disease

Symptoms include headaches that may increase in frequency and severity, nausea, irritability, and clumsiness. Vomiting, hallucinations, coma, and seizures of the jacksonian type occur in more advanced cases. Acute cryptococcal meningitis may occur in patients who are being treated with corticosteroids or who are receiving chemotherapeutic agents for lymphoma or leukemia. *Cryptococcus neoformans* is the fourth most common cause of life-threatening infection in patients with AIDS. Meningitis and meningoencephalitis may be caused by direct extension of orbital or sinus zygomycosis, particularly in patients with diabetes mellitis complicated by acidosis. Cerebral zygomycosis can be rapidly fatal if not treated promptly, particularly if underlying acidosis is also not corrected. Small brain abscesses, usually multifocal, may be seen in patients with systemic aspergillosis. In both cerebral zygomycosis and aspergillosis, hemorrhagic infarctions may occur secondary to hyphal invasion of vessels. Brain abscesses may also be caused by the dematiaceous fungus *Cladosporium trichoides* (*Xylophyla bantiana*).[61]

Genitourinary Tract Disease

The recovery of *Candida* species from urine specimens is difficult to interpret, particularly in female patients, because of the chance for contamination from the vagina and periurethral area. *Candida* infections of the urinary tract, when confirmed, are usually ascending, resulting in acute pyelonephritis and papillary necrosis. Most urinary tract fungal infections are caused by *C. albicans*; *Torulopis* (*Candida*) *glabrata* is also a relatively frequent isolate, particularly in young women. Genitourinary infections with the other agents more commonly results from hematogenous spread as part of disseminated disease. Urine colony counts of yeast colonies are not valid indicators of urinary tract infection. Yeast isolates from the urinary tract, particularly in the presence of signs and symptoms of infection, should undergo further evaluation. The urine may also be a prime source for the recovery of yeasts in cases of disseminated fungal infections, often in the absence of urinary tract symptoms. For example, *Cryptococcus neoformans* may be recovered from the urine in cases of disseminated cryptococcosis, even when cerebrospinal fluid and sputum cultures are negative.

Candida species are also common causes of vaginitis, a disease called vaginal thrush in the classic literature. The disease is manifest by the presence of a thick, curdlike discharge, most commonly complicating other conditions such as diabetes mellitus, pregnancy, and prolonged antibiotic therapy. In males with blastomycosis, urinary tract manifestations are not uncommon, presenting as including prostatitis, epididymitis, and orchitis. In these cases, the organism may be recovered from the urine.

Miscellaneous Organ and Tissue Involvement

A variety of fungal species may cause infections of the muscles, tendons, bones, and joints. Patients with blastomycosis often have osteolytic lesions of the bone, primarily of the long bones, vertebrae, and ribs. *Candida* species also cause osteomyelitis of the vertebrae and intervertebral disks, the long bones, bones of the wrist, and ribs, including the costochondral tissue. Osteomyelitis also commonly complicates *Coccidioides immitis* infections, particularly those that occur in the skull, metacarpus, metatarsus, and spine.

Conjunctivitis, corneal infections, and keratoconjunctivitis may be caused by a variety of environmental fungi, such as *Aspergillus, Cladosporium, Acromonium,* and *Fusarium* species. Intraocular infections are most commonly caused by *Candida albicans, Aspergillus* species, or the Zygomycetes, often after eye surgery or trauma.

Fungal otitis externa is most commonly caused by *Aspergillus* species, notably *A. niger*. *Candida albicans* is also a causative agent in cases of chronic cutaneous candidosis.

Endocarditis is caused by a wide variety of fungi. In a review of 46 previously reported cases, Kauf-

mann[35] found the following distribution: 38 were caused by *Candida* species, 6 by *Aspergillus* species, and 1 each by *Hormodendrum* and *Paecilomyces* species. Atkinson and associates[5] reported cardiac fungal infections in 60 autopsied cases: *Aspergillus* species in 18%, Zygomycetes in 12%, and *Cryptococcus neoformans* in 3%. *Histoplasma capsulatum, Curvularia lunata,* and *Helminthosporium* species were found to complicate cardiac surgery in single cases in this series.

Several reports of mycotic sinusitis have been reported; included are six case reports by Morgan and associates[49]—two caused by *Aspergillus fumigatus* and one each by *A. flavus, Sporothrix schenckii, Alternaria* species, and *Pseudallescheria boydii*. Sobol and colleagues[65] report a case of phaeohyphomycosis of the ethmoidal sinus caused by *Drechslera spiciferum*. The propensity of these fungi to invade the tissue deeply and, potentially, to involve the meninges directly and their tropism for blood vessels make these infections potentially dangerous, particularly in immunocompromised hosts.

Fungal ball infections refer to the presence of a growing fungus colony within a preexistent cavity, after inhalation of fungal spores. The developing colony often remains confined to the cavity and does not invade the surrounding tissues. *Aspergillus* species, the Zygomycetes, and *Pseudallescheria boydii* are among the more common fungi involved in fungal ball infections. Symptoms may or may not be present. *Rhinosporidium seeberi* causes rhinosporidiosis, a chronic granulomatous infection of the nasal passages with production of hyperplastic nasal polyps.

Disseminated Disease

The host who has a chronic debilitating disease, who receives prolonged antibiotic or corticosteroid therapy or chemotherapy, or who is immunosuppressed is at high risk for developing disseminated fungal infections.[1,5] Most disseminated fungal infections, particularly those caused by the dimorphic fungi, begin in the lungs after inhalation of aerosolized spores. In most instances, the initial infection is contained and spontaneously resolves. Fever, anemia, leukopenia, weight loss, and lassitude are features that indicate a locally progressive or disseminated infection. Gold[21] has reported that 220 patients die annually of fungal infections at Memorial–Sloan Kettering Cancer Center. *Can-*

dida species, *Aspergillus* species, *Cryptococcus neoformans*, and the Zygomycetes were the most common isolates. Kiehn and Armstrong,[36] reporting from the same institution, found that 50% of cases of fungemia were related to vascular access devices. *Rhodotorula* species, *Torulopsis* species, and *Cryptococcus* species were recovered with increased frequency.

SPECIMEN COLLECTION AND TRANSPORT

Although prompt delivery of specimens to the laboratory is to be encouraged, it has been shown that several fungal species, including *Histoplasma capsulatum*, *Blastomyces dermatitidis*, *Cryptococcus neoformans*, and *Aspergillus* species, can be recovered from samples that have been in transit for as long as 16 days.[60] Sealed, sterile transport containers, however, should be used for all liquid or moist specimens. Skin scrapings, nail fragments, and hairs can be transported in an envelope, Petri dish, or other convenient conveyance. Because many specimens contain contaminating bacteria that may compromise their quality, 50,000 units of penicillin, 100,000 g of streptomycin, or 0.2 mg of chloramphenicol can be added per milliliter of specimen if it is anticipated that transit will be prolonged (such as transport through the mail). Directions for the proper packaging and labeling of specimens for shipping and mailing are discussed in Chapter 1.

The following are recommendations by the American Thoracic Society for the collection of several common specimen types for fungal cultures.[60] As a general rule, specimens should not be frozen or allowed to dry; rather, they should be either refrigerated at 4°C or left at room temperature.

Sputum

The first early-morning sputum sample should be collected after rising but before breakfast. Patients are instructed to rinse their mouths with water vigorously immediately before coughing at least 30 mL of sputum into a sterile, screw-capped container. Sputum induction with a heated aerosol saline suspension may be required if an adequate specimen cannot be obtained.

Bronchoscopy

Bronchial brushings, biopsy, or bronchoalveolar lavage fluid should be transported promptly to the laboratory in sterile, sealed containers. Middlebrook 7H11 broth is used in some laboratories as a transport medium because mycobacteria will also be preserved. A postbronchoscopy sputum sample should be collected when possible.

Cerebrospinal Fluid

As much cerebrospinal fluid as possible should be used for the culture of fungi. If processing is to be delayed, samples should be left at room temperature and not be refrigerated since cerebrospinal fluid is an adequate fluid culture medium in which fungal elements can survive until subcultured.

Urine

The first early-morning urine sample is preferred; random samples are acceptable. Specimens should be collected aseptically in sterile, screw-capped containers and sent immediately for processing. If a delay in processing beyond 2 hours is anticipated, the urine sample should be placed in a 4°C refrigerator to inhibit the overgrowth of rapidly growing bacteria.

Prostatic Secretions

Some deep-seated mycoses, notably blastomycosis and less commonly histoplasmosis or coccidioidomycosis, may be diagnosed by collecting prostatic secretions. The bladder is first emptied, followed by prostatic massage. Secretions should be inoculated directly to appropriate fungal culture media; also, 5 to 10 mL of urine should be collected in a separate container.

Exudates

The skin over pustular lesions should be disinfected and exudates aspirated using a sterile needle and syringe. The syringe also serves as a transport container if the needle is capped. Biopsy of the lesion may be necessary if the aspirate fails to yield fungi.

Skin, Nails, and Hair

The area of skin to be sampled is first swabbed with 70% alcohol to remove surface bacterial contaminants. The peripheral, erythematous, growing margin of a typical "ringworm" lesion is sampled by scraping with the side of a glass microscope slide or the edge of a scalpel blade. Infected nails should be sampled from beneath the nail plate to obtain softened material from the nail bed. If this is not possible, scrape away the surface of the nail before collecting shavings form the deeper portions. Hairs should be collected from areas of scaling or alopecia, and hairs that fluoresce when viewed under a Wood's (long wavelength) ultraviolet lamp should be sampled.

Tissue

Tissue biopsy specimens of suspected sites of infection should be transported in sterile gauze moistened with physiologic, nonbacteriostatic, sterile saline solution in a screw-capped container. The specimen should not be frozen or allowed to dehydrate before culture.

Blood

Biphasic agar/broth bottles designed specifically for fungal cultures are superior to routine bottles used for the recovery of bacterial pathogens. Lysis-centrifugation systems, such as the Isolator (Wampole Laboratories, Cranbury, NJ) are also highly recommended, particularly for the recovery of *H. capsulatum* and other yeasts.

LABORATORY APPROACH TO THE DIAGNOSIS OF FUNGAL INFECTIONS

Specimen Processing

Once received in the laboratory, a specimen should be examined as soon as possible. Swab specimens are generally inadequate for the recovery of fungi;

attempts should be made to receive aspirated material or tissue biopsy specimens. Direct wet mounts or smears should be prepared if appropriate, and a portion of the specimen transferred to appropriate fungal culture media. This last step is also important in the ultimate recovery of fungi and cannot be slighted or delegated to marginally trained personnel.

Direct Examination

A direct microscopic examination is highly recommended for most specimens submitted for fungal culture. Not only may this provide an immediate presumptive diagnosis for the physician, but it may also aid in the selection of appropriate culture media. The following are procedures for the direct examination of different specimen types and what one may potentially see microscopically. Table 16-1 provides clues to the presumptive identification of various fungi based on the observation of characteristic forms.

SPUTUM. The most purulent-appearing parts of the sample should be selected. Depending on the viscosity of the sample, homogenization should occur after adding a small pinch of crystalline N-acetyl-L-cystine to the specimen. Sodium hydroxide or other digesting agents that are employed for the processing of specimens for the recovery of mycobacteria should not be used. A wet mount of the homogenized sample is prepared for direct microscopic examination and about 0.5 mL is inoculated to each of the culture media to be used.

In direct mounts or smears prepared from the sample or the homogenate, one should look for the yeast forms of dimorphic fungi—the broad-based buds of *Blastomyces dermatitidis*, spherules of *Coccidioides immitis*, the tiny yeast forms of *Histoplasma capsulatum* (rarely seen), the hyphal segments suggestive of *Aspergillus* species (hyphae with parallel walls and 45-degree dichotomous branching), or the pseudohyphae and budding blastoconidia characteristic of *Candida* species.

BRONCHOSCOPY. The surface of appropriate culture media is inoculated with about 0.5 mL of the sample. The inoculum is spread over the surface with a sterile swab or inoculating loop. If larger quantities of bronchoalveolar wash fluids are received, the sample can be centrifuged and

Table 16-1
Presumptive Identification of Fungi Based on Direct Microscopic Examination of Material from Clinical Specimens

DIRECT MICROSCOPIC OBSERVATIONS	PRESUMPTIVE IDENTIFICATION
Hyphae relatively small (3–6 μm) and regular in size, dichotomously branching at 45-degree angles with distinct cross-septa	*Aspergillus* species
Hyphae irregular in size, ranging from 6 to 50 μm, ribbon-like, and devoid of septa	Zygomycetes (Phycomycetes) *Rhizopus-Mucor-Absidia*
Hyphae small (2–3 μm) and regular, some branching, with rectangular arthroconidia sometimes seen; found only in skin, nail scrapings, and hair	Dermatophyte group *Microsporum* species *Trichophyton* species *Epidermophyton* species
Hyphae regular in diameter, 3–6 μm, parallel walls, irregular branching, septate, dark yellow, brown, or hyaline	*Phaeohyphomyces* species *Hyalanohyphomyces* species
Hyphae, distinct points of constriction simulating link sausages (pseudohyphae), with budding yeast forms (blastospores) often seen	*Candida* species
Yeast forms, cells spherical and irregular in size (5–20 μm), classically with a thick polysaccharide capsule (not all cells are encapsulated), with one or more buds attached by a narrow constriction	*Cryptococcus neoformans* *Cryptococcus* species non-encapsulated
Small budding yeast, relatively uniform in size (3–5 μm), with a single bud attached by a narrow base, extracellular or within macrophages	*Histoplasma capsulatum*
Yeast forms, large (8–20 μm), with cells appearing to have a thick, double-contoured wall, with a single bud attached by a broad base	*Blastomyces dermatitidis*
Large, irregularly sized (10–50 μm), thick-walled spherules, many of which contain small (2–4 μm), round endospores	*Coccidioides immitis*

0.5 mL of sediment used for preparation of direct mounts and inoculation of culture plates.

CEREBROSPINAL FLUID. Although centrifugation of cerebrospinal fluid and the use of the sediment for preparation of an India ink mount is acceptable, passage of larger volumes (1 mL or more) of fluid through a 0.45-μm membrane filter using a Swinnex syringe attachment is recommended. The filtrate side of the filter paper is placed face down on the surface of appropriate culture media. The paper should be repositioned to other sites on the medium on an every-other-day schedule.

The India ink (nigrosin is an acceptable substitute) technique is a time-honored approach for the direct detection of the encapsulated yeast cells of *Cryptococcus neoformans*. To prepare the mount, the specimen can be centrifuged for 10 to 20 minutes at 1500 *g* and a drop of sediment or the membrane scraping is mixed with a drop of India ink on a microscope slide. A coverslip as applied, and the specimen is observed with a 25 × or 40 × objective for the presence of encapsulated, budding yeast forms. With the ready availability of latex agglutination tests for the detection of cryptococcal polysaccharide antigen, many laboratories have abandoned the India ink procedure because of its relatively low sensitivity. Yeast cells are found in only about 30% of cases of cryptococcosis, using

India ink preparations. The latex agglutination test has a reported sensitivity of 90% to 100% if samples are treated to remove interfering substances and if proper controls are used with each test procedure.[7]

URINE, PROSTATIC SECRETIONS, AND OTHER FLUIDS. About 10 mL of sample is centrifuged and 0.5 mL of sediment is used to inoculate the surface of appropriate culture medium. Thick exudates aspirated from closed lesions can be inoculated directly to a culture medium without prior treatment. Direct mounts can be prepared and examined microscopically for yeast or hyphal forms.

SKIN, NAILS, AND HAIR. Skin scales, nail scrapings, and hairs should be examined after preparation with potassium hydroxide (KOH). The KOH preparation is made by emulsifying the specimen in a drop of 10% KOH on a microscope slide. The purpose of the KOH is to clear out any background scales or cell membranes that may be confused with hyphal elements. Clearing can be accelerated by gently heating the mixture over the flame of a Bunsen burner. A coverslip is applied and the specimen examined for the presence of narrow, regular hyphae that characteristically break up into arthroconidia. The visualization of hyphae is improved by adding calcofluor white to the potassium hydroxide reagent. Any fungal elements present will show a brilliant green-yellow or white fluorescence when examined with a fluorescent microscope depending on the wavelength of the exciter light used[25] (Fig. 16-1).

Selection and Inoculation of Culture Media

Two general types of culture media are essential to ensure the primary recovery of all clinically significant fungi from clinical specimens. One medium should be nonselective, that is, one that will permit the growth of virtually all fungal species. The use of Sabouraud's dextrose agar as a primary recovery medium is discouraged, except for the recovery of dermatophytes from cutaneous samples or yeasts from vaginal cultures.[40] Instead, either inhibitory mold agar or Sabhi agar is recommended to improve the recovery of certain of the more fastidious or slow-growing fungi. Sabouraud's dextrose agar

(2%) can be used to subculture fungi recovered on enriched medium to enhance sporulation and provide the more characteristic colonial morphology. Czepak's agar should be used for the subculture of *Aspergillus* species if colonial morphology is an important identifying criterion for any given unknown isolate.

A second medium more selective for the recovery of fungi should also be used. Combinations of antibiotics, including penicillin (20 IU/mL) and streptomycin (40 IU/mL), gentamicin (5 g/mL), and chloramphenicol (16 g/mL), can be used to inhibit the growth of bacteria. Cycloheximide (Actidione) in a concentration of 0.5 mg/mL may be added to prevent the overgrowth of certain rapidly growing environmental molds that may contaminate the culture plates. Opportunistic pathogenic fungi, including *Cryptococcus neoformans* and *Aspergillus fumigatus*, may, however, be partially or totally inhibited by cycloheximide. For the recovery of the more fastidious dimorphic fungi, such as *Blastomyces dermatitidis* and *Histoplasma capsulatum*, an enriched agar base such as brain-heart infusion must be used. For optimal recovery of these organisms, the addition of 5% to 10% sheep blood is also recommended.

All fungal cultures should be incubated at a controlled 30°C. Incubation of a second set of plates at 35°C for the recovery of the yeast forms of dimorphic fungi is not cost-effective. Any mold recovered in primary culture that is suggestive of a dimorphic species can be subcultured to brain-heart infusion agar containing 10% sheep blood or to cottonseed conversion medium (if *Blastomyces dermatitidis* is suspected) (Traders Protein Division, Fort Worth, TX) and incubated for 7 to 10 days at 35°C to accomplish in vitro yeast conversion. The exoantigen extraction test is recommended in lieu of the in vitro conversion procedure for confirming the identification of *B. dermatitidis*, *Histoplasma capsulatum*, *Coccidioides immitis*, and *Paracoccidioides brasiliensis*.[33,34]

Exoantigen test reagents are also available for the identification of a variety of fungi, including *Aspergillus* species, *Penicillium marneffi*, *Pseudoallescheria boydii*, *Sporothrix schenckii*, and dematiaceous fungi belonging to the *Cladosporium*, *Exophiala*, and *Wangiella* genera. The commercial availability of reagents (Nolan Biologicals, Tucker, GA) provides clinical laboratories with the capability to identify these species of dimorphic fungi

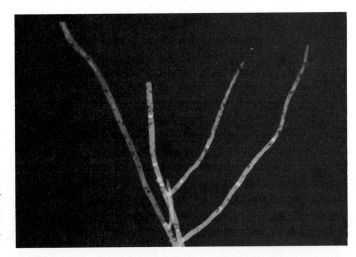

Figure 16-1. Oil immersion photomicrograph of a fungus colony mount treated with calcofluor white and observed with fluorescence microscopy. The hyphae have a brilliant green fluorescence. The septa appear as sharp, narrow, white bands. (Courtesy of G.D. Roberts)

without the need for the more time-consuming mold conversion studies.[33] Nucleic acid probes for the culture confirmation of *Blastomyces dermatitidis*, *Histoplasma capsulatum*, and *Coccidioides immitis* are also available (Gen-Probe, Inc, San Diego, CA); this procedure requires special equipment and a relatively large volume of testing to be economical

All fungal cultures should be incubated for a minimum of 30 days before being discarded as negative, even if plates appear contaminated with bacteria or other fungi. We have seen colonies of *Histoplasma capsulatum*, for example, growing on the surface of colonies of *Candida albicans* or contaminating molds.

Taxonomy and Classification of Mycoses and Medically Important Fungi

Clinical Classification

Table 16-2 is the classic clinical categorization of human mycoses and the various causative agents of each. Although this approach still offers a valuable point of reference, many human fungal infections can no longer be separated into the neatly defined categories of "deep-seated" or "systemic," "opportunistic," "subcutaneous," and "superficial" mycoses. Fungal species that formerly were considered as contaminants or confined to the realm of the natural environment are now known to cause human infections. For example, the fungal agent *Malassezia furfur*, which formerly caused only the superficial dermatomycosis tinea versicolor, is now an agent of disseminated infections in patients receiving parenteral nutrition through indwelling catheters.[22,43]

The term *deep-seated* has referred to a group of fungal infections caused by agents that inherently can be highly virulent, can invade deeply into tissues and organs, and have the capability of spreading widely throughout the body. As seen in Table 16-2, this group of fungi (with the exception of the yeast *Cryptococcus neoformans*) have the common characteristic that they are dimorphic; that is, they exist in the mold form in the environment ("room temperature incubation") but as yeasts when incubated at 35° to 37°C (body temperature). The mold form is the infective form; humans and animals become infected either by inhaling or being injected with conidia or hyphal elements of these fungi. For the dimorphic fungi, the yeast form is the invasive form that produces infection when present in tissues. For other fungi, notably *Aspergillus* and *Zygomycetes* species, the mold form is both infective and invasive.

The term *opportunistic* has been used to designate those infections caused by fungi that are inherently of limited virulence but that can cause either local or disseminated disease in persons who are debilitated, who are immunosuppressed, or who have intravascular or prosthetic devices. *Aspergillus* species, *Candida* species, and Zygomycetes species are the three groups of fungi that classically were considered opportunistic. Localized and deep-seated infections have been ascribed to several species of light (hyaline) and dark (de-

Table 16-2
Classification of the More Commonly Encountered Human Mycoses and Their Etiologic Agents

DEEP-SEATED MYCOSES	OPPORTUNISTIC MYCOSES	SUBCUTANEOUS MYCOSES	SUPERFICIAL MYCOSES
Blastomycosis *Blastomyces dermatitidis* Coccidioidomycosis *Coccidioides immitis* Cryptococcosis *Cryptococcus neoformans* Histoplasmosis *Histoplasma capsulatum* Paracoccidioidomycosis (South American blastomycosis) *Paracoccioides brasiliensis* Sporotrichosis (unusual) *Sporothrix schenckii*	Aspergillosis *Aspergillus fumigatus* *Aspergillus flavus* *Aspergillus niger* *Aspergillus terreus* Candidosis *Candida albicans* *Candida* species Geotrichosis *Geotrichum candidum* Phaeohyphomycosis *Alternaria* species *Curvularia* species *Drechslera/Bipolaris* species *Exophiala* species *Wangiella* species Hyalohyphomycosis (rare) *Acremonium* species *Fusarium* species *Paecilomyces* species *Penicillium* species *Scedosporium* species (*Pseudallescheria* species) Zygomycosis *Rhizopus* species *Mucor* species *Cunninghamella* species	Maduromycosis (Mycetoma) *Acremonium* species *Exophiala jeanselmei* *Pseudallescheria boydii* *Nocardia* species Chromoblastomycosis *Cladosporium carrionii* *Fonsecaea* species *Phialophora* species Phaeohyphomycosis (cutaneous) *Alternaria* species *Cladosporium* species *Xylohypha emmonsii* *Exophiala* species *Phialophora* species *Wangiella dermatitidis* Sporotrichosis *Sporothrix schenckii*	Black piedra *Piedraia hortae* Tinea nigra *Phaeoannelomyces wernickii* Tinea versicolor *Malassezia furfur* Dermatomycoses *Microsporum* species *Trichophyton* species *Epidermophyton floccosum* Mycotic keratitis *Fusarium* species *Aspergillus* species *Candida* species Onychomycosis *Candida* species *Aspergillus* species *Trichosporon beigelii* *Geotrichum candidum* Tinea unguium *Trichophyton* species *Epidermophyton floccosum*

matiaceous) rapidly growing molds that formerly were considered contaminants. The term *phaeohyphomycosis* now refers to those mycoses (both systemic and subcutaneous) caused by fungi that appear dark or black from the production of a yellow- or brown-pigmented mycelium. *Hyalohyphomycosis* refers to fungal infections caused by several fungal species that produce colorless, transparent (hyaline) hyphae.[45]

The *subcutaneous* mycoses are caused by fungal agents that typically cause deep infections of the skin. Mycetoma and chromoblastomycosis (chromomycosis) are the classic diseases caused by several species of soil fungi that gain access to the body through penetrating injuries of the skin. Mycetomas are deeply penetrating infections of the subcutaneous tissue characterized by granulomatous inflammation, varying stages of fibrosis and scarring, and the production of sinus tracts that

exude pus from openings in the skin. Actinomycotic mycetomas are caused by bacteria, notably those species belonging to the family Actinomycetaceae (*Actinomyces, Nocardia, Streptomyces, Actinomadura, Nocardiopsis*) in contrast to the "eumycotic" mycetomas that are caused by fungi (see Chapter 10). *Chromomycosis* is the term used to describe the exophytic, fungating infections of the skin caused primarily by slowly growing dematiaceous fungi belonging to the genera *Cladosporium, Phialophora,* and *Fonsecaea*. Several species of more rapidly growing dematiaceous fungi have been incriminated in subcutaneous infections, now termed *cutaneous phaeohyphomycosis*. In rare instances, deep organ or disseminated disease with these agents have been reported that will be discussed in more detail below.

Superficial mycoses are infections that classically were caused by a group of fungi that infect only the skin, hair, and nails. Included are the three genera of dermatophytes, *Microsporum*, *Trichophyton*, and *Epidermophyton*, that have an obligate requirement of keratin to initiate and maintain growth. These fungi cause the classic skin infections commonly known as ringworm (tinea corporis), jock itch (tinea cruris), athlete's foot (tinea pedis), infections of the hair and skin of the scalp (tinea capitis), and infection of the nails (tinea unguium). The fungus *Malassezia furfur*, the cause of tinea versicolor, has an obligate requirement of fatty acids for growth and thus inhabits the sebum-rich areas of the skin, causing a more generalized cutaneous eruption in persons with poor body hygiene. As mentioned earlier, disseminated disease has been reported, particularly in neonates who receive parenteral fluids (which are often rich in lipid nutrients). Other species of hyaline and dematiaceous fungi can also cause infections of the cornea (keratitis), hair (piedra), and nails (onychomycosis) as listed in Table 16-2.

Taxonomy of Fungal Species

Table 16-3 is a revised taxonomy of medically important fungi (abridged to the "class" division) derived from the simplified taxonomic scheme presented by Dixon and Fromtling.[16] The simplified taxonomy as presented can be better understood if the meaning of each of the terms in the nomenclature is derived. The term *mycology* itself is derived from the Greek word *mykes*, a direct counterpart of the Latin word, *fungus*, in turn believed to be a modification of the Greek word *sponges*, from which our word *sponge* is derived.

The first class of fungi listed in Table 16-3 is the Zygomycetes. The term *zygo* is derived from the Greek *zygon*, meaning "a fusion or joining in the manner of a yoke." This derivation refers to the sexual phase of reproduction in which there is a joining or fusion of the two independent sex cells to form a zygospore. The previous designation, "phycomycete" (from the Greek *phykos*, meaning "seaweed") for this group of fungi has been more correctly replaced by the term *zygomycete*. The term for the order Mucorales is derived from the Latin *mucere*, meaning "to be moldy or musty." The order Mucorales includes those zygomycetes that can reproduce both asexually by forming spores within saclike sporangia and sexually by forming zygospores. Thus the frequently used term *mucor-*

Table 16-3
The Major Groups of Medically Important Fungi: A Simplified Taxonomic Scheme

Class: Zygomycetes
  Order: Mucorales
    Genera: *Rhizopus, Mucor, Rhizomucor, Absidia, Cunninghamella, Saksenaea*
  Order: Endomophthorales
    Genera: *Basidiobulus, Conidiobolus*
Class: Ascomycetes
  Order: Endomycetales
    Genera: *Saccharomyces, Pichia*
    Telomorphs of some *Candida* species
  Order: *Onygenales*
    Genera: *Arthroderma* (telomorphs of *Trichophyton* and *Microsporum* species)
    Ajellomyces (telomorphs of *Histoplasma* and *Blastomyces* species)
    Telomorphs of some *Aspergillus* and *Penicillium* species
Class: Deuteromycetes
  Order: Cryptococcales
    Genera: *Candida, Cryptococcus, Trichosporon, Pityrosporum*
  Order: Moniliales
    Family: Moniliaceae
    Genera: *Epidermophyton, Coccidioides, Paracoccidioides, Sporothrix, Aspergillus*
    Family: Dematiaceae
    Genera: *Phialophora, Fonsecaea, Exophiala, Wangiella, Xylohypha, Bipolaris, Alternaria*
  Order: Sphaeropsidales
    Genera: *Phoma*
Class: Oomycetes
  Genera: *Pythium*

mycosis refers to a mycosis that can be caused by any of the fungal species included in the Mucorales, not just to infections caused by the species *Mucor*. Most human zygomycoses are caused by fungi belonging to the order Mucorales.

The order Endomycetales (*endo*: "within"; *myces*: "fungus") includes those zygomycetes that produce only sexually, with the production of ascospores. The only medically significant member of this order is *Saccharomyces* species. The word *telomorph*, as used in Table 16-3, refers to the sexual form of a fungus. Most mycologists believe that every fungus has a sexual phase that may manifest if the correct environmental conditions and nutritional requirements are provided.

The class Basidiomycetes includes the mushrooms, which are only indirectly of medical importance because of the mycotoxins they produce. The term *basidio* is directly from the Latin, referring to a clublike organ in which spores are formed by both mitosis and meiosis, resulting in four spores called basidiospores.

The class Deuteromyces (Latin *deutero*: "second") refers to the "fungi imperfecti," that is, those fungi in which only an asexual phase of reproduction has been observed. Included are most species of fungi of medical importance. The subclass Blastomycetes (Gk., *blasto*: "budding") includes the order Cryptococcales (Gk., *kryptos*: "hidden" or "covered") or those fungi that are yeastlike throughout most of their life cycle. In contrast, the subclass Hyphomycetes (Gk., *hyphe*: "web") includes those fungi in which a mycelium is produced. The order Moniliales (L., *monile*: "necklace") includes those fungi imperfecti in which spores are borne directly off the hyphae (conidia) and not aggregated within fruiting bodies. This includes most of the important hyaline and dematiaceous molds. In older usage, the term *monilia* or *moniliasis* referred specifically to infections with *Candida* species, probably because early workers recognized the formation of pseudohyphae giving rise to blastoconidia. The archaic term *torula* (L., *torus*: "protuberance" or "bulge"), in contrast, referred to infections with cryptococci, which only formed buds ("bulges") and not pseudohyphae.

The order Sphaeropsidales (Gk., *sphairo*: "sphere") includes the single medically important genus *Phoma* (there are hundreds of species of Sphaeropsidales that inhabit and cause disease in plants). This order of fungi has the characteristic of forming large, spherical spore-bearing structures called pycnidia (Gk., *pykno*: "skin"). Pycnidia are asexually derived fruiting bodies and contain conidia, in contrast to the sexually derived cleistothecia and perithecia, which contain asci and ascospores. In practice, one can distinguish these in microscopic mounts by pressing down on the coverslip with the tip of a pencil to "pop open" the spherical fruiting body and looking to see if the single, spherical or elliptical conidia or the clusters of four or eight irregular shaped ascospores are released.

Identification of Fungal Cultures

The identification of an unknown fungal isolate recovered from a clinical specimen need not be difficult if a few preliminary observations are made. In most instances it is not difficult to distinguish the smooth, pasty to mucoid colony of a yeast growing on the surface of primary isolation media from the cottony or woolly presentation of a mold. The immediate task for the clinical microbiologist or mycologist when an unknown fungus is encountered is to determine the potential pathogenicity of the isolate. Every isolate must be considered potentially pathogenic; certain groups, including the dimorphic fungi, the dermatophytes, and some of the slow-growing dematiaceous molds, are almost always associated with disease when recovered from clinical specimens. Therefore, these fungi must be identified without fail and answers must be forthcoming as soon as possible so that antifungal therapy can be instituted.

Following are observations that may be helpful in making this initial decision:

Appearance of the growth. The dimorphic fungi and the dermatophytes in particular produce delicate hyphae, no more than 1 to 2 mm in diameter, which gives the mold form of the colonies a cobweb or hairlike appearance. Therefore, whenever delicate hyphae are observed, either visually or microscopically, the possibility of an obligate pathogen should be considered. The jet black reverse surface of a colony can be used to distinguish the dematiaceous group of fungi from their hyaline counterparts. This can be an important first step in making an identification. Certain fungi produce colonies that are characteristic of the genus.

Rate of growth. How quickly an unknown colony appears in primary isolation from clinical specimens may be of some help in making a preliminary identification. The saprobic molds that may on occasion cause opportunistic infections, generally produce mature colonies within 3 to 5 days, a rate of growth that is more rapid than the dimorphic fungi. In cases of heavy infections, however, when the concentration of organisms in tissues and secretions may be high, times of recovery for the dimorphic molds may be considerably shortened as well. Therefore, rapid rate of growth is merely a guide, not an absolute criterion.

Colony pigmentation. Many strains of the hyaline group of saprobic molds produce pigmented conidia that impart a brightly colored surface to the colony, ranging from pastel to dark green, blue, yellow, orange, and red. The more profuse the sporulation, the more granular or sugary the colony surface appears. Although the vegetative hyphae of certain strains of the dimorphic molds, particularly *Coccidioides immitis*, may appear lightly pigmented, the deeper, granular pigmentation of the colony surface rarely develops. Certain fungi produce water-soluble pigments that diffuse into the agar color the reverse of the colony. The wine-red diffusible pigment produced by *Trichophyton rubrum* is a helpful clue in making an identification.

Growth on media containing antifungal agents. Most strains of the dimorphic fungi can grow in the presence of antifungal agents, specifically on culture media containing cycloheximide. Most strains of the rapidly growing saprobes are inhibited.

Dimorphic growth. The dimorphic fungi are characterized by their unique capability of growing in two forms: (1) a mold form (the environmental and infective form) when incubated at ambient or room temperature (below 30°C) and (2) a yeast form (invasive form) when incubated at body temperature 30° to 35°C. The presumptive identification of a dimorphic mold that has been recovered at ambient temperature must be confirmed by demonstrating conversion to the yeast form when incubated at 35°C on appropriate culture media. This exercise is necessary because each of the dimorphic molds has a monomorphic saprobic look-alike (eg, *Sepodonium* species produce rough-walled macroconidia that appear similar to those of *Histoplasma capsulatum*; *Chrysosporium* species produce single-celled "lollipop" conidia similar to those of *Blastomyces dermatitidis*). Because yeast conversion may be difficult, particularly with some strains of *Histoplasma capsulatum*, exoantigen extraction or DNA probes, as previously mentioned, may be used to provide an early identification of a dimorphic mold.

Observation of other colony characteristics may provide an early clue to making a presumptive identification. Following are guidelines:

1. A white or gray-brown, woolly or cottony mold that grows from border to border in the Petri dish without producing a colony margin is characteristic of one of the Zygomycetes. Growth is sometimes so profuse that the name "lid lifter" has been applied to this group of fungi.

2. A mold that grows from border to border in the Petri dish in the form of a green or green-yellow lawn is typical of *Trichoderma* species or *Gliocladium* species.

3. A hyaline mold that produces a distinctive rose-red, lavender, or red-purple diffusable pigment is highly suggestive of *Fusarium* species.

4. A hyaline mold that produces a cottony colony with a house mouse gray surface is highly suggestive of *Pseudallescheria boydii* (specifically, the anamorph *Scedosporium apiospermum*).

5. A hyaline mold producing a marginated colony with a blue-green, granular surface surrounded by a white apron is suggestive of *Penicillium* species or *Aspergillus fumigatus*.

6. A dematiaceous mold producing a play of colors, ranging through hues of red, yellow, black, and white is suggestive of *Epicoccum* species.

7. A dematiaceous mold that grows very slowly, producing a small, button-like colony with a delicate hairlike surface, is suggestive of *Cladosporium carrioni*, *Phialophora* species, or *Fonsecaea* species.

8. A black yeast is most suggestive of *Aureobasidium pullulans* Young colonies of *Exophiala* species, *Wangiella* species, and *Sporothrix schenckii* may also present as black yeasts.

9. A yeast colony that is distinctly mucoid indicates the presence of capsular material and is suggestive of *Cryptococcus* species. An orange pigmented yeast (that may also appear mucoid) is suggestive of *Rhodotorula* species.

10. A slower growing colony that appears to have both mold and yeast components or has a prickly appearance suggests one of the dimorphic molds.

With experience, microbiologists and mycologists begin to learn the colonial presentations of the various yeasts and molds that are endemic in any given locale. Because colonial characteristics may vary depending on the environmental conditions, the culture media used, and the strain differences, microscopic confirmation is obviously necessary before a final report can be issued.

Identification of Filamentous Molds

PREPARATION OF MOUNTS FOR STUDY. The tease mount, the Scotch tape preparation, and the microslide technique are three commonly used methods for the microscopic examination of filamentous molds. In each instance a portion of the mold colony is mounted in a drop of lactophenol aniline (cotton) blue stain or calcofluor white reagent on a microscope slide. A coverslip is positioned over the drop and gently pressed to disperse the sample more evenly throughout the mounting fluid to facilitate microscopic examination. Following are brief descriptions of each type of mount.

The Tease Mount. A small portion of the colony to be examined is removed from the agar and transferred to a glass slide in the center of a drop of lactophenol aniline blue stain. The mount is teased apart with a pair of dissection needles, overlaid with a coverslip, and examined microscopically.

Transparency Tape Preparation. The cellophane tape method of preparing cultures for microscopic examination is often helpful because the spore arrangements of the more delicate filamentous molds are better preserved. Unfrosted, clear cellophane tape is used and the sticky side is pressed gently but firmly to the surface of the colony, picking up a portion of the aerial mycelium. This operation should always be performed under a biologic safety hood. A drop of lactophenol aniline blue stain or calcofluor white reagent is placed on a microscope slide. One end of the tape is stuck to the surface of the slide adjacent to the drop of stain. Then the tape is stretched over the stain, gently lowering it so that the mycelium becomes permeated with stain. The opposite end is then stuck to the glass, avoiding as much as possible the trapping of air bubbles. Examine microscopically.

The Microslide (Slide Culture) Technique. In instances when neither the tease mount nor the cellophane tape preparations establish an accurate identification or when permanent slide mounts are desired for further study or for use of student study, the microslide culture technique is recommended. A round piece of filter paper or gauze is place into the bottom of a sterile Petri dish and saturated with sterile water. Thin glass rods or applicator sticks are cut to length to fit on top of the filter paper. A clean glass slide is placed on these supports. A 1-cm square block of cornmeal or potato dextrose agar is placed onto the surface of the microscope slide. Each corner of the block is inoculated with a small portion of the colony to be studied, using a straight inoculating wire or the tip of a dissecting needle.

A coverslip is gently heated by passing it quickly through the flame of a Bunsen burner and then it is immediately placed directly on the surface of the inoculated agar block. The lid is placed on the Petri dish and the assembly is incubated at room temperature (or 30°C) for 3 to 5 days. When growth visually appears to be mature, the coverslip is gently lifted from the surface of the agar with a pair of forceps and placed over a drop of lactophenol aniline blue dye on a separate glass slide. The slide is then examined microscopically. The mount can be preserved for future study by rimming the outside margins of the coverslip with mounting fluid or clear nail polish.

DEFINITION OF TERMS USEFUL IN THE IDENTIFICATION OF FUNGI. The fundamental microscopic unit of a fungus is the threadlike structure called a *hypha*. Several hyphae combine to form the mat of growth known as the *mycelium*. Hyphae that are subdivided into individual cells by transverse walls or septa are called *septate*; those without walls are *aseptate*. The portion of the mycelium that extends into the substratum of the culture medium and is responsible for absorbing water and nutrients is the *vegetative mycelium*; the portion that projects above the substrate is the *aerial mycelium* and is also called the *reproductive mycelium* since special spore or conidia-bearing fruiting bodies are produced from this portion. The identification and classification of fungi is primarily based on the morphologic differences in reproductive structures and the manner in which spores or conidia are formed from specialized cells called *conidiogenous cells*.

Three general types of reproduction are commonly observed in the fungal species of medical importance: vegetative sporulation, aerial sporulation, and sexual sporulation.

Vegetative Reproduction. Three types of spores or conidia may form directly from the vegetative mycelium: *blastoconidia*, *chlamydoconidia*, and *arthroconidia*. The term *spore* should be reserved only for those reproductive elements that arise from meiosis (sexual reproduction) such as ascospores, oospores, or zygospores or from mitosis (asexual reproduction) within a sporangium (as with the

Zygomycetes). All other asexual "spores" are conidia. Therefore, the terms *blastoconidia* and *arthroconidia* are correct; the designations blastospores and arthrospores are incorrect. Although chlamydoconidia is the correct terminology, the common usage, chlamydospores is retained in most circles. Blastoconidia are the familiar budding forms characteristically produced by yeasts. A bud scar (dysjuncter) often remains at the point where the conidium becomes detached. Chlamydoconidia (chlamydospores) are formed from preexistent cells in the hyphae, which become thickened and often enlarged. Chlamydoconidia may be found within (intercalary), along the side (sessile), or at the tip (terminal) of the hyphae. This type of conidiation is characteristic of *Candida albicans*. Arthroconidia are also formed from preexistent cells in the vegetative hyphae, which become enlarged and thickened. On maturity, these conidia are released by lysis of adjacent hyphal cells. This type of sporulation is characteristic of the mold form of *Coccidioides immitis* and *Geotrichum* species, among others.

Aerial Reproduction. Emanating from the hyphae and extending from the mycelial surface are specialized fruiting bodies that give rise to a variety of spores or conidia. Fruiting bodies may form closed sacs called *sporangia*, within which spores called *sporangiospores* are produced. The specialized hyphal segment that holds up or supports the sporangium is called the *sporangiophore* (the suffix "phore" [Gk., *phoros*] means "bearing"). This type of sporulation is characteristic of the Zygomycetes. Many other fungi produce elaborate fruiting bodies that give rise to conidia. The specialized hyphal segment that supports a conidia-bearing fruiting head is called a *conidiophore*. The conidiophore may branch into secondary segments, called *phialides*, which in turn produce the conidia. A phialide by definition is a conidiogenous cell that produces conidia from a locus inside its apex, which does not increase in width or length during conidiogenesis (in contrast to an annellide, which increases in length and may constrict as conidia are formed, leaving a succession of scars or rings). This property of branching into phialides is characteristic of the finger-like fruiting body of *Penicillium* species. Conidia may be borne singly, in long chains, or in tightly bound clusters. Tiny one-celled conidia, usually borne either directly from the sides of the hyphae or supported by a hairlike conidiophore, are called *microconidia*, in contrast to the much larger, multicellular *macroconidia*.

When conidia form in chains, those that are formed at the apex of a chain are known as *acropetal* and those forming at the base of a chain are *basipetal*.

Sexual (Perfect) Sporulation. Sexual sporulation requires the merging and nuclear recombination of two specialized fertile cells (each having undergone meiosis) arising on the aerial hyphae. If the reproductive cells that fuse are identical and arise from the same hyphae (homothallic), the spore that forms is called a *zygospore*. This mode of sporulation is seen in the Zygomycetes. If the fusing reproductive cells are derived from two different cells, often derived from separate hyphal segments, the resulting spore is called an *oospore*. The sexual spores of several members of the class Ascomycetes, previously mentioned, which are of medical importance, are called *ascospores*. The sexual form of a fungus is known as a *telomorph*, in contrast to the term *anamorph*, which refers to the various asexual reproductive form or structure produced by an imperfect fungus (eg, phialides, annellides, branching chains). Thus, for example, *Pseudallescheria boydii* is the telomorph of this species, and various "perfect" forms such as cleistothecia, asci, and ascospores may be observed. *Scedosporium monosporium* is the imperfect form of this species, producing primarily single-celled conidia as the chief anamorphic (imperfect) structure.

LABORATORY IDENTIFICATION OF MEDICALLY IMPORTANT FUNGI AND CLINICAL CORRELATION

A full description of the morphologic features by which each of the 75 or so medically important fungi can be differentiated is given elsewhere.[40] Several color reproductions depicting the colonial morphology of these fungi are presented in a series of color plates. To present the microscopic morphology here, the eight black and white composite photographs together with the accompanying legends are included. Following is a brief review of the microscopic features of the fungi included in each of these composites, together with a summary of the important clinical infections caused by these agents.

Zygomycetes

The colonies grow very rapidly, forming a white to gray-brown cottony aerial mycelium that soon fills the Petri dish. Microscopically, this group of fungi is characterized by the production of broad, aseptate hyphae and the bearing of spores in closed sacks called sporangia.

Rhizopus and *Mucor* species are the two most frequent isolates from clinical specimens. They can be differentiated because *Rhizopus* species form rootlike structures called rhizoids and *Mucor* species are devoid of rhizoids. *Absidia*, *Syncephalastrum*, *Circinella*, and *Cunninghammella* species are other genera within this group that rarely cause human infections. (See Composite 16-1 for photomicrographs depicting the differential features of this group of fungi.)

Rhinocerebral, pulmonary, cutaneous, and disseminated forms of disease are most commonly encountered with the Zygomycetes. Patients with diabetes, particularly during periods of acidosis, are particularly at risk for developing invasive rhinocerebral infection, with the real danger of developing invasive meningitis and encephalitis by direct invasion from the primary infection in the sinus. The propensity for the hyphae to invade blood vessels, causing thrombosis and infarction, tends to give the infected tissues a red-black, hemorrhagic appearance.

Aspergillus

Aspergillus species can be suspected in culture if a rapidly growing (3 to 5 days), usually yellow, yellow-green, yellow-brown, or green, granular colony with a distinct margin and a white peripheral apron is observed on an agar plate containing fungal culture medium. Microscopically, *Aspergillus* species are characterized by the production of uniform, 4- to 6-μm, hyaline, septate hyphae with parallel walls. Conidiation occurs through a specialized fruiting body composed of a swollen vesicle situated at the terminus of a conidiophore, from the surface of which are borne one or two rows of phialides, giving rise to chains of pigmented conidia (see Composite 16-2*A*). The length and width of the conidiophores, the size and contour of the vesicle, the arrangement of the phialides, and the color, size, and length of chains of the conidia are the structures used in making species identifications.[54]

Four species are recovered with any frequency from hospitalized patients: *Aspergillus fumigatus* (the species causing most allergic pulmonary and invasive diseases), *Aspergillus flavus*, *Aspergillus niger*, and *Aspergillus terreus*. The differential features are described in Composite 16-2. Clinically, aspergillosis may present as well-defined clinical syndromes involving a variety of sites and organ systems: pulmonary,[14] disseminated,[55,56] central nervous system,[8,70,73] cutaneous,[6] endocardial,[11] and nasoorbital.[13,47,72] Pulmonary aspergillosis can be further divided into allergic bronchopulmonary,[41,62] colonizing (fungus ball),[51,55,56] and invasive forms.[14,76] The propensity for the hyphae to invade into blood vessels in deep-seated infections results in mycotic thrombi with a propensity of the disease to disseminate to multiple distant organs.

Agents of Hyalohyphomycosis

Ajello[2,3] has suggested that infections caused by a variety of unrelated hyaline Hyphomycetes be categorized under the general umbrella "hyalohyphomycosis." Hundreds of recognized species of hyaline saprobes exist in nature; only a few are encountered with any frequency in clinical laboratories. Of these, only isolated cases of human infections have been reported. Following is a list of the hyaline hyphomycetes most commonly encountered in clinical laboratories:

Hyaline Hyphomycetes Forming Conidia in Chains
Aspergillus species
Penicillium species
Paecilomyces species
Scopulariopsis species

Hyaline Hyphomycetes Forming Conidia in Clusters
Gliocladium species
Trichoderma species
Acremonium species
Fusarium species

Hyaline Hyphomycetes Forming Conidia Borne Singly
Beauveria species
Pseudallescheria boydii (*Scedosporium apiospermum*)
Chrysosporium species

Colonies of the hyaline Hyphomycetes typically mature within 3 to 5 days on culture media free of antifungal agents. Most colonies have distinct margins except for *Gliocladium* species and *Trichoderma* species, which tend to grow from rim to rim in the Petri dish as a green or yellow lawn. As the colonies mature and sporulation takes place, the surface of the colonies become sugary, powdery, or granular. The colonies of *Penicillium* species and *Paecilomyces* species are generally various shades of green, although yellow and yellow-brown variants are encountered. *Scopulariopsis* species produce a yellow-brown, granular, radially rugose colony. *Acremonium* species produce colonies that in general are less woolly and granular but glabrous, owing to the production of a very delicate mycelium. Colonies may be white or various shades of light green and yellow. Colonies that have a distinct lavender, rose-red, or magenta surface pigmentation point immediately to *Fusarium* species. *Beauvaria* species usually produce delicate, cottony, white colonies. *Pseudallescheria boydii* (*Scedosporium apiospermum* is the name of the asexual anamorph) also has a distinct colony characterized by a mouse-gray, silky surface on which tiny water droplets tend to aggregate.

The microscopic morphology of these hyaline fungi is described in Composite 16-3. As indicated by the previous list, conidia form either in long chains, in clusters, or singly from a variety of distinctive conidiophores. The hyphae are clear (hyaline) and distinctly septate.

Several literature reports of infections with the Hyphomycete group of fungi have been cited by Rippon[56] and by Rogers and Kennedy.[57] Five cases of penicilliosis caused by *Penicillium marneffei* were reported from Thailand in patients with a variety of underlying disorders, including tuberculosis, lupus erythematosus, and lymphoreticular neoplasms.[28] Infections with *Penicillium* species have also been reported in patients with AIDS[4,27,53] and in a patient with osteomyelitis.[10] Vajpayee and colleagues[71] found *Fusarium* species to be the most common cause of mycotic keratitis among 156 patients with mycotic corneal ulcer disease, most commonly complicating allergic conjunctivitis and a combination of antibiotic and corticosteroid therapy. *Scedosporium apiospermum* (telomorph *Pseudallescheria boydii*) has been incriminated in cases of subcutaneous mycetomas and involved in a variety of infections, including pulmonary infections, sinusitis, fungus ball infections, meningitis, osteomyelitis, endocarditis, mycotic keratitis, endophthalmitis, and otomycosis.[56]

Agents of Chromomycosis, Eumycotic Mycetomas, and Phaeohyphomycosis

Ajello[2,3] coined the term *phaeohyphomycosis* to include infections caused by a diverse group of rapidly growing, dark, dematiaceous molds.[44] Phaeohyphomycosis is to be distinguished from chromomycosis and eumycotic mycetoma, which are caused by the slower growing dematiaceous molds. Following is a genus and species list of commonly encountered agents for these diseases:

Agents of Chromomycosis and Mycetoma
Phialophora verrucosum
Cladosporium carrioni
Fonsecaea pedrosi
Fonsecaea compacta
Exophiala jeanselmei
Wangiella dermatitidis

Agents of Phaeohyphomycosis
Alternaria species
Aureobasidium pullulans
Bipolaris species (formerly mistakenly called *Drechslera* species)
Cladosporium species
Curvularia species
Exophiala jeanselmei
Exserohilum species
Phaeoannellomyces species
Phoma species
Xylohypha emmonsii

The dematiaceous fungi can be suspected in culture by observing the dark gray, brown, or black, woolly, hairy, or velvety surface colonies that have a black pigmentation on the reverse. Although it may no longer be appropriate to subdivide the dematiaceous fungi into "pathogenic" and "saprobic" groups, the agents causing classic cases of chromoblastomycosis, namely *Cladosporium carionii*, *Phialophora verrucosum*, and *Fonsecaea pedrosi*, grow more slowly than several more rapidly growing molds that are commonly recovered as environmental contaminants in clinical laboratories but that can on occasion cause phaeohyphomycosis.

Microscopically, the dematiaceous molds are characterized by a dark yellow-brown mycelium composed of uniform hyphae with parallel walls and distinct septations. The various genera and species are identified based on morphologic differences in fruiting bodies and conidiation. Photomicrographs of select species are shown in Composite 16-4.

Chromoblastomycosis was the term originally used to describe a cutaneous and subcutaneous infection characterized by the formation of elevated, roughened verrucoid vegetations, most commonly spreading over the dorsal surfaces of the feet and lower legs. This infection is caused by a group of slow-growing, dematiaceous fungi belonging to the genera *Phialophora*, *Cladosporium*, and *Fonseceae*. These agents gain entrance to the skin through traumatic wounds and penetrating injuries. Dematiaceous hyphal elements may be seen in the tissues; more diagnostic is the presence of muriform, light yellow-staining yeast bodies grouped in clusters or in short chains known as "Medlar bodies" or "copper pennies" (Composite 16-5*F*). Microabscesses, granulomatous nodules, extreme acanthosis, and pseudoepitheliomatous hyperplasia with varying degrees of fibrosis and scarring are the common histologic changes. Local spread of the infection is common, and prognosis for complete cure is poor. Combinations of heat treatment (pocket warmers) and a regimen of 5-fluorocytosine have been efficacious.[66]

Mycetoma refers to subcutaneous infections in which the tissue is markedly swollen with the formation of deeply penetrating sinus tracts that break through the superficial skin and discharge purulent material. The feet (Madura foot) and hands are most commonly involved, becoming markedly swollen and deformed in serious infections. Mycetomas have two primary causes: those caused by bacteria belonging to the family *Actinomycetes* (*Actinomyces*, *Nocardia*, and *Streptomyces* species) and the true fungi (eumycotic mycetomas), primarily caused by the dematiaceous fungus *Exophiala jeanselmei* and the hyaline mold *Pseudallescheria boydii* in sporadic cases encountered in the United States. Suppurating abscesses, purulent draining sinus tracts, and varying degrees of granulomatous inflammation are seen histologically. Often white, gray, brown, or yellow "grains" or granules ("sulfur granules") including necrotic debris admixed with either branching filamentous bacteria (actinomycotic mycetomas) or true hyphal elements, which are usually clubbed or swollen at their tips.

Phaeohyphomycosis is the accepted clinical designation for a variety of superficial, cutaneous, subcutaneous, and systemic fungal infections caused by several species of dematiaceous saprobic fungi.[44,45] Rippon[56] has divided the clinical spectrum of phaeohyphomycosis into superficial, cutaneous, mycotic keratitis, subcutaneous, and invasive or systemic forms of infection. The superficial infections include black piedra, caused by *Piedraia hortae*, and tinea nigra, caused by *Phaeoannellomyces* (formerly *Cladosporium*) *wernickii*. Onychomycosis is the most common form of cutaneous phaeohyphomycosis. Central nervous system phaeohyphomycosis in the form of cerebral abscesses has been caused by *Cladosporium trichoides* (*Xylohypha bantiana*).[17]

The Dermatophytes

The dermatophytes are a distinct group of fungi that infect the skin, hair, and nails of humans and animals, producing a variety of cutaneous infections, colloquially known as "ringworm." Although more than 30 species of dermatophytes are described, the following six cause the majority of human dermatophyte infections in the United States:

Microsporum canis
Microsporum gypseum
Trichophyton mentagrophytes
Trichophyton rubrum
Trichophyton tonsurans
Epidermophyton floccosum

Any mold recovered in culture from specimens labeled skin, nail, or hair should be suspected of being one of the dermatophyte species. One must be alert, however, that other pathogenic fungi, including the dimorphic molds, can also involve the skin and in early culture may have microscopic features similar to the dermatophytes. Making a misidentification could have adverse consequences. Typical hyphal segments in direct KOH mounts of skin scales and either ectothrix or endothrix invasion of infected hairs are helpful preliminary findings. A few colony characteristics, when present, may be helpful in identifying a given species. The colonies of *Epidermophyton floccosum* growing on Sabouraud's dextrose or Mycosel agars are typically khaki or green-yellow and have a low aerial mycelium, giving a "suede" appearance to the surface. Gentle folds are usually seen. *Microsporum canis* is cottony or woolly and may be suspected when a lemon-yellow pigmentation around the growing periphery or the reverse of the colony is observed. *M. gypseum* typically sporulates heavily, imparting a sugary, granular surface that is cinnamon brown to buff. *Trichophyton rubrum* generally produces a deep, water-soluble burgundy-red pigment that diffuses into the agar, particularly when grown on potato dextrose or cornmeal agars. *T. mentagrophytes* can also form a similar pigment; it is usually less intense than *T. rubrum* and is usually minimally evident on potato dextrose and cornmeal agars. *T. mentagrophytes* produces a variety of colonial variants; only two basic patterns are generally recognized: fluffy and granular.

Microscopically, the dermatophytes produce delicate, narrow, hyaline, septate hyphae. The three genera are morphologically separated by the relative production of macroconidia and microconidia: *Microsporum* species is characterized by the production of roughened, thick-walled macroconidia and few or absent microconidia; the genus *Trichophyton* produces many microconidia but few or absent thin-walled, pencil-shaped, multicelled macroconidia and *Epidermophyton floccosum* produces only three- or four-celled, smooth-walled macroconidia in clusters of two or three, and no microconidia. These structures are illustrated in Composite 16-6.

A commonly encountered superficial infection of the skin is tinea (pityriasis) versicolor caused by *Malassezia furfur*, a lyophilic yeast that is a commensal of normal skin. The organism proliferates during times of poor hygiene when washing and bathing are not possible for prolonged periods, owing to the accumulation of sebum and skin oils. The infection is manifest early on by irregular patches of apigmented or untanned skin, particularly noticeable on exposure to sunlight. Intermittent areas of scaling with variegated hues varying between light yellow and dark brown may be observed as the infection progresses, accounting for the term *versicolor*. Folliculitis may be seen in more severe cases where the infection extends into the hair shafts and sebaceous glands. The skin of the chest, back, and upper arms is most commonly involved. Irritation and inflammation are usually absent; mild pruritus may be experienced in some cases.

The diagnosis can usually be readily established by directly observing the skin for a characteristic yellow fluorescence when viewed with a Wood's lamp or by microscopically observing for tight clusters of spherical yeast cells admixed with hyphal fragments (a picture colloquially known as "spaghetti and meatballs") in KOH or lactophenol aniline or methylene blue-stained preparations made from superficial skin scrapings taken from areas of involvement. The organism can be recovered in culture on Sabouraud's dextrose agar that has been overlain with long-chain fatty acid, such as contained in olive oil. Yeastlike creamy colonies develop slowly after 2 to 4 days of incubation at 30°C (growth at 25°C does not occur). Microscopically, 12 by 24 μm in diameter, broadly budding yeast cells are observed, which are described as being bottle shaped, with a collarette-like thickening seen at the junction of the mother and daughter cells.

Several cases of *Malassezia furfur* and *M. pachydermatis* systemic infections and septicemia have been reported, most commonly associated with deep-line vascular catheters in patients receiving parenteral therapy.[22,43,63] Many of the emulsions used for parenteral therapy are rich in long-chain fatty acids. An ideal microenvironment is established at the catheter site where a small amount of the oily emulsion can pool, supporting growth of the endogenous lipophilic organisms present on the skin surface. The catheter provides a barrier break in the skin through which the proliferating organisms can enter the bloodstream.

The Dimorphic Molds

Dimorphism refers to the ability of certain species of fungi to grow in two forms, depending on the environmental conditions: (1) as a mold when growing or incubated at 25° to 30°C and (2) as a yeast when incubated at 35° to 37°C. The mold form is the infective form, and humans contract disease by inhaling airborne spores or by having direct penetration of skin or mucous membranes with soil contaminated with environmental conidia. Infection in organs and tissues is produced by the yeast form. Following are the dimorphic fungi that are responsible for specific mycotic diseases:

Blastomyces dermatitidis
Histoplasma capsulatum
Coccidioides immitis
Sporothrix schenckii
Paracoccidioides brasiliensis

One of the dimorphic fungi may be suspected in culture if (1) it is slow growing, usually requiring 7 to 14 days in primary isolation (although in heavy infections, growth may be as soon as 3 to 5 days); (2) growth is not inhibited by culture media containing cycloheximide; (3) the colonies have hairlike or cobweb-like texture; (4) the hyphae appear thin and arranged in parallel, ropelike masses when examined microscopically; and (5) conversion from the mold to the yeast form can be demonstrated or the exoantigen test reveals a specific precipitin.

The differential microscopic morphologic features, both for the yeast form and the mold form, are illustrated in Composite 16-7. An isolate of one of the dimorphic fungi can be suspected if extremely narrow, hyaline, septate hyphae are observed (the reason why the colonies have a hairlike or cobweb appearance).

A brief review of the clinical manifestations of the infections caused by the five dimorphic fungi follows. Infections almost always begin in the lungs as the primary pulmonary form of the disease, which occasionally may be progressive and severe but most commonly resolves spontaneously after a brief flulike syndrome. Dry cough, low-grade fever, and myalgia may be presenting features early in acute infections. Persistent localized chest pain, weight loss, night sweats, and malaise may indicate progression into a chronic form of disease. Multiple organ systems may be involved in disseminated disease, which in rare instances may assume a rapidly fatal course. Even in disseminated cases, recovery of yeast forms from blood cultures is extremely rare, except for *Histoplasma capsulatum* in patients with AIDS when blood cultures are not infrequently positive.[50]

Blastomycosis

Blastomycosis is caused by the dimorphic mold *Blastomyces dermatitidis*, a natural inhabitant of moist, warm soil. Most cases in the United States occur sporadically in regions around the Great Lakes, adjacent to the upper Mississippi river and its tributaries, and in the Southeast. Endemic regions are also located in southern Canada.[31] Inhalation of conidia from infected soil probably represents the mode of human infection. A soil of high organic or humus content (60% to 70%), an alkaline *p*H, and critical concentrations of moisture from recent rains, dew, or mist are the conditions optimal for recovery of the organism from dirt, wood, or other environmental sources. The tissue (incubator) form of the organism is the large broad-based budding yeast cell; the mold form features single elliptical conidia, each supported by a delicate conidiophore ("lollipops"). Skin or mucous membrane involvement usually indicates systemic disease and in many instances may be the initial lesions. Blastomycosis should be considered in the differential diagnosis of any patient with nonhealing skin lesions associated with risk factors such as living in an endemic area and having an occupation or vocation involving frequent contact with soil.[74]

Histoplasmosis

Histoplasmosis, caused by the dimorphic fungus *Histoplasma capsulatum*, is the most common systemic fungal disease in the United States. The mycelial form is present in warm, moist soil rich in organic content, particularly where there are heavy accumulations of bird or bat excreta. Bird roosts, chicken houses, caves, or old buildings frequented by bats are potentially highly infective areas. Disruption of these areas by bulldozing or clean-up efforts may expose humans to large numbers of airborne spores. The major endemic areas in the United States are the drainage basins of the Ohio, Mississippi, and Missouri River valleys.

Most cases of histoplasmosis resolve after an acute pulmonary illness of varying degrees of severity, characterized by fever, headache, chills, cough, and chest pain. Underlying pneumonia and enlargement of the mediastinal lymph nodes often occur. In less than 1% of cases, a chronic pulmonary form may develop, characterized by persistent cough, low-grade fever, and occasional episodes of hemoptysis. Cavitary lesions may develop in adults; or, one or more thick, laminated, calcified "histoplasmomas" may be seen on a roentgenogram. Mediastinal granuloma formation followed by fibrosing mediastinitis and esophagitis are rare complications.

Because *H. capsulatum* is an obligate intracellular organism residing in macrophages of the reticuloendothelial system, varying degrees of hepatomegaly, splenomegaly, and lymphadenopathy may be seen in cases of acute and chronic disseminated disease, which usually occurs in immunosuppressed hosts. Of concern is the increased incidence of histoplasmosis in patients with AIDS.[29,30] The production of large, roughened or spiked macroconidia is the key identifying feature of the mold form. Regular sized, 2- to 4-μm in diameter yeast cells are characteristic of the yeast form.

Coccidioidomycosis

Coccidioides immitis, the causative agent of coccidioidomycosis, is endemic in hot, dry, alkaline soil in the lower Sonoran, western, and southwestern desert regions of the United States. The arthroconidia that develop from the mycelial form of the fungus mature under the intense heat of the subsurface desert sand and easily become windborne. These conidia, being small and light, are highly infectious for humans, resulting in primary pulmonary disease when inhaled.

The microscopic observation of delicate hyphae that break up into alternately staining arthroconidia is sufficient to suspect *C. immitis*. Typically, mature arthroconidia are thick-walled and barrel shaped and appear alternate-staining owing to empty cells between adjacent cells (see Composite 16-7). The diagnostic "yeast" form are spherules ranging from 10 to 200 μm, enclosing uniform three to four endospores, seen only in tissue sections.

The clinical manifestations of coccidioidomycosis and progression of disease differ in patients who are immunocompetent and in persons with AIDS. Most primary infections are of the classic disease and are confined to the lungs and self-limited. Sixty percent of infected persons are asymptomatic; many patients with positive skin tests do not remember having symptoms. Those who are symptomatic experience an acute, short-term flulike, lower respiratory tract infection with varying degrees of cough, sputum production, chest pain, fever, and arthralgia. Only 2% of infected persons ultimately develop chronic pulmonary disease with sequelae. Solitary "coin lesions" or granulomas that may cavitate, usually located peripherally within the lung parenchyma, are common residual findings in previously infected persons, particularly those not living in endemic areas.

Sporotrichosis

Sporotrichosis, caused by the dimorphic fungus *Sporothrix schenckii*, is primarily a subcutaneous mycosis found worldwide. The disease is most prevalent in the midwestern United States, particularly in the states bordering the Missouri and Mississippi River valleys. The mycelial form of the fungus from which the infective conidia are produced resides in the soil and lives on plants and plant debris. Sporotrichosis has also been known as the rose gardener's disease because the primary lesion often presents as a nonhealing ulcer of the skin of the fingers, hands, forearm, or feet that develops 1 or 2 weeks after skin puncture by an infected rose thorn or other contaminated vegetation.

Microscopically, small, one-celled, round or oval microconidia (3 to 6 μm in diameter) develop laterally along the hyphae in a sleevelike pattern. The arrangement of the conidia in flowerettes atop a long, slender conidiophore, simulating daisy petals, may be seen in the mature colony (see Composite 16-7G). By focusing up and down with the microscope and using an oil immersion objective, the characteristic hairlike attachments between the conidia and the conidiophore (from which the species name is derived) can be observed. The yeast forms of *S. schenckii* are 2 to 4 μm and tend to be oval or elliptical, often with a single bud. Most helpful in making the microscopic identification of *S. schenckii* yeast cells is the observation of cigar-shaped forms measuring 3 to 10 μm (see Composite 16-7H).

Clinically, the appearance of a small, red, painless pustule on an extremity together with multiple, linearly placed secondary pustular or ulcerating lesions along the proximal lymphatics is sufficient to suspect sporotrichosis. The primary pustule may slowly enlarge, ulcerate, and discharge a small amount of serosanguineous exudate. Varying degrees of cellulitis with swelling and redness of the surrounding subcutaneous tissue may be observed. The secondary satellite lesions present initially as verrucous, erythematoid plaques or scaly patches, often developing into ulcers that also exude purulent material.

Paracoccidioidomycosis

The dimorphic fungus *Paracoccidioides brasiliensis* causes South American blastomycosis, a subacute and chronic progressive infectious disease that begins in the lungs and disseminates to other organs. The disease is limited to areas of Latin America, including southern Mexico, Brazil, and Argentina, excluding countries such as San Salvador and Chile. The disease most frequently involves adults older than 30 years of age and occurs more often in men than women in a ratio of 15:1. Agricultural workers in particular are susceptible to infection.

Microscopically, delicate hyphae are noted, on which the characteristic singly borne, oval, 2- to 3-μm conidia are borne in a "lollipop" fashion, similar in appearance to those of *Blastomyces dermatitidis*. Conversion to the yeast form is slow. The yeast cells of *P. brasiliensis* are 6 to 15 μm in diameter and also similar to those of *B. dermatitidis*; in contrast, they produce multiple buds from the outer circumference (known as "mariner's wheel").

Yeasts: Clinical Diseases and Laboratory Identification

One approach to the identification of yeast isolates is shown in Figure 16-2. Most yeasts grow well on routine blood agar isolation plates, and special fungal media are not required. The colonies generally are entire, slightly domed or flat, and smooth and buttery or roughened and pasty as the colony matures. An aerial mycelium does not develop, although spider-like extensions may radiate from the periphery of the colony in some cases. If a distinct aerial mycelium is observed, the possibility of a dimorphic fungus must be considered. A colony with a mucoid appearance and consistency suggests capsule formation and may provide an initial clue to the identification of *Cryptococcus neoformans*.

The first step in the identification of an unknown yeast isolate is to perform a germ tube test. A germ tube is defined as a filamentous extension from a yeast cell that is about one half the width and three to four times the length of the cell (Fig. 16-3). If present, the presumptive identification of *Candida albicans* can be made. If germ tubes are not observed, a report "*Candida* not *C. albicans*" may be issued; one must realize, however, that about 5% of *C. albicans* are germ tube–negative.[69] False-negative results may also occur if too heavy an inoculum

of yeast cells is used. Again, if a definitive identification is clinically indicated, further testing must be done. Christensen's urea agar slant (or one of the rapid urease tests) should be performed. *Cryptococcus neoformans* can be presumptively identified since it quickly converts urea agar to a pink color.

A portion of the unknown colony should be inoculated to a cornmeal agar plate. After 24 to 48 hours of incubation, the cornmeal preparations should be examined for the presence of hyphae, blastoconidia, chlamydoconidia, or arthroconidia. The cornmeal morphology of several species of yeasts is shown in Composite 16-8. If hyphae are present, it should first be determined whether they are pseudohyphae, resulting from the pinching off process of blastoconidiation (and therefore have regular points of constriction) or whether they are true hyphae breaking up into arthroconidia. If the cornmeal growth reveals pseudohyphae and blastoconidia, the unknown yeast belongs to the genus *Candida*. It may be possible in many instances to make a species identification based on the morphology and specific arrangement of the blastoconidia. The production of chlamydospores is diagnostic of *C. albicans* (see Composite 16-8*A*). *C. albicans* may also be tentatively identified if compact clusters of blastoconidia are formed at regular intervals along the pseudohyphae (see Composite 16-8*B*). Smaller numbers of blastoconidia, widely spaced singly or in small clusters along the hyphae, are more consistent with *C. tropicalis* (see Composite 16-8*C*). The formation of spider or "matchstick" colonies that satellite along the streak lines is suggestive of *C. parapsilosis* (see Composite 16-8*D*); certain strains may also produce giant hyphae (see Composite 16-8*E*). A "long-in-stream" arrangement of the blastoconidia leads to a presumptive identification of *C. pseudotropicalis* (see Composite 16-8*F*).

If the previously discussed procedures do not establish the identification of an unknown yeast isolate, carbohydrate assimilation tests may be required for final species identification. Carbohydrate assimilation tests measure the ability of different species of yeasts to assimilate and grow in various single carbohydrate substrates. The auxotrophic test, utilizing carbohydrate-free yeast nitrogen base and dried filter paper disks previously saturated with 1% carbohydrate solutions, is the least expensive to perform. Alternatively, several commercial yeast identification kits and semiauto-

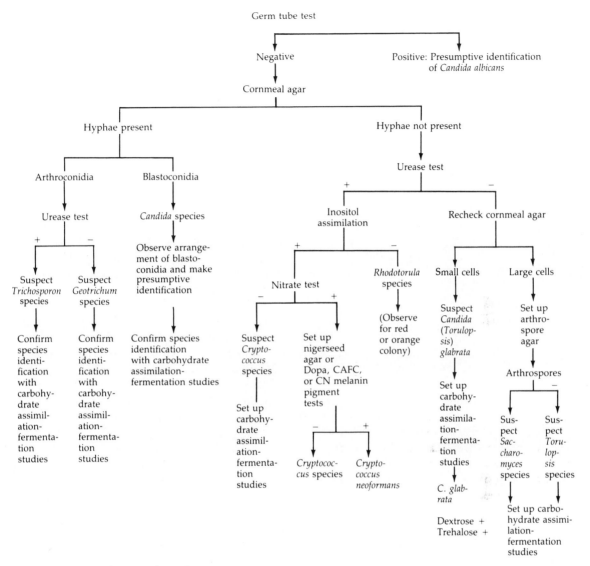

Figure 16-2. Identification schema for common yeasts.

mated instruments are available. These are more costly but have the advantage of providing a large data base by which identifications can be compared with results from other laboratories where a similar system is being used. Characteristics required for the identification of medically important yeasts are included in most current textbooks and will not be reproduced here.

The infectious disease manifestations of yeast infections are varied. *Candida albicans* produces three primary types of diseases: mucocutaneous, cutaneous, and systemic. Candidiasis of the mucous membranes may involve the oral cavity (a condition known as thrush), the vaginal canal, the trachea and bronchi, and the alimentary canal, manifesting as esophagitis, gastritis, or enteric and perianal disease.[23] Infections of the skin commonly involve the moist, intertriginous areas such as in the webs of the fingers and toes, beneath the female breasts, in the axillae, and in the folds of the groin. Infection of the nails is known as onychomycosis or as paronychia if the folds of skin encasing the nails are involved. Diaper rash infection of neonates is also a common manifestation.

Vaginal candidiasis in women without AIDS, which is characterized by the production of a thick

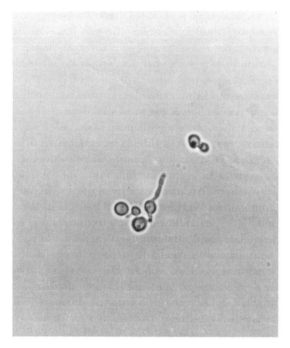

Figure 16-3. Photomicrograph of a germ tube, characteristic of *Candida albicans* (oil immersion).

yellow, milky discharge, is often associated with diabetes, pregnancy, and the use of oral contraceptives. Candidiasis of the urinary tract is relatively rare, manifesting as cystitis (more commonly caused by *Torulopsis* [*Candida*] *glabrata*) and pyelonephritis, either ascending from a bladder infection or from hematogenous spread from a distant primary site of infection. *T. glabrata* is an agent of urinary tract infections, comprising about 20% of all yeast isolates from urine specimens.[20] Endocarditis is most often noted in patients with preexisting valvular disease, particularly after episodes of septicemia associated with the use of indwelling catheters, prolonged intravenous infusions, and intravenous drug abuse. Candidal septicemia may also be found in patients receiving long-term antibiotic and corticosteroid therapy. Cases of endocarditis caused by *T. glabrata* have been reported.

Human cryptococcosis generally manifests clinically as pulmonary, central nervous system, and disseminated or visceral forms of disease. Cutaneous and osseous forms of disease are less common occurrences. It should be remembered that central nervous system disease may occur without evidence of disease elsewhere; likewise, lungs and other organs can be involved in the absence of central nervous system disease.

Infections with other yeasts are less common. Edwards[19] has presented the various clinical forms of candidiasis and has cited the following species as important pathogens for humans: *C. tropicalis*, *C. parapsilosis*, *C. pseudotropicalis*, *C. lusitaniae*, *C. kruzei*, *C. guilliermondii*, and *Torulopsis* (*Candida*) *glabrata*. *C. lusitaniae* has emerged as an important human pathogen.[24]

Trichosporon beigelii, classically the cause of white piedra, is the species most commonly encountered in clinical laboratories. Disseminated disease may occur in patients with a variety of neoplastic diseases.[26] Disseminated infections have also been seen with *Trichosporon capitatum*, recently renamed *Blastoschizomyces capitatus*.[59] The clinical presentation in patients with *B. capitatus* infections did not differ among these patients from those with other fungal infections, with evidence of hepatosplenic and pulmonary involvement evident in most cases.

Pulmonary and disseminated infections with *Geotrichum* species are less commonly encountered. Tawfik and coworkers[67] report a case of polymicrobial pneumonia including *Saccharomyces cerevisiae* in a patient with AIDS.

SEROLOGIC DETECTION OF FUNGAL DISEASE

The details of serologic diagnosis of fungal infections are beyond the scope of this book. They have been reviewed by Kaufman and Riess[32] and are detailed elsewhere.[40] The general principles of serologic diagnosis and interpretations of the more common pathogenic fungi have also been prepared in an official statement by the American Thoracic Society.[60] A review of the role of serodiagnostic tests in the diagnosis of fungal disease by Davies and Sarosi[12] is worthy of attention by those who wish to pursue the subject.

A few general comments are in order. For antibody testing, single serologic reactions in titers of 1:32 or greater generally indicate disease; demonstrating a rising titer fourfold or greater in samples drawn 3 weeks apart has greater significance. Titers of less than 1:32 or less than a fourfold increase between the paired samples usually indicate the presence of either early infection or nonspecific cross-reactivity with other antigens. Antibodies of the IgM class (using tube precipitin, latex agglutination, or immunodiffusion methods) are commonly detectable about 2 weeks after the disease is acquired and indicate recent infection. Usually IgM antibodies are no longer detectable after 6 months. The presence of IgG antibodies (detected by complement fixation tests or by immunodiffusion) appear shortly after the rise in IgM titer, do not peak until about 6 to 12 weeks, and may remain elevated for many months after infection. Thus, a single elevated IgG antibody titer cannot be used to distinguish between recent and remote infections.

The serodiagnosis for opportunistic infections, in particular candidiasis and aspergillosis, remains disappointing.[15] Immunosuppressed patients may have a poor immune response or defects in cell-mediated immune functions that compromise antibody production. Many of the opportunistic organisms, particularly *Candida* species, are ubiquitous in the environment and commonly colonize the mucous membranes of humans. Establishing antibody threshold levels to distinguish invasive disease from mucous membrane colonization has been difficult.

More promising is the focus on identifying fungal antigens in blood and body fluids using the new enzyme immunoassay and nucleic acid probe technologies. The detection of cryptococcal capsular antigen with specificities approaching 100% in cerebrospinal fluid and other body fluids has been the most dramatic application of this approach. Antigen detection is particularly useful in establishing the diagnosis of histoplasmosis, coccidioidomycosis, and blastomycosis. Thus, the ability to detect antigen may provide an early diagnosis, even in patients who are severely immunodepressed. Wheat and colleagues,[75] applying radioimmunoassay techniques, were able to detect *H. capsulatum* antigen in the urine and serum of 22 episodes of disseminated histoplasmosis in 16 patients. Antigen was detected, however, in only 6 of 32 patients with self-limited infection and in only 2 of 32 patients with cavitary histoplasmosis, indicating that radioimmunoassay for *H. capsulatum* antigen may be a useful method only for diagnosing disseminated histoplasmosis.

Prepared kits are commercially available but do not preclude the need for proper specimen collection and processing and the exercise of careful techniques in performing the tests. The manufacturer's instructions must be followed carefully to obtain reliable results, and positive controls must be included with each sample run. When properly performed, however, commercial kit tests make fungal serologic testing possible in virtually any laboratory.

REFERENCES

1. Abe F, Teteyama M, Shibuya H, et al. Disseminated fungal infections: a review of 20 autopsy cases. Acta Pathol Jpn 1984;34:1201–1208.
2. Ajello L. Hyalohyphomycosis: a disease entity whose time has come. Newsl Med Mycol Soc NY 1982;10:305.
3. Ajello L. Hyalohyphomycosis and phaeohyphomycosis: two global disease entities of public health importance. Eur J Epidemiol 1986;2:243–251.
4. Alvarez S. Systemic infection by *Penicillium decumbens* in a patient with acquired immunodeficiency syndrome. J Infect Dis 1990;162:283.
5. Atkinson JB, Connor DH, Robinowitz M. Fungal infections: a review of autopsy findings in 60 patients. Hum Pathol 1984;15:935–942.
6. Bohler K, Metze D, Poitschek C, Jurecka W. Cutaneous aspergillosis. Clin Exp Dermatol 1990;15:446–450.
7. Boom WH, Piper DJ, Rouff KL, et al. New cause for false-positive results with the cryptococcal antigen test by latex agglutination. J Clin Microbiol 1985;22:856–857.
8. Boon AP, Adams DH, Buckels J, McMaster P. Cerebral aspergillosis in liver transplantation. J Clin Pathol 1990;43:116–118.
9. Bronnimann DA, Adams RD, Galgiani JN. Coccidioidomycosis in the acquired immunodeficiency syndrome. Ann Intern Med 1987;106:372–379.
10. Chan YF, Woo KC. *Penicillium marneffei* osteomyelitis. J Bone Joint Surg 1990;72:500–503.
11. Cox JN, Di Dio F, Pizzolato GP, et al. *Aspergillus* endocarditis and myocarditis in a patient with the immunodeficiency syndrome: a review. Virchows Arch 1990;417:255–259.
12. Davies SF, Sarosi GA. Role of serodiagnostic tests and skin tests in the diagnosis of fungal disease. Clin Chest Med 1987;8:135–146.
13. Defoier C, Fossion E, Vaillant JM. Sinus aspergillosis. J Craniomaxillofac Surg 1990;18:33–40.
14. Denning DW, Williams AH. Invasive pulmonary aspergillosis diagnosed by blood culture and successfully treated. Br J Dis Chest 1987;81:300–304.
15. De Repintigny L, Reis E. Current trends in immunodiagnosis of candidiasis and aspergillosis. Rev Infect Dis 1984;6:301–312.

16. Dixon DM, Fromtling RA. Morphology, taxonomy and classification of the fungi. In: Balows A, ed. Manual of clinical microbiology. 5th ed. Washington, DC, American Society for Microbiology, 1991.

17. Dixon DM, Walsh TJ, Merz WG, McGinnis MR. Infections due to *Xylohypha bantiana* (*Cladosporium trichoides*). Rev Infect Dis 1990;11:515–525.

18. Dumich PS, Neel HB. Blastomycosis of the larynx. Laryngoscope 1983;93:1266–1270.

19. Edwards JE. *Candida* species. In: Mandell GL, Douglas RG Jr, Bennett JE, eds. Principles and practice of infectious diseases. 3rd ed. New York, Churchill Livingstone, 1990:1943–1958.

20. Frye KR, Donovan JM, Drach GW. *Torulopsis glabrata* urinary tract infections. J Urol 1988;139:1245–1249.

21. Gold JMW. Opportunistic fungal infections in patients with neoplastic disease. Am J Med 1984;76:458–463.

22. Gueho E, Simmons RB, Pruitt WR, et al. Association of *Malassezia pachydermatis* with systemic infections of humans. J Clin Microbiol 1987;25:1789–1790.

23. Gupta TP, Ehrinpreis MN. *Candida*-associated diarrhea in hospitalized patients. Gastroenterology 1990;98:780–785.

24. Hadfield TL, Smith MB, Winn RE, et al. Mycoses caused by *Candida lusitaniae*. Rev Infect Dis 1987;9:1006–1012.

25. Hageage GJ Jr, Harrington BH. Use of calcofluor white in clinical mycology. Lab Med 1984;15:109–111.

26. Hoy J, Hsu KC, Rolston K, et al. *Trichosporon beigilii* infection: a review. Rev Infect Dis 1986;8:959–967.

27. Hulshof CM, Vanzanten RA, Sluiters JF, et al. *Penicillium marneffei* infection in an AIDS patient. Eur J Clin Microbiol Infect Dis 1990;9:370.

28. Jayanetra P, Nitiyanant P, Ajello A, et al. *Penicillium marneffei* in Thailand: report of five human cases. Am J Trop Med Hyg 1984;33:637–644.

29. Johnston PC, Khardori N, Najjar AF, et al. Progressive disseminated histoplasmosis in patients with acquired immunodeficiency syndrome. Am J Med 1988;85:152–158.

30. Jones PG, Cohen RL, Bates DH, et al. Disseminated histoplasmosis, invasive pulmonary aspergillosis and other opportunistic infections in a homosexual patient with acquired immune deficiency syndrome. Sex Transm Dis 1983;10:202–204.

31. Kane J, Richter J, Krajden S, et al. Blastomycosis — a new endemic focus in Canada. J Can Med Assoc 1983;129:728–731.

32. Kaufman L, Reece E. Serodiagnosis of fungal diseases. In: Lennette EH, ed. Manual of clinical microbiology. 4th ed. Washington, DC, American Society for Microbiology, 1985:924–944.

33. Kaufman L, Standard PG. Specific and rapid identification of medically important fungi by exoantigen detection. Annu Rev Microbiol 1987;41:209–221.

34. Kaufman L, Standard PG, Weeks RJ, et al. Detection of two *Blastomyces dermatitidis* serotypes by exoantigen analysis. J Clin Microbiol 1983;18:110–114.

35. Kaufman SM. *Curvularia* endocarditis following cardiac surgery. Am J Clin Pathol 1971;56:466–470.

36. Kiehn TE, Armstrong D. Changes in the spectrum of organisms causing bacteremia and fungemia in immunocompromised patients due to venous access devices. Eur J Clin Microbiol Infect Dis 1990;9:869–872.

37. Kirkpatrick CH, Rich RR, Bennett JE. Chronic mucocutaneous candidiasis: model-building in cellular immunity. Ann Intern Med 1971;74:955–978.

38. Klein BS, Vergeront JM, DiSalvo AF, et al. Two outbreaks of blastomycosis along rivers in Wisconsin: isolation of *Blastomyces dermatitidis* from riverbank soil and evidence of transmission along waterways. Am Rev Respir Dis 1987;136:1333–1338.

39. Klein BS, Vergeront JM, Roberts RJ, et al. Isolation of *Blastomyces dermatitidis* in soil associated with a large outbreak of blastomycosis in Wisconsin. N Engl J Med 1986;314:529–534.

40. Koneman EW, Allen SD, Janda WM, Schreckenberger PC, Winn WC Jr. Color atlas and textbook of diagnostic microbiology. 4th ed. Philadelphia, JB Lippincott, 1992.

41. Lee TM, Greenberger PA, Patterson R, et al. Stage V (fibrotic) allergic bronchopulmonary aspergillosis: a review of 17 cases followed from diagnosis. Arch Intern Med 1987;147:319–323.

42. Mamikunian C, Gatti WM, Reyes CV. Subcutaneous blastomycosis: diagnosis by fine-needle aspiration cytology. Otolaryngol Head Neck Surg 1989;101:607–610, 1989

43. Marcon MJ, Powell DA. Epidemiology, diagnosis and management of *Malassezia furfur* systemic infection. Diagn Microbiol Infect Dis 1987;7:161–175.

44. McGinnis MR. Chromoblastomycosis and phaeohyphomycosis: new concepts, diagnosis and mycology. J Am Acad Dermatol 1983;8:1–15.

45. McGinnis MR, Ajello L, Schell WA. Mycotic diseases: a proposed nomenclature. Int J Dermatol 1986;24:9–15.

46. McKensie R, Khakoo R. Blastomycosis of the esophagus presenting with gastrointestinal bleeding. Gastroenterology 1984;88:1271–1273.

47. Milroy CM, Blanshard JD, Lucas S, Michaels L. Aspergillosis of the nose and paranasal sinuses. J Clin Pathol 1989;42:123–127.

48. Minamoto G, Armstrong D, Fungal infections in AIDS: histoplasmosis and coccidioidomycosis. Infect Dis Clin North Am 1988;2:447–456.

49. Morgan MA, Wilson WR, Neel HB III, et al. Fungal sinusitis in healthy and immunocompromised individuals. Am J Clin Pathol 1984;82:597–601.

50. Musial CE, Cockerill FR III, Roberts GD. Fungal infections of the immunocompromised host: clinical and laboratory aspects. Clin Microbiol Rev 1988;1:349–364.

51. Nolan MT, Long JP, MacRean DP, Fitzgerald MX. Aspergillosis and lung fibrosis. Ir J Med Sci 1985;154:336–342.

52. Page LR, Drummond JF, et al. Blastomycosis with oral lesions: report of two cases. Oral Surg 1979;47:157–160.

53. Piehl MR, Kaplan RL, Haber MH. Disseminated penicilliosis in a patient with acquired immunodeficiency syndrome. Am J Clin Pathol 1988;112:1262–1264.

54. Raper KB, Fennel DL. The genus *Aspergillus*. Baltimore, Williams & Wilkins, 1965.

55. Rinaldi MG. Invasive aspergillosis. Rev Infect Dis 1983;5:1061–1077.

56. Rippon JW. Medical mycology: the pathogenic fungi and the pathogenic actinomycetes. 3rd ed. Philadelphia, WB Saunders, 1988:482.

57. Rogers AL, Kennedy MJ. Opportunistic hyaline hyphomycetes. In: Balows A, ed. Manual of clinical microbiology. 5th ed. Washington, DC, American Society for Microbiology, 1991:659–673.

58. Rolston KV, Radentz S, Rodriquez S. Bacterial and fungal infections in patients with acquired immunodeficiency syndrome. Cancer Detect Prev 1990;14:377–381.

59. Salkin IF, Gordon MA, Samsonoff WM, Rieder CL. *Blastoschizomyces capitatus*, a new combination. Mycotaxon 1985;22:373–380.

60. Sarosi GA, et al. Laboratory diagnosis of mycotic and specific fungal infections. Am Rev Respir Dis 1985;132:1373–1379.

61. Seaworth BJ, Kwon-Chung KJ, Hamilton JD, et al. Brain abscess caused by a variety of *Cladosporium trachoides*. Am J Clin Pathol 1983;79:747–752.

62. Shah A, Khan ZU, Chaturvedi S, et al. Allergic bronchopulmonary aspergillosis with coexistent aspergilloma: a long-term followup. J Asthma 1989;26:109–115.

63. Shek YH, Tucker MC, Viciana AL, et al. *Malassezia furfur*–disseminated infection in premature infants. Am J Clin Pathol 1989;92:595–603.

64. Simon GB, Bersonet SD, et al. Blastomycosis of the tongue. S Afr Med J 1977;52:82–83.

65. Sobol SM, Love RG, Stutman HR, et al. Phaeohyphomycosis of the maxillary ethmoid sinus caused by *Drechslera spicefera*: a new fungal pathogen. Laryngoscope 1984;94:620–627.

66. Tagami H, Ginoza M, Imaizumi S, Urano-Suehisa. Successful treatment of chromoblastomycosis with topical heat therapy. J Am Acad Dermatol 1984;10:615–619.

67. Tawfik OW, Papasian CJ, Dixon AY, Potter LM. *Saccharomyces cerevisiae* pneumonia in a patient with acquired immune deficiency syndrome. J Clin Microbiol 1989;27:1689–1691.

68. Thomson RB Jr, Roberts GD. A practical approach to the diagnosis of fungal infections of the respiratory tract. Clin Lab Med 1982;2:321–242.

69. Tierno PM Jr, Milstoc M. Germ tube–positive *Candida tropicalis*. Am J Clin Pathol 1977;68:284–295.

70. Tong QJ, Chai WX, Wang ZF, et al. A case of cerebral aspergillosis caused by *Aspergillus nidulans*. Chin Med J (Engl) 1990;103:518–522.

71. Vajpayee RB, Gupta SK, Bareja U, Kishore K. Ocular atopy and mycotic keratitis. Ann Ophthalmol 1990;22:369–372.

72. Vollier AF, Peterson DE, DeJongh CA, et al. *Aspergillus* sinusitis in cancer patients. Cancer 1986;58:366–371.

73. Walsh TJ, Hier DB, Caplan LR. Aspergillosis of the central nervous system: clinicopathological analysis of 17 patients. Ann Neurol 1985;18:574–582.

74. Weingardt J, Li YP. North American blastomycosis. Am Fam Physician 1991;43:1245–1248.

75. Wheat LJ, Kohler RB, Tewari RP. Diagnosis of disseminated histoplasmosis by detection of *Histoplasma capsulatum* antigen in serum and urine specimens. N Engl J Med 1986;314:83–88.

76. Yu VL, Muder RR, Poorsattar A. Significance of isolation of *Aspergillus* from the respiratory tract in diagnosis of invasive pulmonary aspergillosis: result from a three-year prospective study. Am J Med 1986;81:249–254.

Microscopic Features of the Zygomycetes

The zygomycetes are a group of rapidly growing fungi that are microscopically characterized by the formation of broad, irregular sized, ribbon-like, aseptate hyphae and the production of spores, called sporangiospores, that are borne within closed saclike encystments called sporangia. Certain of the zygomycetes also produce rootlike formations called rhizoids, the structure and arrangement of which are useful in establishing genus identifications. *Mucor* species is characterized by the failure to produce rhizoids.

A
Lactophenol aniline blue mount of a zygomycete illustrating broad, aseptate, ribbon-like hyphae, sporangiophores, and immature and mature sporangia.

B
Illustration of rootlike rhizoids that are characteristic of certain of the zygomycetes.

C
Illustration of *Rhizopus* species in which sporangiophores are borne from the stolon adjacent to the rhizoids (seem centrally in this photograph), termed "nodal derivation." *Rhizopus* species are most frequently recovered from cases of human infections.

D
Shown here is *Absidia* species in which the sporangiophores are borne from the stolon at some distance from the rhizoids, a so-called internodal derivation. *Absidia* species are only rarely encountered in clinical laboratories.

E
A microscopic view of *Syncephalastrum* species illustrating a broad, aseptate hypha from which is borne a fruiting head consisting of a spherical columella, from which radiate elongated, cylindrical sporangia. This fruiting head can be confused with those of *Aspergillus* species; however, the rapidly growing gray-white, cottony colony and the aseptate hyphae provide sufficient differential criteria so that misidentifications are rarely made.

F
Circinella species with broad, aseptate hyphae in the background from which are borne curved sporangiophores that support large, spherical sporangia packed with sporangiospores. Note that the sporangiophore in the lower right field of view is interrupted by several septations. Occasional septa may be seen in older colonies of most of the zygomycetes, particularly in the sporangiophores. This aberrant feature rarely causes a problem with misidentifications, as the other features of rapid colony growth, aseptate hyphae, and the presence of sporangia are sufficient to categorize an unknown fungus as a zygomycete.

G
Close-in view of spherical columella of *Cunninghamella* species, from which are borne numerous spherical spores known as sporangiola. Although not well illustrated in this photomicrograph, each sporangiola is attached to the columella by a delicate strand called a denticle.

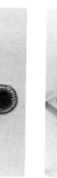

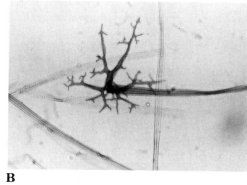

A

B

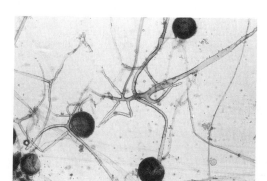

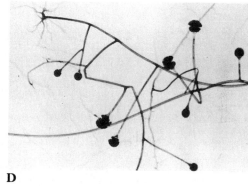

C

D

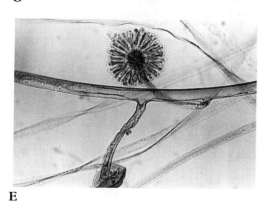

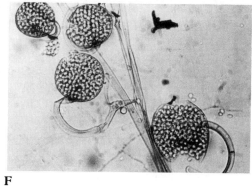

E

F

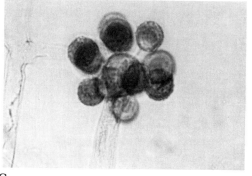

G

Microscopic Features of Aspergillus Species

Aspergillus species are characterized by the formation of regularly septate hyphae that are uniform in diameter with parallel walls. Certain hyphal segments, known as foot cells, become thickened and give rise to conidiophores of varying length that support fruiting heads from which spores, called conidia, are borne from the surface. Each conidiophore terminates in a vesicle that may be spherical, club shaped, large, or small, depending on the species. From the surface of the vesicle are derived one (uniseriate) or two (biseriate) rows of phialides from which, in turn, are borne short or long rows of spherical or oval conidia that may have a variety of pigments that give a characteristic hue to the gross colony. The variations in the various structures of the fruiting head are used to make species identifications. In practice, fewer than two dozen of the several hundred named *Aspergillus* species are of medical importance, and of these only four, *A. fumigatus*, *A. flavus*, *A. niger*, and *A. terreus*, cause the great majority of human infections.

A
Typical fruiting head of *Aspergillus* species illustrating the swollen vesicle, row of phialides, and chains of conidia.

B
Aspergillus species illustrating a foot cell, conidiophore, and vesicle, components of the specialized supporting structures for the fruiting head. (Photograph courtesy of Glenn D. Roberts, PhD)

C
Typical fruiting head of *Aspergillus fumigatus*. The vesicle is typically club-shaped and only a single row of phialides are seen, giving rise to long chains of conidia that often sweep inward as illustrated in this photograph. Conidiation is typically only from the top half of the vesicle.

D
Close-in view of a fruiting head of *Aspergillus flavus*. The vesicle is typically large and spherical and conidiation covers the entire circumference. Two rows of phialides are usually present (difficult to show in photographs because they interdigitate), those in the proximal row being longer than the distal ones. The conidia generally only form short chains. The terminal conidiophore immediately below the vesicle often is roughened.

E
Fruiting heads of *Aspergillus niger*. Sporulation is usually so heavy, as shown here, that the vesicles and phiadides are obscured. *A. niger* is among the easier molds to recognize because of the distinct appearance of the colony.

F
Close-in view of a fruiting head of *Aspergillus terreus*. The vesicles are relatively small and spherical, giving rise to two rows of phialides, the terminal longer than the proximal row. Together with the long chains of conidia borne from the surface, the fruiting head has an elongated, sweeping appearance.

G
Close-in view of substratum hyphae of *Aspergillus terreus* revealing a chlamydospore and two small, spherical, sessile aleureospores. Aleureospore formation is an additional feature helpful in making the identification of *A. terreus*.

H
Photomicrograph illustrating the anamorph (asexual) form of *Aspergillus* species (left) consisting of the fruiting head described above, and the telomorph (sexual) form (right), consisting of a baglike structure called a cleistothecium, within which are borne ascospores in turn enclosed within smaller sacs called asci.

A

B

C

D

E

F

G

H

Microscopic Features of Select Hyaline Hyphomycetes

The hyaline hyphomycetes are rapidly growing molds comprising several taxonomically unrelated genera with the common characteristic of producing septate hyphae that are transparent when microscopically viewed in unstained wet mounts. Although these species are less commonly associated with human infections than other groups of molds, cases of mycotic keratitis, onychomycosis, cutaneous infections, and, less commonly, pulmonary disease have been reported.

A

Penicillium species are characterized by the production of fruiting heads composed of conidiophores that branch into primary matulae and secondary phialides forming a brush or "penicillus" structure. Spherical or oval conidia 1 to 2 μm in diameter are borne in long chains from the tips of phialides that are blunt and appear to be cut off at right angles.

B

The fruiting heads of *Paecilomyces* species are similar to those of *Penicillium* species except that the phialides are long and tapered. The chains of conidia tend to be shorter than those seen in *Penicillium* species, they are more elliptical, and the terminal conidium (*arrow*), the first formed, tends to be larger than those lying proximally in the chain.

C

The fruiting head of *Scopulariopsis* species are also branched, and the conidia are formed in chains; however, each individual conidium is two to three times larger than those of *Penicillium* species and are lemon shaped. The conidia appear to be connected by a delicate filament and may become delicately spiked (echinulate) as the colony ages. (Photograph courtesy of Glenn D. Roberts, PhD)

D

Shown here is *Gliocladium* species revealing a fruiting head in which the conidiophore is also branched; however, the conidia 2 to 3 μm in diameter are borne in tight clusters. The green-lawn type of colony is the initial clue to making the identification.

E

Shown here is *Acremonium*, the fruiting heads of which are composed of elongated conidia that arrange in diphtheroid-like clusters, having some resemblance to the surface of the cerebral cortex. It is this "headlike" appearance of the conidia that led to the previous genus designation, *Cephalosporium*. The conidiophores tend to be long and delicate, and the clusters of conidia are commonly dislodged when making microscopic mounts.

F

Fusarium species are unique among the hyaline hyphomycetes because they form both macroconidia and microconidia. The microconidia often arrange in formations identical to the fruiting heads of *Acremonium* species (*arrow*); however, the elongated, multicelled, sickle-form macroconidia, observed near the top of the larger cluster of conidia in this photograph, establish the identification. An initial clue to the identification is the rose-red or lavender-red colonies.

G

This photomicrograph shows the fruiting structures of *Beauveria* species, a rapidly growing mold that is not uncommonly recovered in clinical laboratories. Tiny 1 to 2 μm conidia are formed in loose clusters, with each conidium attached to the hyphae by a delicate, hairlike, bent, or "zigzag" conidiophore.

H

This photomicrograph shows the singly borne, pyriform conidia of *Scedosporium apiospermum*, which represents the anamorph (asexual) form of *Pseudallescheria boydii*. Each conidium is attached to the hypha by a short, delicate conidiophore, giving an appearance that is colloquially known as "lollipop." This mold can be suspected if the colony has a mouse-gray appearance.

A

B

C

D

E

F

G

H

Microscopic Features of the Dematiaceous Hyphomycetes

The dematiaceous hyphomycetes are rapidly growing molds comprising several taxonomically unrelated genera with the common characteristic of producing septate hyphae that innately have a yellow-brown appearance when viewed microscopically in unstained wet mounts. A variety of infections, notably subcutaneous mycetomas, collectively known as phaeohyphomycosis, are caused by many species of these dematiaceous molds.

A
The conidia of *Alternaria* species stain dark brown and are drumstick shaped, with the blunt end of one attached to the thin end of the next. The conidia are multicelled, with septations running both longitudinally and transversely (muriform).

B
The mold shown in this photomicrograph is called *Ulocladium* species. As with *Alternaria* species, the conidia are separated into several segments by septations that run both longitudinally and transversely; however, here they are more oval in outline and do not arrange in chains. *Ulocladium* species can be confused with *Stemphilium* species; however, in the former, conidia are borne sympodially (from geniculate or "bent-knee" conidiophores), as illustrated here.

C
Close-in view of *Stemphilium* species. The muriform conidia appear similar to those of *Ulocladium* species; however, as shown here, the conidia of *Stemphilium* species are borne terminally from straight, nongeniculate conidiophores, simulating a bale of cotton on a stick. (Photograph courtesy of Glenn D. Roberts, PhD)

D
The twisted, geniculate nature of a conidiophore is well illustrated in this photomicrograph of *Bipolaris* species. The sympodial conidiation is also well demonstrated here. Note that the conidia are produced circumferentially in several planes. As each conidium is formed, the conidiophore takes an angle turn, before producing the next conidium in a different direction. *Bipolaris* species have been confused with *Drechslera* species, which produce conidia that appear structurally similar, but without the production of geniculate conidiophores and sympodial conidiogenesis.

E
Helminthosporium species is another mold that has been confused with both *Bipolaris* species and *Drechslera* species. Note in this photomicrograph of *Helminthosporium* species that the conidiophore is straight, bearing multicelled, elongated, outwardly pointing conidia laterally, in what is known as the rhinocladiella type of sporulation. (Photograph courtesy of Glenn D. Roberts, PhD)

F
Demonstrating the formation of germ tubes from both sides of the conidium in an incubated mount of *Bipolaris* species is another helpful feature to differentiate *Bipolaris* species from *Drechslera* and *Helminthosporium* species. The genus name *Bipolaris* is derived from this feature, as illustrated in this photomicrograph. Note the germ tube emanating from both poles of the single, multicelled, smooth-walled conidium shown here.

G
The conidia of *Curvularia* species are also dark yellow-brown and multicelled but subdivided only by transverse septations. The center cells grow more rapidly than those at the periphery of each conidium, producing a distinctive boomerang-like bend.

H
Shown here are the elongated, pencil-shaped, smooth-walled, multicelled conidia of *Exserohilum* species. Note the distinct, dark-staining protrusion at the base of the conidium designated by the arrow.

A

B

C

D

E

F

G

H

Microscopic Features of the Causative Agents of Mycetoma and Chromomycosis

Three genera of slow-growing, dematiaceous molds are agents of chromomycosis and mycetoma: *Cladosporium* species, *Pialophora* species, and *Fonsecaea* species. These genera can be differentiated microscopically, based on whether sporulation is of the cladosporium, phialophora, or acrotheca (rhinocladiella) type. These differences will be demonstrated in the photomicrographs included in this composite.

A

The cladosporium type of sporulation, as shown in this photomicrograph of a mount prepared from a culture of *Cladosporium carrionii* is characterized by the production of elliptical, 2 to 3 μm × 4 to 7 μm conidia borne in long chains from branched phialides. When conidia break off, a prominent scar or disjunctor is typically seen.

B

The phialophora type of sporulation is characterized by the production of urn-shaped or flasklike phialides, as seen in this photomicrograph of a mount prepared from a culture of *Phialophora verrucosum*. The conidia are typically borne in tight clusters from the open tips of the phialides. The flare at the tip of the phialides is known as a collarette.

C

Photomicrograph of a mount prepared from a culture of *Phialophora richardsiae*. The phialides tend to be longer and more flask shaped than those seen in *Phialophora verrucosum*. Also, the collarettes with *P. richardsiae* are flatter and more dish shaped than the bottle-lip collarettes seen with *P. verrucosum*. Again, elongated conidia are formed from the open terminus of the phialide that have some tendency to fall down the sides of both the phialides and the hyphae.

D

Photomicrograph of the acrotheca-type sporulation characteristic of *Fonsecaea pedrosoi*. Short chains of conidia are formed from the tips of phialides that typically are in sympodial arrangements.

E

Photomicrograph of the tip of a phialide of *Exophiala jeanselmei*. Clusters of elongated conidia are borne from the tip of the phialide, which is derived from a conidiophore that forms an obtuse or right angle with the supporting hypha. Note that the tip of the phialide here is pointed, a distinguishing feature from the look-alike *Wangiella* species, which is more blunt. The phialides of *Exophiala* species elongate and contract as conidia are formed, producing annelids, which typically are difficult to identify with light microscopy and can be best seen in scanning electron micrographs.

F

High-power photomicrograph of a tissue section demonstrating a giant cell that has engulfed several multicelled grains ("copper pennies") that may be seen in cases of chromoblastomycosis.

G

The hyphae of *Aureobasidium* species are broad and, when mature, divided into deeply yellow-brown arthroconidia-like segments. Myriads of tiny, elliptical, nonpigmented microconidia are borne from the points of junction of the hyphal segments.

H

Photomicrograph of the one- and two-celled yeastlike forms of *Phaeoannelomyces* species, a cause of black piedra. (Photograph courtesy of Glenn D. Roberts, PhD)

A

B

C

D

E

F

G

H

Microscopic Features of Select Dermatophytes

Three genera of dermatophytes are the agents of cutaneous dermatophytosis in humans: *Microsporum* species, *Trichophyton* species, and *Epidermophyton* species. These genera are distinguished microscopically by observing the morphology and arrangement of macroconidia and microconidia. The genus *Microsporum* is characterized by the production of many thick, rough-walled, multicelled macroconidia and few or absent microconidia. In contrast, *Trichophyton* species produce many microconidia but few or absent, thin, smooth-walled macroconidia. *Epidermophyton floccosum*, the only species within the genus, is characterized by the production of club-shaped, thin-walled, three- or four-celled macroconidia that cluster in twos or threes. Microconidia are not produced.

A

Oil-immersion photomicrograph of a KOH preparation of skin scales illustrating a hyphal segment of one of the dermatophytic fungi. Note that the hyphal fragment is breaking up into tiny arthroconidia.

B

The macroconidia of *Microsporum canis* typically have a thick, rough wall, have six to eight cells, and are spindle shaped, each with a pointed terminus that slightly deviates to one side.

C

The macroconidia of *Microsporum gypseum* are also thick and rough walled but are more club shaped with a rounded terminal end.

D

Trichophyton mentagrophytes produces many microconidia that tend to arrange in loose clusters. Note in this photomicrograph that two elongated, pencil-shaped, thin, and smooth-walled macroconidia are also present. *T. mentagrophytes* also tends to produce spiral hyphae (not shown in this photograph), although this is not a unique feature.

E

Photomicrograph of a mount of *Trichophyton rubrum*, demonstrating tear-shaped microconidia that are borne laterally and singly from the hyphae, in what has been called a "bird on the fence" arrangement. (Photograph courtesy of Glenn D. Roberts, PhD)

F

The conidia of *Trichophyton tonsurans* are also borne singly and laterally from the hyphae; however, in contrast to those of *T. rubrum*, they are irregular in size, with many enlarged and either club shaped and/or balloon shaped. The microscopic features may not always be distinctive, and observation of the colony morphology and the inability to grow in the absence of thiamine are other helpful characteristics in making a definitive identification. (Photograph courtesy of Glenn D. Roberts, PhD)

G

Photomicrograph of a cluster of large, three- or four-celled, club-shaped, smooth-walled macroconidia of *Epidermophyton floccosum*. Microconidia are not produced by this species. (Photograph courtesy of Glenn D. Roberts, PhD)

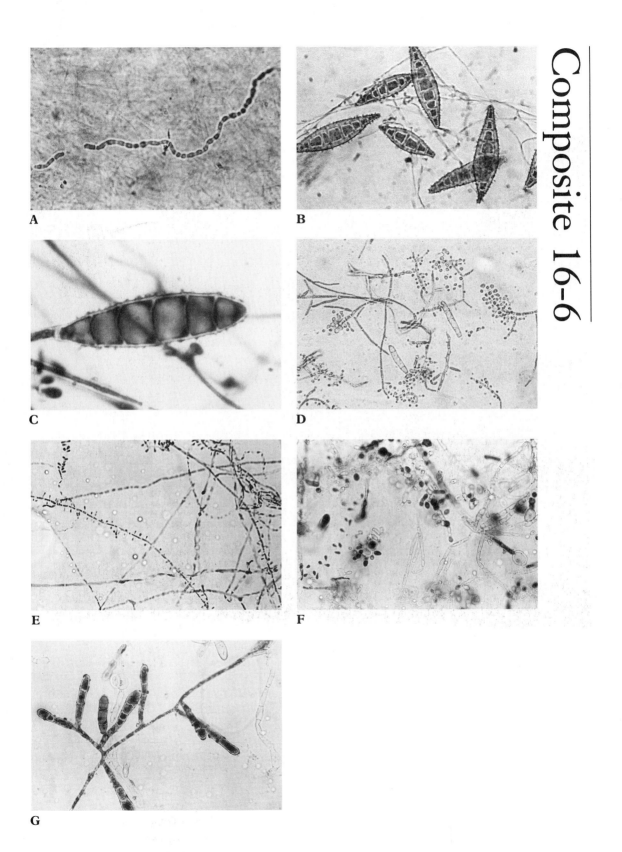

A

B

C

D

E

F

G

Microscopic Features of the Dimorphic Molds

The dimorphic molds are so called because they grow as yeasts (the invasive form in humans) when incubated at 37°C (body temperature) and as molds (the infective form in humans, usually through inhalation of conidia) when grown at 25°C (room or environmental) temperature. The property of dimorphism is in some manner related to the innate capability of these organisms to cause disease when introduced into the tissues of the human host. *Blastomyces dermatitidis*, *Histoplasma capsulatum*, *Coccidioides immitis*, and *Sporothrix schenckii* are the more common species recovered in the United States. *Paracoccidioides brasiliensis* is common in South America. Microscopically, the hyphae tend to be thin and delicate, producing the characteristic cobweb or hairlike colonies.

A

Blastomyces dermatitidis mold form is characterized by the formation of very delicate hyphae that give rise to single, pyriform-shaped, small microconidia, each supported laterally from the hyphae by a delicate conidiophore (so-called lollipop formation).

B

The yeast forms of *Blastomyces dermatitidis* are large (8 to 15 μm in diameter), have a thick refractile wall away from which the central part of the cell often contracts, and produce a single bud attached by a broad base. This photomicrograph illustrates an incomplete conversion of a culture from mold to yeast form. Because *Crysosporium* species appear microscopically similar, conversion of an unknown isolate to the yeast form by incubating a subculture at 35°C may be required if the clinical manifestations are not typical. Exoantigen extraction tests and DNA probe techniques may also be applied.

C

The diagnostic structure seen in the mold form of *Histoplasma capsulatum* is the large, thin-walled macroconidia. Early in culture, only microconidia, often closely simulating those seen in *Blastomyces dermatitidis* may be observed. After an additional few days of incubation, occasional smooth-walled macroconidia may begin to appear. Only in more mature cultures will the macroconidia show the characteristic spikes. *Sepodonium* species is the saprobic counterpart of *H. capsulatum*; therefore, yeast conversion or exoantigen extraction tests of an unknown clinical isolate may be required to confirm an isolate if the clinical history is atypical.

D

The yeast forms of *Histoplasma capsulatum* are small, 2 to 4 μm in diameter, and spherical. When seen in tissue sections, these yeast cells are clustered within the cytoplasm of reticuloendothelial cells and appear to be surrounded by a capsule. Electron micrographic studies, however, have revealed that no capsules exist and that the species name is a misnomer.

E

The mold form of *Coccidioides immitis* is characterized by septate, hyaline hyphae that become enlarged and thick walled as the culture matures. In time, barrel-shaped arthroconidia, separated by empty segments giving an alternate staining effect provide the morphologic support for making an identification. Because *Malbranchia* species and *Gymnoascus* species may also produce alternate staining arthroconidia, confirmation of clinical isolates with atypical clinical histories by exoantigen studies may be in order.

F

Close-in view of a Gomori methenamine silver preparation of lung tissue showing a single spherule of *Coccidioides immitis*, packed with endospores 2 to 4 μm in diameter.

G

Mold form of *Sporothrix schenckii* revealing delicate hyaline hyphae from which are borne tiny conidia, typically clustering in a daisy-petal arrangement at the tips of delicate, straight conidiophores. The genus name is derived from the hairlike attachment of the conidia to the conidiophore, a structure that can only be seen by focusing up and down under oil-immersion magnification.

H

Yeast forms of *Sporothrix schenckii* revealing elongated, "cigar-body," 2 × 3 to 6 μm yeast cells.

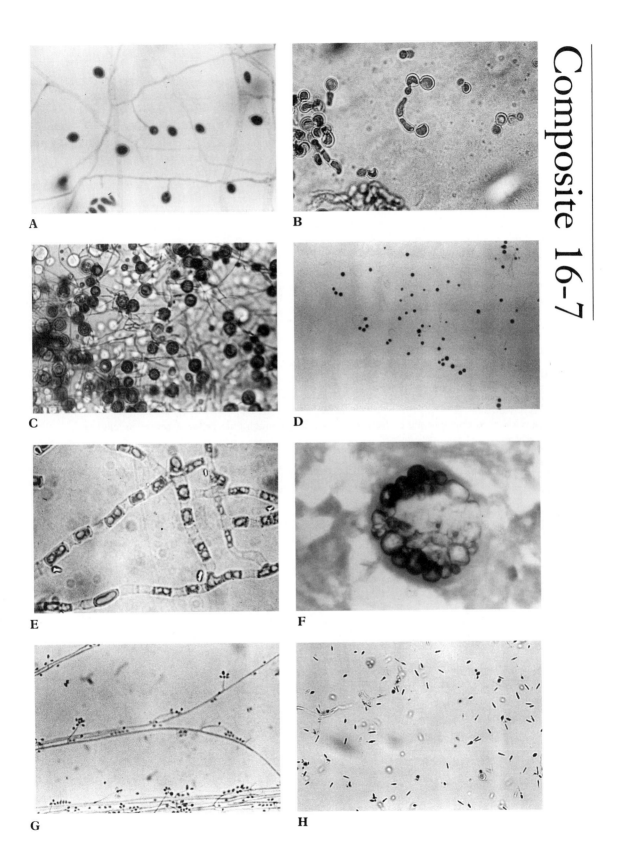

A

B

C

D

E

F

G

H

Cornmeal Morphology of Select Yeasts

The microscopic observation of the morphologic formations produced by yeasts grown in cornmeal or rice extract preparations can be a helpful guide in making presumptive identifications of unknown clinical isolates. The formation of pseudohyphae is characteristic of *Candida* species; *Cryptococcus* species, *Torulopsis glabrata*, and *Rhodotorula* species do not form pseudohyphae, rather they produce only blastoconidia. *Arthroconidia* are formed by *Geotrichum* species and *Trichosporon* species. It is recommended that cornmeal agar preparations be set up on all germ-tube–negative yeast isolates, particularly those identified by one of the commercial systems, as a quality control check on the final identifications being suggested by reading the various biochemical reactions into the data base.

A
Typical cornmeal agar morphology produced by *Candida albicans*. Both clusters of blastoconidia and large, spherical chlamydospores are typically seen.

B
Another cornmeal agar preparation of *Candida albicans* showing the alternate distinguishing morphologic forms, notably the production of blastoconidia in dense clusters regularly along the hyphae.

C
So-called spider, sagebrush, or matchstick colonies of *Candida parapsilosis*. Multiple spider colonies are formed adjacent to, but distant from, the inoculation streak.

D
Single colony of *C. parapsilosis*.

E
Giant hyphae characteristic of *Candida parapsilosis*, although only rarely visualized in clinical isolates.

F
Typical "log in stream" arrangement of elongated, detached blastoconidia of *Candida pseudotropicalis*.

G
Careful examination must be made of any yeastlike colony producing hyphal forms on cornmeal agar. Look for the formation of arthroconidia. Illustrated here is a cornmeal agar mount of *Geotrichum* species revealing the formation of blastoconidia from one corner of the arthroconidia, forming what have been called "hockey sticks." *Trichosporon* species typically produce blastoconidia from two corners of the arthroconidia. Most strains of *Trichosporon* species are urease positive.

H
Photomicrograph of a cornmeal agar preparation of *Cryptococcus* species, revealing the lack of pseudohyphae. Notice that the cell bodies are spherical, varying in size, and separated one from the other by the production of capsular material. The irregularity in size of the cell bodies is a helpful clue in differentiating non–capsule-producing strains of *Cryptococcus* species from the smaller and more uniformly sized and compactly clustered yeast cells of *Torulopsis glabrata*.

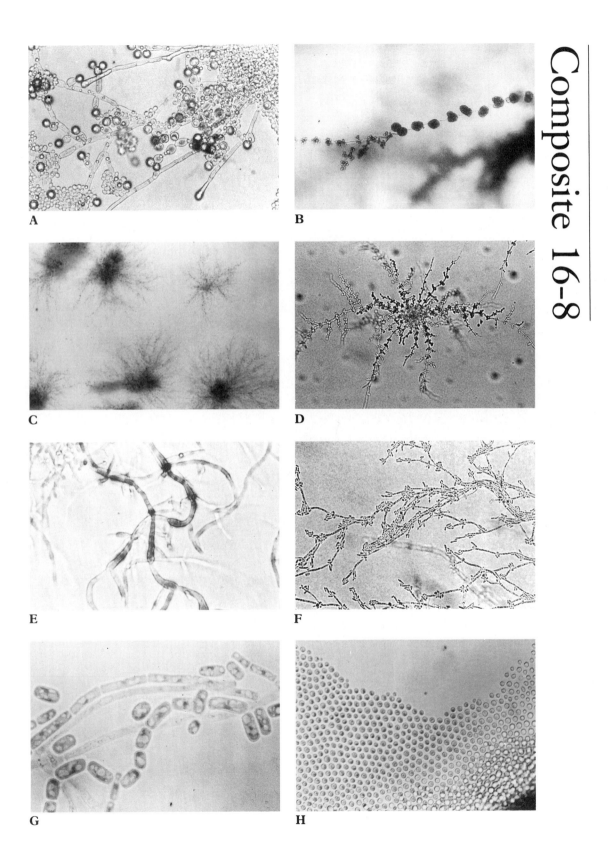

A

B

C

D

E

F

G

H

17

Parasitology

The published prevalence numbers of parasitic infections worldwide are astounding. Human parasites still account for inestimable loss of life, widespread morbidity, and the retardation of economic development in many countries. To quote one report,[66] "prevalence rates (of parasitic diseases) are of such staggering magnitude that the mind has difficulty in conceiving the descriptive statistics." To continue from this report, "the total number of protozoan and helminthic infections currently existing worldwide far outnumbers the total world population since multiple infections are the rule rather than the exception."

Following are estimates of the worldwide prevalence of certain parasitic diseases:

Ascariasis — 800 million to 1.3 billion
Hookworm — 700 to 900 million, most of whom are anemic
Schistosomiasis — 100 to 200 million
Malaria — 100 million, 1 million of whom die annually in Africa alone
Filariasis — 81.6 million, with 905 million at risk
Chagas' disease — 15 million, with 65 million at risk

In the United States, certain parasite species are encountered more frequently than others, and expertise in their identification must remain foremost. In an early CDC intestinal parasite surveillance study[11] cited earlier, parasitic forms were found in 64,901 (15.6%) of the more than 400,000 stool samples examined. *Giardia lamblia* was found in 3.8% of all stool specimens, *Trichuris trichiura* ova in 2.7%, *Ascaris lumbricoides* ova in 2.3%, *Enterobius vermicularis* ova in 1.6% (not a true reflection of the incidence of this disease, since stool specimen examination is not the most sensitive method for establishing a diagnosis), and *Entamoeba histolytica* in 0.6% of all stool specimens.

Following is a summary of the percentages of positive parasites found by Bruckner and associates in a 6-month survey of 1350 stool specimen examinations on outpatients treated at Olive View Medical Center and Harbor General Hospital in Los Angeles:[10]

G. lamblia — 14.5%
Endolimax nana — 13%
Entamoeba coli — 10.5%
E. histolytica — 4.5%
A. lumbricoides — 3.9%
Hymenolepis nana — 3.3%
Dientamoeba fragilis — 2.1%

Other protozoa were identified in about 3% of all stool specimens in this study with other nematodes in 3% and cestodes in 0.5%. These statistics reasonably reflect the species of parasites encountered in most practice settings in the United States, although the percentages of prevalence may vary.

RISK FACTORS AND PREVENTION OF PARASITIC INFECTIONS

Following are risk factors for acquiring parasitic infections, as reviewed by Warren and Mahmoud.[63] As a general statement, at lowest risk is the businessman who stays in first-class hotels in large cities for short periods of time. At the opposite end of the spectrum are volunteers and missionaries who live in tents or native dwellings in rural settings.

- Ingestion of raw, undercooked, or poorly preserved food or water contaminated with infective forms (drinking untreated water, including ice water, or brushing teeth with contaminated water can be particularly hazardous)
- Sting or bite of an arthropod vector carrying the infective forms
- Swimming in fresh water lakes, rivers, and canals in areas endemic for schistosomiasis
- Immunosuppression, particularly from the acquired immunodeficiency syndrome (AIDS), in which infections with *Pneumocystis carinii*, *Toxoplasma gondii*, *Cryptosporidium* species, *Isospora belli*, and *Strongyloides stercoralis* are particularly troublesome and potentially lethal.[28,35]
- Organ transplantation, particularly in the period after bone marrow transplantation

Depending on the prevalence of parasitic diseases in certain locales, the examination of stool specimens may be necessary before a patient is placed on anticancer therapy or given immunosuppressive drugs.

CLINICAL MANIFESTATIONS OF PARASITIC DISEASES

The most common symptom of intestinal parasitic infection is diarrhea, which may be bloody or purulent. Cramping abdominal pain may be a prominent feature in which the bowel mucosa or wall is invaded, such as in infections with hookworms, Manson's or Oriental schistosomes, or intestinal flukes. Heavy infection with *A. lumbricoides* can result in small bowel obstruction. Patients with tapeworms may be symptomatic except for weight loss despite increased appetite and food intake. Bloating, belching, and steatorrhea may be seen in patients with giardiasis.

Hepatosplenomegaly is a common manifestation of liver fluke infection. Portal hypertension, in particular, can be caused by *Schistosoma japonicum*, and jaundice is a common presenting sign. Space-occupying cystic lesions of the liver, brain, and other organs can be found in amebiasis, echinococcosis, and cysticercosis (larval stage of *Taenia solium* infections).

Suprapubic pain, frequency of urination, and hematuria are highly suggestive of *Schistosoma haematobium* infection. Transient pneumonitis may be experienced during the larval migratory phases of *Ascaris* or hookworm infections. Cough, chest pain, and hemoptysis, together with the formation of parabronchial cysts, are common manifestations of infection by the lung fluke *Paragonimus westermani*. Reinfection strongyloidiasis may present as asthma. Low-grade fever, weight loss, facial edema, and skeletal muscle pain indicate possible infection with *Trichinella spiralis*. Focal itching of the skin may occur at the sites of penetration of hookworm larvae or schistosome cercariae.

Peripheral blood eosinophilia (15% to 50%) is one of the more important signs that parasitic infestation may be present. A generalized urticarial rash, believed to be a hypersensitivity reaction secondary to metabolic or lytic products of dead organisms that are absorbed into the circulation, may also suggest parasitic infection.

Generalized constitutional symptoms are more commonly experienced after infections with the blood parasites. Fever, chills, night sweats, lassitude, myalgias, and weight loss are common manifestations of malaria, leishmaniasis, and trypanosomiasis. Varying degrees of hepatosplenomegaly and lymphadenopathy are also seen with these diseases. Neurologic signs and symptoms secondary to encephalitis, meningitis, or space-occupying cysts may be seen in a variety of parasitic diseases. Central nervous system involvement is commonly diffuse in African trypanosomiasis (sleeping sickness), falciparum malaria, and toxoplasmosis, while space-occupying abscesses or cysts are more com-

mon with *E. histolytica*, the larval forms of *T. solium* (cysticercosis), and *Echinococcus granulosis* infections. Cardiac myopathy is one of the most serious complications of South American trypanosomiasis (*Trypanosoma cruzi*). Huge swellings of the legs, arms, and scrotum (elephantiasis) are common symptoms of filariases because the adult worms block the lymphatic vessels, resulting in extensive chronic inflammation and fibrosis. Localized subcutaneous nodules or serpiginous inflammatory areas in the skin may be seen in diseases such as onchocerciasis, dracunculiasis, or cutaneous larval migrans from hookworms of dogs and other animals.

One of the most interesting aspects of parasitic infections is the propensity of certain species to invade and infect a specific organism or tissue. This "organotropism," in which there are complex larval migrations from the site of primary inoculation to a specific distant end organ where the adult forms develop and mature, is poorly understood. Many of the parasites can complete their life cycles only in specific animal or arthropod hosts, whereas others infect a broad range of hosts. A better understanding of host specificities for various parasites has been important in the epidemiology of parasitic diseases and in developing a prophylactic approach to their control. A succinct overview of several common and uncommon parasitic diseases has been published by Tan.[60]

LIFE CYCLES OF PARASITES IMPORTANT TO HUMANS

Microbiologists must gain sufficient understanding of the various life cycles so that the infective and diagnostic forms of human parasites and the role of intermediate hosts can be recognized. To assist in this endeavor, Figure 17-1 has been designed for new students and for readers whose knowledge of parasitic diseases is limited. Parasites can be divided into three major groups on the basis of their life cycles: (1) those having no intermediate hosts, (2) those having one intermediate host, and (3) those for which two intermediate hosts are necessary.

Parasites having no intermediate hosts are transmitted directly between humans (or animal to animal) through fecally contaminated food or water. Parasites requiring one intermediate host commonly select either a large mammal, crustacean, or

No Intermediate Host	One Intermediate Host	Two Intermediate Hosts

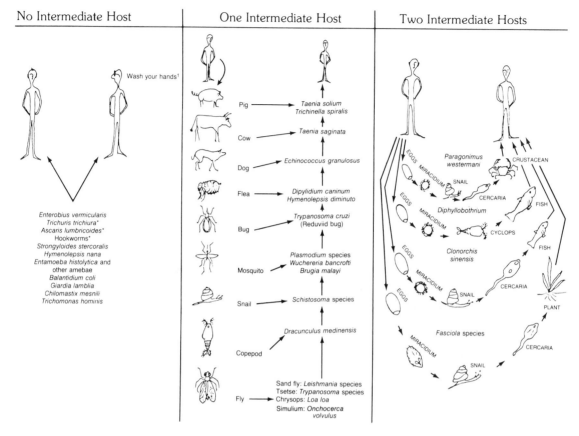

*Require a period of maturation after passage before they are infective.

Figure 17-1. An overview of the life cycles of parasites of importance to humans.

insect vector within which they complete their life cycle, a process that can be either simple or complex. For example, the human intestine serves as the primary site for the adult worms of *T. solium* and *T. saginata*. The pig and cow, respectively, are secondary hosts for these tapeworms in which larvae reside in skeletal muscle. The larval form of the disease (cysticercosis) may develop in humans, however, if ova of *T. solium* are ingested, leading to the formation of cysts in the liver, brain, and other organs. Parasites involving crustaceans and insects usually go through a complex series of developmental stages before the infective form is released. In malaria, for example, the plasmodia undergo sexual gametogenesis within the mosquito before infective sporozoites are injected back into a human host. With the schistosomes, the snail serves as an intermediate host within which a series of maturation stages (rediae) occur. Thus, a single miracidium (a free-swimming ciliated form that infects the snail) is multiplied into numerous free-swimming, infective cercariae.

Parasites that require two intermediate hosts follow essentially the same life cycles. Eggs that are passed from the primary host hatch in a suitable aqueous environment and release miracidia. These are usually ingested by a snail (a crustacean cyclops with *Diphyllobothrium latum*), which, in turn, produces numerous cercariae. The cercariae, in turn, invade crustaceans or fish, in which they become encysted as metacercariae in the somatic musculature. A second host becomes infected by ingesting the metacercariae in raw or inadequately cooked crab or fish. In the life cycle of *Fasciola* species and *Fasciolopsis* species, the cercariae become attached as metacercariae to water plants and humans become infected by ingesting these plants incorporated in raw or poorly cooked food.

Therefore, the use of Figure 17-1 precludes, to some extent, the need to memorize a large number of detailed facts about the life cycles of individual parasites and allows one to develop a broader perspective of the developmental stages common to various groups. For an in-depth review of the life cycles of the common parasites of humans, the reader is referred to the work of Melvin and associates.[42,43]

COLLECTION, TRANSPORT, AND PROCESSING OF SPECIMENS

The diagnosis of parasitic infections relies in large part on macroscopic and microscopic examination of feces, urine, blood, sputum, and tissues. The implementation of reliable laboratory processing techniques is an integral step. It is not possible to review more than a few of the commonly used laboratory procedures that can aid in the recovery and identification of parasitic forms in clinical specimens. For a succinct and practical overview of these procedures, the reader is referred to the textbook by Garcia and Bruckner.[21]

Fecal Specimens

Stool specimens should be collected in a clean, wide-mouthed container with a tightly fitting lid. Specimens that are admixed with water (eg, contamination from the toilet bowel or bed pan) or urine are unsuitable because trophozoites may lose their motility or undergo lysis. Medications containing mineral oil, bismuth, antibiotics, antimalarials, or other chemical substances may compromise the detection of intestinal protozoa. Thus, examination of specimens must be delayed for 1 or more weeks after diagnostic procedures (eg, barium enema) or therapy is stopped. Patients who have received a barium enema may not excrete organisms in their stools for at least 1 week after the enema.[21,64] The lid should be tightly fitted to the container immediately after collection of the sample to maintain adequate moisture. Every specimen container must be properly labeled, as outlined in Chapter 1.

The collection of three fecal specimens usually suffices to make the diagnosis of intestinal parasitic diseases—two obtained on successive days during normal bowl movement and a third after a Fleet's phospho-soda or magnesium sulfate purge. Cathartics with an oil base should be avoided, since oils retard motility of trophozoites and distort the morphology of the parasites. A total of six specimens, collected on successive days, may be required if intestinal amebiasis or giardiasis is suspected. Examination of more than six samples in a 10-day period rarely yields additional information. Post-therapy specimens should be examined 3 to 4 weeks after treatment of patients with protozoan infections and 5 to 6 weeks after therapy for *Taenia* infections.

Preservation of Stool Specimens

Optimally, liquid specimens should be examined within 30 minutes after collection (not 30 minutes after receipt in the laboratory) to detect motile trophozoites, particularly in suspected infections with *E. histolytica*. Formed stools, in which trophozoites are not expected, may be examined up to 24 hours after passage. If timely examination is not possible, portions of specimens should be placed into a suitable fixative, such as merthiolate-iodine-formalin (MIF) or polyvinyl alcohol (PVA). Stool specimens should never be frozen and thawed or placed in an incubator because parasitic forms may deteriorate rapidly. Several preservatives are available for permanent fixation of stool specimens that must be sent to reference laboratories for analysis. Ten-percent formalin-saline (100 mL formaldehyde in 900 mL 0.85% sodium chloride) is a time-honored fixative. One disadvantage is the unsuitability of formalin-fixed stool specimens for the preparation of permanent-stained smears. PVA is widely used because the performance of concentration procedures and the preparation of permanent-stained smears are both possible. MIF solution can also be used as a fixative.[38]

Permanent stained smears are poor at best when prepared from fixed fecal suspensions, and only examination of direct wet mounts or the sediment from centrifuged concentrates is advised. The two solutions must be prepared and stored separately and mixed together only immediately before use. Sodium acetate formalin can be used, from which concentrated mounts and stained smears can be prepared. This fixative has the advantage of not containing the toxic chemical mercuric chloride. Staining of parasitic forms tends to be lighter, however, particularly with the trichrome stain. The preparation of these preservatives can be found in other suitable textbooks.[21,34]

Visual Examination

Freshly passed stool specimens submitted for parasitologic study should be visually examined for the presence of barium, oils, or other materials that may render them unacceptable for further processing. Patches of blood or mucin should be specifically selected for microscopic study because they may be derived directly from ulcers or purulent abscesses where the concentration of amebae may be highest.

Visual examination can also be used to determine the appropriate procedures to perform, as outlined by Melvin and Smith.[44] Formed stools are unlikely to contain trophozoites; thus, wet mounts are usually unnecessary and only concentrates need to be prepared. Helminth eggs and larvae and protozoan cysts can be seen in the sediment of concentrates. The preparation of stained smears is helpful in identifying cysts found in wet mounts.

Wet mounts, concentrates, and permanent stains should all be prepared for the examination of soft stools because all forms of parasites may be present. For fecal specimens that are watery or liquid, it may be sufficient simply to centrifuge the specimens, since trophozoites do not concentrate and cysts that may be present can be seen in the sediment. In the examination of preserved specimens in which motile trophozoites cannot be visualized, the direct examination may be omitted since any forms present will still be detected in the concentrated preparation. Final identifications of parasites should not be made on the basis of the direct mounts alone; rather, permanent stained smears should be examined to confirm the characteristic morphologic features.

Preparation of Direct Wet Mounts

The saline mount is made by emulsifying a small portion of fecal material in a drop of physiologic saline on a microscope slide and overlaying the mixture with a coverslip. Mounts should be just thick enough that newspaper print can be read through the slide. If the mounts are too thick, particularly iodine preparations, parasitic forms often stain poorly and may be difficult to differentiate from background debris. If the smear is too thin,

parasitic forms in low numbers may be diluted out and missed during routine microscopic examination. Saline mounts have the advantage over fixed and stained smears in that the motility of trophozoites can be observed. Protozoan cysts also appear more refractile on saline preparations than on iodine preparations. Definitive identification of either trophozoites or protozoan cysts is difficult in saline mounts because the internal structures are often poorly delineated.

Concentration Methods

Eggs, cysts, and trophozoites are often in such low numbers in fecal material that they are difficult to detect in direct smears or mounts; therefore, concentration procedures should always be performed. The two commonly used concentration procedures are flotation and sedimentation. When fecal material is concentrated by the flotation technique, eggs and cysts float to the top of the zinc sulfate solution, which has a specific gravity of 1.18. The specific gravity of protozoa and many of the helminth eggs is lower; for example, the specific gravity of hookworm eggs is 1.055, that of *Ascaris* eggs is 1.110, that of *Trichiura* eggs is 1.150, and that of *G. lamblia* cysts is 1.060. After these cysts and eggs float to the top of the heavier zinc sulfate suspension, they can be collected by placing a coverslip on the surface of the meniscus. The oocysts of *Cryptosporidium* species can be concentrated using Schaeffer's flotation technique.[6]

Operculated trematode and cestode eggs may not be detected because the high concentration of the zinc sulfate suspension causes the operculum to pop open, fill with fluid, and sink to the bottom of the tube. Bartlett and associates[6] described a modified zinc sulfate flotation technique that may be adapted for use with specimens that have been fixed in formalin. The formalin fixation not only prevents operculated eggs from popping so that they can be detected in flotation eluates but also prevents the distortion of parasitic forms caused by salt solutions of high specific gravity. All flotation techniques have the advantage that most of the interfering background debris is eliminated.

Concentration of intestinal parasites by sedimentation techniques, using either gravity or centrifugation, leads to a good recovery of protozoa, eggs, and larvae, although they may be more difficult to detect in microscopic mounts and in stained smears because of the comparatively large amount of background debris. Ethyl acetate has been substituted for diethyl ether in the formalin concentration procedure. Young and associates[67] have demonstrated that ethyl acetate is less flammable and less hazardous to use than diethyl ether and that the capability to concentrate cysts and eggs is not compromised. Care must be taken during the washing steps in the procedure to decant the supernatant carefully; otherwise, a significant number of parasitic forms can be lost.

Permanent Stained Smears

The morphology of cysts and trophozoites is better visualized in stained smears that can be used as permanent mounts for future study, for use in teaching collections, and for consultation with experts when unusual forms are observed. Because smaller protozoan organisms may be missed if only direct smear and concentration methods are employed, Garcia and colleagues[20,21] have recommended that permanent stains be prepared as part of the examination of every stool specimen submitted for parasitologic examination.

Permanent stained smears are prepared by spreading a thin film of fecal material on the surface of a glass slide. Smears should be prepared from fresh specimens if possible and immediately placed in fixative. An old, thick smear that has been inadequately fixed may result in failure of the organisms to stain. Two permanent stains commonly used to visualize intestinal protozoa in fecal smears are (1) the iron hematoxylin stain and (2) the modified (Wheatley's) Gomori's trichrome stain. The iron hematoxylin stain is the time-honored technique used for the most exacting definition of the morphology of intestinal parasites. The staining procedure is somewhat difficult to control and is best performed by an experienced person to achieve optimum results. The trichrome stain is widely used in diagnostic laboratories because it is easy to perform and good results are obtained with both fresh and PVA-preserved fecal material. Shetty and Prabhu[56] have demonstrated that, although the trichrome and the iron hematoxylin stains were comparable for the detection of cysts and trophozoites of the entamoebas, the trophozoites of *G. lamblia* stained better with iron hematoxylin. These staining procedures are described in detail in other standard parasitology textbooks.[21]

Other Intestinal Specimens

Parasites such as *G. lamblia* and *Strongyloides stercoralis* commonly inhabit the duodenum and jejunum. Samples of duodenal contents may be required to demonstrate these organisms. A saline mount can be prepared from the aspirated material and microscopically examined. If motile organisms are seen, a second preparation in a drop of iodine may be helpful to highlight the characteristic internal structures so that a definitive identification can be made.

Duodenal contents can be examined by the string test.[29] The implement used is a weighted gelatin capsule containing a coiled length of nylon string (commercially available as Enterotest from HEDECO, Palo Alto, CA). One end of the string protrudes from an end of the capsule, and the other end of the string is taped to the face of the patient. The capsule is swallowed and peristalsis carries the weighted string into the duodenum. After 4 to 6 hours, the string is removed and any bile-stained mucus adhering to the distal end is used to prepare direct mounts and stained smears for microscopic study. The examination of duodenal contents should be performed only on patients with signs and symptoms suggestive of giardiasis.

Enterobius vermicularis infection of the rectal canal is best detected using cellulose tape. The adhesive surface of a 3- or 4-inch strip of clear cellulose tape is applied to the perianal folds of a patient suspected of having pinworm infection. A tongue blade can be used to provide a firm backing for the tape. The tape is then placed adhesive side down on a glass microscope slide and examined for the characteristic ova of *E. vermicularis*. Optimal recovery of eggs is achieved if specimens are collected in the early morning soon after the patient arises and before bathing. A commercially available "paddle" with a flat, sticky surface ("Swube"-Falcon 2012 disposable applicator, Falcon, Oxnard, CA) can be used to obtain the specimen.

Extraintestinal Specimens

Sputum

On rare occasions, the larval stages of hookworm, *A. lumbricoides* or *S. stercoralis*, or the eggs of *P. westermani* may be seen in sputum samples. The preparation of a direct saline mount is usually sufficient. If the sputum is unusually thick or mucoid, an equal quantity of 3% *N*-acetyl-L-cysteine or 3% sodium hydroxide (or undiluted chlorine bleach) can be added to liquefy the specimen, which is then mixed for 2 or 3 minutes and centrifuged. After centrifugation, a wet mount of the sediment is prepared for microscopic examination. If for any reason examination of the sputum specimen is delayed, 10% formalin should be added to preserve helminth eggs and larvae.

Urine and Body Fluids

Depending on the volume of fluid obtained, it may be necessary to let the specimen settle for 1 or 2 hours. About 50 mL of the bottom sediment can then be centrifuged and the highly concentrated sediment examined in wet mount preparations. If objects suggestive of parasites are seen, examination of an iodine preparation may be helpful in highlighting the diagnostic internal structures.

Tissue Biopsy Specimens and Aspirates

Cutaneous ulcers (as seen in leishmaniasis), skin nodules (seen in onchocerciasis and in *Mansonella streptocerca* infections), and lymph nodes may be either aspirated or biopsied. In suspected cases of cutaneous leishmaniasis, material should be aspirated with a needle and syringe from beneath the ulcer bed. Skin biopsy specimens can be obtained by either cutting with a razor a small fold of skin pinched between the thumb and forefinger or slicing from a small "cone" produced by elevating the skin with the tip of a needle. The biopsy should be sufficiently deep to include the dermal papillae but not so deep as to produce free bleeding. Biopsies of rectal and bladder mucosa may be indicated to identify the characteristic ova in cases of suspected intestinal or urinary schistosomiasis. Impression smears should also be prepared by pressing a freshly cut surface of the tissue against the surface of a glass slide and placing the slide immediately into a fixative, such as Schaudinn's solution. Trichrome and other stains can be applied. The remaining portion of the biopsy material should then be submitted for histologic examination.

Corneal Scrapings

In cases of suspected *Acanthamoeba* keratitis, the microscopic examination of corneal scrapings may be helpful in making a diagnosis. The corneal scrapings are placed on a slide and fixed in methyl alcohol for 3 to 5 minutes. Garcia and Bruckner[21] suggest that staining should be done using calcofluor white, a textile whitener that is commercially available. A solution of 0.1% calcofluor white and 0.1% Evans blue can be dissolved in distilled water. A few drops of this solution are placed on the methanol-fixed smear for 5 minutes. The slide is then tipped and the fluid drained into an absorbent paper towel, a coverslip is added, and the slide is examined for apple-green amebic cysts (trophozoites do not stain), which will have an apple-green or blue-white fluorescence depending on the exciter light–filter combination used.

Muscle

The characteristic spiral larval forms of *T. spiralis* are best demonstrated in a tease mount made from a skeletal muscle biopsy specimen (Fig. 17-2). Garcia and Bruckner[21] suggest that the biopsy material be treated with a digestion fluid before examination. The digestion fluid is prepared by adding 5 g of pepsin to a mixture of 1000 mL of distilled water and 7 mL of concentrated hydrochloric acid. The tissue is placed in a wide-mouthed Erlenmeyer flask, and digestion fluid is added in a ratio of 1 part tissue to 20 parts fluid. The digestion mixture is held at 37°C for 12 to 24 hours. A few drops of the eluate are examined under the microscope for the presence of larvae. If none are seen, a 15-mL aliquot of the mixture is centrifuged and the sediment reexamined.

Blood

A drop of anticoagulated blood can be placed on a microscope slide, a coverslip added, and the specimen microscopically examined for large, often motile, extraerythrocytic forms, such as trypanosomes and microfilaria. The morphology of intraerythrocytic plasmodia (malaria, babesiosis, theileriasis) is best observed on Wright or Giemsa-stained peripheral blood films. Both thick and thin smears should be prepared.

The thin blood smear, used primarily for specific species identification of plasmodia and other intraerythrocytic parasites, is prepared exactly as for performing a differential blood cell count. The thin, feathered end should be at least 12 mm long, show no overlapping of erythrocytes, and be cen-

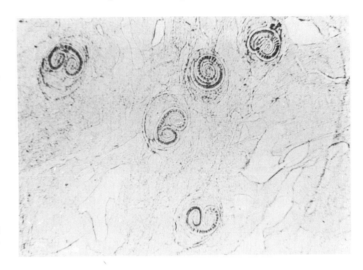

Figure 17-2. High-power view of tease preparation of skeletal muscle showing infestation with *Trichinella spiralis* larvae.

trally placed with free margins on either side. Care must be taken in preparing the thin film to see that the feathered edge is evenly spread and free of holes, streaks, or other artifacts.

Thick blood smears, which allow examination of a large quantity of blood, are especially useful in detecting small concentrations of malarial parasites in light infections. Two or three drops are placed to cover an area the size of a dime. Blood should be obtained from a finger stick and allowed to flow freely; "milking" of the finger should be avoided. The drop should be stirred continually for about 30 seconds to prevent formation of fibrin clots. If anticoagulated blood is used, stirring is not necessary because fibrin strands are prevented from forming. The film is allowed to air dry in a dust-free area. Once the film is dry, the blood should be "laked" by placing the slide in water or a buffer solution immediately before staining. At least three specimens should be taken on successive days if initial samples are negative for parasites.

Both thin and thick smears should be stained as soon as possible after preparation (always within 48 hours) with Giemsa or Wright stain. Thick smears may require a slightly longer exposure to the stain than the time used for the thin smear preparations.

It is recommended that at least 200 oil fields be microscopically examined at $\times 1000$ magnification on the thin film and about 100 fields be examined on the thick film. The number of organisms may be very few in patients in relapse, in those who have an early infection, or in those who have received inadequate treatment or partial prophylaxis. In these instances, the number of fields examined should be doubled. Proper interpretation of the thick smear requires considerable experience, and positive controls for comparison should be made available.

IDENTIFICATION AND DIFFERENTIATION OF PARASITES

Although certain clinical signs and symptoms may suggest the possibility of a parasitic disease, the final diagnosis is made by demonstrating the causative organism in properly collected specimens. Because many artifacts resemble parasite forms, the final identification must always rest on well-established morphologic criteria. Microscopic interpretations, in particular, cannot be left to guesswork, and a laboratory diagnosis of a parasitic disease should not be rendered until adequate identifying features can be clearly and objectively demonstrated. There are a number of publications that provide alternate approaches and valuable guidelines to the detection and identification of unknown parasites in clinical materials.[4,7,21,34,57,63]

Space in this text does not permit a full description of the morphologic criteria by which the medically important parasites can be identified in the laboratory. This information can be found in several current texts and monographs.[21,34,42,43,57,63] For visualization and comparison purposes, the key features for the laboratory identification of parasites are included in tables and color photographs found elsewhere.[34]. These tables are organized around the traditional morphologic grouping of parasites as mentioned previously.

Intestinal Protozoa

Four broad groups of intestinal protozoa are recognized: the amebae, the flagellates, the ciliates, and the coccidia.[36] The task of learning the differential features of these protozoa is somewhat lessened when one recognizes that only a few species are of medical importance within each of these major groups.

Intestinal Amebae

The following are the species of amebae that are discussed in this text:

Entamoeba histolytica
Entamoeba coli
Iodamoeba bütschlii
E. nana

One valuable observation when a form observed in a stool specimen is confirmed to be an ameba, either a trophozoite or a cyst, is to determine whether the nucleus is of the "entamoeba type." The trophozoite is the active, motile feeding stage of an amoeba; the cyst is the resting nonmotile, encysted stage. One should look for the ring of chromatin deposited on the outer membrane, which gives the appearance of a densely stained ring. The nuclei of amebae belonging to the other genera, *Iodamoeba* and *Endolimax*, are devoid of this peripheral placement of chromatin and appear more as a "ball in socket." Once it is determined that indeed the ameba being observed in a stool specimen is an entamoeba, the remaining task is then to differentiate *E. histolytica* from *E. coli*.

Only two of these features definitively separate the two: The trophozoites of *E. histolytica* have a unidirectional motility; that is, they extend pseudopods only along one plane and actually will walk off the edge of the field of focus when observed in a microscopic mount. The trophozoites of *E. coli*, on the other hand, extend pseudopods in multiple planes and wander aimlessly in one direction then the other. The trophozoites of *E. histolytica* also have the unique capability of ingesting erythrocytes; it is extremely rare that ingested red blood cells will be seen in *E. coli* trophozoites.

E. coli trophozoites have nuclei with relatively large, eccentrically placed karyosomes with an uneven, blotchy distribution of chromatin around the nuclear membrane; the karyosomes of *E. histolytica* are small and centrally located, and the chromatin is evenly distributed along the nuclear membrance. The cytoplasm of *E. histolytica* is finely granular; that of *E. coli* is coarse and "junky." The chromatoidal bars of *E. coli* have splintered ends; those of *E. histolytica* are rounded. The cysts of *E. histolytica* never possess more than 4 nuclei; those of *E. coli* typically have 8 and occasionally 16. The same differences in nuclear structure as described for the trophozoites pertain to the cysts as well.

The trophozoites of *Endolimax nana* are small (5 to 12 μm in diameter, with an average of 6 to 7 μm) and possess a nucleus with a large karyosome and absence of nuclear chromatin along an otherwise faintly visible nuclear membrane, giving a ball-in-socket appearance. The cysts are also small, 5 to 6 μm in diameter, and contain four nuclei, also with the ball-in-socket appearance. The small race of *E. histolytica* called *E. hartmanii* are of similar small size, but they can be differentiated from *E. nana* because they possess an entamoeba-type nucleus. *Iodamoeba butchlii* also has a ball-in-socket type of nucleus. Both the trophozoites and the cysts are larger (8 to 20 μm), and the presence of a distinct, large glycogen vacuole that stains brown in iodine preparations are usually sufficient to distinguish it from the smaller forms of *E. nana*.

FREE-LIVING AMEBAE.   One additional group of amebae, not listed previously, must be briefly mentioned. Small free-living water and soil amebae of the genera *Naegleria* and *Acanthamoeba* are capable of producing opportunistic infections in humans. These species and other genera of free-living amebae, have a worldwide distribution in various freshwater habitats, including rivers, lakes, ponds, hot springs and spas, domestic water systems, air-conditioning systems, humidifiers, and cooling towers. They are ubiquitous in soils, dust, air, and composts; have been found on the surfaces of vegetables; and have been isolated from sewage sludge and fresh water polluted by domestic or industrial waste.

The major diseases produced by this group are forms of devastating, usually fatal meningoencephalitis and *Acanthamoeba* keratitis. *Naegleria fowleri* produces a diffuse and fulminant meningoencephalitis characterized by the presence of trophozoites but no cysts in large areas of hemorrhagic necrosis, especially involving the olfactory bulbs, frontal lobes, base of the brain, proximal spinal cord, and temporal lobes of the brain. *Acanthamoeba* species may produce perivascular granulomatous lesions in the brain containing both trophozoites and cyst forms, the latter being diagnostic.

Acanthamoeba keratitis is a serious, often devastating infection of the cornea involving certain species of *Acanthamoeba*.[5,12,46,59] Until about 1984, most infections were associated with trauma to the cornea and exposure to contaminated water; more recently, many cases have been associated with the use of contact lenses, especially daily-wear or extended-wear soft contact lenses. Other factors involved in *Acanthamoeba* keratitis include trauma to the cornea and the use of contaminated homemade saline or tap water rinses to clean lenses, the failure to disinfect lenses properly or as often as recommended by manufacturers, and wearing lenses while swimming.[59]

When amebic disease is suspected, fresh cerebrospinal fluid or tissue (eg, corneal biopsy, corneal scrapings, central nervous system tissue) should be collected aseptically and examined immediately. For direct microscopic examination, small drops of cerebrospinal fluid, other body fluids, or tissue suspensions should be examined in wet mounts (on slides under coverslips) by light microscopy, under reduced light, or by phase microscopy for motile trophozoites (using a 40× objective). Keeping the microscope stage warmed to 30° to 37°C may enhance motility. Material to be stained on slides should first be fixed in 10% neutral buffered formalin. After the slide is air dried it can then be stained with trichrome, the Papanicolaou stain, or hematoxylin and eosin. Tissue sections should be stained with hematoxylin and eosin.

Intestinal Flagellates

The following is a list of the intestinal flagellates discussed in this text:

G. lamblia
Chilomastix mesnili
Trichomonas species
Dientamoeba fragilis

The flagellates are a subclass of protozoa that possess one or more flagella. A flagellum is a motile, whiplike projection from a cell that serves as the locomotor organelle. The axostyle is the central supporting rod running through the body of flagellates that protrude from the posterior. One or more parabasal bodies, representing the energy center of the flagellum, and one or more nuclei may be present.

GIARDIA LAMBLIA. The trophozoite is bilaterally symmetric and has two nuclei, one on either side of a central axostyle (giving the appearance of a "monkey face"). In wet preparations, a graceful "falling leaf" motility can be a helpful identifying feature, distinguishing it from *C. mesnili*, which has a slower, stiff motion, and from *T. hominis*, which is quick, jerky, and darting. *G. lamblia* cysts are distinctly oval; measure 8 to 12 μm; have a thin, smooth membrane; and contain four nuclei clustered at one end, a longitudinal parabasal body near the center of the cell, and fibrils. Light bile staining is often seen, and there is a tendency for the cytoplasm to retract slightly from the cell wall.

Because of irregular shedding of organisms in the feces, several samples obtained on nonsuccessive days may be required to establish a diagnosis in suspected cases, particularly in chronic disease. The yield can be improved by preparing stained smears from concentrated fecal specimens, since organisms may often be missed if only saline mount procedures are performed.[21,56] Success has been reported in the use of several immunologic methods to directly detect *G. lamblia* antigen in fecal specimens.[27] Enzyme-linked immunosorbent assay using antibodies prepared against a variety of *G. lamblia* antigens has been the technology most often used.[33]

Symptoms of giardiasis include acute diarrhea, abdominal pain, and, in some cases, constitutional features such as weight loss and lassitude. In chronic cases, malabsorption and steatorrhea simulating sprue may be experienced. The exact mechanism by which *G. lamblia* causes disease is not completely known. Physical occlusion of the mucosa, bile salt deconjugation, enterotoxin excretion, prostaglandin release, and injury to the mucosal epithelial cell brush border are among the hypotheses that have been advanced. Most infections are sporadic, contracted after exposure to contaminated food or water under a variety of circumstances. Water-borne outbreaks in locales as diverse as Colorado, Russia, and New York have been reported. Campers who ingest native stream water are at risk; as are residents of communities where leakage of sewage-effluent irrigation systems may communicate with potable water systems. Both wild and domestic animals may serve as reservoirs and contaminate streams and lakes.

Children attending day care centers are perhaps at greatest risk for contracting giardiasis, proportional to factors such as increasing duration of attendance, time per week attending, low family income, large family size, and frequency of travel to the Colorado mountains.

CHILOMASTIX MESNILI. The most helpful feature in identifying *C. mesnili* is the large anterior nucleus placed immediately beneath the outer membrane and the presence of a prominent cytosome. Three anterior flagellae can often be seen by lowering the condenser and sharpening the focus. The cysts may be difficult to identify because the internal structures are not always well defined; the lemon shape and presence of a hyaline knob are helpful features. In well-preserved specimens, a cytosome giving the appearance of a safety pin may be seen adjacent to a single nucleus. This flagellate is not pathogenic to humans, and persons harboring this flagellate do not require treatment.

TRICHOMONAS HOMINIS. *T. hominis* may be somewhat more difficult to identify definitively because it is fragile and does not stain well. An undulating membrane that extends the full length of the organism is a helpful feature. *T. vaginalis*, which can contaminate fecal specimens from its normal habitat in the vaginal canal, has an undulating membrane that extends only one half of the distance of the body. These membranes and multiple flagellae of *Trichomonas* species are best observed in stained smears prepared from cultures. This flagellate is not pathogenic in humans.

DIENTAMOEBA FRAGILIS. Because the cytoplasm is so delicate, *D. fragilis* may be difficult to identify in wet mounts, and study of a permanent stained preparation is virtually mandatory if morphologic details are to be studied. The trophozoite typically has two nuclei with karyosomes fragmented into four to eight granules (about 20% have a single nucleus). Single-nucleated forms of *D. fragilis* may be difficult to differentiate from the trophozoites or early cysts of *E. nana*. Relatively broad-lobed, clear pseudopods provide purposeful motility. A cyst stage has not been identified.

D. fragilis produces a syndrome characterized by diarrhea, abdominal pain, and anal pruritus. Microbiologists in clinical laboratories must be aware that *D. fragilis* is being recovered from stool specimens with increasing frequency, particularly among individuals living in close quarters, such as inmates in institutions.

Intestinal Ciliates

The ciliates are characterized by the presence of cilia that surround the outer cell membrane. They usually possess a large, kidney-shaped macronucleus and one or more micronuclei. Cilia are motile, hairlike projections, larger and more complex than a microvillus. Most are 0.2 μm in diameter and 5 to 10 μm in length. The trophozoites possess a prominent cytosome, which is an opening in the membrane to one side that serves as a portal for ingestion of food. *Balantidium coli* is the species of human importance.

BALANTIDIUM COLI. *B. coli* is the only member of the ciliates known to infect humans. It is easy to recognize because of its large size (up to 100 μm in diameter), an outer membrane covered with short cilia, and its large, kidney-shaped macronucleus. The cyst measures 50 to 65 μm in diameter and can be recognized by the single large macronucleus.

Human balantidiosis is most prevalent where pigs are raised and slaughtered. Light infections tend to be asymptomatic; heavy infections in debilitated patients may cause bloody diarrhea, dehydration, and, in rare instances, death. Ulcers may occur in the intestine, accompanied by mesenteric lymphadenitis. Rare cases of extraintestinal extension to liver, lung, and other organs have been reported.[32]

Coccidia

The coccidia are a subgroup of protozoa within the subphylum Sporozoa that lack organelles for locomotion and that are obligate tissue parasites with sexual (schizogomy) and asexual (sporogony) stages in their life cycles. Included in this group are the malarial parasites in the blood, *Plasmodium* species, the tissue protozoan *T. gondii*, and the following intestinal coccidia, which are associated with diarrhea in immunosuppressed patients:

Cryptosporidium species
Isospora belli
Sarcocystis species

CRYPTOSPORIDIUM SPECIES. Cryptosporidia are minute coccidian protozoa that have been

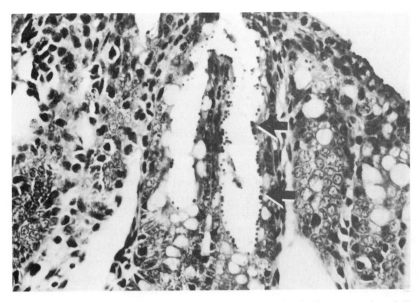

Figure 17-3. Section of mouse intestinal mucosa infected with *Cryptosporidium* illustrating the tiny oocysts on the surface epithelium (*arrows*) (original magnification × 320). (Courtesy of Bruce C. Andersen)

known to be associated with enterocolitis in a variety of domestic animals, including calves, pigs, and chickens.[2] This microorganism can be added to the list of agents of human diarrheal disease, which primarily affect persons with immunodeficiency, especially patients with AIDS.[16,47,58] Humans become infected either from direct contact with infected animals or from ingestion of fecally contaminated food or water. Human-to-human transmission has been particularly prevalent in day care centers.[1] The diagnosis is made by observing the 4- to 5-μm in diameter, spherical, acid-fast oocysts either along the brush border of the epithelial cells lining the small bowel mucosa (Fig. 17-3) or in stool specimens excreted between 7 and 28 days after infection (Fig. 17-4).

ISOSPORA BELLI. Isosporiasis, an illness characterized by diarrhea and malabsorption, was formerly only rarely encountered and was considered to be of limited clinical significance. Currently, *I. belli* is being seen in increasing frequency as one of the causes of the diarrheal syndrome in patients with AIDS.[18] Fever, headache, steatorrhea, and weight loss may occur in protracted cases; deaths due to water loss and electrolyte imbalance have been reported in overwhelming infections.[32] The

20- to 30-μm in diameter, elliptical, thin-walled oocysts are the diagnostic forms seen in human fecal specimens (Fig. 17-5). Immature oocysts contain only one sporocyst; more typically, mature oocysts contain two sporocysts. The drug of choice is trimethoprim-sulfamethoxazole.

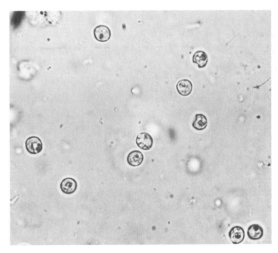

Figure 17-4. Cryptosporidial oocysts as observed in a fecal flotation preparation (original magnification × 1280). (Courtesy of Bruce C. Andersen)

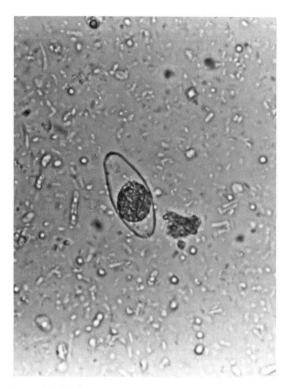

Figure 17-5. Immature oocyst of *Isospora belli*. These oocysts average 25 to 30 μm × 15 to 20 μm, are typically ellipsoidal and nonmotile, and have a smooth, thin wall and a single granular zygote within. Mature oocysts contain two granular zygotes.

SARCOCYSTIS SPECIES. *Sarcocystis* species use two mammals for the sexual and asexual phases of their life cycles. Humans may serve as either the intermediate or the definitive host. As intermediate host, encysted sporozoites from various *Sarcocystis* species have been identified in skeletal and cardiac muscle at autopsy.[8] This form is usually asymptomatic, although a history of polymyositis and eosinophilia have been reported. Humans acquire the intestinal form of sarcocystosis by ingesting poorly cooked, infected beef or pork. Patients may be asymptomatic but may on occasion manifest a diarrheal syndrome similar to that produced by *I. belli*. The diagnostic forms in stool specimens are mature, 25- to 33-μm oocysts containing two sporocysts, appearing similar to those of *I. belli*.

Blastocystis hominis and *Microsporidium* Species

Two other organisms of undetermined taxonomic status and clinical significance are *B. hominis* and

Microsporidium species. *B. hominis* can be found in a high percentage of stool specimens but have been incriminated as the causative agent in a few reported cases. The organisms are irregular in size, ranging between 5 and 30 μm, and are characterized by a large central, homogeneous staining body or vacuole with a thin rim of cytoplasm at the periphery, in which are scattered granules and evenly spaced nuclei. When seen in low numbers in stool specimens, the presence of these organisms is usually ignored; because their role as agents of diarrheal disease has not been established, however, the presence of five or more *B. hominis* forms per high-powered field is reported from many laboratories, leaving the clinical significance and the decision whether to treat up to the consulting physician, based on clinical evidence.

The role of *Microsporidium* species as agents of diarrheal disease and as extraintestinal pathogens as well is emerging. Included are obligate intracellular parasites, ranging from about 1.5 to 5 μm wide and 2 to 7 μm long. These tiny organisms have been found in virtually all animal groups, including birds, lower vertebrates, and invertebrates. Only a few human infections have been reported, with only members of the genus *Enterocytozoon* being involved. The principal feature distinguishing *Microsporidium* species from other protozoa is the production of spores, each with a complex system of polar tubules. These tubules have an extrusion mechanism that is used to inject sporoplasm into the host cell, preparatory to extensive multiplication within the cytoplasm. Further description of these organisms is beyond the scope of this text; identification in human tissues is dependent on the electron microscopic study of ultrastructures. Until laboratory workers become more familiar with the light microscopic features of these infections and until electron microscopic studies become more readily available, microsporidiosis will remain under diagnosed.

Nematodes

Nematodes are a class of helminths that includes the roundworms, the adults of which possess a tapered, cylindric body with longitudinally oriented muscles and a triradiate esophagus. In addition to the adults, two other forms may be encountered in the clinical laboratories—larvae and ova, or eggs. The larvae are independently functioning, immature stages in the life cycle of an animal that undergoes one or more stages of metamorphosis to become an adult. In some nematodal diseases, such as hookworm infections, it may be the infective form.

Eggs, or ova, represent the mature female gamete, a resting form designed to survive adverse environmental conditions, that serves as both the diagnostic and infective forms. The diagnosis of many nematode infections is first made by observing characteristic ova in feces or other material.

The species of intestinal nematodes that most commonly infect humans include the following:

Ascaris lumbricoides
Trichuris trichiura
Hookworms
    Necator americanus
    Ancylostoma duodenale
Strongyloides stercoralis
Enterobius vermicularis
Capillaria philippinensis
Trichostrongylus species

Life Cycles and Modes of Infection

The life cycles of this group of helminths vary considerably in complexity. Many of these nematodes do not have an intermediate host in their life cycle (*A. lumbricoides, T. trichuria, E. vermicularis*), as shown in Figure 17-1; most require a stage outside the human host to develop into an infective form. The ova of most nematode species require an intermediate time of development in the external environment to develop into a larval and often infective stage, depending on the temperature, moisture, and nature of the soil into which they are passed.

The mode of infection with *N. americanus, A. duodenale, S. stercoralis,* and *Trichostrongylus* species is somewhat more complex, involving direct penetration of the skin with filariform larva. For example, hookworm eggs that are passed in the feces are already in an early cleavage stage and soon hatch into the *rhabditiform* larval stage. In 5 to 7 days, the muscular esophagus is lost and the filariform larval stage is formed. Well-aerated, moist soil in a temperature range of 23° to 33°C is optimal for development of the filariform larvae, which may remain viable for several weeks. Filariform larvae represent the infective stage for humans and are able to penetrate the skin of a bare foot when contact is made with infected dung or soil. These larvae enter the circulation and pass through the right side of the heart and lungs. They are coughed up and swallowed and then take up final residence in the small intestine where they develop into adult worms.

The life cycle of *S. stercoralis* is similar to that of hookworms except that the eggs have usually hatched by the time they are passed in the feces, so that the rhabditiform larvae are the common diagnostic form observed in stool specimens. In immunosuppressed hosts, the rhabditiform larvae of *S. stercoralis* may transform into filariform larvae that can, in turn, invade the bowel mucosa, causing a hyperinfection syndrome. In severe cases, these larvae can circulate widely to many organs, which can be fatal.

Ascaris lumbricoides

The laboratory diagnosis of ascariasis is made either by observing the adult worms as they protrude from body orifices or in situ in the intestine or contiguous duct systems (as seen at surgery or at autopsy) or, more commonly, by detecting the characteristic 45- by 60-μm, spherical, thick-walled, scalloped, bile-stained ova in stool specimens. Patients with light infections may be asymptomatic. In heavy intestinal infections, abdominal pain, discomfort, and diarrhea are common findings. *Ascaris* adults have the propensity to migrate and wander into the bile ducts, pancreatic, duct or lumen of the appendix. Appendicitis, pancreatitis, biliary obstruction, and hepatic abscess formation are all potential complications.

Trichuris trichiura

The adult *Trichuris* worms measure between 30 and 50 mm in length, with males being slightly smaller than females. The *Trichuris* adult worm derives its colloquial name, "whipworm," from the thin, anterior, whiplike head. The ova measure approximately 54 by 22 μm and are easy to recognize in microscopic preparations by their distinct barrel shape and refractile hyaline polar plugs at either end. In light infections, patients are generally asymptomatic. In heavy infections, diarrhea, dysentery, and abdominal discomfort may be experienced. Varying degrees of malabsorption may also be observed, and, because the diarrhea tends to be watery, sodium and potassium electrolyte imbalances may be a problem. Rectal prolapse in children is one of the complications of heavy infection.

Ancylostoma duodenale and *Necator americanus*

The adult hookworms, which measure up to 1.5 cm in length, reside in the upper intestine, where they are firmly attached to the mucosa by the biting action of cutting mouth parts. The male worms are distinguished by their frayed, posterior bursa. Observation of the mouth parts can be used to distinguish between the two species. *A. duodenale* has two pairs of chitinous teeth; the mouthpart of *N. americanus* is fitted with a pair of cutting plates. The laboratory diagnosis is usually made by observing the characteristic thin-walled, transparent, unpigmented, 40- by 65-μm ova in stool specimens. The yolk cells retract, leaving a clear space beneath the shell. In a heavy infection of 500 or more worms the host could be bled the equivalent of 1 pint of blood per week, producing severe hypochromia, iron deficiency anemia, and marked erythroid hyperplasia of the bone marrow. Weakness, fatigue, growth retardation, peripheral edema, and congestive heart failure may be complications in severe infections. Diarrhea, abdominal pain, and nausea are manifestations of the intestinal phase of infection.

Strongyloides stercoralis

The laboratory diagnosis of strongyloidiasis is usually made by observing for motile rhabditiform larvae in stool specimens. The rhabditiform larvae of *S. stercoralis* have a short buccal cavity in contrast to a long buccal cavity for the rhabditiform larvae of the hookworms.

The intestinal manifestations of *Strongyloides* infections vary from few if any symptoms in light infections to severe necrotizing bowel disease in heavy infections. Symptoms may suggest peptic ulcer disease in some patients; in others, involvement of the small intestine may radiographically mimic Crohn's disease. As mentioned earlier, immunosuppressed hosts are particularly vulnerable to disseminated *Strongyloides* infections.[9] The propensity for *S. stercoralis* eggs to hatch quickly and to produce intraintestinal filariform larvae makes patients vulnerable to autoinfection, resulting in a condition known as hyperinfection syndrome.[26]

Once immunity is compromised or abrogated, hyperinfection with dissemination of larvae to many organs and tissues is likely to occur in patients harboring the parasite. Mortality rates as high as 50% have been reported in naturally or iatrogenically compromised patients with hyperinfection strongyloidiasis.[25]

Enterobius vermicularis

The adult female worm measures 8 to 13 mm long by 0.4 mm in diameter. It can be recognized by the cuticular, winglike alar expansion at the anterior end and the long pointed tail ("pin"). The diagnosis of *E. vermicularis* (pinworm) infection is most commonly made by identifying the characteristic thin-walled, smooth, 30- by 50-μm ova that are flattened on one side, in a cellulose acetate ("Scotch tape") preparation, in which the sticky side of a piece of transparent tape is pressed on the perianal skin. Yield is best in children if the test is performed early in the morning when worm migration is maximal, immediately on waking before bowel movement. The gravid female deposits eggs in the folds of the perianal skin during the late evening hours. Nocturnal pruritus ani is the usual presenting symptom because of the irritation caused by the deposition of eggs on the perianal skin.

Cestodes

The cestodes are a subclass of helminths comprising true tapeworms. The cestodes of human importance include the following:

Taenia saginata
Taenia solium
Diphyllobothrium latum
Hymenolepis nana
H. diminuta
Dipylidium caninum

The body of an adult cestode or tapeworm, called the strobila, consists of two parts, a scolex and the proglottids. The scolex is the anterior portion with hooklets or suckers by which the worm can attach and anchor to the intestinal mucosa. The crown of the scolex, called the rostellum, may be fitted with hooklets (armed) or may be devoid of hooklets and smooth (unarmed). These morphologic differences are helpful in establishing a species identification.

The major portion of the body of a tapeworm is composed of a long series of segments called proglottids. Each proglottid possesses male and female reproductive structures, the uterine branches of which are packed with ova when mature. The ova are passed in the feces, where they are observed in microscopic mounts to establish a laboratory diagnosis. Subtle differences in the size, shape, and internal structures of proglottids serve as aids in establishing a species identification.

With the exception of *H. nana*, when human-to-human transmission of infections may occur through ingestion of fecally contaminated food or water that contains infective eggs, the life cycle of the cestodes requires one or more intermediate hosts to support stages of larval development. For example, humans with an intestinal tapeworm infection pass feces containing mature ova that can contaminate vegetative matter, soil, or fresh water. Tapeworm eggs ingested by cows, pigs, and fish, for example, hatch in the intestines of these intermediate hosts, liberating larvae that penetrate the bowel mucosa and migrate into the skeletal muscle or flesh. The larvae become encysted in a form called cysticercus, or bladder worm. Humans become infected by eating raw or poorly cooked beef, pork, or fish infested with the cysticerci.

Taenia solium and Taenia saginata

The strobila of *T. saginata* can reach as long as 10 meters and contain as many as 2000 proglottids; *T. solium* is somewhat smaller, reaching up to 4 meters long and up to 1000 proglottids. The scolex of *T. solium* has an armed rostellum with a double row of hooklets; the scolex of *T. saginata* is unarmed. The laboratory diagnosis of *Taenia* tapeworm infections is usually made by observing in microscopic mounts of fecal material the characteristic spherical, thick-shelled, 30- by 45-μm ova with radial striations. Three pairs of hooklets may be observed internally within the yolk substance.

Symptoms are generally minimal. Abdominal discomfort and mild diarrhea may be experienced; rarely, in the presence of a large worm, intestinal obstruction may occur. The treatment of choice for intestinal disease is niclosamide in a single 2-g dose; for cysticercus disease, praziquantel,

16.6 mg/kg three times a day for 14 days, is recommended.

Differentiation of *T. saginata* from *T. solium* is more than an academic exercise. In addition to serving as the definitive host and harboring the adult tapeworm, humans may also serve as the intermediate host if the ova of *T. solium* are ingested, leading to a potentially lethal larval form of extraintestinal disease called cysticercosis. Cysticercosis does not occur with *T. saginata*. Although larvae may migrate to and be found in virtually any organ, the central nervous system is involved in 60% to 96% of patients, a condition known as neurocysticercosis.[41,51] Most patients with neurocysticercosis have more than one cyst, with as many as 200 cysts found in one autopsy case.[41] Symptoms vary considerably from patient to patient. Lesions in the cerebral cortex may result in seizures or localizing neurologic deficits. Cranial nerve palsies, in particular involving the fifth and seventh nerves, and abnormal reflexes are commonly found. Personality changes, intracranial hypertension (headache, vertigo, nausea, vomiting), and sudden death from obstruction of the fourth ventricle are other symptoms that have been reported.

Diphyllobothrium latum

D. latum, the human giant fish tapeworm, has a strobila that measures from 3 to 10 meters and has more than 3000 proglottids. Although the proglottids are rarely passed in the stool, they are distinctive because the individual segments are broader than they are long (from L., *latum*, meaning "broad"). The laboratory diagnosis of *D. latum* infection in humans is commonly made by identifying the characteristic 55- by 75-μm, smooth-shelled, "nonshouldered" operculated eggs in stool specimens. Humans become infected by ingesting these plerocercoid larvae in raw or poorly cooked fish, from which an adult worm develops in the intestine. Patients may harbor an adult worm for up to 20 years. Symptoms are usually minimal. Large adult worms may cause mechanical bowel obstruction, accompanied by abdominal pain and diarrhea. In a minority of patients, particularly in northern Europe, megaloblastic anemia may develop secondary to the selective competition of the parasite for intraintestinal vitamin B_{12}. A single 2-g dose of niclosamide is the treatment of choice.

Hymenolepis nana and *Hymenolepis diminuta*

The adult worms of *H. nana*, the dwarf tapeworm, are small, measuring no longer than 1.5 inches when mature, and often simulate mucous threads; those of *H. diminuta* are longer, measuring between 20 and 60 cm. Neither of the adults is commonly found in stool specimens. The laboratory diagnosis of human *Hymenolepis* infection is usually made by microscopically detecting the characteristic spherical, double-membrane, 45- by 60-μm (70- by 85-μm for *H. diminuta*), hexacanth (possessing three pairs of hooklets) ova in mounts or stained smears of fecal specimens. The ova of *H. nana* are smaller than those of *H. diminuta* but are better distinguished by observing slender polar filaments arising from thickenings on either side of the inner membrane of the hexacanth embryo and extending into the space beneath the shell. *H. diminuta* is devoid of these polar filaments.

Humans become infected with *H. nana* most commonly by ingesting embryonated eggs in contaminated food or water. *H. diminuta* infections occur after ingestion of the infective pleocercoids that are present in infected larval rat and mouse fleas or adult meal beetles that inhabit various cereals and grains. *H. nana* infections are most common in children and are prevalent in the southeastern United States. In heavy infections, often due to the propensity for internal hyperinfection, up to 1000 *H. nana* worms may be present. Symptoms in light infections may be absent; anorexia, abdominal pain, diarrhea, headache, and nervousness may be seen in heavy infections. Peripheral eosinophilia is mild to moderate (4% to 16%).

Dipylidium caninum

D. caninum, the most common tapeworm of dogs and cats, may also infect humans, particularly children who have more intimate contact with household pets. The strobila ranges from 15 to 70 cm in length and possesses 60 to 175 proglottids. The scolex is rhomboidal, possessing a retractile, conical, armed rostellum. The proglottids average 12 by 2.7 mm and are distinctive in that each possesses a double genital pore. Humans become infected by ingesting food, water, or matter contaminated with dog, cat, or human fleas.

The laboratory diagnosis in human infections is usually made by microscopically observing the characteristic egg packets. Each packet contains 15 to 25 globular eggs, each measuring 35 to 60 μm in diameter containing an oncosphere with six hooklets. Infected persons usually have minimal or no symptoms. In heavy infections, symptoms are usually limited to indigestion, appetite loss, and vague abdominal discomfort. Niclosamine in a single 2-g dose is the treatment of choice.

Trematodes

The trematodes are a class of helminths including all the flukes that are parasites in humans. Flukes are leaflike and flat, are hermaphroditic except for the schistosomes, and possess two suckers—one oral, through which the digestive tract opens, and the other ventral, for attachment. The trematodes of human importance include the following:

Liver flukes: *Fasciola hepatica* and *Clonorchis sinensis*
Giant intestinal fluke: *Fasciolopsis buskii*
Schistosomes: *S. mansoni*, *S. haematobium*, *S. japonicum*
Lung fluke: *P. westermani*

The initial stages of the life cycles of the trematodes are virtually identical; that is, eggs are passed with feces into water and hatch either immediately or after a short period of embryonation. Free-swimming miracidia are released, which are either ingested or penetrate into the flesh of the first intermediate host—a snail. Within the snail, the miracidia transform into a second larval stage known as a sporocyst (schistosomes) or a redia (the trematodes). This developmental period may be as short as 3 weeks for *C. sinensis* and as long as 12 weeks for *F. hepatica*. The purpose of this larval stage in the snail is to provide an environment for replication of hundreds of cercariae.

The mode of infection for various cercariae varies with the species. For example, mature schistosome cercariae, with characteristic forked tails, after release from the snail, infect humans who wade or swim in infested waters. Cercariae directly penetrate the water-softened skin without requiring a second intermediate host. A mild inflammatory response may occur at the sites of cercarial penetration. *C. sinensis* cercariae infect freshwater fish; those of *P. westermani* use various species of crustaceans (crabs or crayfish); and those with

F. hepatica and *F. buski* attach to a variety of water plants (water chestnut or watercress), where they form encysted structures known as metacercariae. These metacercariae are more resistant to environmental stresses than free-swimming cercariae and can survive for several weeks or months. Humans become infected by ingesting the metacercariae that are contained in the raw or undercooked flesh of fish or crustaceans or that are attached to the leaves or stems of water plants.

Schistosoma Species

The name *schistosome* is derived from the appearance of the adult male, the body of which has a longitudinal genital groove, or canal, serving as a receptacle for the female during copulation. Three *Schistosoma* species, *S. mansoni*, *S. haematobium*, and *S. japonicum*, cause most human infections. Depending on the species, schistosome adults are found in various locations in the portal vein system: (1) in the portal veins of the large intestine for *S. mansoni* and *S. intercalatum*, (2) in the small intestine for *S. japonicum* and *S. mekongi*, and (3) in the veins of the urinary bladder for *S. haematobium*.

The laboratory diagnosis is made by detecting the characteristic ova in stool or, in cases of *S. haematobium* infections, in the urine. The ova are very large, measuring 80 to 150 μm in diameter. The ova for each species are morphologically distinct: *S. mansoni* possesses a prominent lateral spine, *S. haematobium* has a delicate terminal spine. The ova of *S. japonicum* are broadly oval to semispherical with a small rudimentary, lateral, knoblike spine.

After transmigrating the wall of the veins in which the adult female resides, the ova penetrate into the adjacent viscera, eliciting a severe suppurative and granulomatous inflammation, ultimately resulting in fibrosis and scarring. Bloody diarrhea, vague abdominal pain, and, in severe cases, bowel obstruction may be observed with *S. mansoni* and *S. japonicum*, infections; *S. haematobium* produces inflammation of the urinary bladder, resulting in intermittent hematuria, lower abdominal pain, and, ultimately, contraction.

Fasciola hepatica and Fasciolopsis buski

F. hepatica is a large fluke measuring about 2.5 by 1.5 cm that primarily infects the liver of sheep.

Humans become an accidental definitive host when they ingest uncooked water plants such as water chestnuts or watercress that are infected with *Fasciola* metacercariae. Human fascioliasis is manifested by headache, chills, fever, and right upper quadrant pain. Hepatomegaly, jaundice, diarrhea, and anemia may occur in severe infections; hepatic biliary cirrhosis is a late complication. Laboratory diagnosis is made by identifying the large eggs in the feces, which are identical in appearance to those of *F. buskii*. They are large, averaging 130 to 150 μm by 60 to 90 μm, and they have a smooth, thin shell and an indistinct operculum at one of the long ends.

F. buski is a fluke similar to *F. hepatica* except that it is somewhat larger (20 to 75 mm by 8 to 20 mm) and has a rounded instead of a conical anterior portion. These flukes reside in the small intestine and attach by means of a small oral sucker to the intestinal mucosa. Local mucosal ulcers produce varying degrees of epigastric pain, nausea, and diarrhea, especially in the morning. Ascites and intestinal obstruction may be seen in heavy infections.

Clonorchis sinensis

C. sinensis, the Chinese liver fluke, is a relatively small fluke that varies in size (12 to 20 mm by 3 to 5 mm) when mature and resides within the biliary ducts or in the gallbladder of humans. In light infections, the parenchymal liver cell damage is minimal and cirrhosis does not occur; in heavy infections, the bile ducts may become thickened and dilated. Biliary obstruction and jaundice are rare; several reports indicate an increase in cholangiocarcinoma.[54,55]

Humans become infected with *C. sinensis* by ingesting infected raw or poorly cooked freshwater fish. The laboratory diagnosis is made by identifying the characteristic, small, urn-shaped eggs in stool specimens. These ova average 30 by 15 μm and have a prominent operculum at the narrow, constricted end. They generally are yellow and bile stained when seen in unstained fecal mounts.

Paragonimus westermani

P. westermani and other *Paragonimus* species are lung flukes that represent a classic example of organotropism, which is the special affinity a parasite has to seek out and reside within a given organ. Humans become infected after ingestion of raw or poorly cooked crab meat or crayfish, the flesh of which contains encysted metacercariae. After ingestion, the metacercariae hatch in the duodenum, releasing larvae that penetrate the full thickness of the bowel wall, enter the abdominal cavity, transmigrate the diaphragm, and enter the pleural space. The larvae then bore into the peripheral lung tissue and ultimately reside within a pseudocyst. The cyst enlarges as the adult fluke grows and may break into an adjacent bronchiole. When a pseudocyst ruptures into a bronchus, coughing and hemoptysis are common symptoms. Eggs produced by mature flukes are discharged into the bronchi and are ultimately swallowed by the patient from secretions coughed into the oropharynx. The laboratory diagnosis is made by observing the characteristic ova in stool specimens. They average 65 to 120 μm long and 40 to 70 μm wide, with an operculum at one end that is demarcated on either side by a lateral protrusion ("shouldered").

Blood and Tissue Parasites

In general, the life cycles of the blood and tissue parasites are more complex than those of their intestinal counterparts. Most of the blood parasites are transmitted to humans by an arthropod vector within which the sexual phase of the life cycle develops. Many parasites causing tissue infections use various insects for the development of intermediate stages in their life cycles. Tissue parasites may be either intracellular or extracellular, depending on the species and the phase of the parasitic cycle. The following is an outline of human blood and tissue parasites and infections that are briefly discussed here:

Malaria
P. falciparum
P. vivax
P. malariae
P. ovale

Tissue Coccidia Infection
T. gondii
P. carinii

Leishmaniasis
L. donovani
L. tropica complex
L. brasiliensis complex
L. mexicana complex

Trypanosomiasis
T. brucei gambiense
T. brucei rhodesiense
T. cruzi
T. rangeli

Filarial Nematodes
Wuchereria bancrofti
Brugia malayi
Loa loa
Mansonella ozzardi
Mansonella perstans
Onchocerca volvulus
Dirofilaria immitis

Tissue Nematodes
T. spiralis
Toxocara canis (visceral larva migrans)
Ancylostoma braziliensis or A. caninum (cutaneous larva migrans)
Dracunculus medinensis
Anisakis species
Gnathostoma species

Tissue Cestodes
Echinococcus granulosis
Echinococcus multilocularis
Multiceps species (coenurosis)
Spirametra mansonoides (sparganosis)

Tissue Protozoa

PLASMODIUM SPECIES. The life cycle of the *Plasmodium* parasite has two phases: a sexual cycle, known as sporogony, which takes place within the intestinal tract of the mosquito; and an asexual cycle, known as schizogony, occurring in the human host. Humans become infected when they are bitten by a female *Anopheles* mosquito that contains the infective sporozoites in the salivary secretions. Laboratory identification of the malarial parasites in humans is made by studying stained thin and thick peripheral blood smears. Table 17-1 lists the differential features by which the three common species, *P. vivax*, *P. falciparum*, and *P. malariae*, can be identified.

Temperature spike, up to 105°C, is the constant presenting symptom of infections with all *Plasmodium* species, beginning up to 10 days after the bite of an infected mosquito. Prodromal symptoms of headache, myalgia, malaise, and fatigue suggestive of a flulike syndrome may be experienced early in the infection. Later, the temperature spikes become regularly spaced every other day, tertian (*P.*

Table 17-1
Plasmodia: Key Features for Laboratory Identification

SPECIES	APPEARANCE OF ERYTHROCYTES	TROPHOZOITES	SCHIZONTS	GAMETOCYTES	SPECIAL FEATURES
Plasmodium vivax	Enlarged and pale; Schüffner's dots usually prominent	*Early:* ring relatively large (one third the size of red blood cell). Rings with two nuclei or cells with two or three rings may be seen. *Mature:* ameboid, with delicate pseudopodia that flow to fill the entire red blood cell.	12 to 24 segments (merozoites); pigment fine grained and inconspicuous.	Round to oval and almost completely fill red blood cell. Large chromatin mass. Pigment is coarse and evenly distributed.	Length of asexual cycle (fever cycle) is 48 hours (benign tertian). Be alert for possibility of mixed species infection when *P. vivax* forms are identified.
Plasmodium falciparum	Normal size; Maurer's dots or clefts are rarely seen.	Ring forms extremely small, occupying no more than one fifth of red blood cell. Double nuclei are common, and multiple rings per red blood cell are usual. Appliqué forms plastered on the red blood cell membrane are virtually diagnostic.	Not normally seen except in fulminant disease; 24 or more segments are characteristic.	Characteristic crescent or banana-shaped forms are virtually diagnostic. Microgametocytes stain lighter blue than macrogametocytes.	The ratio of infected to normal red blood cells is high. Intermediate ring forms or schizonts are not commonly seen in the peripheral blood. Length of asexual cycle is 48 hours (malignant tertian).
Plasmodium malariae	Normal size; no dots or clefts form.	*Early:* similar to *P. vivax*, except staining is deeper blue and the cytoplasma of the ring is broader. Double rings are rare. *Mature:* less tendency to become ameboid; rather, it forms a ribbon or band.	More than 12 segments rarely seen. Merozoites arrange in rosettes. Pigment is abundant and coarse, often in aggregates within "hoff" of rosettes.	Not distinctive and resemble those of *P. vivax*. Red blood cells are not enlarged. Pigment usually more abundant in *P. vivax* and tends to be coarse and unevenly distributed.	Asexual cycle lasts 72 hours (quartan). Identification of *P. malariae* is often made after either *P. vivax* or *P. falciparum* have been excluded by their more distinctive morphologic features.

vivax and *P. falciparum* malaria), every third day, or quartan (*P. malariae*), every fourth day. The periodicity of each episode of high fever is related to the rupture of erythrocytes as merozoites are released into the circulation. Infections with *F. falciparum* may be severe and fulminant, owing to small areas of hemorrhagic infarction caused by the plugging of capillary vessels by "sticky" infected erythro-

cytes. Persons planning travel to parts of the world endemic for malaria should consult with local public health authorities for advice on protection and prophylaxis.

TOXOPLASMA GONDII. *T. gondii* is a protozoan parasite that has particular predilection for infecting the central nervous system in humans. As is

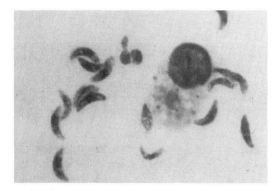

Figure 17-6. High-power view of Giemsa-stained impression smear demonstrating *Toxoplasma* trophozoites. Note characteristic bow shape and central, dark-staining nucleus (× 1000).

characteristic of other coccidia, the life cycle of *T. gondii* has both sexual and asexual stages. The sexual stage occurs in the intestine of cats, where infective oocysts 10 to 12 μm in diameter are excreted in the feces. The asexual stage commonly occurs in a variety of herbivorous and carnivorous animals and also in humans.

Three modes of transmission lead to most human infections: (1) directly from ingestion of infective oocysts in food (eg, unwashed leafy vegetables) or water contaminated with cat feces; (2) indirectly from ingestion of the raw or undercooked meat of animals that had ingested oocysts (it is estimated that 25% of lamb and pork sold at supermarkets contain viable tissue cysts); and (3) transplacental transfer to the fetus from a mother infected during pregnancy.

The diagnosis of acute toxoplasmosis can be made by demonstrating clusters of bow-shaped, 3- to 4-μm by 6- to 7-μm tachyzoites in stained tissue sections or impression smears (Fig. 17-6). The diagnostic form in patients with chronic and usually inactive toxoplasmosis are cysts measuring up to 200 μm in diameter (Fig. 17-7). The presence of cysts is probably one source of acute reactivation toxoplasmosis. Serologic tests for the detection of specific *Toxoplasma* antibody has been the mainstay of diagnosing active infections for years.[40] Several tests are available to measure serum *Toxoplasma* antibodies. In brief, acute acquired toxoplasmosis can be suspected if a seroconversion from negative to positive is demonstrated, if there is a twofold increase in titer of a sample drawn 3 weeks after a baseline level, or if there is a high IgM titer. A full presentation of serologic findings in other types of congenital and chronic toxoplasmosis can be found elsewhere.[34]

A broad spectrum of signs and symptoms may be encountered in cases of human toxoplasmosis. Symptomatic acute toxoplasmosis in immunocompetent humans presents as generalized lymphadenopathy, particularly of the cervical area of the neck, often accompanied by sore throat, fever, and myalgias.

Immunosuppressed persons are highly susceptible to infection with *T. gondii*. A marked increase in incidence of symptomatic disease has been found among homosexual men and intravenous-drug users.[65] The disease often localizes in the central nervous system with symptoms of encephalitis or meningoencephalitis or manifests as a space-occu-

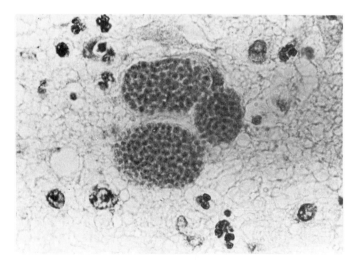

Figure 17-7. High-powered view of the *Toxoplasma* pseudocysts illustrated in Figure 17-6. Each pseudocyst contains several scores of trophozoites. These pseudocysts are most commonly seen in patients with latent disease. Note the absence of an inflammatory reaction adjacent to these pseudocysts (H & E, × 1000).

pying lesion.[37,52] The disease can progress rapidly and usually results in death if the compromised immune status remains unchanged. Pulmonary, cardiac, and lymphoreticular disease may also be present. The cerebrospinal fluid typically shows high protein levels and an increase in mononuclear inflammatory cells.

Premature or antibody-deficient infants are more susceptible to developing congenitally acquired disease. General symptoms include splenomegaly, jaundice, fever, and lymphadenopathy. The central nervous system is particularly susceptible, with features including impaired vision, convulsions, mental retardation, spasticity, hydrocephalus, microcephalus, and deafness. Neonates who are asymptomatic at birth may develop late-onset disease; spinal or subarachnoid punctures should be performed in suspected cases to make the diagnosis.

PNEUMOCYSTIS CARINII. Pneumocystosis is among the more common causes of nonbacterial pneumonia in immunocompromised hosts in the United States[3,19] and is a leading cause of death in patients with AIDS.[39,45] Pifer and associates[50] also found *P. carinii* to be a common agent of pneumonia in pediatric patients with AIDS, many of whom acquired the disease through blood transfusions. Dyspnea, fever, nonproductive cough, cyanosis, rales, and hepatosplenomegaly are the most common clinical signs and symptoms of pulmonary pneumocystosis. The disease may be fulminant and rapidly fatal, particularly in the sporadic form.[62]

The diagnosis can be made by demonstrating in tissue sections the presence of cysts measuring 5 to 8 μm in diameter, either using the Gomori methenamine silver (GMS) stain or the rapid toluidine blue stain described by Chalvardjian and Grawe.[13] With the silver stain, the organisms appear deep blue-black. Alternatively, for demonstrating organisms in bronchial washings or bronchoalveolar lavage specimens, the long staining time required for performing silver stains can be reduced by using either the traditional Giemsa stains, which take 45 to 60 minutes, or the very rapid and commercially marketed Diff-Quick stain (Baxter Care Corp, Scientific Products Division, McGraw Park, IL), which can be performed in 10 minutes.[15] These stains demonstrate the trophozoites, which measure 1.5 to 4 μm in diameter and stain with red

nuclei and light blue cytoplasm. A rapid modified toluidine blue O stain and direct immunofluorescence assays using monoclonal antibodies[64] have also been successfully used.

Hemoflagellates

The protozoan family Trypanosomatidae includes members from the genera *Leishmania* and *Trypanosoma*, which are flagellates that inhabit the blood and tissues of humans. Four stages of development of the parasites may be observed. The adult or trypanosomal forms have an elongated body with a whiplike posterior flagellum that is attached by a delicate undulating membrane that runs the length of the body. Three species are associated with human disease: *T. gambiense* and *T. rhodesiense* cause African sleeping sickness, whereas *T. cruzi* is responsible for South American trypanosomiasis. The least developed form of these protozoa, called the amastigote or leishmanial forms, are devoid of a flagellae and are found as intracellular parasites in reticuloendothelial cells.

LEISHMANIA SPECIES. Human leishmaniasis may take two forms, a disseminated disease, kala-azar, involving the liver, spleen, and other parts of the reticuloendothelial system, and a primary cutaneous form, clinically manifesting as ulcers or "sores" of the skin and mucous membranes. Humans become infected through the bites of several species of *Phlebotomus* sandflies. Visceral leishmaniasis is caused by several species belonging to the *L. donovani* complex, namely, *L. donovani donovani*, *L. donovani infantum*, and *L. donovani chagasi*. A small skin papule develops at the site of the bite but rarely progresses to an ulcer. The amastigotes proliferate locally in the subcutaneous tissue but soon disseminate throughout the reticuloendothelial system to involve the spleen, liver, bone marrow, and lymph nodes where the organisms are found as obligate intracellular parasites.

Symptoms may be mild and self-limited in light, contained infections; or there may be the sudden onset of spiking fevers (a pattern of two or three peaks per day), anorexia, malaise, and a feeling of ill health, simulating typhoid fever or malaria. If the disease progresses and becomes chronic, persistence of low-grade fever, vague abdominal pain, enlargement of the abdomen from hepatomegaly and splenomegaly (which can become enormous), generalized lymphadenopathy, anemia, and leuko-penia may become pronounced.

Primary cutaneous leishmaniasis includes both Old World and New World diseases. The Old World disease, or oriental sore, is most commonly caused by members of the *L. tropica* complex (including *L. major*, *L. tropica minor*, and *L. aethiopica*). New World cutaneous leishmaniasis is caused by the *L. braziliensis* complex (also including *L. braziliensis gyanensis* and *L. braziliensis panamensis*), which is endemic in almost all countries in South America and in several regions in Latin America, and by the *Leishmania mexicana* complex, including several separate species endemic in various regions in Mexico, Guatemala, Venezuela, and the Amazon River basin of Brazil.[30,49] The *L. braziliensis* complex of organisms cause aggressive, chronic cutaneous ulcers, with mucous membrane (oral, nasal, pharyngeal) spread, a clinical picture called espundia.[30] Organisms of the *L. mexicana* complex are more likely to produce self-limiting cutaneous ulcers (60% of lesions occur on the earlobes, producing what are known as "chiclero ulcers"). The mucous membranes are less commonly involved, although *L. peruviana* is likely to produce a more diffuse cutaneous disease known as "uta" in Peru. Stibogluconate sodium is the treatment of choice.

The laboratory diagnosis is made by demonstrating amastigotes in stained smears, imprints, or biopsy specimens of infected tissues. The organisms are oval, intracellular, and very small, averaging 2 to 4 μm and simulating the yeast cells of *Histoplasma capsulatum*). The *Leishmania* amastigotes possess a barlike kinetoplast adjacent to the nucleus, a structure that is helpful in distinguishing these organisms from *H. capsulatum*.

TRYPANOSOMA SPECIES. Human trypanosomiasis is caused by a flagellate protozoan that inhabits the blood and tissues. The adult form, which measures 1.5 to 30 μm long by 1.5 to 3.5 μm wide, has an elongated body with a whiplike posterior flagellum that is attached by a delicate undulating membrane that runs the length of its body. A central nucleus and a posterior kinetoplast are usually easily seen. These forms can be readily identified in stained smears of peripheral blood and in the cerebrospinal fluid in cases of active infection. Two distinct forms of disease occur, one endemic in Africa, the other in South America.

African trypanosomiasis, also known as sleeping sickness, is caused by one of two species, *T. brucei rhodesiense*, endemic in the savannah and woodland regions of central and east Africa, and *T. brucei gambiense*, endemic in the tropical rain forests of Central and Western Africa. Humans become infected through the bites of infected *Glossina* tsetse flies that harbor the infective procyclic trypanomastigotes in their salivary glands. The clinical disease caused by *T. brucei rhodesiense* tends to be of more rapid onset with a greater tendency to become rapidly progressive, even leading to death. Intermittent recurring fever associated with lymphadenopathy (involvement of the posterior cervical region of the neck is referred to as Winterbottom's sign) and hepatosplenomegaly are among early signs of infection. As the disease becomes chronic, organism invasion of the central nervous system results in the sleeping sickness stage of the disease, characterized initially by behavioral and personality changes, leading to apathy, fatigue, confusion, and somnolence, which are signs of progressive meningoencephalitis. Emaciation and profound coma ultimately lead to death, often secondary to superinfections. Suramin or pentamidine are the drugs of choice.

South American trypanosomiasis, also known as Chagas' disease, caused by *T. cruzi*, is found from the southern United States through Latin and South America to Argentina. The life cycle of *T. cruzi* differs from the African species of trypanosomes in that a species of the triatomid or reduviid bug serves as the arthropod vector. Humans become infected when the trypanosomal-infected fecal matter is discharged into the wound when the bug feeds. The bite is quite painful, and the infected feces are rubbed into the wound. In the human host, the C-shaped trypanosomes circulate in the bloodstream during the early acute phase of the disease and intermittent febrile episodes are experienced.

In the acute form of disease, an inflamed and edematous chagoma may develop at the site of the bug bite. Local lymph nodes are commonly involved. Involvement of the conjunctiva is known as Romana's sign. Fever, malaise, anorexia, generalized lymphadenopathy, edema of the face and lower extremities, and hepatosplenomegaly of varying degrees of severity may be observed.

The chronic form of disease is caused by invasion of the reticuloendothelial system or heart muscle with the leishmanial form of the organism. Cardiomyopathy with an accompanying interstitial myocarditis is the leading cause of death.

Megaesophagus and megacolon are other complications of the chronic form of the disease. Although central nervous system involvement is atypical, meningoencephalitis progressing through confusion, apathy, stupor, coma, and death may occur.

Filarial Nematodes

The filarial parasites discussed here are an order of nematodes consisting of adult threadlike worms that inhabit primarily the circulatory and lymphatic channels but may also be found in muscles, connective tissues, and serous cavities. Three species commonly cause disease in humans: *Wuchereria bancrofti*, *Brugia malayi*, and *Loa loa*.

Humans acquire filariasis after the bite of an infected mosquito (*W. bancrofti* and *B. malayi*) or of a tabanid fly for *Loa loa*. Biting midges serve as the intermediate hosts for *M. perstans* and *M. ozzardi*, which are two species considered to be of minor clinical significance. When the insect bites a human, these infective larvae move down the proboscis to penetrate the skin. These infective larvae reproduce locally in the subcutaneous tissue and ultimately enter the peripheral lymphatics, where they find their way to lymph nodes. Over a period of several weeks, the larvae develop into white, threadlike adult worms. The lymphatics of the lower extremities and the epitrochlear and femoral lymph nodes are the sites most commonly involved.

The chronic form of the disease is initiated as the adult worms produce lymphatic obstruction, inflammation, and swelling of the surrounding tissues, a condition known as elephantiasis. The characteristic clinical manifestation of *W. bancrofti* is genital disease with funiculitis, epididymoorchitis, and hydrocele and less often elephantiasis.[17,45] In brugian filariasis, adenolymphadenitis of the inguinal region and elephantiasis, predominantly involving the leg below the knee, are more common.[48] *Loa loa* causes a disease in which the adult worms migrate through the subcutaneous tissue and may be observed as a small, serpiginous elevation of the thin parts of the skin or beneath the conjunctival lining of the eye ("eyeworm"). The skin reaction at the site of worm migration produces what are known as Calabar swellings.

The laboratory diagnosis is made by observing circulating microfilaria in stained peripheral blood smears. Mature female worms produce myriads of prelarvae known as microfilariae that circulate in the blood and serve as the mode of transmission when the mosquito vector takes a blood meal. Microfilariae measure between 240 and 300 μm in length and about 7 μm in width. A prominent sheath that extends beyond the tail section may be observed. Identification of the three pathogenic species can be made by observing the size and the pattern of extension of nuclei into the tail sections. In the microfilaria of *W. bancrofti*, nuclei do not extend into the tail section; those of *B. malayi* have two nuclei extending into the tail, spaced about 10 μm apart, and an uninterrupted column of nuclei extends into the tail with *Loa loa*. The "nonpathogenic" species, *M. perstans* and *M. ozzardi*, are unsheathed. Microfilariae circulate in the peripheral blood with a regular periodicity. Those of *W. bancrofti* and *B. malayi* are nocturnal; those of *Loa loa* are diurnal. Therefore, to diagnose bancroftian filariasis, it is best to examine blood smears obtained between midnight and 2 AM.

Onchocerca volvulus

O. volvulus is another tissue nematode related to the filarial worms. Microfilariae of this species do not circulate in the peripheral blood, however. The parasite is transmitted to humans through the bite of *Simulium* blackflies where the infected larval forms are deposited in the subcutaneous tissue, ultimately producing a dense, fibrous nodule. The adult worms then develop within this fibrous nodule, forming an entangled mass.

Microfilariae are produced by the female worms, which then wander through the skin, and often migrate to the tissues of the eye. Blindness may eventually ensue. Diagnosis is established by demonstrating microfilariae in teased snips of skin. Surgical removal of detectable nodules may be efficacious. Diethylcarbamazine, beginning with small doses, plus suramin are the drugs of choice if surgical excisions are not feasible. Cutaneous and systemic side effects from death of the microfilariae may require coverage with antiinflammatory drugs. Mebendazole and benzimidazole derivatives are alternatives with fewer side effects.

Dracunculus medinensis

D. medinensis is another tissue roundworm often grouped with the filariae. *D. medinensis* is the guinea worm that probably represents the "fiery serpent" of biblical lore.[24] Humans acquire the infection through ingestion of infected copepods.

The larvae develop into adult worms in the serous cavities, and the gravid females migrate to the subcutaneous tissue. These female worms can measure as long as 100 cm and cause a burning sensation and ulceration of the skin at the sites of infection. They can be removed surgically from the subcutaneous tissue by winding them slowly on a stick. The life cycle of the parasite is complete when the larvae produced by the female escape from the skin blister and are discharged into water in which the copepods live.

Dirofilaria immitis

Dirofilaria species, transmitted by mosquitos, are filarial parasites commonly infecting animals. *D. immitis*, the common dog heartworm, may occasionally infect humans who serve as accidental hosts. When this happens, the life cycle cannot be completed because the filarial worm is in an inappropriate host. Granulomatous nodules, containing immature adult worms, may be seen in the subcutaneous tissue or in the lungs of humans. Microfilariae are not produced in humans.

Miscellaneous Larval Tissue Parasite Infections

Humans may be inadvertent intermediate or accidental hosts for several nematodes and cestodes that have life cycles in other animals. The adults of these species normally reside in the intestinal tract of the definitive hosts. Humans become infected by ingesting either the larvae in poorly cooked meat or the fertile ova. Of particular concern in the United States is the potential increased exposure to a variety of helminthic parasites through the ingestion of uncooked seafood in the form of dishes such as sushi, sashimi, lomi lomi salmon, and pickled herring. Because humans are not the natural definitive host for certain of these parasites, the larvae often aimlessly wander among tissues and organs, either forming cysticercoid lesions or areas of granulomatous inflammation.

TRICHINOSIS. Trichinosis is a disease of carnivores caused by infection with the nematode *T. spiralis*, resulting from ingestion of raw or poorly cooked meat. Humans are accidental hosts and are most commonly infected through ingestion of pork or pork products that contain encysted larvae.[22]

Infections have also been reported after ingestion of poorly cooked bear meat.[14]

When a person ingests the poorly cooked meat, the larvae are released in the intestine, where they burrow into the villi. After molting, the trichinellae develop into adult male and female worms, measuring from 2 to 4 mm. The average life span of the adults in the intestine is about 4 months; during that time, however, each female releases as many as 3000 larval offspring. These larvae enter the circulation and are deposited throughout the tissues of the body, where most are killed. Many of those that reach the skeletal muscle become encysted and survive.

In the laboratory, trichinosis is diagnosed by detecting the spiral larvae in biopsy specimens of muscle tissue, usually the deltoid or the gastrocnemius. The specimen may be examined by first digesting the muscle fibers with trypsin and then mounting some of the digested tissue on a microscope slide or by preparing a tease preparation of the muscle tissue in a drop of saline solution and squeezing it between two microscope slides. These larval forms coil two and a half times on themselves and form the granulomatous foci of infection within muscle fibers.

Most infections are subclinical. The minimal number of ingested larvae required to produce symptoms is about 100, and a fatal dose is estimated to be 300,000.[22] Fever, muscle pain and aching, periorbital edema, and peripheral blood eosinophilia are the cardinal features by which a clinical diagnosis can be made.

VISCERAL LARVA MIGRANS. *Toxocara canis*, the dog intestinal roundworm, with a life cycle similar to that of human *A. lumbricoides*, is the most common cause of larva migrans. Larva migrans is a condition in which the larvae of nematode parasites of lower animals migrate into the tissues of humans without further development. In *T. canis* infection, humans become an accidental host through ingestion of unwashed food or soil contaminated with embryonated eggs. The disease is most common in children because of their close association with dogs and their inadvertent ingestion of soil. Because humans are abnormal hosts, the lung cycle is not completed; rather, the larvae are filtered out in various organs, chiefly the liver. They may cause local tissue reactions or granulomas, but the larvae eventually die out with no sequelae. The infection can be suspected in a child with hepatomegaly, nonspecific pulmonary disease, and a high peripheral blood eosinophilia.

CUTANEOUS LARVA MIGRANS. The filariform larvae of dog and cat hookworms, commonly of the species *Ancylostoma braziliense* and *A. caninum*, are capable of penetrating the exposed skin of humans producing a pruritic, papular condition known as "creeping eruption." The larvae penetrate deeply into the subcutaneous tissue and produce linear tracts that extend for several millimeters each day. The diagnosis is made by a history of exposure and the presence of subcutaneous linear tracts. Biopsies of suspicious lesions are of little help in establishing a diagnosis, showing only an eosinophilic cellular infiltrate.

ANISAKIASIS. Anisakiasis is a zoonotic disease in which humans, through the ingestion of raw, pickled, smoked, or poorly cooked seafood (such as sushi, sashimi, pickled herring, and the like) become an accidental host for the larval nematodes belonging to the genera *Anisakis*, *Phocanema*, and *Contracaecum*. On entering the stomach with the raw fish meal, the larvae penetrate into the wall, forming small tunnels and burrows amid a dense granulomatous inflammatory reaction.[53] Larvae may on occasion migrate beyond the stomach producing metastatic infections in the omentum liver, pancreas, and lungs.

GNATHOSTOMIASIS. *Gnathostoma spinigerum* is a nematode that normally infects the intestinal tract of cats and dogs; humans may become accidental hosts by ingesting poorly cooked or pickled seafood. In the cat or dog, ingested larvae develop in the stomach or intestinal wall into adults that produce granulomatous lesions. In humans, however, the larvae do not mature but rather penetrate the gastric wall and migrate throughout the tissues. Deep cutaneous or subcutaneous tunnels may develop, simulating cutaneous larva migrans, or hard, nonpitting painful swellings may occur. A case of intestinal gnathostomiasis was reported by Hira and coworkers.[23]

ANGIOSTRONGYLIASIS. Angiostrongyliasis, caused by the larvae of nematodes with rats as the definitive host, presents in humans in two clinical forms depending on the species: *A. cantonensis*, endemic in Thailand, Tahiti, and Taiwan among other South Pacific locales, causes a syndrome of meningitis, eosinophilic pleocytosis in the cerebrospinal fluid (known as eosinophilic meningitis), and peripheral blood eosinophilia; and *A. costaricensis*, endemic primarily in Costa Rica with reported cases also in Mexico and in Central and South America, causes abdominal disease primarily of the distal small intestine and ascending colon, the sites of penetration by the developing larvae. Humans acquire the infection by ingesting foods, usually leafy vegetables, contaminated with infected snails and slugs. After ingestion by humans, the larvae migrate to the brain, causing eosinophilic meningitis.

ECHINOCOCCOSIS (HYDATID DISEASE). Echinococcosis, or hydatid disease, is a disease in nature passed between dogs (also wolves and foxes) and sheep or cattle. Two species with somewhat different morphology and patterns of behavior may be encountered, *E. granulosis* and *E. multicellularis*. The normal life cycle of *E. granulosa* involves dogs or foxes as the definitive hosts, within the intestines of which the adult tapeworms reside. Sheep, cattle, or swine serve as the intermediate hosts and develop cystic larval disease. *E. multilocularis* differs slightly in this regard since the definitive hosts are dogs, foxes, wolves, and cats, while the intermediate hosts are small rodents, including squirrels, field mice, and voles. Humans serve as accidental intermediate hosts in whom the larval form of the parasite is harbored.

Hexacanth eggs, closely resembling those of *Taenia* species, are passed from the adult female worm in dog feces and become embryonated in the soil. Under normal circumstances, these eggs are ingested by the natural intermediate hosts—sheep, cattle, or swine—or by the small rodents mentioned earlier in the case of *E. multilocularis*. The larvae are released from the eggs in the intestines of the intermediate hosts and, by means of their hooklets, bore through the bowel wall and enter the circulation.

Human infection is similar to that found in the herbivorous animals, and the disease is acquired through ingestion of vegetative material or soil infested with egg-contaminated dog feces. The circulating embryos are filtered out in the capillaries of various organs (usually the liver because it is the first organ to drain the mesenteric blood). Within the organ, *E. granulosis* produces a single multilayered cyst or small cysts called *bladder worms* may form. The cysts of *E. multilocularis*, as the species name would imply, have multiple locules. Multiple cysts up to 5 cm in diameter resemble what Aristotle called hailstones.

The inner lining of the cyst is a germinal membrane from which numerous daughter embryos develop. These form as tiny polypoid structures (brood capsules) that line the inner membrane. When the embryos break free from the membrane and float in the fluid within the cyst, they are known as *hydatid sand*. If examined under the microscope, each grain of sand is, in fact, a tiny embryonic beginning of a new tapeworm, complete with an inverted scolex with a rostellum armed with hooklets (Fig. 17-8). The laboratory diagnosis is made by demonstrating hydatid sand in surgically removed tissue.

COENUROSIS. Coenurosis is another human disease related to a dog tapeworm, a *Taenia*-like cestode of the genus *Multiceps*, in which the normal intermediate hosts are sheep, cattle, horses, and other herbivorous animals. Humans become infected by ingesting food or water contaminated with dog feces containing *Multiceps* eggs. The disease in humans primarily involves the central nervous system, where the migrating larvae develop into echinococcal-type cysts individually known as a coenurus, producing symptoms of a space-occupying lesion.

SPARGANOSIS. Dogs and cats serve as the definitive host for several species of diphyllobothroid tapeworms belonging to the genus *Spirametra*. Two intermediate hosts are required to complete the life cycle. *Spirametra* eggs passed in dog or cat feces into fresh water hatch and are ingested by minute *Cyclops* crustaceans, within which they develop into procercoid larvae. These larvae in turn develop into pleurocercoid larvae, individually known as sparganum, in the flesh of a second intermediate host (fish, snakes, frogs) that feed on the *Cyclops*. Humans become infected either by ingesting an infected *Cyclops*; by eating the raw, infective flesh of the second intermediate host; or from the practice in certain cultures of applying raw fish to the skin, eyes, or vagina to heal other maladies. On ingestion, sparganum larvae penetrate the bowel wall and enter the circulation. Most lesions in humans are subcutaneous, where slow-growing, painful, red, edematous nodules develop. The diagnosis is made on surgical removal of a sparganum and identifying the slender, delicate, white worm that measures 60 to 80 mm long and 1 to 2 mm wide.

SEROLOGIC DIAGNOSIS OF PARASITIC INFECTIONS

A discussion of the serologic diagnosis of parasitic diseases is beyond the scope of this book. The serologic approach to the evaluation of parasitic diseases is most applicable when invasive techniques other than the routine examination of blood, feces, or other body fluids are required to establish a diagnosis.[31] For example, the infective parasitic forms in toxoplasmosis, extraintestinal amebiasis, trichinosis, and cysticercosis are often lodged deep within tissues and organs and either deep-needle or open-surgical biopsies are needed to confirm the diagnosis. In such cases, serologic diagnosis may be possible. Readers are requested to consult with the Serology Unit, Parasitology Section, at the Centers forDisease Control in Atlanta, Georgia, or with the corresponding sections in the local state health laboratories for details on what tests are available and how and when to send specimens. The various serodiagnostic tests for parasitic diseases have been reviewed by Walls and Smith,[61] and, based on their experience, the levels presented in Table 17-2 have been published as representing significant titers.

Physicians must be informed of the potential limitations of the serologic approach to parasitic diseases. The interpretation of serologic test results must be made in conjunction with informa-

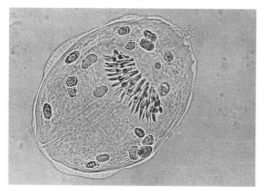

Figure 17-8. Photomicrograph of a single grain of "hydatid sand" illustrating a protoscolex with a prominent row of hooklets, representing the anlage of the armed rostellum of the adult worm.

Table 17-2
Serodiagnostic Tests for Parasitic Diseases

DISEASE	TEST	DIAGNOSTIC TITERS
African trypanosomiasis	IFA	≥1:16
Amebiasis	IHA	≥1:256
Ascariasis	ELISA	≥1:32
Chagas' disease	CF, IHA	≥1:8; 1:64
Cysticercosis	IHA	≥1:64
Echinococcosis	IHA	≥1:256
Fascioliasis	IHA	≥1:128
Filariasis	IHA	≥1:128
Leishmaniasis	IIF	≥1:16
Malaria	IIF	≥1:64
Paragonimiasis	CF	≥1:8
Pneumocystosis	IIF	≥1:16
Schistosomiasis	IIF	≥1:16
Strongyloidiasis	IHS	≥1:64
Toxocariasis	ELISA	≥1:32
Toxoplasmosis	IIF, IgM-IIF	≥1:256; 1:16
Trichinosis	Bentonite Floc	≥1:16

tion derived from the clinical history, physical examination, and other laboratory data. Delays in obtaining test results may be incurred if samples must be sent to reference laboratories; and, in certain cases, it may be necessary to institute empiric therapy before having presumptive diagnosis confirmed.

REFERENCES

1. Alpert G, Bell LM, Kirkpatrick CE, et al. Outbreak of cryptosporidiosis in a day-care center. Pediatrics 1986;77:152–157.
2. Anderson BX. Cryptosporidiosis. Lab Med 14: 1983;55–56.
3. Armstrong D, Rosen PP, et al. *Pneumocystis carinii* pneumonia: a cluster of eleven cases. Ann Intern Med 1975;82:772–777.
4. Arrowood MJ, Sterling CR. Comparison of conventional staining methods and monoclonal antibody-based methods for *Cryptosporidium* oocyst detection. J Clin Microbiol 1989;27:1490–1495.
5. Auran JD, Starr MB, Jakobiec FA. *Acanthamoeba* keratitis: a review of the literature. Cornea 1987; 6:2–26.
6. Bartlett MS, Harper K, Smith N, et al. Comparative evaluation of a modified zinc sulfate flotation technique. J Clin Microbiol 1977;7:524–528.
7. Beal CB, Viens P, Grant RGL, Hughes JM. A new technique for sampling duodenal contents. Am J Trop Med Hyg 1970;19:349–352.
8. Beaver PC, Gadgel PK, Morera P. Sarcocystis in man: a review and report of five cases. Am J Trop Med Hyg 1979;28:819–844.
9. Bradley SL, Dines DE, Brewer NS. Disseminated *Strongyloides stercoralis* in an immunosuppressed host. Mayo Clin Proc 1978;53:332–335.
10. Bruckner DA, Garcia LS, Voge M. Intestinal parasites in Los Angeles, California. Am J Med Technol 1979;45:1020–1024.
11. Centers for Disease Control. Intestinal parasite surveillance: United States 1976. MMWR 1978; 27:167.
12. Centers for Disease Control. *Acanthamoeba* keratitis associated with contact lenses—United States. MMWR 1986;35:405–408.
13. Chalvardjan AM, Grawe LA. A new procedure for the identification of *Pneumocystis carinii* cysts in tissue sections and smears. J Clin Pathol 1963; 16:383–384.
14. Clark PS, Brownsberger KM, Saslow AR, et al. Bear meat trichinosis: epidemiologic, serologic, and clinical observations from two Alaskan outbreaks. Ann Intern Med 1972;76:951–956.
15. Cregan P, Yamamoto A, Lum A, et al. Comparison of four methods for rapid detection of *Pneumocystis carinii* in respiratory specimens. J Clin Microbiol 1990;28:2432–2436.
16. Current WL. The biology of *Cryptosporidium*. ASM News 1988;54:605–611.
17. Davis BR. Filariasis. Dermatol Clin 1989;7: 313–321.
18. De Hovitz JA, Pape JW, Boncy J, Johnson WD Jr. Isosporiasis in AIDS. N Engl J Med 1986;315:87.
19. Gajdusek EC. *Pneumocystis carinii* as the cause of human disease: historical perspectives and magnitude of the problem—introductory remarks. NCI Monogr 1976;43:1–10.
20. Garcia LS, Ash LR. Diagnostic parasitology: clinical laboratory manual. 2nd ed. St Louis, CV Mosby, 1979.
21. Garcia LS, Bruckner DA. Diagnostic medical parasitology. New York, Elsevier, 1988.
22. Gould SE. The story of trichinosis. Am J Clin Pathol 1970;55:2–11.
23. Hira PR, Neafie R, Prakash B, et al. Human gnathostomiasis: infection with an immature male *Gnathostoma spinigerum*. Am J Trop Med Hyg 1989;41:91–94.
24. Hoepli R. Parasites and parasitic infection in early

medicine and science. Singapore, University of Malaya Press, 1959.

25. Holcombe DJ. A case of *Strongyloides stercoralis* in central Louisiana. J La State Med Soc 1989; 141:22–24.

26. Ingra-Siegman Y, Kapila R, Sen P, et al. Syndrome of hyperinfection with *Strongyloides stercoralis*. Rev Infect Dis 1981;3:397–407.

27. Isaac-Renton JL. Immunological methods of diagnosis in giardiasis: an overview. Ann Clin Lab Sci 1991;21:116–122.

28. Janda WM. The acquired immunodeficiency syndrome. Clin Microbiol Newsl 1982;4:169–171.

29. Jones JE. String test for diagnosing giardiasis. Am Fam Physician 1986;34:123–126.

30. Jones TC, Johnson WD Jr, Barretto AC, et al. Epidemiology of American cutaneous leishmaniasis due to *Leishmania braziliensis*. J Infect Dis 1987;156:73–83.

31. Kagan IG, Normal L. Serodiagnosis of parasitic diseases. In Rose NR, Freidman HG, eds. Manual of clinical immunology. Washington, DC, American Society for Microbiology, 1976:382–409.

32. Knight R. Giardiasis, isosporiasis and balantidiasis. Clin Gastroenterol 1978;7:31–47.

33. Knisley CV, Englekirk PG, Pickering LK, et al. Rapid detection of *Giardia* antigen in stool with the use of enzyme immunoassays. Am J Clin Pathol 1989;91:704–708.

34. Koneman EW, Allen SD, Janda WM, Schreckenberger PC, Winn WC Jr. Color atlas and textbook of diagnostic microbiology. Philadelphia, JB Lippincott, 1992.

35. Levine GI. Parasitic diseases: diseases associated with acquired immunodeficiency syndrome. Prim Care 1991;18:129–152.

36. Levine ND, Corliss JO, Cox FEG, et al. A newly revised classification of the protozoa. J Protozool 1980;27:37–58.

37. Luft BJ, Brooks RG, Conley FK, et al. Toxoplasmic encephalitis in patients with acquired immune deficiency syndrome. JAMA 1984;252:913–917.

38. Markell EK, Quinn PM. Comparison of immediate polyvinyl alcohol (PVA) fixation with Schaudinn's fixation for the demonstration of protozoa in stool specimens. Am J Trop Med Hyg 1977;26:1139–1142.

39. Masur H, Lane HC, Kovacs JA, et al. NIH Conference: *Pneumocystis* pneumonia: from bench to clinic. Ann Intern Med 1989;111:813–826.

40. McCabe RE, Remington JS. *Toxoplasma gondii*. In: Mandell GL, Douglas RG Jr, Bennett JE, eds. Principles and practices of infectious diseases. New York, Churchill Livingstone, 1989.

41. McCormick GF, Chi-Shing ZEE, Heiden J. Cysticercosis cerebri: review of 127 cases. Arch Neurol 1982;39:534–539.

42. Melvin DM, Brooke MM, Healy GR. Common blood and tissue parasites of man: life cycle charts. DHEW Publication No. 1234. Washington, DC, US Government Printing Office, 1969.

43. Melvin DM, Brooke MM, Sudan EH. Common intestinal helminths of man: life cycle charts: DHEW publication No. 1234, Washington, DC, US Government Printing Office, 1974.

44. Melvin DM, Smith JW. Intestinal parasitic infections: problems in laboratory diagnosis. Lab Med 1979;10:207–210.

45. Mills J. *Pneumocystis carinii* and *Toxoplasma gondii* infections in patients with AIDS. Rev Infect Dis 1986;8:1001–1011.

46. Moore MB, McCulley JP. *Acanthamoeba* keratitis associated with contact lenses: six consecutive cases of successful management. Br J Ophthalmol 1989;73:271–275.

47. Navin TR, Juranek DD. Cryptosporidiosis: clinical, epidemiological and parasitic review. Rev Infect Dis 1984;6:313–317.

48. Partona F. The spectrum of disease in lymphatic filariasis. Ciba Found Symp 1987;127:15–31.

49. Pearson RD, De Queiroz Sousa A. *Leishmania* species: visceral (kala-azar), cutaneous and mucosal leishmaniasis. In: Mandell GL, Douglas RG Jr, Bennett JE, eds. Principles and practices of infectious diseases. New York, Churchill Livingstone, 1990.

50. Pifer LL, Woods DR, Edwards CC, et al. *Pneumocystis carinii* serologic study in pediatric acquired immunodeficiency syndrome. Am J Dis Child 1988;142:36–39.

51. Polly SM. Neurocysticercosis. Infect Dis Newsl 1986;5(December):89–91.

52. Rossitch E Jr, Carrazana EJ, Samuels MA. Cerebral toxoplasmosis in patients with AIDS. Am Fam Physician 1990;41:867–873, 1990.

53. Sakanari JA, McKerrow JH. Anisakiasis. Clin Microbiol Rev 1989;2:278–284.

54. Schwartz DA. Cholangiocarcinoma with liver fluke infection: a preventable source for morbidity in Asian immigrants. Am J Gastroenterol 1986;81:76–79.

55. Sher L, Shunzaburo I, LeBeau G, Zajko AB. Hilar cholangiocarcinoma associated with *Clonorchis*. Dig Dis Sci 1989;34:1121–1123.

56. Shetty N, Brabhu T. Evaluation of faecal preservation and staining methods in the diagnosis of acute amoebiasis and giardiasis. J Clin Pathol 1988;41:694–699.

57. Smith JW, Gutierrez Y. Medical parasitology. In: Henry JB, ed. Clinical diagnosis and management by laboratory methods. Philadelphia, WB Saunders, 1991.

58. Soave R. Cryptosporidiosis and isosporiasis in patients with AIDS. Infect Dis Clin North Am 1988;2:485.

59. Stehr-Green JK, Bailey TM, Visvesvara GS. The epidemiology of *Acanthamoeba* keratitis in the United States. Am J Ophthalmol 1989;107: 221–336.

60. Tan JS. Common and uncommon parasitic infections in the United States. Med Clin North Am 1978;62:1059–1081.

61. Walls KW, Smith JW. Serology of parasitic infections. Lab Med 1979;10:329–336.

62. Walzer PD. *Pneumocystis carinii*. In: Mandell GL, Douglas RG Jr, Bennett JE, eds. Principles and practices of infectious diseases. New York, Churchill Livingstone, 1990.

63. Warren KS, Mahmoud AAF. Tropical and geographical medicine. 2nd ed. New York, McGraw-Hill, 1990.

64. Wolfson JS, Waldron MA, Sierra LS. Blinded comparison of a direct immunofluorescent monoclonal antibody staining method and a Giemsa staining method for identification of *Pneumocystis carinii* in induced sputum and bronchoalveolar lavage specimens of patients infected with human immunodeficiency virus. J Clin Microbiol 1990; 28:2136–2138.

65. Wong B, Gold JWM, Brown AE, et al. Central nervous system toxoplasmosis in homosexual men and parenteral drug abusers. Ann Intern Med 1984;100:36–42.

66. World Health Organization. Parasitic diseases programme: major parasitic infections: a global view. World Health Stat Q 1986;39:145–160.

67. Young DK, Bullock SL, Milvin DM, et al. Ethyl acetate as a substitute for diethyl ether in the formalin-ether sedimentation technique. J Clin Microbiol 1979;10:852–853.

18

Virology

EVOLUTION OF DIAGNOSTIC VIROLOGY

The first stage of historical interest in the evolution of diagnostic microbiology spanned the years during which the very existence of infection by submicroscopic particles was established. For many decades after Carlos Finlay hypothesized that yellow fever was transmitted by the bite of a mosquito, the only means available for isolation of viral agents was the inoculation of animals or embryonated eggs.

The next major breakthrough in diagnostic virology was provided by Enders and colleagues, who demonstrated that the virus that caused poliomyelitis could be isolated in nonneural cells in vitro.[66] In the 1950s and 1960s there was a rapid expansion of knowledge about clinical features, epidemiology, and diagnosis of common viral infections, largely provided by the expanding use of cell culture.

In the past 15 years, several events have promoted and facilitated the provision of diagnostic virology services by laboratories of different sizes and backgrounds:

1. Situations have arisen in which important clinical decisions depend on prompt and accurate viral diagnosis. The risk for the newborn of maternal herpes simplex infection was recognized in the early 1970s.[181] Investigators who recognized the association of neonatal herpes with active herpetic infection of the maternal genital tract developed protocols to screen mothers for herpesvirus shedding.[16] Careful study, however, documented serious problems with the screening protocols.[7] The American College of Obstetrics and Gynecology no longer advocates routine genital cultures for herpes simplex virus in pregnant women.[6] This impetus to the development of diagnostic virology services in many hospitals has, nevertheless, left an enduring legacy.

2. The availability of effective antiviral chemotherapy for herpes simplex encephalitis[262] and for respiratory syncytial virus infection[227] has further emphasized the importance of reliable laboratory diagnostic support. Antiviral chemotherapy is also useful for influenza A virus infection in selected patients.[63,233] Although ganciclovir therapy for cytomegalovirus infections is not curative, it has provided a first tool for combatting potentially lethal or blinding infections in immunosuppressed patients.[67]

3. A ready commercial supply of diverse mammalian cell cultures has made isolation of viruses feasible for many laboratories.

4. An expanding list of reliable immunologic reagents has also enhanced the ability of laboratories to identify many viruses rapidly and definitively. Increasingly, kits for direct identification of specific agents in clinical specimens or for isolation and identification of the agent in culture are being marketed commercially.

Economic pressures are making it imperative to provide clinically useful and cost-effective results. The time is right for virology to enter the diagnostic laboratory.

Levels of Service

Each laboratory director or supervisor must decide the level of service that is appropriate for local clinical needs. It is far better to limit the scope of effort to those tests that can be performed with high proficiency than to attempt broad coverage when resources are insufficient.

For most diagnostic laboratories the most frequently requested service will be isolation of herpes simplex virus. Direct detection of certain viruses, particularly respiratory syncytial virus, has become increasingly important, because of the availability of reliable reagents for rapid detection and the need to provide immediate guidance for clinical decisions.

In this chapter, a brief discussion is presented of common viral illnesses and general principles of viral isolation and detection are outlined. Isolation of herpes simplex virus and direct detection of respiratory syncytial virus are discussed in detail as examples of the general principles.

TAXONOMY

Many viral infections, such as influenza, chickenpox, measles, and hepatitis, were well characterized clinically long before the etiologic agent was recognized. Once isolated, the virus was given the name of the corresponding clinical condition. In an attempt to bring order to the scheme of classification, taxonomists have used modern knowledge of viral structure and antigenic composition when naming viruses.[178] Names have a Latin stem, but the conventions of bacterial nomenclature have not been followed completely. Families and genera have been delineated, but the designation of viruses at the species level has not yet been accomplished. Rather, the vernacular names are used most commonly as species designations. In the absence of formal binomial nomenclature, the vernacular names should not be capitalized or italicized. For instance, the name herpes simplex virus should be used, not *Herpes simplex*. In some instances, the traditional names, derived from clinical usage, have been incorporated into the official nomenclature. For example, the smallpox and cowpox viruses have been assigned to the family Poxviridae.

Much of viral taxonomy derives from detailed knowledge of viral structure. Viruses are among the smallest of infectious agents (Fig. 18-1). The poxviruses, which are the largest members of the

virus family and very similar in size to the smallest bacteria, are close to the resolution of the light microscope; an electron microscope is necessary to visualize all other viruses.

Almost without exception, viruses contain either DNA or RNA, but not both. The center of any viral particle, the ribonucleoprotein core, contains coiled nucleic acid and protein.[110] Around the core is a protective shell composed of repeating protein units called capsomeres, which, in the aggregate, make up the capsid shell. With the nucleoprotein core, the nucleocapsid unit is complete. The architecture of most viruses has a symmetry that is either helical, similar to nucleic acid, or icosahedral, the architecture of a geodesic dome. These two symmetries, illustrated in Figure 18-2, provide the most efficient means for assembling the structural shells, an economy that is essential for these very small particles with limited genetic resources.

As a general rule, DNA viruses replicate and are assembled in the nucleus; RNA viruses are assembled in the cytoplasm. The complex events that

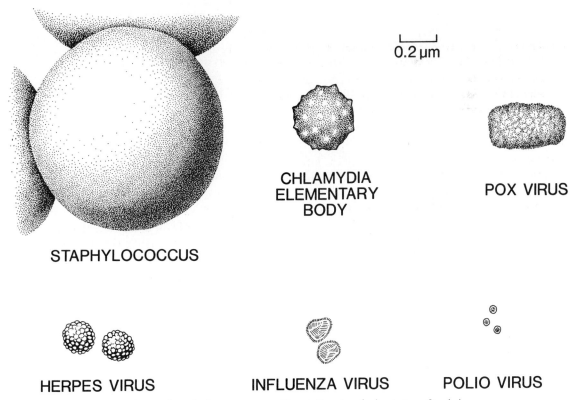

STAPHYLOCOCCUS

CHLAMYDIA ELEMENTARY BODY

0.2 μm

POX VIRUS

HERPES VIRUS

INFLUENZA VIRUS

POLIO VIRUS

Figure 18-1. Viruses are the smallest of infectious agents. The relative size of a bacterium, *Staphylococcus*, is compared with *Chlamydia*, with the largest virus group (poxvirus), and with one of the smallest viruses (poliovirus, a member of the enterovirus group).

A

B

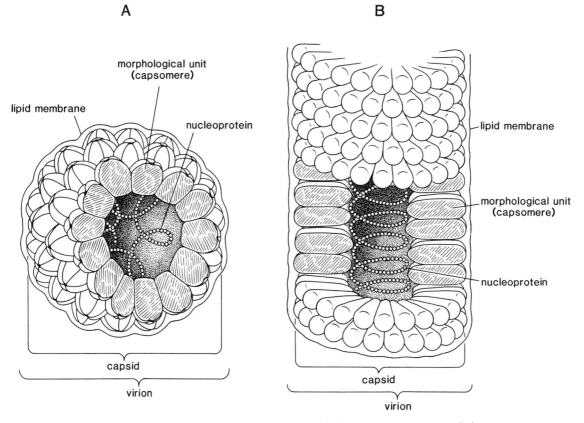

lipid membrane

morphological unit
(capsomere)

nucleoprotein

lipid membrane

morphological unit
(capsomere)

nucleoprotein

capsid

virion

capsid

virion

Figure 18-2. Viruses are constructed with great economy. A central nucleoprotein core is surrounded by a protein capsid, which is made up of individual capsomeres. Some viruses also have a lipoprotein membrane around the nucleocapsid. The two most common organizational patterns of symmetry are icosahedral (**A**) and helical (**B**). Ultrastructurally, the icosahedral viruses appear round, although the facets may occasionally be visualized (see the illustration of adenovirus in Table 18-2).

occur after a virus infects a cell are reflected only incompletely in the morphologic cellular changes. In some instances, however, one can see clearly how the virus has appropriated the genetic resources of the cell (Fig. 18-3*A* and *B*). The final assembly of some viruses occurs at the nuclear or cytoplasmic membrane. As the virion moves from the nucleus to the cytoplasm or passes from the cytoplasm to the extracellular space, an external lipid-containing envelope is added to the nucleocapsid (see Figs. 18-2 and 18-3*A* and *F*). Lipid solvents inactivate such enveloped viruses, whereas their nonenveloped counterparts are not affected. Replication of some viruses results in death of the cell with release of the assembled nucleocapsids. The enveloped viruses that mature at the cytoplasmic membrane are released from the cell by "budding" through the membrane (see Fig. 18-3*F*). In this

process, the envelope accumulates portions of the lipid membrane, as well as virus-specified glycoproteins that have been inserted into that membrane.

The major groups of viruses are summarized in Tables 18-1 and 18-2. Illustrative electron micrographs of negatively stained viral particles (kindly provided by Frederick A. Murphy, School of Veterinary Medicine, University of California at Davis) are juxtaposed with a brief description of the families and genera. The list is not exhaustive but includes the most important human pathogens. In this chapter general principles of diagnostic virology are discussed. Clinical features and diagnosis of selected viral infections are used as examples, in particular, herpes simplex virus, respiratory syncytial virus, rotavirus, human immunodeficiency virus, and hepatitis virus infections.

(*text continues on page 448*)

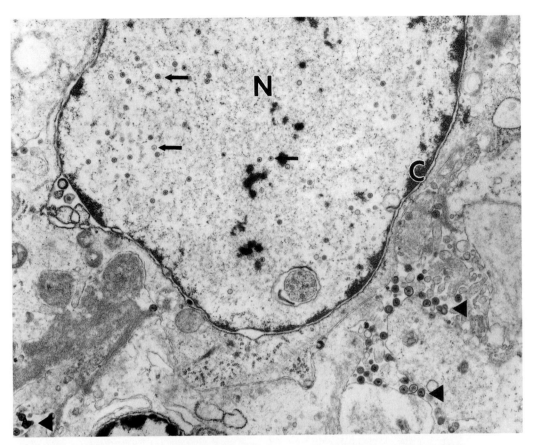

Figure 18-3. (**A**) Ultrastructure of viruses. Herpes simplex virus. The herpesviruses are assembled in the nucleus of the cell (N). The cellular chromatin (C) is pushed to the edge of the nucleus by the viral deoxyribonucleoprotein, which stains lightly in the micrograph. This material corresponds to the eosinophilic intranuclear inclusion seen with the light microscope. Naked (nonenveloped) virions (*arrows*) are assembled in the nucleus. Outside the cell, some mature virions that have acquired a lipid envelope from the cell (*arrowheads*) are visible (MRC-5 cells, infected with herpes simplex virus, type 1, × 22,400). (**B**) Adenovirus. Adenoviruses are assembled in the nucleus (N). They have icosahedral symmetry and are not enveloped. They are often closely packed in paracrystalline arrays (*arrows*). As the viruses accumulate, the whole nucleus may become filled with virions, producing the inclusions seen with the light microscope (infected HEp-2 cells, × 22,400). (**C**) Respiratory syncytial virus is assembled in the cytoplasm and matures at the cell membrane. Inclusions may be seen in the cytoplasm of infected cells, both in vivo and in vitro. The inclusions (*arrows*) are intracytoplasmic and are composed of fibrillar ribonucleoprotein. Contrast the density of the nucleolus (*arrowhead*) with that of the inclusions (infected HEp-2 cells, × 3,150). (**D**) Coxsackievirus B. The enteroviruses are small RNA-containing viruses that have icosahedral symmetry and are often packed in a paracrystalline array (*arrows*). They are assembled in the cytoplasm. Inclusions are not seen with the light microscope (infected rhesus monkey kidney cells, × 56,000). (**E**) Rabies virus. This bullet-shaped rhabdovirus is assembled in the cytoplasm. The fibrillar nucleoprotein (P) and the elongated viruses (*arrows*) are found together. The mass of viral material corresponds to the Negri body, which is seen with the light microscope. The internal structure that may be seen in classic Negri bodies comes from the incorporation of cytoplasmic material into the body of the inclusion (infected human brain, × 25,000). (**F**) Eastern equine encephalitis virus. This togavirus illustrates the maturation of virus particles at the surface of the cell. Mature virions (*arrows*) are present in the extracellular space. A maturing (budding) virion is denoted by the dense nucleoprotein core and a condensation of the cellular membrane where the envelope is forming (*arrowhead*). Some viruses, such as the myxoviruses, insert their hemagglutinins into the membrane at this stage; they can be detected by the adherence of red blood cells to the viral hemagglutinin in the cell membrane (hemadsorption) (infected mouse brain, × 60,000). (**E** courtesy of Daniel Perl; **F** courtesy of Frederick Murphy)

(continued)

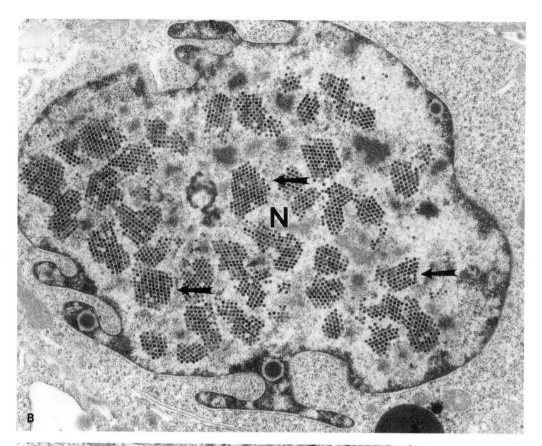

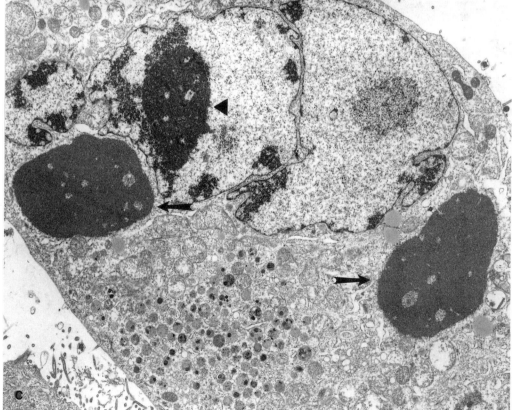

Figure 18-3
(continued)

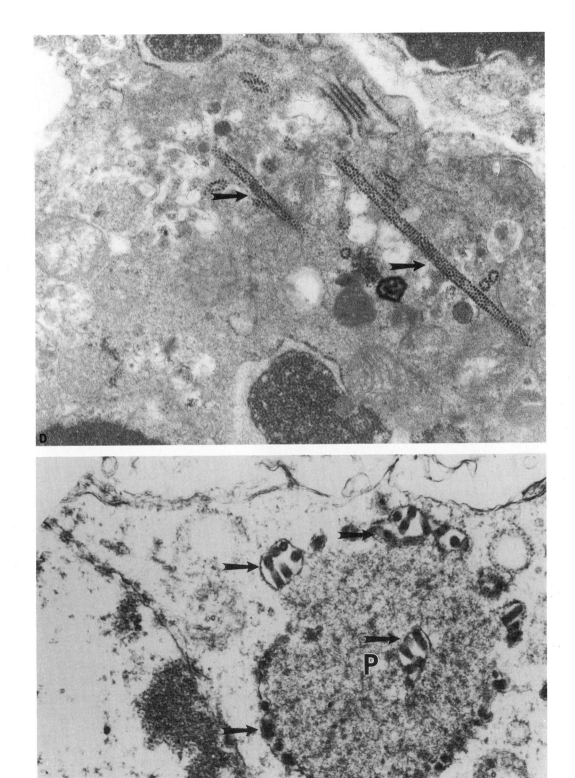

Figure 18-3
(continued)

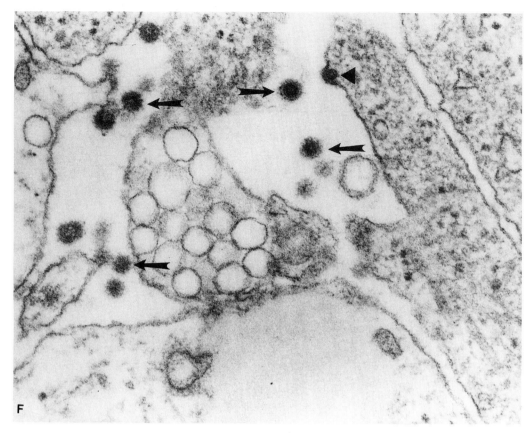

Figure 18-3
(continued)

CLINICAL MANIFESTATIONS OF VIRAL INFECTIONS

The clinical manifestations of viral infection are legion. General symptoms include fever with or without chills, malaise, and myalgias. Specific symptoms derive primarily from the propensity of the virus to infect various cells and tissues (tropism) but may also depend on the route of infection, the virulence of the strain, the immunologic status of the patient, and other predisposing factors, such as underlying pulmonary or cardiac disease. The reader is referred to several excellent textbooks for additional details.[71,75]

Respiratory Syncytial Virus

Respiratory syncytial virus causes recurrent respiratory infections from infancy through adult life. Epidemics are common and may be hospital asso-

ciated.[68,105] There are two distinct serologic groups of respiratory syncytial virus (A and B). One group predominates in most epidemics.[175] Waris reported that the two groups produced epidemics in Finland in an alternating cycle.[257] Epidemics in nurseries have been recognized for many years, and outbreaks of respiratory syncytial virus infection have been described in nursing homes.[73]

Infection is spread by large particle droplets and by fomites (contaminated environmental particles, such as dust), rather than by small particle aerosols.[104,106] Almost all seronegative infants who are exposed to their first epidemic become infected, but immunity is incomplete. As a result, the rate of nosocomial infection may be almost 50% unless active measures to control transmission are undertaken.[105] Wearing gowns and masks does not prevent transmission.[177]

Respiratory syncytial virus may produce croup, bronchitis, bronchiolitis, or interstitial pneumonia.

(text continues on page 457)

Table 18-1
Classification of RNA Viruses

Family: **Orthomyxoviridae**

Size: 100 nm, spherical or pleomorphic

Symmetry: Helical

Lipid envelope: Present

Antigens: Hemagglutinin and neuraminidase

Genus: Influenzavirus
  Types: Influenza A
         Influenza B

Genus: Unnamed
  Type: Influenza C

Natural habitat: Humans and animals

Distribution: Worldwide

Mode of transmission: Aerosol droplet spread from person to person; rarely animal to person

Route of infection: Respiratory

Diseases: Respiratory infections including coryza (common cold), tracheobronchitis, and pneumonia. Extrapulmonary symptoms are prominent in the influenza syndrome; rarely, extrapulmonary disease such as myocarditis may be present.

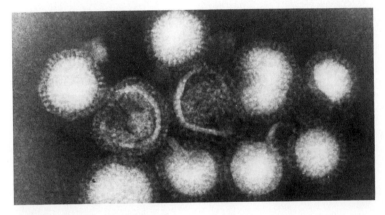

Influenzavirus A. The particles are roughly spherical but irregular. The internal helical structure is difficult to appreciate, but the fringelike projections of hemagglutinin and neuraminidase are shown well ($\times$ 135,000).

Family: **Paramyxoviridae**

Size: 150 to 300 nm, spherical or pleomorphic

Symmetry: Helical

Lipid envelope: Present

Genus: Paramyxovirus
  Types: Parainfluenza viruses 1 through 4
         Mumps virus
  Antigens: Hemagglutinin and neuraminidase

Genus: Morbillivirus
  Type: Measles virus

Antigens: Nucleocapsid; envelope hemagglutinin; no strain variation

Genus: Pneumovirus
  Type: Respiratory syncytial virus (RSV)
  Antigens: No hemagglutinin or neuraminidase

Natural habitat: Humans

Distribution: Worldwide

Mode of transmission: Droplet aerosol or direct inoculation

Route of infection: Respiratory

Diseases: Common cold, tracheobronchitis, rarely pneumonia (parainfluenza); tracheobronchitis and pneumonia especially in young children (RSV); parotitis, pancreatitis, orchitis, meningitis (mumps); rash, pneumonia, encephalitis, subacute sclerosing panencephalitis (measles).

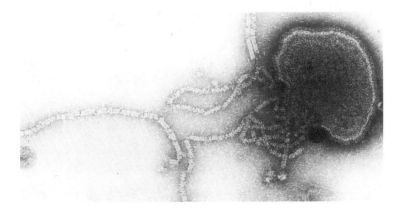

Parainfluenzavirus 1. The irregular virion has been disrupted, releasing a long strand of uncoiled RNA. The hemagglutinin fringes on the virion are evident ($\times$ 72,000).

(continued)

Table 18-1 (continued)

Family: Rhabdoviridae

Size: 50 to 95 nm × 130 to 389 nm, bullet shaped

Symmetry: Helical

Lipid envelope: Present

Genus: Vesiculovirus
  Type: Vesicular stomatitis virus (VSV)

Genus: Lyssavirus
  Type: Rabies virus
Natural habitat: Wild and domestic animals
Distribution: Worldwide

Mode of transmission: Infected secretions, rabies usually transmitted by bite

Route: Cutaneous or respiratory

Diseases: Encephalitis (rabies); veterinary diseases (VSV)

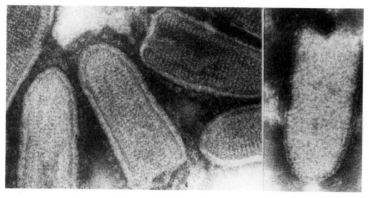

Vesicular stomatitis virus. The bullet shape of the virion is evident. The coiled helical nature of the internal ribonucleoprotein is reflected in the striations (× 216,000).

Family: Proposed Family: Filoviridae

Size: 80 × 800 nm to 1000 nm, filamentous

Symmetry: Helical

Lipid envelope: Present

Genus: None established
  Types: Marburg virus
         Ebola virus
Natural habitat: Unknown

Distribution: Africa

Mode of transmission: Unknown but close contact required

Diseases: Hemorrhagic fever with fatality rates as high as 90%

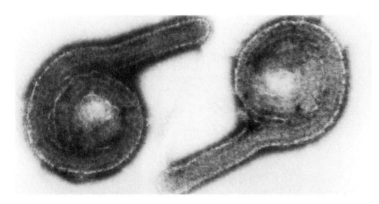

Ebola virus. Long, filamentous form has assumed a "crook" shape (× 59,000).

(continued)

Table 18-1 (continued)

Family: **Bunyaviridae**

Size: 90 to 120 nm
Symmetry: Helical
Lipid envelope: Present
Antigens: Surface hemagglutinin
Genus: Bunyavirus

Types: California encephalitis virus
LaCrosse virus
Natural habitat: Small mammals
Distribution: Worldwide; in U.S. primarily in midwest and north central regions

Mode of transmission: Bite of infected mosquitoes
Diseases: Febrile illness; aseptic meningitis

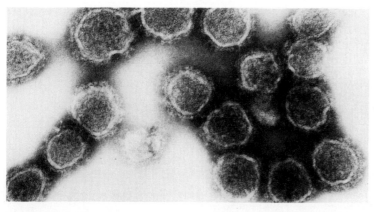

LaCrosse virus. Irregular virus particles; the lipid envelope and surface projections are evident ($\times$ 117,000).

Family: **Coronaviridae**

Size: 80 to 130 nm, pleomorphic with large, clubbed projections
Symmetry: Helical
Lipid envelope: Present

Genus: Coronavirus
Natural habitat: Humans and animals
Distribution: Worldwide
Transmission: Person to person, presumably by aerosol

Route of infection: Respiratory
Diseases: Common cold, rarely lower respiratory disease

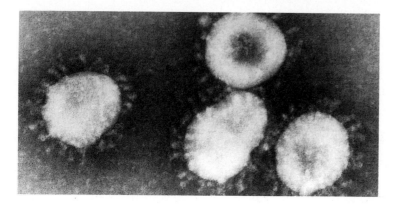

Human coronavirus OC43. The club-shaped projections are the most distinctive features of these pleomorphic particles ($\times$ 180,000).

(continued)

Table 18-1 (continued)

Family: Picornaviridae

Size: 22 to 30 nm, 60 subunits
Symmetry: Icosahedral
Lipid envelope: Absent
Genus: Enterovirus
  Types: Poliovirus 1, 2, 3
  Coxsackievirus A, 23 types
  Coxsackievirus B, types 1–6
  Echovirus, 31 types
  Enterovirus 68–71
  Enterovirus 72 (hepatitis A)

Genus: Rhinovirus
  Types: Rhinovirus, 100 types
Natural habitat: Human gastrointestinal tract; survives in environment (enterovirus); human upper respiratory tract (rhinovirus)
Distribution: Worldwide
Transmission: Fecal-oral from human to human or contaminated water (enterovirus); human respiratory tract by aerosol or on hands (rhinovirus)

Route of infection: Gastrointestinal (enterovirus); respiratory (rhinovirus)
Diseases: Febrile illness, meningitis, encephalitis, myocarditis (enteroviruses); common cold (rhinoviruses)
Poliovirus 1. The particles are small, regular, and nonenveloped (× 180,000).

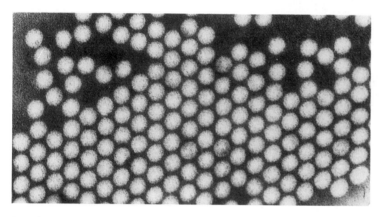

Poliovirus 1. The particles are small, regular, and nonenveloped (× 180,000).

Family: Caliciviridae

Size: 35 to 39 nm
Symmetry: Icosahedral
Lipid envelope: Absent
Genus: Calicivirus
  Types: Possibly Norwalk agent
  Other gastroenteritis agents

Natural habitat: Human gastrointestinal tract; other agents infect animals
Distribution: Worldwide

Transmission: Fecal-oral; contaminated water
Portal of entry: Gastrointestinal
Diseases: Gastroenteritis

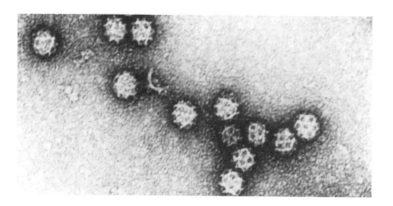

Swine exanthemata virus. Very small regular particles with prominent cup-like depressions. The surface depressions of the human Norwalk-like viruses are not as pronounced.

(continued)

Table 18-1 (continued)

Family: Reoviridae

Size: 60 to 80 nm, variable morphology
Symmetry: Icosahedral
Lipid envelope: Absent
Genus: Reovirus

Genus: Rotavirus
Natural habitat: Gastrointestinal tract of humans (reovirus and rotavirus) and animal (rotavirus)
Distribution: Worldwide

Transmission: Fecal-oral by direct contact; possibly animal to human
Portal of entry: Gastrointestinal tract
Diseases: Gastroenteritis (rotavirus); none (reovirus)

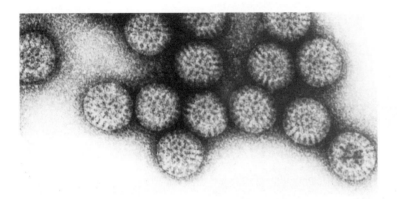

Human rotavirus. The distinctive feature of the reoviridae is the presence of a double shell, each with icosahedral symmetry (× 135,000).

Family: Togaviridae

Size: 40 to 70 nm
Symmetry: Icosahedral
Lipid envelope: Present
Genus: Alphavirus
   Type: Group A arboviruses
Genus: Flavivirus
   Type: Group B arboviruses

Genus: Rubivirus
   Type: Rubella virus
Natural habitat: Small mammals and insects (arboviruses); humans (rubella)
Transmission: By mosquito or tick vectors (arboviruses); aerosols or transplacental (rubella)

Portal of entry: Cutaneous (arboviruses); respiratory or vascular (rubella)
Diseases: Hepatitis, meningitis, encephalitis, arthritis, febrile illness (arboviruses); rash illness, congenital infection (rubella)

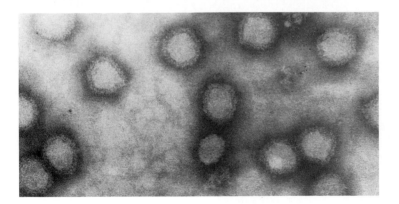

Rubella virus. The spherical virions have a lipid membrane and surface hemagglutinin projections (× 135,000).

(continued)

Table 18-1 (continued)

Family: Retroviridae

Size: 80 to 100 nm
Symmetry: Unknown
Lipid envelope: Present
Subfamily: Oncovirinae
   Types: Human T-cell leukemia/lymphoma virus (HTLV), types 1–2

Human immunodeficiency virus (HIV), types 1–2
Natural habitat: Humans
Distribution: Worldwide
Transmission: Unknown (HTLV); transfusions or contaminated needles, sex acts (HIV)

Portal of entry: Unknown (HTLV); intravenous or venereal (HIV)
Diseases: T-cell leukemia and lymphoma (HTLV); acquired immunodeficiency syndrome (AIDS) (HIV)

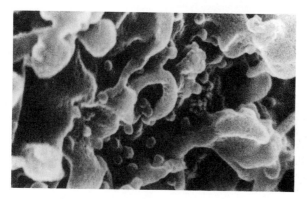

Human immunodeficiency virus. Scanning electron micrograph of human T-lymphocyte with virus particles budding from surface.

Family: Arenaviridae

Size: 50 to 300 nm
Symmetry: Unknown
Lipid envelope: Present
Genus: Arenavirus
Types: Lassa virus
   Lymphocytic choriomeningitis virus

Machupo virus (Bolivian hemorrhagic fever)
Junin virus (Argentinian hemorrhagic fever)
Natural habitat: Small mammals
Distribution: Worldwide (LCM)

South America (Machupo and Junin); Africa (Lassa)
Transmission: Secretions from infected rodents or patients
Portal of entry: Respiratory
Diseases: Febrile illness, meningitis (LCM); hemorrhagic fever (others)

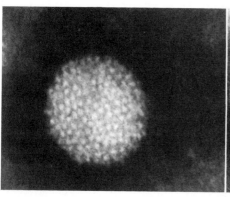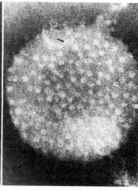

Lymphocytic choriomeningitis virus. The spherical virus has large surface projections. The name is derived from the Latin word *arena* (sand), which was suggested by the internal ribosome-like particles that are seen by transmission electron microscopy ($\times$ 225,000).

Table 18-2
Classification of DNA Viruses

Family: Herpesviridae

Size: 100 to 200 nm

Symmetry: Icosahedral

Lipid envelope: Present

Subfamily: Alphaherpesvirinae
Types: Herpes simplex virus 1
and 2
Varicella-zoster virus (VZV)

Subfamily: Betaherpesvirinae
Type: Cytomegalovirus (CMV)

Subfamily: Gammaherpesvirinae
Type: Epstein-Barr virus (EBV)

Natural habitat: Humans; related viruses are found in animals

Distribution: Worldwide

Transmission: By infected oral or genital secretions, by blood, or transplacentally

Portal of entry: Respiratory, cutaneous, intravascular, transplacental

Diseases: Neonatal sepsis, pharyngitis, cervicitis, local skin lesions, pneumonia, esophagitis (herpes simplex), congenital infection, hepatitis, mononucleosis, pneumonia (CMV); chickenpox (VZV); pharyngitis, mononucleosis, hepatitis (EBV)

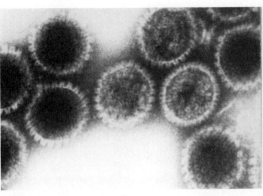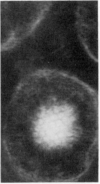

Herpes simplex virus. (*Left*) Naked nucleocapsids demonstrate the regular structure of the virion. Clearly defined structural units appear to have a central depression. (*Right*) Enveloped particle has, in addition, a lipid membrane derived from the infected cell (× 189,000).

Family: Adenoviridae

Size: 70 to 90 nm; 252 capsomeres

Symmetry: Icosahedral

Lipid envelope: Absent

Genus: Mastadenovirus
Types: Adenovirus, types 1 to 37
Noncultivatable adenovirus, types
40–41

Natural habitat: Humans (other genera of adenoviridae infect animals)

Distribution: Worldwide

Transmission: Fecal–oral, possibly aerosol droplet

Portal of entry: Gastrointestinal, respiratory

Diseases: Conjunctivitis, keratitis, pharyngitis, tracheobronchitis, pneumonia, cystitis; gastroenteritis (types 40 and 41)

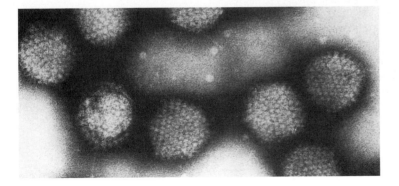

Adenovirus, type 5. The regular arrangement of the structural units of the virion is clearly evident (× 234,000).

(continued)

Table 18-2 (continued)

Family: Papovaviridae

Size: 45 to 55 nm
Symmetry: Icosahedral
Lipid envelope: Absent
Genus: Papillomavirus
    Types: Human wart viruses
Genus: Polyomavirus
    Types: BK virus
           JC virus
           SV 40 virus

Natural habitat: Humans and animals; the viruses are largely species-specific
Distribution: Worldwide
Transmission: By contact with infected secretions; viruses remain dormant in tissue

Portal of entry: Cutaneous, genital, or respiratory (papilloma); possibly respiratory (polyoma)
Diseases: Cutaneous, genital and laryngeal warts (papilloma); progressive multifocal leukoencephalopathy (polyoma)

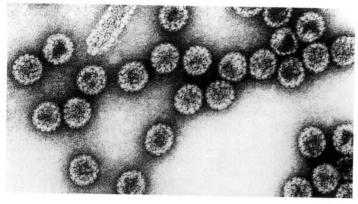

Human wart virus. These viruses have never been propagated successfully in cell cultures. The diseases have been associated by demonstration of virions, viral antigens or nucleic acid in lesions (× 135,000).

Family: Parvoviridae

Size: 18 to 26 nm
Symmetry: Icosahedral
Lipid envelope: Absent
Genus: Parvovirus
    Types: Possibly Norwalk agent; human parvovirus–like agent (HPLA)

Natural habitat: Humans, animals, and insects; viruses are species specific
Distribution: Worldwide

Transmission: Unknown
Portal of entry: Unknown
Diseases: Gastroenteritis, erythema infectiosum (fifth disease) of childhood; hemolytic disease

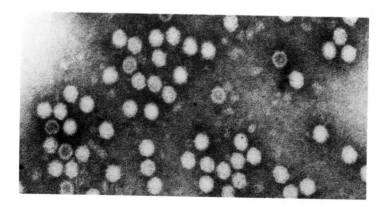

H-1 virus. The virions are very small and regular in size and shape. Parvoviruses are unusual in that they contain single-stranded DNA.

(continued)

Table 18-2 (continued)

Family: Proposed Family: Hepadnaviridae

Size: 42 nm
Symmetry: Unknown
Lipid envelope: Present
Genus: None established
   Types: Hepatitis B–like viruses
Antigens: Surface antigen (HBsAg)

Core antigen (HBcAg)
Early antigen (HBeAg)
Natural habitat: Humans
Distribution: Worldwide
Transmission: Infected secretions and blood

Portal of entry: Transfusions, cutaneous by shared implements, close contact (mechanisms probably various)
Diseases: Hepatitis, cirrhosis, hepatocellular carcinoma

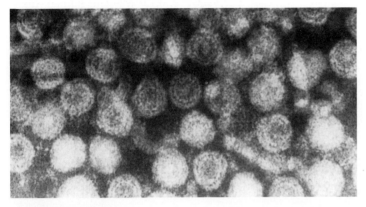

Hepatitis B virus. These 42-nm particles, which are the infectious agent, were originally known as Dane particles (× 225,000).

Family: Poxviridae

Size: 300 to 450 nm × 170 to 260 nm; brick shaped
Symmetry: Unknown
Lipid envelope: Absent
Subfamily: Chordopoxvirinae
   Genus: Orthopoxvirus
      Types: Variola (smallpox)

Vaccinia virus
Cowpox virus
Monkeypox virus
   Genus: Parapoxvirus
   Type: Orf virus
Natural habitat: Humans and animals

Distribution: Worldwide, variola exists now only in two research laboratories
Transmission: From infected humans or animals
Portal of entry: Respiratory
Diseases: Cutaneous ulcerative lesions; smallpox (eradicated)

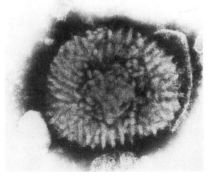

Vaccinia virus. The convoluted outer coat of these large, brick-shaped particles is evident. When smallpox existed, negative stain electron microscopy was a useful tool for differentiation of the pocks from those of varicella (× 49,500).

It is the most common cause of respiratory disease in hospitalized infants who are younger than 1 year of age.[135] Respiratory syncytial virus infections are often severe in young children. If congenital heart disease[162] or immunologic deficiency is present,[107] the disease may be lethal; in one study, 8 (73%) of 11 infants with congenital heart disease and pulmonary hypertension died.[165] Many previously normal children, especially infants, are sufficiently ill that ventilatory support is required. Apnea is a prominent part of the syndrome.[40] As has been mentioned, the availability of ribavirin as effective chemotherapy against this virus has increased the need for effective diagnostic services.[227]

The diagnosis of respiratory syncytial virus infection is best accomplished by direct detection of antigen in clinical specimens. Culture of this labile virus is definitive but difficult to accomplish in a timely fashion. Serology is used primarily for epidemiology studies.

Human Gastroenteritis Viruses

Viral gastroenteritis is second only to viral respiratory disease as a cause of morbidity in the United States. The incidence of viral gastroenteritis has been estimated at about 11% per year.[62] Mortality is very rare. In the past decade much has been learned about the etiologic agents, but only about half the cases of infectious gastroenteritis can be assigned an etiology. Most of these agents have been identified by electron microscopy.

Many aspects of viral gastrointestinal infections caused by a diverse group of agents are similar. They produce acute vomiting and diarrhea, which is usually mild, self-limited, and noninflammatory. Bloody diarrhea does not occur. Diarrhea that lasts more than 7 to 10 days is unlikely to be viral. Treatment is by correction of fluid and electrolyte loss, usually caused by vomiting. Unfortunately, immunity appears to be only partial.[62]

Of note is the absence of conventional intestinal viruses from the list of enteric pathogens. There is little evidence that enteroviruses or respiratory adenoviruses cause gastrointestinal disease.

Laboratory diagnosis of viral gastroenteritis can be accomplished by a variety of means, some of which are commercially available. This subject has been reviewed by Christensen.[37] The first question clinicians and microbiologists must ask is whether diagnosis of individual patients is necessary. It is important to remember that the necessity for having diagnostic tests with which to understand the biology of the disease does not mean that those tests must be employed on individual patients.

Rotaviruses

Rotaviruses are the most important human pathogens in the Reoviridae. The reoviruses themselves are not associated with human disease, but they have been useful in the study of molecular mechanisms of viral pathogenesis.[222] *Reo* stands for *r*espiratory-*e*nteric *o*rphan, from the source of virus isolates and the lack of association with clinical disease. Rotavirus got its name from the wheel-like appearance of the virion in electron micrographs.

The rotaviruses contain both human and animal pathogens, but animal rotaviruses do not infect humans. Human rotaviruses have been classified serologically, with most pathogenic human strains in the United States and Europe falling into group A. Human rotavirus is a common cause of gastroenteritis in infants and young children.[144] The clinical presentation is varied, but vomiting and dehydration are prominent features in comparison with gastroenteritis produced by other viruses. The combination of vomiting and a seasonal occurrence in the winter has led investigators to name the condition "winter vomiting disease."

Chronic rotavirus infection may occur in immunosuppressed children. In adults, rotavirus infection is usually asymptomatic. These viruses are notorious causes of nosocomial infection, including epidemics, in children.[82]

Rotaviruses were discovered, using electron microscopy, and were associated with human disease using immunoelectron microscopy.[144] The most common diagnostic methods employed in clinical laboratories have been the identification of viral antigen with a variety of enzyme immunoassays and latex agglutination tests. False-positive test results have been the primary problem with these assays. The reliability of enzyme immunoassays in diagnosing neonatal infections has been questioned in particular, especially with early versions of the tests.

Commercial products that include confirmatory assays, such as a blocking enzyme immunoassay, are preferred.[143] Many other diagnostic approaches, including molecular probes, have been developed. The reader is referred to the thorough review by Christensen for details of individual tests.[37]

Retroviruses

The retroviruses are RNA viruses; they were so named because they contain an enzyme that transcribes RNA into DNA, a reversal of the normal sequence in which DNA is transcribed into RNA.

For many years, these viruses were known to cause tumors in animals. In the 1970s, two viruses that caused T-cell lymphocytic lymphomas in humans were recognized and named human T-cell lymphoma virus (HTLV-I and HTLV-II). This discovery was extremely important biologically, but the tumors are uncommon.

The retrovirus group assumed sudden prominence and increased notoriety in 1983 when a third human retrovirus was identified as the cause of the acquired immunodeficiency syndrome (AIDS).[91] AIDS had been recognized clinically several years earlier when opportunistic infections were detected in young men who were homosexual, bisexual, or drug addicts but did not have conventional risk factors for *Pneumocystis* pneumonia or candidiasis.[96,168]

Similar viruses were isolated in several laboratories and named variously HTLV-III, lymphadenopathy-associated virus (LAV), and AIDS-related virus (ARV). An expert panel settled on the name, human immunodeficiency virus (HIV).[45] Although HIV virus was first isolated in 1983, retrospective analysis of frozen serum and tissue suggested that a similar virus had infected a sexually active teenaged boy in St. Louis in 1968.[87] Subsequently, a serologically related virus was isolated and named HIV-2. The distribution of HIV-1 is worldwide. HIV-2, found predominantly in West Africa, also produces an acquired immunodeficiency syndrome.[42] Cases of HIV-2 infection have been reported in the United States, but most patients have had some connection with West Africa.[28] There are immunologic cross-reactions between HIV-1 and HIV-2.[246] Specific immunoassays must be performed both to distinguish between the two infections and to detect the type-specific antigens with maximum sensitivity.[92]

There is no question that HIV is the plague of the latter half of the 20th century. It has changed the face of our society and will continue to wreak havoc for many years to come, especially in the third world.[95] The discussion below is a brief attempt to capture some of the most salient features of this multifaceted virus and the diseases it produces. It is a tribute to modern science that an infectious agent was reported only 3 years after the first reports of the clinical syndrome. Without the modern armamentarium of molecular biology and virology we would still be defenseless against this scourge.

The HIV-1 virion is icosahedral and contains 72 external spikes.[98] It is considerably more complex than HTLV-I and HTLV-II, consonant with its more complicated natural history. The gene products can be divided into three groups:

1. The gag proteins (group specific antigen/core) are a part of the viral nucleocapsid, providing stability for the shell and binding directly to the genomic RNA.
2. The pol proteins (polymerase) are enzymatic proteins that are crucial to the life cycle of the virus. The most famous of the pol proteins is the RNA-dependent DNA polymerase or reverse transcriptase.
3. The env proteins (envelope) are envelope glycoproteins that are critical for interactions with the outside world. These proteins are responsible for adhering to target cells (gp 120) and for production of cytopathic cell fusion (gp 41). The envelope also includes host cell components that are picked up as the virus buds through the cell membrane.

The viral proteins that represent the most important diagnostic antigens are summarized in Table 18-3.

The gp 120 envelope protein holds the initial key for entry of HIV-1 virus into the patient. This protein has a remarkable affinity for a receptor on the surface of cells throughout the body, known as the CD4 receptor. The CD4 receptor, which invites the entry of the HIV-1 virus into its cell, is found on T-helper lymphocytes, macrophages, and Langerhans cells in the skin. It has been hypothesized that uncircumcised men are more likely to develop HIV infection because the prepuce is a

Table 18-3
Major Antigens of Human Immunodeficiency Virus, Type I

GENE	GENE PRODUCTS
Group-Specific Antigen/Core (GAG)	p(protein)18, p24, p55
Polymerase (POL)	p31, p51, p66
Envelope (ENV)	gp(glycoprotein)41, 120, 160

(Adapted from Centers for Disease Control. Interpretation and use of the Western blot assay for serodiagnosis of human immunodeficiency virus type 1 infections, MMWR 1989; 38 [Suppl 7]:1–7)

rich source of Langerhans cells as well as macrophages and lymphocytes.[1] The enhanced susceptibility to HIV infection in patients with genital ulcers may result from the accessibility of CD4-positive macrophages and lymphocytes in the inflamed bases of the ulcers.[234] Macrophages provide the vehicle for transport to distant organs, such as the brain.[149] The most important viral targets, however, are the CD4-positive T lymphocytes.[156] These "helper" lymphocytes are the "Times Square" of the cellular immune system. Without them the body is at increased risk for many opportunistic infections. In addition to the T-cell abnormality, defective response of B cells to T-cell–independent antigens has also been documented.[157]

The initial encounter with HIV-1 virus produces a transient febrile disease, which may be accompanied by lymphadenopathy, pharyngitis, or a diffuse rash.[147] During the acute illness high levels of circulating virus are present in the absence of specific antibody.[41,54] In the natural course of the infection antibody develops within several weeks to several months. The duration of the antibody-negative, virus-positive window has been estimated to be a median of 2.1 months with 95% of seroconversions occurring within 5.8 months.[129] The window is important because there are not yet any practical means for detecting infectivity until antibody develops.

The ensuing subclinical phase of the disease is accompanied by antibody, circulating p24 antigen,[72] low levels of circulating virus, and infectious immune complexes.[78] During the chronic viremia, repetitive mutations in the viral genome thwart the attempts of the host immune system to eliminate the infection.[102,214] The onset of clinical illness is associated with an increase in the quantity of virus, both within peripheral blood mononuclear cells and in plasma.[121]

A wide spectrum of clinical conditions may result after HIV-1 infection. The Centers for Disease Control and Prevention classification of HIV disease is summarized in Table 18-4.[120] Longitudinal follow-up of HIV-1 infected men with lymphadenopathy has indicated increasing risk of developing AIDS after the third year of lymphadenopathy.[146] By far the most serious stage is group IV, including AIDS resulting from HIV destruction of helper T-lymphocytes followed by a profound immunosuppression. The patient is then rendered defenseless against many infectious

Table 18-4

Classification of Disease Produced by Human Immunodeficiency Virus

CLINICAL GROUP	CHARACTERISTICS
Group I	Acute infection
Group II	Asymptomatic infection
Group III	Persistent generalized lymphadenopathy
Group IV	Other disease
Subgroup A	Constitutional disease
Subgroup B	Neurologic disease
Subgroup C	Secondary infectious disease
Category C-1	Specified secondary infectious diseases listed in the CDC Surveillance Definition for AIDS
Category C-2	Other specified infectious diseases
Subgroup D	Secondary cancers (including those listed in the CDC Surveillance Definition for AIDS)

(Hirsch MS, Curran J. Human immunodeficiency virus: biology and medical aspects. In: Fields BN, Knipe DM, eds. Virology. 2nd ed. New York, Raven Press, 1990)

agents, especially those that are normally contained by the cellular immune system.

The infectious complications of HIV infection include viral, fungal, mycobacterial, bacterial, and parasitic infections. The practice of infectious disease and clinical microbiology has been irrevocably altered by HIV. Strand has discussed the role of the microbiology laboratory in support of patients with HIV disease.[237] The most common opportunistic infections that afflict patients with AIDS are listed in Table 18-5. Some of the infections are characteristic of a particular phase of the disease.

Not all disease is caused by opportunistic infection. The HIV virus itself is cytopathic and produces clinical disease such as encephalitis.[22] Collapse of the cellular immune system and its surveillance mechanisms leads to neoplastic complications, some of which may be virus induced.[108]

HIV-1 virus is excreted in the saliva,[99] milk,[190] semen,[268] and other body fluids,[85] but transmission of infection has been documented to occur only after exposure to blood or genital secretions. The importance of maternal milk in the transfer of virus from mother to child is unclear.

The most important groups at risk of HIV infection are those who have received blood products (recipients of blood transfusions, hemophiliacs),

Table 18-5
Opportunistic Infections Commonly Associated With Human Immunodeficiency Virus Infection

BACTERIAL	FUNGAL	PARASITIC	VIRAL
Mycobacterium tuberculosis	*Histoplasma capsulatum*	*Pneumocystis carinii*	Cytomegalovirus
Mycobacterium avium-intracellulare	*Candida* species	*Toxoplasma gondii*	Epstein-Barr virus
Mycobacterium kansasii	*Cryptococcus neoformans*	*Strongyloides stercoralis*	Herpes simplex virus
Chlamydia trachomatis	*Coccidioides immitis*	*Cryptosporidium*	
Pyogenic pneumonia		*Microsporidium*	
Mycoplasma fermentans		*Isospora belli*	
Rochalimaea-like organism			

those who have shared contaminated needles (drug addicts), those who have had sexual intercourse with an infected individual, and children of an infected mother.[85] At the outset of the epidemic most of the sexually transmitted infections in the United States and Europe were between homosexual men, but heterosexual transmission was soon documented.[109] Heterosexual transmission of HIV-1 virus has been dominant in Africa from the beginning of the epidemic.[95]

The risk of transmitting HIV virus in blood transfusions has been dramatically reduced by screening all units of blood for antibody and asking members of high-risk groups not to donate blood. In one study it was estimated that the risk of undetected HIV infection in blood units was 1 in every 61,171 units transfused.[23] A previous study had pegged the risk of HIV-1 screened blood at 0.003% per unit (1 in 33,000 units) for HIV-1 and 0.024% (1 in 4000 units) for HTLV-I.[46]

Special concern has been expressed about transfer of HIV to and from health care workers. This virus is transmitted by the same mechanisms as hepatitis B virus. Fortunately, HIV is much less contagious than hepatitis B virus and continuing surveillance has discovered very few cases of nosocomial transmission.[167] High rates of infection in African hospitals appear to reflect community infection rather than nosocomial transmission.[180] Only one instance of transmission from a health care worker to a patient is on record. The mechanisms of a highly publicized transmission from an HIV-1 infected dentist to multiple patients have not been elucidated,[31] but enormous public concern has resulted.

The most recalcitrant problem in AIDS control is the population of drug addicts who share needles. Infected addicts may pass their infections on both with additional contaminated needles and by sexual contact.

Herpesviruses

Viruses of the human herpesvirus group are the most frequent isolates in general laboratories. The group consists of the following:

Herpes simplex virus, type 1
Herpes simplex virus, type 2
Human cytomegalovirus
Epstein-Barr virus
Varicella-zoster virus
Human herpesvirus-6

Most members of the herpesvirus group can integrate their DNA with that of the host cell, produce a latent infection in lymphoid cells or ganglia of the central nervous system, and subsequently reactivate to cause recurrent disease. In general, the primary infections are more severe than are recurrences. The primary infections produced by several viruses of this group are more severe when they occur in adolescence or adult life, rather than childhood. The viruses circulate more freely and early in life among low socioeconomic groups and not until adolescence in more affluent society. The infections in high socioeconomic groups therefore tend to be more severe.

Herpes Simplex Virus

Herpes simplex virus causes a wide variety of infections.[49,239] Two serotypes of the virus infect humans. Shared antigens between types 1 and 2 make serologic differentiation difficult,[100] but reliable monoclonal antibodies for typing isolated viruses have been developed.[194] In healthy persons, infections of the oral cavity and genital tract predominate. Type 1 infections are most common in the upper body, while type 2 infections produce genital lesions; but there are exceptions to the rule. As many as one third of isolates from the genital tract represent type 1 strains. In contrast, very few isolates from the oral cavity are type 2 strains. Typing of herpes isolates from genital sites provides valuable prognostic information, because genital infections caused by type 1 herpes simplex virus are less likely to recur than are those caused by type 2 virus.[153,207] Genital infections with either viral type are more likely to occur than oral infections with the same type.[153]

Herpesvirus is passed from person to person by infected secretions or lesions. Infection is usually sporadic, but an epidemic of cutaneous infection at a wrestling camp (herpes gladiatorum) has been described.[14] The most serious herpes simplex virus infections are encephalitis, which most commonly affects the temporal lobe of the brain in adults, and disseminated infection in neonates, which may be acquired either during or after birth. Herpes simplex virus causes sporadic encephalitis. The diagnosis can only be made definitively by brain biopsy and culture,[263] but the availability of nontoxic antiviral chemotherapy[262] has prompted clinicians to treat patients empirically, thus avoiding an invasive procedure.

Herpes simplex virus is infrequently isolated from cerebrospinal fluid. In the national collaborative study, an isolate was recovered from cerebrospinal fluid in only 2 of 45 (4%) of biopsy-proven cases.[182] Serologic diagnosis is too insensitive, nonspecific, and slow to be of use in therapeutic decisions.[182] Use of molecular techniques to detect antibodies in cerebrospinal fluid has not been successful in correcting specificity problems and does not speed the process.[141]

Herpesvirus remains latent in spinal ganglia after the initial infection. Type 1 virus is recovered from thoracic ganglia, and type 2 virus is recovered from sacral ganglia.[9] Herpetic aseptic meningitis does occur uncommonly, usually caused by type 2 virus.[247]

Neonatal herpes infection is estimated to occur in 1:2,000 to 1:5,000 deliveries.[261] It is almost always symptomatic and frequently fatal.[240] In one collaborative study the mortality was 50% to 60% in infants with disseminated infection who were treated with acyclovir or vidarabine.[260] In contrast, there were no fatalities among infants with disease limited to the nose, eyes, or mouth. The diagnosis is suggested by the development of vesicular skin lesions, but these may be absent in 20% of patients.[240] Poor prognostic factors include disseminated disease, comatose state at admission to the hospital, disseminated intravascular coagulation, or prematurity.[260]

Persons witn compromised defense mechanisms are predisposed to herpes simplex esophagitis,[2] tracheobronchitis,[224] and pneumonia[97,203] and disseminated infection, including hepatitis.[202] Patients with extensive burns are at risk for infection both of the denuded skin and of the lower respiratory tract.[80]

Infection of the eye includes conjunctivitis, which may be accompanied by fever, photophobia, and regional lymphadenopathy. Herpetic keratitis, which has a branching or dendritic appearance, is the second most common cause of corneal blindness (after trauma) in the United States.[261]

Herpes simplex virus is one of the viral causes of pharyngitis and tonsillitis, usually as a primary infection. The mucosa may be ulcerated, and lesions may be limited to the posterior pharynx.[90] Hemorrhagic cystitis has been reported as a part of disseminated infection,[57] and herpetic proctitis may occur in homosexual men.[94]

Epstein-Barr Virus

Epstein-Barr virus is the primary cause of infectious mononucleosis. This versatile virus produces disease that ranges from acute self-limited infection to malignant neoplasms. The mononucleosis syndrome consists of fever, malaise, exudative pharyngitis, lymphadenopathy, and atypical lymphocytes circulating in the peripheral blood. Splenomegaly is common, and rupture of the spleen is a serious complication.[192] Acute hepatitis may also be a part of the syndrome.[50,259]

Epstein-Barr virus was originally recognized during studies of Burkitt lymphoma in Africa[211] and only later associated with mononucleosis.[184] The virus gains entry to the body by infecting the pharyngeal epithelium.[226] Its primary target, however, is the circulating B lymphocyte, which it infects and then immortalizes.[171] The result of this interaction is a polyclonal stimulation of the humoral immune system, which produces an array of antibodies to many antigens. At the same time the cellular immune system is triggered to fight the Epstein-Barr virus infection. It is the activated T lymphocytes that are seen in the peripheral blood smear as atypical lymphocytes.[193,213] The circle is completed when virus is excreted through the oral mucosa into the saliva.[185] Young children usually have an asymptomatic or minimally symptomatic infection, and the diagnostic heterophil antibody test is often negative.[130]

If integration of the Epstein-Barr virus genome into certain types of cells takes place, a neoplasm may result instead of an acute infection. The unregulated growth of Epstein-Barr virus in patients with HIV infection, who have lost the regulatory control of cellular immunity, may lead to increased Epstein-Barr virus–related tumors.[17] Most of these tumors are of B-lymphocyte lineage, such as Burkitt lymphoma and primary lymphoma of the brain,[123] but nasopharyngeal carcinoma has also been associated strongly with Epstein-Barr virus.[211]

The laboratory diagnosis of acute Epstein-Barr virus infection is serologic. The mainstay of diagnosis, the heterophil antibody test, was described decades before the viral etiology was elucidated.[55]

Culture of the virus can be accomplished by infecting and transforming normal lymphocytes, but this complicated procedure is not necessary. The major viral antigens that are useful diagnostically are listed in Table 18-6. The diagnosis of neoplastic manifestations must be by molecular demonstration that the virus has been integrated into the genome of the malignant cells.

Hepatitis Viruses

Many viruses can produce infectious damage to the liver. Epstein-Barr virus and cytomegalovirus occasionally cause symptomatic hepatitis as a part of the mononucleosis syndrome. The primary hepatitis viruses are a diverse group. The "alphabet soup" of hepatitis is summarized in Table 18-7.

HEPATITIS A VIRUS. Hepatitis A virus produces sporadic and epidemic infectious hepatitis. The disease has been known since antiquity, but the virus was not identified until the 1970s. As has been noted, hepatitis A virus is an RNA virus and has been named enterovirus 72, but the common name has the advantage of familiarity and use.

Hepatitis A virus produces acute self-limited hepatitis. The incubation period between exposure and clinical disease is short (less than 1 month). For

Table 18-6
Diagnostic Antigens of Epstein-Barr Virus

PHASE OF REPLICATION	ANTIGEN	COMMENTS
Latent phase	EBNA (EB-nuclear antigen)	Group of neoantigens in infected cells; responsible for immortalization
	LDMA (lymphocyte detected membrane antigen)	Target for the T-cell immune response to the EBV-infected cell
Early replication phase	EA (early antigen); "D" (diffuse); "R" (restricted; ie, localized)	Indicates onset of viral replication
Late replication stage	VCA (viral capsid antigen)	Indicates complete viral particles are being assembled; IgG and IgM responses detected
	MA (membrane antigen)	Responsible for viral neutralization

(Miller G. Epstein-Barr virus. In: Fields BN, Knipe DM, eds. Virology. 2nd ed. New York, Raven Press, 1990)

Table 18-7
Primary Viral Causes of Hepatitis

VIRUS	TAXONOMY	TRANSMISSION	CHRONICITY	NEOPLASIA
Hepatitis A	Enterovirus 72 RNA	Enteric: water, food, shellfish	No	No
Hepatitis B	Hepadnavirus DNA	Parenteral: blood, sexual contact, needles Enteric	Yes	Yes
Hepatitis C	? Togavirus 27-nm virion RNA	Parenteral: blood	Yes	?
Hepatitis D	42–47-nm virion RNA	Parenteral	Yes	No
Hepatitis E	27–34-nm virion	Enteric	? No	? No

7 to 10 days before clinical illness there is non-cytopathic viral replication in hepatocytes, viremia, and fecal shedding of infectious virus.[61] A period of viral replication with hepatocyte damage, including classic ballooning degeneration of liver cells, follows. At this point the communicable period is almost complete. Hepatitis A virus infection is rarely transmitted by blood transfusions because little virus is present in the blood and the duration of viremia is limited. Massive hepatic necrosis and postinfectious cirrhosis are rare. Chronic hepatitis and neoplasia are not complications.

Hepatitis A is transmitted by contaminated food and water.[230] Bivalve shellfish from contaminated waters have produced numerous outbreaks because they are often eaten raw or steamed to a temperature that does not kill the virus.[150] The transmission of hepatitis A virus, like Epstein-Barr virus and poliovirus, is determined by sanitation and socioeconomic condition. Virus circulates freely under conditions of poor sanitation and infects humans at an early age, when the infection is usually asymptomatic. More affluent citizens escape infection until adulthood, when symptomatic hepatitis results.[125]

Hepatitis A virus is the only primary hepatitis virus to have been cultured in vitro. Culture is not a viable diagnostic option, however, because recovery from primary specimens is not reliable. Hepatitis A is diagnosed serologically by detection of specific IgM antibody.[201,230,241] An experimental two-step process, using monoclonal antibodies and DNA hybridization, has been described for detection of hepatitis A.[136]

HEPATITIS B VIRUS.   Hepatitis B virus is a DNA hepadnavirus. It produces acute and chronic hepatitis and is an etiologic agent of hepatocellular carcinoma. Hepatitis B virus has a long incubation period (45 to 120 days) and is transmitted primarily by parenteral means. Until routine screening of blood products for this virus was begun, hepatitis B was the most common cause of transfusion-associated hepatitis. Other parenteral routes have included acupuncture[26] and tattooing.[174] Hepatitis B antigen has been demonstrated in mosquitoes, but transmission of infection by arthropods has not been authenticated.[200] This virus can be transmitted by sexual contact[118] and has produced epidemic disease in male homosexuals. Perinatal infection occurs,[188] but breast milk does not appear to play a role in transmission.[11] In contrast to hepatitis A virus, hepatitis B virus may produce fulminant fatal acute hepatitis, called massive hepatic necrosis. It has been suggested that a mutation in the virus may cause this severe manifestation.[182,189]

Hepatitis B virus is a 47-nm spherical virus that possesses several antigens of importance for diagnosis and pathogenesis. There are three envelope polypeptides that come under the designation HBsAg (hepatitis B surface antigen), HBcAg (hepatitis B core antigen), and HBeAg (hepatitis B e antigen). This virus has not been cultured in vitro, but the variety of antigens and corresponding antibodies provide ample tools for documenting clinical disease. DNA and DNA polymerase are not commonly measured. Although not absolute, the presence of e antigen correlates well with the presence of DNA and DNA polymerase and with viral infectivity.[5] The fascinating story of the discovery of Australia antigen (now known as HBsAg) and its relationship to hepatitis has been reviewed by Blumberg.[18] It serves as a reminder that no one can predict where basic research will have its impact. Who would have predicted that a research group interested in genetic polymorphisms of blood proteins would discover the key to the most important cause of human hepatitis?

For reasons that are unclear some persons who are infected with hepatitis B virus develop antibody and clear the virus from their system whereas others continue to circulate viral antigens. A subset of these chronic carriers develops chronic liver disease. Another serious complication of this infection is the integration of viral DNA into the genome of the liver cells and the development of hepatocellular carcinoma.[221]

Along with the knowledge of hepatitis B biology has come an effective vaccine, which can provide financial savings as well as prevent disease if used wisely.[176] Unfortunately, some populations most in need of protection respond poorly to the vaccine and are incompletely protected.[101]

HEPATITIS C VIRUS. After diagnostic reagents for hepatitis A and B viruses became available it became obvious that there were other causes of transfusion-associated hepatitis.[74] The unknown virus or viruses were dubbed non-A, non-B hepatitis. Thanks to the sophisticated technology of molecular biology we now recognize hepatitis C as the cause of most cases of transfusion-associated non-A, non-B hepatitis.

HEPATITIS D VIRUS. Hepatitis D virus, also known as the delta agent, is a 35-nm double-shelled RNA virus that is incapable of multiplication without the surface antigen of hepatitis B.[127] The maturing delta virus covers itself in the HBsAg coat before infecting other cells. Thus the biology of hepatitis D is inextricably tied to that of hepatitis B. Hepatitis D can produce infection and disease only in patients who are concurrently infected with hepatitis B or who are producing HBsAg from a previous infection. Not surprisingly, hepatitis D virus infection is concentrated in pockets of populations with hepatitis B virus infection, such as drug addicts and homosexual men.[56]

When co-infection takes place, the clinical disease is similar to that of hepatitis B and is usually self-limited.[125] When hepatitis D infects a patient who is a chronic carrier of hepatitis B, the clinical disease is much more severe, disease becomes chronic in as many as 80% of cases, and fatality rates may be dramatically increased to as high as 12%.[27]

HEPATITIS E VIRUS. This newest addition is a 27-nm labile RNA virus.[208] Hepatitis E virus produces an enterically transmitted acute hepatitis that most closely resembles that of hepatitis A. The viral genome has been cloned by techniques similar to those used to identify hepatitis C. Large epidemics of disease are produced under conditions of poor sanitation, but the infection has not yet been recognized in the United States.[124]

CLINICAL CLASSIFICATION OF VIRAL INFECTIONS

Although the virologic taxonomy is important scientifically, clinical schemes of classification have practical validity when considering an individual patient. The clinical syndromes and associated viruses that are most commonly encountered are summarized in Table 18-8. Viruses from varying taxonomic groups may produce the same symptoms.

DIAGNOSIS OF VIRAL INFECTIONS

The primary diagnostic technique for most viral infections is the isolation of the virus in cell culture. Serologic techniques may also be useful, especially if the virus was isolated from a nonsterile site. In some instances, serologic diagnosis is the only practical approach in a clinical laboratory. Direct detection of antigen in body fluids or tissues has also been effective for some viruses. The list of agents for which direct detection of antigen is useful will undoubtedly continue to expand. In Table 18-9, the methods most commonly used in hospital laboratories to diagnose viral infections are summarized. The advantages and disadvantages of each of these approaches are compared in Table 18-10. There are several excellent reference texts on diagnostic virology that should be consulted for additional information.[8,134,159,212,232]

(text continues on page 468)

Table 18-8
Clinical Syndromes Associated With Viral Infections

ORGAN SYSTEM	SYNDROME	MORE LIKELY AGENTS	LESS LIKELY AGENTS
Respiratory	Coryza: "cold"	Rhinovirus Coronavirus Adenovirus Parainfluenza 3	Influenza A or B Parainfluenza 1 or 2 RSV Enterovirus
	Pharyngitis	Adenovirus Herpes simplex Enterovirus Epstein-Barr virus	Influenza A or B RSV Parainfluenza 1 or 2 Rhinovirus Coronavirus
	Croup	Parainfluenza 1–3	Influenza A RSV Measles Coronavirus
	Bronchiolitis	Parainfluenza 3 RSV	Adenovirus Parainfluenza 1–2 Influenza A or B Rhinovirus
	Pneumonia	Influenza A RSV Parainfluenza 3 Adenovirus Cytomegalovirus (immunosuppressed patients)	Parainfluenza 1–2 Rhinovirus Epstein-Barr virus Influenza B
	Pleurodynia	Coxsackievirus B	Coxsackievirus A Echovirus
Central nervous system	Aseptic meningitis	Echovirus Coxsackievirus A Coxsackievirus B Mumps virus	LCM Herpes simplex 2 Varicella-zoster Adenovirus Bunyaviruses
	Encephalitis	None frequent	Herpes simplex 1 Togaviruses Bunyaviruses Epstein-Barr virus Enteroviruses Rabies virus Cytomegalovirus

(continued)

Table 18-8 (continued)

ORGAN SYSTEM	SYNDROME	MORE LIKELY AGENTS	LESS LIKELY AGENTS
Gastrointestinal	Diarrhea (infants)	Rotavirus Adenovirus 40–41	Adenovirus Enterovirus Norwalk-like virus Coronavirus
	Diarrhea (adults)	Norwalk-like virus	Rotavirus Adenovirus Enterovirus
	Hepatitis	Hepatitis A Hepatitis B Hepatitis non A, B	Epstein-Barr virus Cytomegalovirus
	Parotitis	Mumps virus	Parainfluenza viruses
Cutaneous	Vesicular rash	Herpes simplex Varicella-zoster	Echovirus Coxsackievirus A Vaccinia
	Maculopapular rash	Echovirus Coxsackievirus	Adenovirus Epstein-Barr virus Dengue virus Measles virus Rubella virus
	Petechial rash	None frequent	Adenovirus Echovirus Coxsackievirus Hemorrhagic fever viruses
Urogenital	Hemorrhagic cystitis	None frequent	Adenovirus
Cardiac	Myocarditis/pericar- ditis	Coxsackievirus A, B Echovirus	Adenovirus Influenza A Mumps virus
Ocular	Keratitis/conjunctivitis	Herpes simplex Varicella-zoster Adenovirus	Vaccinia Measles virus

RSV, respiratory syncytial virus; LCM, lymphocytic choriomeningitis virus.
(Adapted from McIntosh K. Diagnostic virology. In: Fields BN, Knipe DM, Melnick JL, et al, eds. Virology. 2nd ed. New York, Raven Press, 1990:411–440)

Table 18-9
Methods for Diagnosis of Viral Infections

VIRUS GROUP	ANTIGEN DETECTION	VIRUS ISOLATION	SEROLOGY
Adenoviruses	Described but not generally available	Primary method	Paired sera required
Enteroviruses	Not available	Primary method	Not generally available; viral isolate required
Epstein-Barr virus	Not available	Not generally available	Primary method
Herpesviruses	Useful for varicella-zoster virus; promising for cytomegalovirus; adequacy for herpes simplex varies	Primary method	Not useful except for immune status
Orthomyxoviruses	Described but not generally available	Primary method	Paired sera required
Paramyxoviruses	Described but not generally available	Primary method	Paired sera required
Rotaviruses	Primary method	Not generally available	Not practical for single cases
Rhabdoviruses	Primary method in reference laboratories	Primary method in reference laboratories	Useful for assessment of immunity
Respiratory syncytial virus	Useful for rapid diagnosis	Primary method	Paired sera required
Togaviruses (Arboviruses and rubella)	Not available	Not generally available	Primary method

Collection of Specimens for Diagnosis

In general, an attempt should be made to obtain material from the organ or organs that are infected. For the most common viral infections of the skin, the cutaneous lesions are the best specimens for culture. For diagnosis of infections of the respiratory and gastrointestinal tracts, secretions from those regions should be cultured. Recommended specimens for viral culture are listed in Table 18-11.

Most viruses enter the body through the respiratory or gastrointestinal tracts. Although the most obvious clinical manifestations of disease may occur in a distant organ, it is often appropriate to collect a specimen from the point of entry. Sampling of multiple sites is particularly useful if it is difficult to obtain a specimen from an internal organ or if the virus is difficult to isolate from the target organ. For example, the skin is most dramatically involved in measles infection, but measles virus may be isolated from the respiratory tract or from the urine. Similarly, the cardiac and central nervous systems are commonly affected in serious

Table 18-10
Comparison of Diagnostic Methods

METHOD	TIME	ADVANTAGES	DISADVANTAGES
Culture	Days to weeks	Specificity and sensitivity maximum; isolate available for characterization	Cell culture facilities needed; time for diagnosis may be long
Direct detection	Hours to 1 day	Speed of diagnosis; used for viruses difficult to culture	False-positive and false-negative results; hard to batch tests
Serology	Weeks	Assessment of immunity or response to virus isolated from nonsterile site; used for viruses difficult to culture	Potential cross-reaction; need for acute and convalescent specimens

Table 18-11
Recommended Specimens for Viral Culture

SYNDROME	OPTIMAL SPECIMENS	PERMISSIBLE ALTERNATES AND ADDITIONAL SPECIMENS
Coryza Croup	Nasopharyngeal aspirate	Nasopharyngeal swab
Pharyngitis	Throat washing or swab	
Bronchiolitis Pneumonia	Nasopharyngeal aspirate Tracheal aspirate Lung aspirate or biopsy	Nasopharyngeal swab
Pleurodynia	Nasopharyngeal aspirate *plus* feces	Nasopharyngeal swab Rectal swab
Aseptic meningitis Encephalitis Transverse myelitis	Spinal fluid *plus* feces *plus* nasopharyngeal aspirate	Rectal swab Nasopharyngeal swab Brain biopsy for herpes simplex; urine for measles or mumps
Gastroenteritis	Feces	Rectal swab
Parotitis	Nasopharyngeal aspirate *plus* urine	Nasopharyngeal swab
Vesicular rash	Aspirate or swab of vesicle	
Maculopapular rash	Nasopharyngeal aspirate *plus* feces	Nasopharyngeal swab Rectal swab
Hemorrhagic cystitis	Urine	
Myocarditis Pericarditis	Nasopharyngeal aspirate *plus* feces	Urine for mumps virus Nasopharyngeal swab Rectal swab
Keratitis Conjunctivitis	Conjunctival or corneal scraping *plus* nasopharyngeal aspirate	Conjunctival or corneal swab Nasopharyngeal swab

(Adapted from McIntosh K. Diagnostic virology. In: Fields BN, Knipe DM, Melnick JL, et al, eds. Virology. 2nd ed. New York, Raven Press, 1990:411–440)

enteroviral infection, but the virus may be isolated from the upper airways or from the gastrointestinal tract.

If the virus is rarely isolated from these non-sterile sites (as is the case with measles), recovery of a virus establishes an etiologic diagnosis. If the virus is recovered from sites where it may be found in the absence of disease (eg, the enteroviruses in throat or stool specimens), the recovery of a potentially pathogenic virus provides a presumptive diagnosis.

The optimal specimens for viral culture are aspirates of fluids, exudates, or secretions; tissues; washings of the upper airways; or stool specimens.

Swab specimens, which are very convenient, may also be obtained from these sites. Smith and associates isolated respiratory viruses from 12.5% of throat swabs that had already been processed for bacterial culture.[229] Calcium alginate swabs are toxic to herpes simplex virus,[52] and there is suggestive evidence that calcium alginate is toxic to respiratory syncytial virus also.[83] If the specimen is processed immediately or if the swab is removed from the transport medium, the toxicity of calcium alginate can be minimized, but it is best to avoid this material if possible.[15] Some investigators prefer not to use swabs with wooden shafts.

There are well-documented situations in which swabs are inferior to aspirates.[103] Aspirates or washings are probably optimal for recovery of all respiratory viruses,[252] although it is difficult to separate specimen type from swab characteristics and other variables in published reports.[83] Toxicity of swab material for certain viruses has already been mentioned.

To culture vesicular skin lesions, the skin should be cleansed with an alcohol swab and allowed to dry for at least 1 minute.[231] The vesicle should then be unroofed with a sterile scalpel and a sterile swab touched several times to the base. The swab should be placed in a viral transport medium, as described later. Alternatively, the contents of the vesicle may be aspirated with a tuberculin syringe and 26-gauge needle, if the vesicle is sufficiently large. Material for a Tzanck preparation can be collected by vigorously scraping the base of the lesion with the edge of a scalpel blade; the material on the blade is then touched to a glass slide and allowed to air dry.[231]

As a general rule, the frequency with which viruses are recovered decreases as the duration of illness increases so that every effort should be made to obtain specimens as early in the infection as possible.

Transportation and Storage of Specimens

Aspirates, fluids, and tissues should be transported to the laboratory in a sterile, leakproof container. Every effort should be made to minimize the interval between collection of the specimen and its inoculation into cell culture. Inoculation of cell cultures at the bedside has been recommended for some fragile viruses.[103] Ray and Minnich, however, found no significant effect on the rate of viral isolation

when delays in transport were as great as 24 hours.[205] Bromberg and colleagues found that delays of up to 3 hours did not compromise the isolation of respiratory syncytial virus.[19] At the University of Vermont we have found the recovery of respiratory syncytial virus to be significantly greater in specimens that are inoculated into cell cultures within 1 hour than in specimens that are inoculated after a delay of up to 6 hours. When specimens that contain a labile virus must be transported to a reference laboratory, direct detection of antigen should be considered as an alternative.

Swabs should be placed into a transport medium that includes antibiotics; dry swabs are not acceptable. The type of transport medium is probably not critical. Huntoon and colleagues found comparable performance by Stuart's (as used for bacterial cultures), Hanks', and Leibovitz-Emory media that had been incorporated into Culturette swabs by the manufacturer (Marion Scientific, Kansas City, MO). The sucrose phosphate glutamate (SPG) medium that was designed for *Chlamydia* is an effective transport medium for viral specimens.[256] Commercial viral[138] and chlamydial transport systems have also been reported to be suitable for herpes simplex virus.

Specimens should be refrigerated until they are inoculated into cell cultures. To select the best temperature for storage, one must balance the decrease in viral titer that occurs progressively at 4°C against the sudden decrease that occurs when specimens are frozen and thawed. It is clear that (1) the specimens should be maintained at −70°C if they are to be stored for a very long time (weeks or months); and (2) the best temperature is 4°C if the delay will be short (less than 24 hours). A very reasonable recommendation is that specimens be refrigerated for up to 96 hours and frozen at −70°C if the delay will be longer.[170] The very worst temperature is −20°C, especially in a frost-free freezer, where repeated cycles of defrosting and freezing are extremely traumatic to all forms of life. Specimens should never be frozen in the freezing compartment of a standard refrigerator. Johnson has thoroughly reviewed the transport of specimens for viral diagnosis.[137]

Isolation of Viruses in Culture

Although a few of the largest hospital laboratories may have facilities for inoculation of animals, most diagnostic facilities are restricted to the use of in vitro analogues. For laboratories that cannot perform cell cultures, inoculation of embryonated eggs is a useful means for surveillance of influenza A virus infections.[119] Eggs are less convenient to manipulate than cell cultures and pose a greater potential biohazard.

Preparation and Maintenance of Cell Cultures

Cell culture is the cultivation in vitro of dissociated single cells. Tissue and organ culture is the maintenance in vitro of a portion of an organ, usually for short, delimited periods of time. The use of organ culture has been restricted almost completely to the research laboratory. Other references are available for readers who desire more detailed information than can be provided in this chapter.[84,219]

Cell cultures are of three types (Table 18-12). Primary cell cultures consist of a mixture of cells, usually kidney or lung, obtained by dissociation of cells from the minced organ. These cells can be maintained in culture for a limited time only. Once subcultured in vitro a primary cell culture becomes a cell line. The most commonly employed cell lines are composed of fibroblasts, obtained from skin or embryonic lung. A cell line is diploid if at least 75% of the cells have a normal complement of chromosomes. A cell line is heteroploid if more than 25% of the cells have an abnormal complement of chromosomes.

The life expectancy of normal diploid cells is about 50 serial doublings in vitro;[112] those cell lines that have been transferred at least 70 times are considered to be established cell lines. These established or continuous lines may be derived from normal tissue, as was the Vero cell line from African green monkey renal cells. Alternatively, they may originate from neoplastic epithelium, such as the HeLa cells that came from a cervical adenocarcinoma and the HEp-2 cells that were derived from a carcinoma of the larynx. The appearance of uninoculated cell cultures is illustrated in Figure 18-3. The fibroblastic cells are usually long, spindly, and oriented in parallel, whereas the established cell lines consist of polygonal epithelial cells. The primary cultures naturally contain a mixture of cell types.

Conditions for growth and maintenance of cell cultures vary considerably, and only a few generalizations are possible. The temperature of incubation is optimal at 36° to 37°C but may be lowered to 35°C after confluence of cells is achieved. This maneuver may facilitate isolation of viruses, such as myxoviruses and rhinoviruses, that grow optimally at 33°C. A physiologic *p*H must be maintained. Usually a CO_2–bicarbonate buffering system is employed, with CO_2 being supplied by the metabolizing cells in a closed tube or flask. In an open system, a CO_2–air mixture must be provided. Buffering compounds that do not depend on CO_2–bicarbonate, such as HEPES buffer (N-2-hydroxyethylpiperazine-N/-2-ethanesulfonic acid), may be employed in open systems if an incubator with CO_2 is not available. A *p*H indicator is often included in the media to monitor closely shifts in *p*H during incubation. Phenol red, which is red at physiologic *p*H, turning yellow at acidic *p*H, and purple at alkaline *p*H is frequently used.

Essential vitamins and amino acids must be supplied in viral culture media. These compounds are stable when stored at 4°C, except for L-glutamine, which must be replenished periodically.[173] Eagle's Minimum Essential Medium (MEM) is the most

Table 18-12
Types of Cell Cultures

TYPE OF CULTURE	CHARACTERISTICS	EXAMPLES	PRIMARY USE
Primary	Diploid; mixed cell types; 1 or 2 passages	Primary monkey kidney	Influenza; parainfluenza; some enteroviruses
Cell lines	Diploid; fibroblasts; limited passage (up to 50–70)	Human diploid fibroblast (WI-38, MRC-5)	Herpes simplex; cytomegalovirus; varicella-zoster; rhinovirus
Established cell lines	Heteroploid; continuous passage in vitro	HeLa; HEp-2	Adenovirus; respiratory syncytial virus

commonly used, both for growth and for maintenance of cells. It is usually supplemented with small amounts of serum (up to 5%) for maintenance of a monolayer after cells have reached confluent growth. To enhance initial growth, larger amounts of serum (usually 10%) are used. It is important that the serum be free of infectious agents, including the mycoplasmas, and not contain antibodies to any viruses that might be present in clinical specimens. For this reason, either fetal, newborn, or agammaglobulinemic calf serum is most commonly used. Other formulations, such as Medium 199 or RPMI 1640, contain a richer mixture of nutrients and may be optimal for maintenance of some cell lines. Two forms of balanced salt solution are most frequently used, both for washing of cells and for incorporation into complete media. The formulations of Hanks' and Earle's solutions differ in several respects, notably the amount of buffering capacity. The two solutions are used virtually interchangeably, but Earle's balanced salt solution with its greater buffering power may be desirable for prolonged maintenance of monolayers.

Contamination of Cell Cultures

Contamination of media is reduced by inclusion of antibiotics. Penicillin (200 g/mL) and streptomycin (200 g/mL) or gentamicin (50 g/mL) are commonly used for suppression of bacterial growth; amphotericin B (1.25 g/mL) is used for inhibition of fungal growth.[134] The use of antibiotics does not substitute, however, for careful aseptic technique.

Shell vials, originally employed for isolation of *Chlamydia trachomatis*, have been used to increase the frequency and speed with which viruses are isolated. A cell monolayer is prepared on a round glass coverslip that has been placed on the bottom of a flat-bottomed vial (Fig. 18-4). If the inoculum is centrifuged onto the monolayer, as is essential for the recovery of *C. trachomatis*, and the monolayer is stained with fluorescein-conjugated antiserum or tested with a molecular probe, many viruses can be detected more rapidly.

Selection of Cell Cultures for Isolation of Viruses

The minimum requirements for isolation of viruses in culture are a primary culture of simian kidney cells (for isolation of myxoviruses and enteroviruses) and a diploid cell line of human origin (essential for isolation of cytomegalovirus, rhinovirus, and varicella-zoster virus; useful for isolation of herpes simplex virus). The addition of an established cell line of human origin (eg, HEp-2 or HeLa) is also useful for isolation of adenovirus and respiratory syncytial virus.

Inoculation and Incubation of Cell Cultures

Transport vials that contain swabs should be vortexed and material from the swab expressed into the medium, which contains antibiotics. Tissues are minced and homogenized in a small volume of transport broth. It may be necessary to suspend fecal specimens in 10 volumes of transport medium. Feces, tissues, and respiratory aspirates that contain excessive debris or mucus may be clarified by low speed centrifugation. Antibiotics are pres-

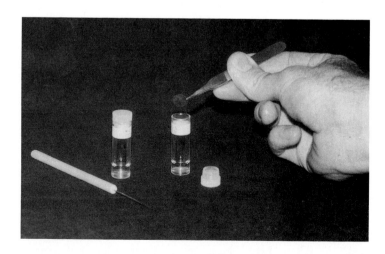

Figure 18-4. Shell vials for isolation of *Chlamydia trachomatis* and viruses. The vials are round with a flat bottom and contain a round coverslip on which the cells are grown. The top may be rubber or plastic as shown here. The coverslip is removed with forceps or with a needle.

ent in most transport and tissue culture media. If bacterial or fungal contamination of the specimen is expected, additional antibiotics should be added to the specimen before inoculation (penicillin and streptomycin or gentamicin plus amphotericin at twice the concentration used in cell culture media).[134]) After processing, the specimen may be inoculated into the culture media. Any remaining specimen should be retained at 4°C or frozen at −70°C in case toxicity or bacterial contamination occurs. If bacterial or fungal growth results, additional antibiotics may be added to the specimen. The specimen may be passed through a 0.45-m micropore filter before additional cultures are inoculated, but viruses that are cell associated, such as cytomegalovirus and varicella-zoster virus, may be lost when infected cells are trapped in the filter.[160] Nonspecific toxicity to the monolayer is usually evident within 24 hours; the specimen may then be reinoculated after making a 1 : 10 dilution in balanced salt solution. The *p*H of the specimen should also be checked and adjusted to neutrality if the specimen is very acid or alkaline. If nonspecific degeneration of the monolayer occurs after incubation for several days, the cells and fluid may be subcultured onto fresh monolayer.

Monolayers should be incubated at 36° to 37°C for recovery of most viruses. The optimal temperature of incubation for respiratory viruses, especially rhinovirus, is 33°C, but recovery of other viruses may be reduced at this temperature. Use of a roller drum (Fig. 18-5) facilitates isolation of pathogens in primary monkey kidney and diploid fibroblast cells, especially from respiratory specimens.

Two weeks of incubation is adequate for the recovery of most viruses. If the recovery of only herpes simplex virus is sought, the period of incubation may be further abbreviated to 7 days. As has been mentioned, centrifugation of the inoculum and detection of antigen will dramatically shorten the detection time for several viruses, including cytomegalovirus.

Detection of Virus and Provisional Identification

Cytopathic Effect

The most common method for detecting a virus is examination of cultures for virus-induced damage to the monolayers or cytopathic effect. Monolayers should be examined daily if herpes simplex virus is

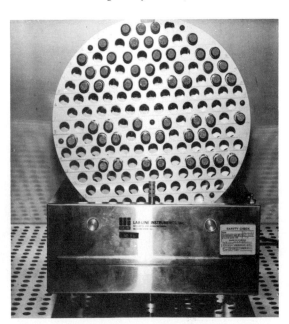

Figure 18-5. Roller drum for viral cultures. The cytopathic effect of many viruses, especially those that cause respiratory infection, is enhanced by slow rotation of the tubes, so that one revolution occurs every 3 minutes.

sought and at least three times a week if more slowly growing viruses are suspected. Glass tubes can be examined with a conventional light microscope, using simple holders to prevent the round tubes from rolling on the microscope stage (Fig. 18-6). If the monolayer is to be examined in shell vials, an inverted microscope must be used.

Provisional identification of the specific virus (or at least the virus group) can often be provided on the basis of the type of cytopathic effect and the type of cell that is affected. Using herpesvirus as an example, Figure 18-7 illustrates the phenomenon of cytopathic effect. The cytopathic effects of other viruses in other cell lines can be found elsewhere.[8]

Detection of Viral Antigens

In addition to confirmation of the identity of a cytopathic agent, demonstration of specific antigens in culture has been used as a method for detecting the presence of a virus, even in the absence of cytopathic effect.[4,70,88,89,172,215] Tests for antigen may be performed after a brief incubation if rapid diagnosis is desired. Alternatively, antigen tests may be performed after a specified incubation before reporting the absence of virus. This technique should work well if the virus can be targeted

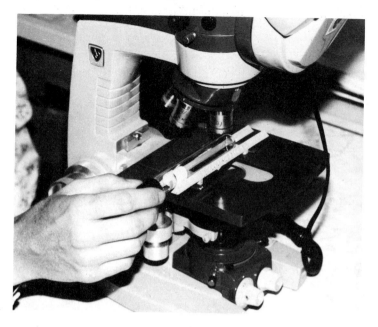

Figure 18-6. Examination of cultures for cytopathic effect can be performed with an inverted or a traditional microscope. A rack, which fits in the specimen holder of the microscope stage, prevents the round tubes from rolling. High magnification is not possible but is not needed for recognition and characterization of cytopathic effect.

precisely on clinical grounds. The most dramatic improvements in the rapidity with which isolates are detected will occur with those viruses that have the slowest growth in conventional systems, such as respiratory syncytial virus, cytomegalovirus, and varicella-zoster virus.

Artifacts and Non–Virus-Induced Changes

As cells age in culture, morphologic changes unrelated to viral infection may occur (see Fig. 18-3). The density of cells in diploid cell lines and, in particular, established cell lines may become very high; dying or dividing cells may appear rounded or granular. Scattered atypical cells occur in any culture and are especially noticeable in less dense areas, such as the edge of the monolayer, where viral cytopathic effect may also become apparent first. It is important, therefore, to maintain uninoculated controls of cells from the same batch as those used for specimens.

Primary monkey kidney cells may be infected with simian viruses that produce a variety of degenerative changes,[134] including a foamy or vacuolated appearance in the monolayer.

A variety of nonviral agents or substances in clinical specimens may be toxic to cell monolayers (see Fig. 18-8*A*). If bacterial or fungal growth occurs (see Fig. 18-8*B*), the nature of the problem is obvious; the specimen must then be treated again

with antibiotics or filtered and inoculated into additional cell cultures.

Usually the nature of the cytotoxicity is unknown. The ordinary remedy is to dilute the specimen and inoculate additional monolayers.

Definitive Identification of Isolates

In a diagnostic laboratory the combination of clinical history and cytopathic effect provides sufficient information to identify some viruses, including herpes simplex, cytomegalovirus, varicella-zoster virus, adenovirus, and respiratory syncytial virus. Enteroviruses can usually be identified to the genus level. Complete identification of isolates, including serotyping, requires immunologic characterization of the viral antigens.

The new monoclonal antibody technology has been aggressively applied to many areas of research, including virology.[267] The reagents have the great advantage that a continuous, unchanging source of antibody is assured. No longer is it necessary to worry that the "new rabbit is not as good as the old rabbit was." The monoclonal reagents also have the capability of recognizing very small segments (epitopes) of the antigen, so that more sophisticated schemes for typing isolates are possible. The monoclonal reagents are not infallible, however, and there are even some potential disadvantages. Although the epitopes with which the

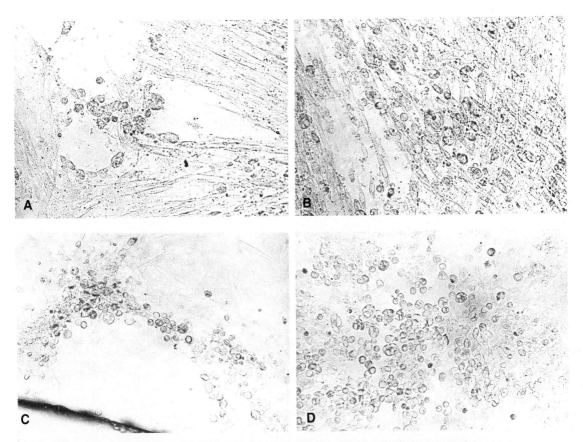

Figure 18-7. Cytopathic effect of herpesviruses. (**A**) MRC-5 fibroblasts infected with herpes simplex virus. There is a focus of enlarged, rounded cells in the monolayer. Many cells have detached from the glass. Such foci will enlarge rapidly, and the entire monolayer is usually involved within a few days (× 180). (**B**) MRC-5 fibroblasts infected with herpes simplex virus. Cytopathic effect has progressed so that virtually every cell in the monolayer is affected. Again, the cells are enlarged, even ballooned, and granular. This type of generalized cytopathic effect can occasionally be seen with cytomegalovirus if very large quantities of virus are present, as in patients with AIDS. Cytomegalovirus can be distinguished from herpes simplex by identification of specific antigens and by demonstration that transfer of cells is necessary to transfer the cytopathic effect to new cultures efficiently (× 180). (**C**) Rhesus monkey kidney cells infected with herpes simplex. As often happens at the outset, this focus of cytopathic effect is at the edge of the monolayer. Enlarged, ballooned cells surround the center of the focus, where the cells have already detached from the glass (× 180). (**D**) HEp-2 cells infected with herpes simplex virus. There is a large focus of swollen cells in the monolayer. Some of the cells have the appearance of multinucleated giant cells, although it is difficult to delineate the cellular structure in an unstained preparation at low magnification (× 180).

monoclonal reagents react are narrowly defined, cross-reactions may still occur if that epitope is shared by other antigens.[163] If the monoclonal reagents are too narrowly defined, they may not detect all isolates.[199,244] (See Chapter 19 for further information.)

For many hospital laboratories, immunofluorescence and immunoenzyme assays provide a viable alternative by which definitive identification of many viruses to the genus level can be made. Fortunately, the expanding catalogue of commercially available reagents, which are of increasingly high quality, simplifies the task. The enteroviruses and rhinoviruses are notable exceptions, because their complicated antigenic composition makes definitive identification difficult without neutralization tests. A full discussion of these techniques is beyond the scope of this text, but more detailed information can be found elsewhere.[152]

Immunofluorescence and immunoenzyme assays are very similar in principle, differing mainly in the detection system. Several variations of the

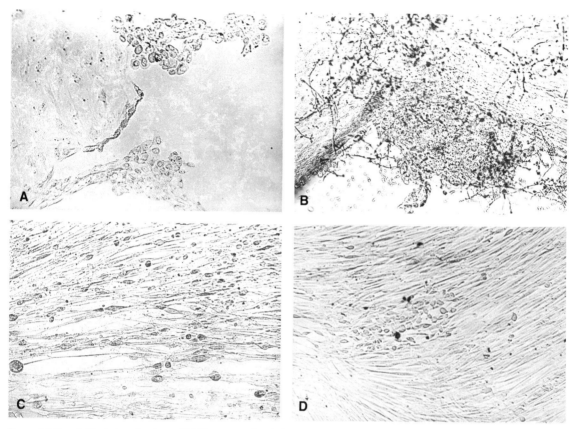

Figure 18-8. Artifacts in cell culture. (**A**) Rhesus monkey kidney cells. The tube has been inoculated with a specimen that contained nonspecific toxic material. Cells in the monolayer have rounded up focally, and many cells have detached from the glass. The nonviral effect can be distinguished from viral cytopathic effect by the overall pattern, by the rapidity of occurrence, and by the inability to reproduce the nonspecific effect after subculture into fresh monolayers (× 180). (**B**) Rhesus monkey kidney cell culture. A stool specimen was inadequately decontaminated before inoculation. Bacteria and fungal hyphae are evident on the monolayer, which is granular and will soon degenerate. The media may become acidic and cloudy. Re-treatment of the specimen with additional antibiotics is necessary. The specimen may also be filtered, but cell-associated viruses may be lost (× 180). (**C**) MRC-5 fibroblasts. A filtrate of stool that contained *Clostridium difficile* was inoculated onto the monolayer 24 hours earlier. The generalized disorganization of the monolayer with rounding and sloughing of cells typical of this toxin. Specific identification of the cause of toxicity is provided by neutralization of the effect with specific antiserum. *C. difficile* toxin may give an initial impression of viral cytopathic effect, but the effect will not be reproduced when material from the suspect tube is subcultured onto additional monolayers (× 180). (**D**) MRC-5 fibroblasts. Focal cell rounding and enlargement appeared on these fibroblasts that had been inoculated with cerebrospinal fluid, suggesting viral cytopathic effect. The atypical progression of the cytopathic effect and observation that some of the foci were superimposed on the fibroblasts suggested cellular contamination. HEp-2 cells were subsequently recovered from the tube and demonstrated to have a karyotype that was identical to that of the HEp-2 cells used in the laboratory. The mechanism by which the contamination occurred was never elucidated (× 180).

procedure are illustrated graphically in Figure 18-9. The direct fluorescent assay test is the simplest to perform, but specific conjugated antisera are required. Indirect immunofluorescent tests—using antiglobulin, staphylococcal protein A, or complement—are more sensitive but often suffer from lower specificity. In contrast to the direct test,

multiple conjugated reagents are not needed to perform the indirect test, but the procedure is more time consuming because of the multiple steps required.

The solid phase of immunoenzymatic tests can be the specimen itself, placed on a glass slide. In this case, the reaction is detected visually with a

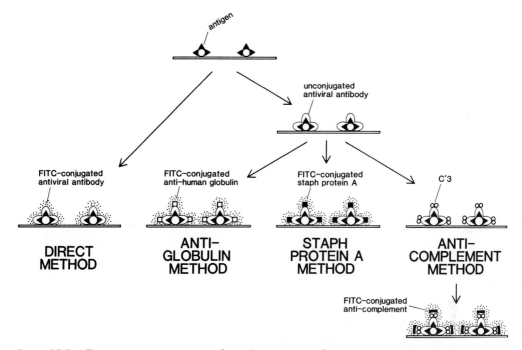

Figure 18-9. Fluorescence assays are performed in a variety of ways. Antigen is first fixed to a microscope slide by treatment with acetone, alcohol, or heat, depending on the nature of the antigen. For direct diagnosis of infections this antigen is, in fact, the clinical specimen. For serologic diagnosis, a known antigen is attached to the solid phase. The simplest method for identifying antigen in clinical specimens is the direct method. The indirect methods are usually more sensitive because they involve several amplification steps; the anticomplement method is probably the most sensitive of these techniques. Along with increased sensitivity, however, goes increased risk of nonspecific reactions. If antibody is to be detected, one of the indirect methods must be used.

microscope. Solid phase immunoassays can also be performed in tubes or microtiter trays. Several of the variations of the serologic enzyme immunoassay are depicted in Figure 18-10. For detection or identification of antigen, the wells are usually coated with an antiserum, which can be IgM as illustrated or can be whole immunoglobulin. For details on the performance of the immunoenzymatic tests, the reader is referred elsewhere.[152]

Enzyme and fluorescence immunoassays can be considered equivalent for most applications, although the fluorescence tests have been slightly more sensitive in some situations.[128,228] Nonspecificity has been a problem in enzyme immunoassays, and controls for specificity should be available. On the other hand, visual assays, such as direct immunofluorescence, are subject to considerable viewer-to-viewer variation. Assays in which a positive reaction is determined microscopically have two advantages: (1) the cellularity (and the quality) of the specimen can be judged and (2) the relation of the antigen to the cells can be assessed.[64]

The decision as to which assay to use will depend on local resources, experience, and the volume of tests. Immunofluorescence is simpler than most immunoassays if a small number of specimens is to be tested. When the number of specimens increases and the tests can be performed in batches, immunoenzyme assays or newer molecular probes become more attractive because automated systems can be used.

Positive and negative controls must be included in these tests. The specificity of the immunoenzyme assay can be enhanced by performing a blocking test.[20]

Identification of viral isolates by nucleic acid hybridization has also been accomplished.[33,36,69,76,186,206,249] The new technique of DNA amplification by the polymerase chain reaction technique has also been applied to many diagnostic problems (see Chapter 19).[48,59,225] We are well into the molecular age but only at the beginning of the application of these tools to diagnostic problems. In the next few years as commercial

INDIRECT METHOD

INDIRECT METHOD FOR IgM ANTIBODY

SANDWICH METHOD

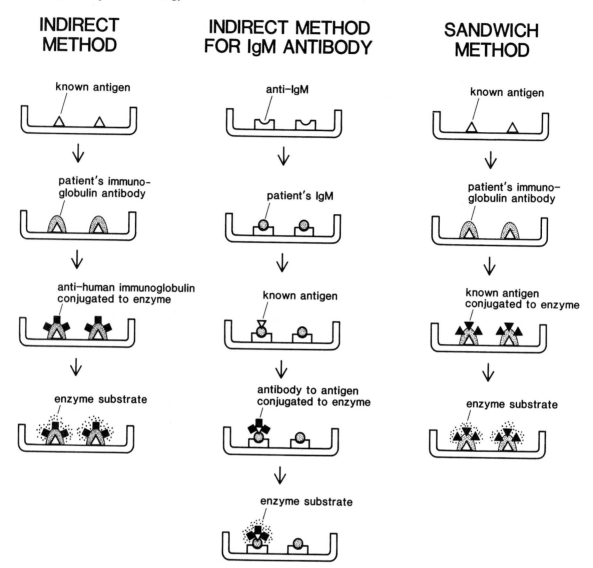

Figure 18-10. Enzyme immunoassays may be performed by a great variety of methods. If antibody is to be measured, antigen is placed on the solid phase as capture layer. After reaction of the antigen with the patient's serum the detection layer may be either an antiglobulin reagent or enzyme-labeled antigen. Although immunoglobulin class-specific (usually IgM or IgG) antiglobulins may be used to detect class-specific antibody responses, the preferred method for detection of IgM responses is to coat the solid phase with anti-IgM to capture any IgM in the patient's serum. Subsequently, the specificity of that captured IgM is tested with specific antigen. If direct detection of the agent in clinical specimens is desired, the first step is usually to coat the solid phase with specific antibody against the antigen to capture the antigen from the specimen. Subsequently, the presence of a reaction is detected by addition of enzyme-conjugated antibody to the antigen of interest.

reagents and kits become increasingly available, the appropriate uses of these sophisticated tools will be clearer.

Storage of Viral Isolates

If the necessity for additional characterization of an isolate seems probable, infected cell culture fluid should be frozen at $-70°C$. If the laboratory has the resources, it is good practice to retain all isolates for a period of time. A general rule is that mammalian cells should be frozen slowly, whereas infectious agents should be frozen quickly. The dramatic decrease in viability that accompanies the freezing process is minimized if the cultures are snap frozen and if a stabilizing agent is included in the medium. A mixture of dry ice and alcohol is a convenient means for snap freezing viral isolates. Many stabilizing agents have been used. Howell and Miller found that the sucrose phosphate broth that is used for transport of swabs for isolation of *Chlamydia* functioned as well as 70% sorbitol for maintenance of some of the most fastidious viruses, including cytomegalovirus and respiratory syncytial virus.[133]

Direct Detection of Viruses in Clinical Specimens

The desire for greater rapidity in diagnosis of viral infections has been stimulated by the availability of rapid diagnostic methods in other areas of the laboratory and by the development of effective antiviral chemotherapy. A variety of methods is available, ranging from the traditional to the experimental.[209,210]

Light Microscopic Detection of Inclusions

The detection of viral inclusions in smears or tissues by light microscopy has been the traditional means of directly demonstrating viral infections.[35,238] In general, those viruses that are assembled in the nucleus (usually DNA viruses) produce intranuclear inclusions, whereas cytoplasmic assembly (predominantly RNA containing viruses) yields cytoplasmic inclusions.

Intranuclear inclusions are produced in cells that have been infected by herpes simplex virus, varicella-zoster virus, cytomegalovirus, adenovirus, and papovaviruses. The inclusions of herpes simplex and varicella-zoster viruses are indistinguishable.

Detection of inclusions provides valuable information in selected clinical situations. The Tzanck test, performed by preparing a Giemsa-stained smear of vesicular scrapings, can be used to document the presence of a herpesvirus by demonstrating multinucleated giant cells. Hematoxylin and eosin or the Papanicolaou stain may also be used. A presumptive diagnosis of herpes infection can be made, although differentiation between herpes simplex virus and varicella-zoster virus is not possible by morphology alone.

Although the direct smears have worked well in the study of skin lesions, the sensitivity has unfortunately been low for other applications. Only a minority of culture-positive specimens from the genital tract or the respiratory tract contain inclusion-bearing cells.

Immunologic Detection of Viral Antigen

Immunologic and, more recently, molecular techniques have been used effectively to expedite diagnoses of certain viral infections. Immunofluorescence or immunoenzyme stains of clinical specimens or tissues and enzyme-linked immunosorbent assays on specimens are frequently used techniques (see Figs. 18-9 and 18-10).

These techniques have many advantages and have functioned well when applied by well-trained persons. The risks of erroneous results are great in the absence of proper equipment and training.[64] For almost all procedures, culture of the infectious agent remains the standard. Whenever possible, cultures should be done in parallel with rapid immunologic tests, until proficiency at the technique is demonstrated.

The diagnosis of infections caused by respiratory syncytial virus has been evaluated most extensively in clinical studies. The sensitivity of either immunofluorescence[128,142,158] or enzyme-linked immunosorbent assay[3,117,128,243] has been 80% to 95%, with immunofluorescence being perhaps slightly more sensitive. Direct antigenic detection of herpes simplex virus in vesicular lesions of the skin has been reliable. Virus was detected in all 15 vesicular lesions of the buttocks[254] and 23 of 24 penile lesions[255] in two studies in which the investigators used a commercial enzyme immunoassay. Lafferty and colleagues found that a combination of culture and direct immunofluorescence provided the maximal yield from lesions on the external genitalia.[154]

Unfortunately, as is the case with light microscopy, results from direct antigen detection procedures have not been entirely satisfactory in the two clinical situations of most concern—diagnosis of herpes encephalitis and evaluation of pregnant women near term.

Human rotavirus is difficult to recover in cell culture.[253] Infections by these viruses can be diagnosed effectively either by an enzyme immunoassay or by latex agglutination. The sensitivity for both methods has ranged from 80% to 90%, while the specificity has been 90% to 100%.[38,39,248]

Molecular Techniques

Nucleic acid hybridization holds great promise in the diagnosis of viral infections because of its molecular specificity. Cloned fragments of DNA or RNA that are complementary to the viral nucleic acid of interest (molecular probe) carrying either an enzyme or a radioactive marker can be reacted directly with a clinical specimen.[65,155,191] The reaction may either be performed in situ on a tissue section or in a test tube. After separating the unreacted nucleic acid from the mixture, the hybridized nucleic acid is quantitated either by measuring radioactivity or the quantity of color generated from the enzyme-labeled substrate. This exciting technique is emerging from research laboratories into the clinical laboratory.[77]

Selection of Tests for Rapid Diagnosis

The choice of a technique for direct detection of virus must depend on the availability of equipment, on the experience of personnel, and on the number of specimens to be tested. Microscopic detection of inclusions is simple and inexpensive but relatively insensitive; it works well for documentation of herpetic skin lesions. Electron microscopy has very restricted indications.

Microscopic solid phase immunoassays (immunofluorescence and enzyme assays) have advantages over assays for soluble antigens: (1) the location and type of staining can be assessed morphologically and (2) small numbers of specimens may be processed quickly. These attributes may be outweighed by the disadvantages of subjectivity in interpretation and the need to acquire an expensive microscope for fluorescence.

Enzyme immunoassay is most useful when a large number of specimens are to be tested or when the specimens can be collected and tested in a batch. The end point can be read with a spectrophotometer, eliminating subjective decisions.

To study tissue sections for viral elements, immunoperoxidase has the advantage over other markers in that viral antigens are generally available for reaction without additional treatment. Endogenous peroxidases in the sections must be blocked completely. Before immunofluorescence for detection of some antigens can be performed, fixed, embedded tissue must be treated with a proteolytic agent, such as trypsin.[32,126]

Well-trained personnel who are familiar with these techniques are essential. It is very important also to have available a gold standard, such as viral culture, at least until experience with the technique has been obtained.

Serologic Diagnosis of Viral Infections

Serologic tests are the mainstay of diagnosis for certain viral infections, such as those caused by hepatitis viruses, Epstein-Barr virus, and rubella virus.

General immunologic principles also apply when establishing a diagnosis of viral disease using serologic methods. Antibodies to many viral antigens remain for months or years after an acute infection. Demonstration of a significant increase (generally considered a fourfold rise) in titer of antibody is considered diagnostic of recent infection with the agent.

If antibodies are not present in the initial specimen, this diagnostic increase in antibody titer is referred to as a seroconversion. In this case, the infection probably represents a primary encounter with the virus. The infection may be either primary or reactivation of a latent infection if antibodies are present, even in low titer, at the time of initial testing.[182]

Serologic cross-reactions within many virus groups and even across groups do exist, notably, among enteroviruses, paramyxoviruses, and togaviruses. All serologic diagnoses must be considered, therefore, to some degree presumptive.

A fourfold or greater decrease in antibody titer suggests an infection at some time in the past. Most antibodies disappear slowly, however, so that it is usually difficult to be sure how recent the infection was.

The clinical setting must be kept in mind when assigning a diagnosis. Even a seroconversion documents only a recent infection with the agent; association with the clinical illness is by inference.

Hepatitis B Virus and Epstein-Barr Virus

There are a few exceptions to the general rule that a seroconversion must be documented to establish a diagnosis. In a few viral infections, antibodies to a variety of antigens appear at different times after infection and persist for varying lengths of time. It may be possible to establish a definitive diagnosis with a single serum when an antibody is detected that appears only acutely. The two prime examples are infectious mononucleosis caused by Epstein-Barr virus (Fig. 18-11) and hepatitis B (Fig. 18-12). infections. In both cases, certain antibodies, such as IgG antibody to Epstein-Barr virus persist for long periods; a seroconversion to these antigens must be detected. Other antibodies, such as those against the early antigen of Epstein-Barr virus, appear transiently and may serve as markers of acute infection.

If the infectious agent is not eliminated by the immune response, the presence of antibody means that the patient may still harbor the microbe. For instance, patients who have antibody to cytomegalovirus, which often produces a latent infection, are more likely to transmit the virus if blood or an organ is transplanted.[122]

Knowledge of the sequence of events is particularly important for the diagnosis of hepatitis B virus infection. Detection of viral antigen, especially the surface antigen (HbsAg), plays an important role in the diagnosis of acute infection. The e antigen of hepatitis B virus is detected at the same time as DNA polymerase activity, which is a marker for infectious virus; the presence of e antigen has correlated with acute, communicable disease in many studies,[179] as discussed earlier. Antibody to the viral core (HBc) is important diagnostically during the time when surface antigen has been cleared from the circulation and antibody to the surface antigen is not yet detectable.

The most common test for detecting infections

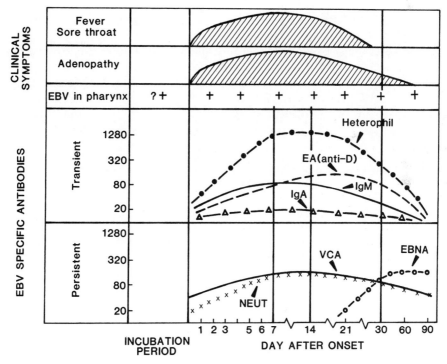

Figure 18-11. The time course of Epstein-Barr virus (EBV) infections and the serologic response. Although virus may be identified in oral secretions, the techniques for culture are difficult and are available only in research laboratories. The heterophil antibody response is the classic means of documenting infectious mononucleosis and is still the most useful test. The transient appearance of heterophil antibody, IgM antibody to viral capsid antigen, and antibody to early antigen (EA) allows one to associate the presence of antibody with the present illness. Neutralizing antibody and IgG antibody to viral capsid antigen (VCA) persist for months or years. These tests are useful to determine that the patient has been infected previously and is therefore immune; they may also be useful diagnostically if the first specimen is collected sufficiently early and a seroconversion is documented. If the patient is seen late in the course of the illness, diagnosis may be made by detection of a seroconversion to viral nuclear antigen (EBNA). (Modified with permission from James C. Niederman, Yale University School of Medicine)

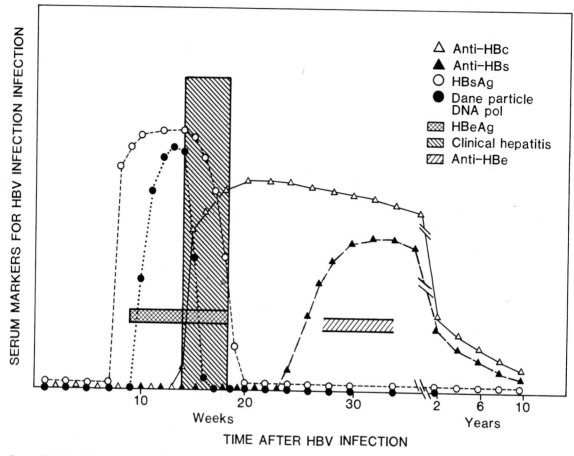

Figure 18-12. The appearance of antigens and antibodies after self-limited infection with hepatitis B virus is an example of how knowledge of the biology of infection led to very effective diagnostic strategies, although the virus itself was difficult or impossible to culture. One must look for both antigen and antibody to detect cases efficiently. Hepatitis B surface antigen (HBs) appears first; after it is cleared from the blood, antibody to that antigen can be detected (anti-HBs). There may be a time, however, when antigen has been cleared but antibody is not detectable; measurement of antibody to the core antigen (anti-HBc) will cover that possibility. The presence of HBs does not equal acute, self-limited infection because some persons become carriers. (Modified with permission from William S. Robinson, MD, Stanford University Medical Center)

by Epstein-Barr virus is the heterophil antibody test. Heterophil antibodies are immunoglobulins that react with substances from another species. In the course of an Epstein-Barr virus infection antibodies are produced to a variety of extraneous antigens. Agglutinins for sheep and horse red blood cells, hemolysins for beef red blood cells, and antibodies to the *Proteus* OX19 antigen of the Weil-Felix test are all produced. The heterophil antibodies that are very specific for infectious mononucleosis are absorbed by beef red blood cells but not by guinea pig kidney. The Paul-Bunnell-Davidsohn differential test for infectious mononucleosis is designed to characterize these heterophil

antibodies; it is highly specific for Epstein-Barr virus and confirmatory for making the laboratory diagnosis of infectious mononucleosis.[55] A variety of simplified tests for detecting the heterophil response in infectious mononucleosis are available commercially; most test agglutination of horse red blood cells after appropriate absorption of the sera.[79,131] Results that do not conform to clinical or hematologic data should be evaluated by performing the differential tube test or testing for Epstein-Barr virus specific antibodies.

Ninety percent of adults with infectious mononucleosis will have a positive test result. The frequency with which young children develop these antibodies is much lower. Only 3 of 11 infants younger than 2 years of age developed heterophil antibodies after a primary Epstein-Barr virus infection, whereas 16 of 21 children between the ages of 2 and 4 years developed such antibodies.[130]

Human Immunodeficiency Virus

Human immunodeficiency virus persists in patients who have developed antibody to the virus. Serologic tests for HIV have been used as a screening tool because isolation of the virus in cell culture is difficult and not readily available. The reference serologic method is a Western blot procedure, in which sera are reacted with viral proteins that have been separated by polyacrylamide gel electrophoresis and transferred onto nitrocellulose paper. This test requires considerable expertise and care in performance. Several other, more easily performed assay systems have been developed. An enzyme immunoassay has been evaluated most extensively[24,86] as a screening test for blood-bank blood and for diagnosis of the infection. The test is both sensitive and specific. In patients with AIDS, the predictive value of a positive result is high. In the general population of blood donors, among whom HIV infection is very infrequent, even a few false-positive test readings result in an unacceptably low predictive value. Numerous versions of the immunoassay have been developed, but a licensed version

that has been validated should be used. In most laboratories, a specimen that contains antibody to HIV by an enzyme immunoassay is first retested in the enzyme assay; if repeated positivity is demonstrated, the specificity of the reaction is documented by performing a Western blot.[47] Not all Western blots produce unequivocal results. The test is not interpreted as positive unless there are multiple protein bands that can be considered truly independent.[29] The criteria suggested by several expert groups for determination of positive Western blots are summarized in Table 18-13. The lack of uniformity among laboratories in applying criteria for interpretation of Western blots makes comparison among test results difficult. In a 1990 survey, 22% of laboratories used multiple sets of criteria. Even among the 78% of laboratories that used a single criterion there were several standards.[30] An example of a positive Western blot is shown in Figure 18-13. Indeterminate Western blots occur in 10% to 20% of sera that are reactive by enzyme immunoassay.[25] The risk of developing AIDS for persons with a repeatedly reactive enzyme immunoassay and an indeterminate Western blot depends on the risk factors of the individual. If there are no risk factors for HIV infection, the patient or donor does not require further follow-up. As noted earlier, there is a finite period of time shortly after infection with HIV when infectious virus may be present in the absence of detectable antibody.

Table 18-13
Criteria for Positive Western Blot for Antibody to Human Immunodeficiency Virus

ORGANIZATION	CRITERIA
Association of State and Territorial Public Health Laboratory Directors/CDC	Any 2 of: p24 gp41 gp120/gp160
FDA-licensed DuPont Test	p24 and p31 and gp41 or gp120/gp160
American Red Cross	3 or more bands—1 from each gene product group: GAG and POL and ENV
Consortium for Retrovirus Serology Standardization	2 or more bands: p24 or p31 plus gp41 or gp120/gp160

(Adapted from Centers for Disease Control. Interpretation and use of the Western blot assay for serodiagnosis of human immunodeficiency virus type 1 infections. MMWR 1989:38[Suppl 7]:1–7)

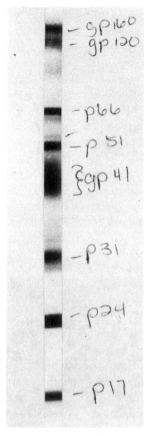

Figure 18-13. Western blot for HIV-1 antibody. Disrupted virus was electrophoresed through polyacrylamide gel after which it was transferred (blotted) onto nitrocellulose paper. Patient's serum was then reacted with the nitrocellulose strips, after which enzyme-labeled anti-human immunoglobulin was added to the strips. Development of the enzyme reaction revealed multiple bands with this serum from an HIV-1–infected patient. The electrophoresis separated the various proteins and glycoproteins by molecular weight. The bands are labeled here according to the viral protein they have detected.

Anti-IgM Antibodies

In general, IgM antibody appears earlier than IgG after an acute infection and is more transient. Additionally, IgM does not readily cross the placenta, so that demonstration of this antibody in a neonate indicates a congenital or perinatal infection, rather than passive transfer of antibody from the mother.

Demonstration of IgM antibody to any antigen suggests a recent infection. The test should be used only in laboratories, in which the results have been carefully evaluated, because there are several theoretic and practical pitfalls that may produce an erroneous interpretation. Most importantly, criti-

cal clinical decisions are often dependent on accurate results.

It is extremely important that the procedure for detection of the IgM class be demonstrably specific. The presence of IgM antibody is usually tested by demonstration of a decrease in titer after removal of IgM, by documenting residual activity after removal of IgG, by using specific antiglobulins directed against IgM, or by a combination of these approaches.

If an anti-IgM antibody is used to determine the acuteness of an infection, the specificity of the antiglobulin must be documented. False-negative results may be generated if there are very high levels of IgG, which may block the sites that would have reacted with IgM. False-positive results may be encountered if antiglobulins, such as rheumatoid factor, are present in the patient's serum. If a serum reacts with multiple antigens (ie, rubella, cytomegalovirus, herpes simplex virus, and *Toxoplasma gondii*), an antiglobulin should be suspected.

Finally, although IgM antibody in serum is usually transient, there are well-documented instances in which IgM antibody has persisted for months or even years. Furthermore, it is recognized that IgM can be detected when a latent infection is reactivated.[64]

A summary of the serologic diagnosis of viral infections is presented in Table 18-14.

Diagnosis of Other Viral Infections

Diagnosis of some viral infections is beyond the scope of most hospital laboratories, because the infections are rare or exotic, the etiologic agents are hazardous, or special diagnostic facilities are necessary. Tests for rabies, arboviral infections, and viral hemorrhagic fevers are usually performed in a reference laboratory, such as those in state departments of health or at the Center for Disease Control and Prevention.

INFECTIONS WITH *CHLAMYDIA*

Clinical Features and Epidemiology

Chlamydiae are obligately intracellular bacterial pathogens. Three species of *Chlamydia* produce human disease. *C. psittaci* causes acute respiratory

Table 18-14
Serologic Diagnosis of Viral Infections

VIRUS	TESTS PERFORMED	COMMENTS
Respiratory Infections		
Influenza A and B	CF; HAI	CF used for stable type-specific antigen; HAI used for strain-specific antigen
Parainfluenza virus	HAI; CF; EIA	Cross-reactions common with other paramyxoviruses
Respiratory syncytial	CF; EIA	EIA most sensitive method
Adenovirus	CF; EIA	Group-specific antigen
Central Nervous System Infections		
Enteroviruses	CF; NT; EIA	Not generally available; used in conjunction with isolation of virus
Mumps virus	HAI; IFA; EIA	Cross-reactions with other paramyxoviruses
Herpes simplex virus	CF; IHA; EIA; IFA	Not useful for diagnosis
Rabies virus	RFFIT; IFA	For diagnosis or confirmation of immune status
Hepatitis		
Hepatitis A	RIA; EIA	IgM antibody for diagnosis
Hepatitis B	RIA; EIA	IgM anti-HBc (core antigen) diagnostic; antigen detection preferred
Cutaneous Infections		
Measles virus	HI; IFA; EIA; CF	For immune status or diagnosis
Varicella-zoster virus	CF	For diagnosis only
	IFA; FAMA	For immune status
Other Infections		
Cytomegalovirus	CF; IHA; EIA; IFA	Limited value except screening of blood or organ donors
Rubella	HI; EIA; IFA; LA	Preferred method of diagnosis
Epstein-Barr virus	Heterophil test	Preferred method; may be negative, especially in children
	IFA for various antigens	For diagnosis of problem cases

CF, complement fixation; HAI, hemagglutination inhibition; EIA, enzyme immunoassay; NT, viral neutralization; IFA, immunofluorescence; RFFIT, rabies fluorescent focus test; RIA, radioimmunoassay; IHA, indirect hemagglutination; FAMA, fluorescent antibody to membrane antigen assay

(Adapted from Herrmann KL. Viral serology. In: Lennette EH, Balows A, Hausler WJ Jr, et al, eds. Manual of clinical microbiology. 4th ed. Washington, DC, American Society for Microbiology, 1985:921–923)

infections, usually transmitted from infected birds.[218] Infections by *C. trachomatis*, which includes 15 serologic variants (serovars), are much more common.[216] Serovars L1, L2, and L3 produce a sexually transmitted disease, lymphogranuloma venereum. Trachoma, a chronic conjunctivitis often complicated by blindness, is associated with serovars A, B1, B2, and C. The newest member of the genus, *C. pneumoniae*, was originally referred to as the TWAR bacillus, using the initials of two patients from whom the bacterium was isolated.

Inclusion conjunctivitis (an infection distin-guished from trachoma by the absence of corneal scarring), pneumonia in neonates,[12] and sexually transmitted infections in adults, all of which are caused by serovars D through K, are the chlamydial diseases of most importance for diagnostic laboratories. It has been suggested on serologic grounds that community-acquired pneumonia in adults may also be caused by *C. trachomatis*.[151] The antibodies detected in this study, however, may have been directed against the newly recognized species, *C. pneumoniae*, the apparent reactivity with *C. trachomatis* representing an unsuspected cross-reaction. The sexually transmitted infections include urethritis,[169] mucopurulent cervicitis,[21] and salpingitis.[242] The sexually transmitted and neonatal infections are, in fact, directly connected. Schachter and colleagues followed 131 infants born to mothers from whose cervix *C. trachomatis* was cultured.[217] Eighteen percent of the infants developed culture-confirmed inclusion conjunctivitis, and 16% had neonatal chlamydial pneumonia.

All of the chlamydia may be isolated in embryonated eggs and cell culture. Recovery of *C. psittaci* in cell culture should not be attempted unless stringent isolation facilities are available for protection of laboratory personnel. Care to prevent laboratory-acquired infections should also be exercised if the serovars that cause lymphogranuloma venereum are suspected.

Collection of Specimens

Cervical and ocular specimens are best collected by scraping the mucosa. Swabs are readily available and minimally traumatic. Wooden-tipped swabs and swabs made of calcium alginate should be avoided; some cotton swabs have been toxic to *Chlamydia*; Dacron or rayon material is preferred.[44] Despite the use of acceptable types of swabs, some lots may be toxic to *Chlamydia*, so that pretesting of lots is recommended.[197] Urethral and nasopharyngeal specimens may be collected with a fine swab on a flexible wire. The swab should be inserted 3 to 5 cm into the urethra. Urine, semen, and purulent urethral discharge are not considered adequate specimens for culture.[44]

Cervical specimens are collected from the endocervix after carefully removing mucus. The isolation rate is increased if a urethral and a cervical swab are placed in the same transport vial. The cytobrush, used for collection of Papanicolaou smears, has been reported to be superior to swabs by some investigators[140] but not others.[258] The cytobrush cannot be used in pregnant women. Lesions in the rectum and fallopian tube should be sampled under direct visualization by anoscopy or laparoscopy.

Direct detection of *C. trachomatis* by immunofluorescence is done after application of the specimen to a clean glass slide. The type and manner of collection of specimens is the same as for diagnosis by culture. The slide should be fixed according to the manufacturer's instructions as quickly as possible. For the commonly used Microtrak reagent (Syva Co., Palo Alto, CA), fixation in methanol enhanced detection of organisms in comparison to fixation in acetone.[140]

Isolation of *Chlamydia trachomatis* in Cell Culture

Although chlamydiae are bacteria, they are obligate intracellular pathogens. Methods for isolation in culture are similar to those employed in the virology laboratory. It is essential, however, that the infective elementary bodies of chlamydiae be centrifuged onto the monolayer in a shell vial (see Fig. 18-4). Inclusion bodies of *C. trachomatis* contain glycogen, which may be stained with iodine. After incubation for 48 to 72 hours, the coverslips are removed and stained with iodine or, for somewhat greater sensitivity, with a fluoresceinated monoclonal antibody[236] prepared against a species-specific antigen. Chlamydial inclusions are well demarcated, cytoplasmic structures. Culture for chlamydiae has become a specialized procedure as methods for direct detection have been developed and improved.

Direct Detection of *Chlamydia* in Clinical Specimens

If large numbers of chlamydial inclusion bodies are present, a diagnosis may be established easily by staining smears by the Giemsa or Gimenez methods.[116] The advent of commercially available monoclonal antibodies to species-specific antigens of *C. trachomatis* has revolutionized the rapid diagnosis of this infection. The monoclonal antibodies detect the elementary particle and inclusions of all serovars with considerably greater sensitivity than histochemical stains.

Immunofluorescence

A direct immunofluorescence test (Microtrak; Syva Co., Palo Alto, CA) has been evaluated most extensively. The sensitivity of the test for detection of genital infections has ranged from 60% to 100%, and the specificity has been very high.[51,81,93,163,198,235,245] The large variation in sensitivity may reflect, in part, differences in the prevalence of chlamydial infection in various populations.[10,81] The direct test may be particularly valuable when long delays are inevitable between the collection of a specimen and the initiation of culture.[264] Interpretation of the test requires well-trained personnel and high-quality (ie, expensive) equipment. Although the antibody is of monoclonal origin, at least one of the antigens of *C. trachomatis* resembles the lipopolysaccharide of enteric bacteria[187] and probable cross-reactions with other bacteria have been reported.[163] Many different immunofluorescence reagents are on the market. In general, the fluorescence of reagents that are directed against the major outer membrane proteins is brighter and the bacterial morphology is more consistent.[43] Antibodies to *C. trachomatis* lipopolysaccharide cross react with other *Chlamydia* species, which may be an advantage or disadvantage, depending on the objective of the user.

Elementary bodies are the infectious form that is seen in clinical specimens. They are small (0.25 to 0.35 μm) and round with sharp, well-defined margins. Smears should be examined with a 40× or 63× objective, and the identity of fluorescing particles should be confirmed with a 100× objective. At the higher magnification, a central, more darkly staining region can often be discerned in the structures. Although the elementary bodies are very small, they often occur in small clusters, even when only few in number. When the infection is very heavy, there is greater variation in the size and shape of elementary bodies and inclusion bodies may be seen occasionally.

Distinguishing the morphology of the tiny, fluorescing particles from debris is of prime importance. Particulate debris often has a yellowish color and can be visualized as refractile structures with incident white light. In contrast, specific fluorescence has an apple-green color and the elementary bodies cannot be seen with white light. The color of the specific fluorescence, however, may appear yellow-green if there is abundant background material that fluoresces red in the presence of a counterstain. A minimum number (defined by the manufacturer) of well-defined elementary bodies should be observed before the smear is reported as positive. The smear should be examined completely for at least 3 minutes before a negative interpretation is reported. Genital specimens that are acellular or contain only mature squamous cells are suboptimal. Brunham and colleagues studied the correlation of inflammatory exudate and recovery of *C. trachomatis* in 100 randomly selected women.[21] More than 10 polymorphonuclear neutrophils per oil immersion field were observed in 17 (89%) of 19 women from whom *C. trachomatis* was isolated. The presence of at least five columnar epithelial cells on a slide increased the sensitivity of the test from 70% to 92% in one study.[197] Unfortunately, the scanty cellular content of the specimen will not be known until after the test has been performed, but the information should be conveyed to the clinician.

The direct immunofluorescence procedure is even more sensitive for detection of inclusion conjunctivitis than for genital infection, as might be expected from the experience with Giemsa-stained smears. Two groups of investigators identified all infants with neonatal chlamydial conjunctivitis using the direct procedure.[13,204] In contrast, the sensitivity of Giemsa-stained smears was only 42%.

In a very small number of patients, the direct immunofluorescence test has been used to diagnose neonatal chlamydial pneumonia.

The direct immunofluorescence test has almost achieved the status of another diagnostic gold standard when performed by highly trained personnel who use high-quality fluorescence microscopes. The influence of inadequate skill and training on the results of this reliable but subjective test can be devastating.[164]

Enzyme Immunoassay

Howard and colleagues studied the effect of specimen quality on detection of elementary bodies.[132] If the slide contained no columnar or transitional epithelial cells, only 0.78% of slides were positive for *C. trachomatis*. If fewer than 25 columnar/transitional cells were present, 2.8% of slides were positive; 8.8% of slides were positive when more than 25 columnar/transitional cells were present.

Enzyme immunoassays for *C. trachomatis* are also available. The original commercial assay has been evaluated most thoroughly (Chlamydiazyme; Abbott Laboratories, North Chicago, IL). The sensitivity of the enzyme assay has varied from 70% to 100%, partially depending on the source of the specimen.[34,139,161] The specificity of a modified test appears to have been improved,[34,139] although one collaborative study documented a sensitivity of only 57% in comparison to culture.[166] The correlation of culture and enzyme immunoassay decreased in subgroups at low risk of disease. A disturbingly low specificity was observed with the original assay and with a modified assay also.[161,166] Most of the positive results that were not supported by culture occurred with cervical specimens from asymptomatic women.

Some investigators have recommended that urine sediments from male patients with urethritis be examined for *C. trachomatis* by the enzyme immunoassay.[220] The advantage of this noninvasive procedure to the patient is obvious. Unfortunately, not all investigators have had success with urine specimens and problems with nonspecificity of the enzyme immunoassay may be magnified.[58]

Serologic Diagnosis

Antibodies to *C. psittaci* and the lymphogranuloma venereum serovars of *C. trachomatis* can be detected by the complement-fixation test. A microimmunofluorescence test for antibodies to *C. trachomatis* is more sensitive for diagnosis of lymphogranuloma venereum infections and can also be used to document infections by other serovars. This test is less widely available, and multiple antigens must be tested. It is most useful for seroepidemiologic studies of populations at high risk of chlamydial infection.

Molecular Techniques

A nonradiometric commercial DNA probe against rRNA of *C. trachomatis* is available. The initial version was relatively insensitive and nonspecific,[195,266] but a revised procedure appears to provide excellent specificity and reasonable sensitivity.[148,265]

INFECTIONS WITH *RICKETTSIA* AND RELATED ORGANISMS

The order Rickettsiales includes the genera *Rickettsia*, *Coxiella*, *Rochalimaea*, *Ehrlichia*, *Bartonella*, and several newly identified pathogens. The most numerous and important genus is *Rickettsia*, and the most important pathogen in the genus is *Rickettsia rickettsii*. In this chapter the discussion centers on

the diagnosis of Rocky Mountain spotted fever, which is caused by *R. rickettsii*.[250]

Rickettsia species infect vascular endothelial cells. The clinical manifestations of infection are consequently protean and may reflect damage to any organ system. Rocky Mountain spotted fever is a multisystemic febrile disease. It is usually accompanied by a rash that begins on the extremities.[113] The infection is widely distributed throughout the country, wherever the tick vectors exist. Paradoxically, the infection is more common in the midwestern and south central states than in the western and mountain states.[53,111]

Collection of Specimens

Culture of *Rickettsia* is performed only in reference laboratories. Blood or biopsy tissue from a lesion should be frozen at −70°C. Direct immunofluorescence may be performed on a frozen or formalin-fixed biopsy or autopsy specimen. Rickettsial infections are usually diagnosed serologically, using acute and convalescent sera.

Serologic Diagnosis

Most diagnoses of rickettsial infections are made by serology. In recent years, the microimmunofluorescence assay has become the reference test.[196] This procedure appears to be the most sensitive and specific method for the diagnosis of rickettsial infections.[145] The degree of cross-reaction among rickettsial species varies from patient to patient.[196] Cross-reactions are strongest within the rickettsial subgroups. It may be difficult to distinguish between epidemic and endemic typhus or between Rocky Mountain spotted fever and rickettsialpox.[251] Antibodies first appear 7 to 10 days after infection. A fourfold rise in serum antibody is desired for diagnosis, but a single titer of more than 1:64 is highly suggestive.

The microimmunofluorescence test requires highly trained personnel and a fluorescence microscope. Latex agglutination tests, which are commercially available for Rocky Mountain spotted fever, are in more general use. The latex tests appear to produce positive reactions only during an acute infection, so a single positive test is diagnostic.[114] The sensitivity has ranged from 70% to

95%.[114,145] The complement-fixation test was once the diagnostic standard,[223] and it remains a valid very specific serologic tool. As the newer tests have been developed, however, it has become apparent that the complement-fixation test is insensitive for rickettsial diagnosis.[145,183]

Historically, the most common diagnostic test for rickettsial disease has been the Weil-Felix test, in which antirickettsial antibodies that cross-react with strains of *Proteus* species are detected. The test originated from the chance observation that sera from patients with typhus agglutinated strains of *Proteus vulgaris*. As experience with immunologically specific serologic tests has been accumulated, it has become apparent that the Weil-Felix test is both insensitive and nonspecific.[115,145,251] In some populations, a positive Weil-Felix test result has been more common in those who did not have Rocky Mountain spotted fever than in those who were infected.[251] All of these facts argue strongly for the relegation of this test to the archives.

REFERENCES

1. Ackerman SJ. HIV-1 link prompts circumspection on circumcision. J NIH Res 1991;3:44–46.
2. Agha FP, Lee HH, Nostrant TT. Herpetic esophagitis: a diagnostic challenge in immunocompromised patients. Am J Gastroenterol 1986;81:246–253.
3. Ahluwalia GS, Hammond GW. Comparison of cell culture and three enzyme-linked immunosorbent assays for the rapid diagnosis of respiratory syncytial virus from nasopharyngeal aspirate and tracheal secretion specimens. Diagn Microbiol Infect Dis 1988;9:187–192.
4. Alpert G, Mazeron MC, Colimon R, Plotkin S. Rapid detection of human cytomegalovirus in the urine of humans. J Infect Dis 1985;152:631–633.
5. Alter HJ, Seeff LB, Kaplan PM, et al. Type B hepatitis: the infectivity of blood positive for e antigen and DNA polymerase after accidental needlestick exposure. N Engl J Med 1976;295:909–913.
6. American College of Obstetrics and Gynecology. Perinatal herpes simplex virus infections. ACOG Tech Bull 1988;122:1–5.
7. Arvin AM, Hensleigh PA, Prober CG, et al. Failure of antepartum maternal cultures to predict the infant's risk of exposure to herpes simplex virus at delivery. N Engl J Med 1986;315:796–800.
8. Balows A, Hausler WJ Jr, Herrmann KL, Isenberg HD, Shadomy HJ. Manual of Clinical Microbiology. 5th ed. Washington, DC, American Society of Microbiology, 1991.
9. Baringer JR. Recovery of herpes simplex virus from human sacral ganglions. N Engl J Med 1974;291:828–830.
10. Barnes RC, Katz BP, Rolfs RT, Batteiger B, Caine V, Jones RB. Quantitative culture of endocervical *Chlamydia trachomatis*. J Clin Microbiol 1990;28:774–780.
11. Beasley RP, Stevens CE, Shiao I, Meng H. Evidence against breast-feeding as a mechanism for vertical transmission of hepatitis B. Lancet 1975;2:740–741.
12. Beem MO, Saxon EM. Respiratory-tract colonization and a distinctive pneumonia syndrome in infants infected with *Chlamydia trachomatis*. N Engl J Med 1977;296:306–310.
13. Bell TA, Kuo CC, Stamm WE, et al. Direct fluorescent monoclonal antibody stain for rapid detection of infant *Chlamydia trachomatis* infections. Pediatrics 1984;74:224–228.
14. Belongia EA, Goodman JL, Holland EJ, et al. An outbreak of herpes gladiatorum at a high-school wrestling camp. N Engl J Med 1991;325:906–910.
15. Bettoli EJ, Brewer PM, Oxtoby MJ, Zaidi AA, Guinan ME. The role of temperature and swab materials in the recovery of herpes simplex virus from lesions. J Infect Dis 1982;145:399.
16. Binkin NJ, Koplan JP, Cates WJ. Preventing neonatal herpes: the value of weekly viral cultures in pregnant women with recurrent genital herpes. JAMA 1984;251:2816–2821.
17. Birx DL, Redfield RR, Tosato G. Defective regulation of Epstein-Barr virus infection in patients with acquired immunodeficiency syndrome (AIDS) or AIDS-related disorders. N Engl J Med 1986;314:874–879.
18. Blumberg BS. Australia antigen and the biology of hepatitis B. Science 1977;197:17–25.
19. Bromberg K, Daidone B, Clarke L, Sierra MF. Comparison of immediate and delayed inoculation of HEp-2 cells for isolation of respiratory syncytial virus. J Clin Microbiol 1984;20:123–124.
20. Bromberg K, Tannis G, Daidone B, Clarke L, Sierra MF. Comparison of ortho respiratory syncytial virus enzyme-linked immunosorbent assay and HEp-2 cell culture. J Clin Microbiol 1985;22:1071–1072.
21. Brunham RC, Paavonen J, Stevens CE, et al. Mucopurulent cervicitis: the ignored counterpart in women of urethritis in men. N Engl J Med 1984;311:1–6.
22. Budka H, Costanzi G, Cristina S, et al. Brain pathology induced by infection with the human immunodeficiency virus (HIV): a histological,

immunocytochemical, and electron microscopical study of 100 autopsy cases. Acta Neuropathol 1987;75:185–198.

23. Busch MP, Eble BE, Khayam-Bashi H, et al. Evaluation of screened blood donations for human immunodeficiency virus type 1 infection by culture and DNA amplification of pooled cells. N Engl J Med 325:1991;1–5.

24. Carlson JR, Bryant ML, Hinrichs SH, et al. AIDS serology testing in low- and high-risk groups. JAMA 1985;253:3405–3408.

25. Celum CL, Coombs RW, Lafferty W, et al. Indeterminate human immunodeficiency virus type 1 Western blots: seroconversion risk, specificity of supplemental tests, and an algorithm for evaluation. J Infect Dis 1991;164:656–664.

26. Centers for Disease Control. Hepatitis B associated with acupuncture—Florida. MMWR 1981;30:1–3.

27. Centers for Disease Control. Delta hepatitis—Massachusetts. MMWR 1984;33:493–494.

28. Centers for Disease Control. Update: HIV-2 infection—United States. MMWR 1989;38:572–580.

29. Centers for Disease Control. Interpretation and use of the Western blot assay for serodiagnosis of human immunodeficiency virus type 1 infections. MMWR 1989;38(Suppl 7):1–7.

30. Centers for Disease Control. Interpretive criteria used to report Western blot results for HIV-1 antibody testing—United States. MMWR 1991;40:692–695.

31. Centers for Disease Control. Update: transmission of HIV infection during an invasive dental procedure—Florida. MMWR 1991;40:21–33.

32. Chandler FW, GOrelkin L. Immunofluorescence staining of adenovirus in fixed tissues pretreated with trypsin. J Clin Microbiol 1983;17:371–373.

33. Chapman NM, Tracy S, Gauntt CJ, Fortmueller U. Molecular detection and identification of enteroviruses using enzymatic amplification and nucleic acid hybridization. J Clin Microbiol 1990;28:843–850.

34. Chernesky MA, Mahony JB, Castriciano S, et al. Detection of *Chlamydia trachomatis* antigens by enzyme immunoassay and immunofluorescence in genital specimens from symptomatic and asymptomatic men and women. J Infect Dis 1986;154:141–148.

35. Cheville NF. Cytopathology in viral diseases. Basel, S Karger, 1975.

36. Chou S. Reactivation and recombination of multiple cytomegalovirus strains from individual organ donors. J Infect Dis 1989;160:11–15.

37. Christensen ML. Human viral gastroenteritis. Clin Microbiol Rev 1989;2:51–89.

38. Christy C, Vosefski D, Madore HP. Comparison of three enzyme immunoassays to tissue culture for the diagnosis of rotavirus gastroenteritis in infants and young children. J Clin Microbiol 1990;28:1428–1430.

39. Chudzio T, Kasatiya S, Irvine N, Sankar-Mistry P. Rapid screening test for the diagnosis of rotavirus infection. J Clin Microbiol 1989;27:2394–2396.

40. Church NR, Anas NG, Hall CB, Brooks JG. Respiratory syncytial virus-related apnea in infants: demographics and outcome. Am J Dis Child 1984;138:247–250.

41. Clark SJ, Saag MS, Decker WD, et al. High titers of cytopathic virus in plasma of patients with symptomatic primary HIV-1 infection. N Engl J Med 1991;324:954–960.

42. Clavel F, Mansinho K, Chamaret S, et al. Human immunodeficiency virus type 2 infection associated with AIDS in West Africa. N Engl J Med 1987;316:1180–1185.

43. Cles LD, Bruch K, Stamm WE. Staining characteristics of six commercially available monoclonal immunofluorescence reagents for direct diagnosis of *Chlamydia trachomatis* infections. J Clin Microbiol 1988;26:1735–1737.

44. Clyde WA, Kenny GE, Schachter J. Diagnosis of *Chlamydia* infection. Cumitech. Washington, DC, American Society for Microbiology, 1984.

45. Coffin J, Haase A, Levy JA, et al. Human immunodeficiency viruses. Science 1986;232:697.

46. Cohen ND, Munoz A, Reitz BA, et al. Transmission of retroviruses by transfusion of screened blood in patients undergoing cardiac surgery. N Engl J Med 1989;320:1172–1176.

47. Consensus Conference. The impact of routine HTLV-III antibody testing of blood and plasma donors on public health. JAMA 1986;256:1778–1783.

48. Cone RW, Hobson AC, Palmer J, Remington M, Corey L. Extended duration of herpes simplex virus DNA in genital lesions detected by the polymerase chain reaction. J Infect Dis 1991;164:757–760.

49. Corey L, Spear PG. Infections with herpes simplex viruses (2). N Engl J Med 1986;314:749–757.

50. Corey L, Stamm WE, Feorino PM, et al. HBsAg-negative hepatitis in a hemodialysis unit: relation to Epstein-Barr virus. N Engl J Med 1975;293:1273–1278.

51. Coudron PE, Fedorko DP, Dawson MS, et al. Detection of *Chlamydia trachomatis* in genital specimens by the Microtrak direct specimen test. Am J Clin Pathol 1986;85:89–92.

52. Crane LR, Gutterman PA, Chapel T, Lerner AM. Incubation of swab materials with herpes simplex virus. J Infect Dis 1980;141:531.

53. D'Angelo LJ, Bregman DJ, Winkler WG. Rocky Mountain spotted fever in the United States: use of age-specific incidence to determine public health policy for a vector-borne disease. South Med J 1982;75:3–5.

54. Daar ES, Moudgil T, Meyer RD, Ho DD. Transient high levels of viremia in patients with primary human immunodeficiency virus type 1 infection. N Engl J Med 1991;324:961–964.

55. Davidsohn I, Lee CL. The laboratory in the diagnosis of infectious mononucleosis with additional notes on epidemiology, etiology and pathogenesis. Med Clin North Am 1962;46:225–244.

56. Decock KM, Govindarajan S, Chin KP, Redeker AG. Delta hepatitis in the Los Angeles area: a report of 126 cases. Ann Intern Med 105: 1986;108–114.

57. Dehertogh DA, Brettman LR. Hemorrhagic cystitis due to herpes simplex virus as a marker of disseminated herpes infection. Am J Med 1988; 84:632–635.

58. Demaio J, Boyd RS, Rensi R, Clark A. False-positive chlamydiazyme results during urine sediment analysis due to bacterial urinary tract infections. J Clin Microbiol 1991;29:1436–1438.

59. Demmler GJ, Buffone GJ, Schimbor CM, May RA. Detection of cytomegalovirus in urine from newborns by using polymerase chain reaction DNA amplification. J Infect Dis 1988;158: 1177–1184.

60. Desigan G, Schneider RP. Herpes simplex esophagitis in healthy adults. South Med J 1985;78: 1135–1137.

61. Dienstag JL, Feinstone SM, Kapikian AZ, Purcell RH, Boggs JD, Conrad ME. Faecal shedding of hepatitis-A antigen. Lancet 1975;1:765–767.

62. Dolin R, Treanor JJ, Madore HP. Novel agents of viral enteritis in humans. J Infect Dis 1987;155: 365–376.

63. Douglas RG Jr. Prophylaxis and treatment of influenza. N Engl J Med 1990;322:443–450.

64. Drew WL. Controversies in viral diagnosis. Rev Infect Dis 1986;8:814–824.

65. Edberg SC. Principles of nucleic acid hybridization and comparison with monoclonal antibody technology for the diagnosis of infectious diseases. Yale J Biol Med 1985;58:425–442.

66. Enders JF, Weller TH, Robbins FC. Cultivation of the Lansing strain of poliomyelitis virus in cultures of various human embryonic tissues. Science 1949;109:85–87.

67. Erice A, Jordan MC, Chace BA, Fletcher C, Chinnock BJ, Balfour HH Jr. Ganciclovir treatment of cytomegalovirus disease in transplant recipients and other immunocompromised hosts. JAMA 1987;257:3082–3087.

68. Eriksson M, Forsgren M, Sjoberg S, Von Sydow M, Wolontis S. Respiratory syncytial virus infection in young hospitalized children: Identification of risk patients and prevention of nosocomial spread by rapid diagnosis. Acta Paediatr Scand 1983;72:47–51.

69. Espy MJ, Smith TF. Detection of herpes simplex virus in conventional tube cell cultures and in shell vials with a DNA probe kit and monoclonal antibodies. J Clin Microbiol 1988;26:22–24.

70. Espy MJ, Smith TF, Harmon MW, Kendal AP. Rapid detection of influenza virus by shell vial assay with monoclonal antibodies. J Clin Microbiol 1986;24:677–679.

71. Evans AS, ed. Viral infections of humans. Epidemiology and control. 2nd ed. New York, Plenum Publshing Corp, 1982.

72. Eyster ME, Ballard JO, Gail MH, Drummond JE, Goedert JJ. Predictive markers for the acquired immunodeficiency syndrome (AIDS) in hemophiliacs: persistence of p24 antigen and low T4 cell count. Ann Intern Med 1989;110:963–969.

73. Falsey AR, Walsh EE, Betts RF. Serologic evidence of respiratory syncytial virus infection in nursing home patients. J Infect Dis 1990;162: 568–569.

74. Feinstone SM, Kapikian AZ, Purcell RH, Alter HJ, Holland PV. Transfusion-associated hepatitis not due to viral hepatitis type A or B. N Engl J Med 1975;292:767–770.

75. Fields BN, Knipe DM, Chanock RM, et al, eds. Virology. 2nd ed. New York, Raven Press, 1990.

76. Fife KH, Ashley R, Shields AF, Salter D, Meyers JD, Corey L. Comparison of neutralization and DNA restriction enzyme methods for typing clinical isolates of human adenovirus. J Clin Microbiol 1985;22:95–100.

77. Figueroa ME, Rasheed S. Molecular pathology and diagnosis of infectious diseases. Am J Clin Pathol 1991;95:S8–21.

78. Fiscus SA, Wallmark EB, Folds JD, Fryer J, Van der Horst CM. Detection of infectious immune complexes in human immunodeficiency virus type 1 (HIV-1) infections: correlation with plasma viremia and CD4 cell counts. J Infect Dis 1991;164:765–769.

79. Fleisher GR, Collins M, Fager S. Limitations of available tests for diagnosis of infectious mononucleosis. J Clin Microbiol 1983;17:619–624.

80. Foley FD, Greenawald KA, Nash G, Pruitt BAJ. Herpesvirus infection in burned patients. N Engl J Med 1970;282:652–656.

81. Forbes BA, Bartholoma N, McMillan J, Roefaro

M, Weiner L, Welych L. Evaluation of a monoclonal antibody test to detect *Chlamydia* in cervical and urethral specimens. J Clin Microbiol 1986;23:1136–1137.

82. Ford-Jones EL, Mindorff CM, Gold R, Petric M. The incidence of viral-associated diarrhea after admission to a pediatric hospital. Am J Epidemiol 1990;131:711–718.

83. Frayha H, Castriciano S, Mahony J, Chernesky M. Nasopharyngeal swabs and nasopharyngeal aspirates equally effective for the diagnosis of viral respiratory disease in hospitalized children. J Clin Microbiol 1989;27:1387–1389.

84. Freshney RI. Culture of animal cells: a manual of basic technique. New York, Alan R. Liss, 1983.

85. Friedland GH, Klein RS. Transmission of the human immunodeficiency virus. N Engl J Med 1987;317:1125–1135.

86. Gallo D, Diggs JL, Shell GR, Dailey PJ, Hoffman MN, Riggs JL. Comparison of detection of antibody to the acquired immune deficiency syndrome virus by enzyme immunoassay, immunofluorescence, and Western blot methods. J Clin Microbiol 1986;23:1049–1051.

87. Garry RF, Witte MH, Gottlieb AA, Alexander SS, Cole WR, Drake WL Jr. Documentation of an AIDS virus infection in the United States in 1968. JAMA 1988;260:2085–2087.

88. Gleaves CA, Smith TF, Shuster EA, Pearson GR. Comparison of standard tube and shell vial cell culture techniques for the detection of cytomegalovirus in clinical specimens. J Clin Microbiol 1985;21:217–221.

89. Gleaves CA, Wilson DJ, Wold AD, Smith TF. Detection and serotyping of herpes simplex virus in MRC-5 cells by use of centrifugation and monoclonal antibodies 16 h postinoculation. J Clin Microbiol 1985;21:29–32.

90. Glezen WP, Fernald GW, Lohr JA. Acute respiratory disease of university students with special reference to the etiologic role of herpesvirus hominis. Am J Epidemiol 1975;101:111–121.

91. Gluckman JC, Klatzmann D, Montagnier L. Lymphadenopathy-associated-virus infection and acquired immunodeficiency syndrome. Annu Rev Immunol 1986;4:97–117.

92. Gnann JW Jr, McCormick JB, Mitchell S, Nelson JA, Oldstone MBA. Synthetic peptide immunoassay distinguishes HIV type 1 and HIV type 2 infections. Science 1987;237:1346–1349.

93. Godfrey E, Winn W Jr, Keathley JD. Performance of microtrak direct test for *Chlamydia trachomatis* in a prevalence study. Diagn Microbiol Infect Dis 1986;5:313–316.

94. Goodell SE, Quinn TC, Mkrtichian E, Schuffler MD, Holmes KK, Corey L. Herpes simplex virus proctitis in homosexual men: clinical, sigmoidoscopic, and histopathological features. N Engl J Med 1983;308:868–871.

95. Goodgame RW. AIDS in Uganda: clinical and social features. N Engl J Med 1990;323:383–389.

96. Gottlieb MS, Schroff R, SchankeR HM, et al. *Pneumocystiscarinii* pneumonia and mucosal candidiasis in previously healthy homosexual men: evidence for a new acquired cellular immunodeficiency. N Engl J Med 1981;305:1425–1431.

97. Graham BS, Snell JDJ. Herpes simplex virus infection of the adult lower respiratory tract. Medicine 1983;62:384–393.

98. Greene WC. The molecular biology of human immunodeficiency virus type 1 infection. N Engl J Med 1991;324:308–317.

99. Groopman JE, Salahuddin SZ, Sarngadharan MG, et al. HTLV-III in saliva of people with AIDS-related complex and healthy homosexual men at risk for AIDS. Science 1984;226:447–449.

100. Guinan ME, Wolinsky SM, Reichman RC. Epidemiology of genital herpes simplex virus infection. Epidemiol Rev 1985;7:127–146.

101. Hadler SC, Francis DP, Maynard JE, et al. Long-term immunogenicity and efficacy of hepatitis B vaccine in homosexual men. N Engl J Med 1986;315:209–214.

102. Hahn BH, Shaw GM, Taylor ME, et al. Genetic variation in HTLV-III/LAV over time in patients with AIDS or at risk for AIDS. Science 1986;232:1548–1553.

103. Hall CB, Douglas RG Jr. Clinically useful method for the isolation of respiratory syncytial virus. J Infect Dis 1975;131:1–5.

104. Hall CB, Douglas RG Jr, Geiman JM. Possible transmission by fomites of respiratory syncytial virus. J Infect Dis 1980;141:98–102.

105. Hall CB, Douglas RG Jr, Geiman JM, Messner MK. Nosocomial respiratory syncytial virus infections. N Engl J Med 1975;293:1343–1346.

106. Hall CB, Geiman JM, Douglas RG. Modes of transmission of respiratory syncytial virus. J Pediatr 1981;99:100–103.

107. Hall CB, Powell KR, MacDonald NE, et al. Respiratory syncytial viral infection in children with compromised immune function. N Engl J Med 1986;315:77–81.

108. Hamilton-Dutoit SJ, Pallesen G, Franzmann MB, et al. AIDS-related lymphoma: histopathology, immunophenotype, and association with Epstein-Barr virus as demonstrated by in situ nucleic acid hybridization. Am J Pathol 1991;138:149–163.

109. Harris C, Small CB, Klein RS, et al. Immuno-

deficiency in female sexual partners of men with the acquired immunodeficiency syndrome. N Engl J Med 1983;308:1181–1184.

110. Harrison SC. Principles of virus structure. In: Fields BN, Knipe DM, Chanock RM, et al, eds. Virology. 2nd ed. New York, Raven Press, 1990.

111. Hattwick MAW, O'Brien RJ, Hanson BF. Rocky Mountain spotted fever: epidemiology of an increasing problem. Ann Intern Med 1976;84: 732–739.

112. Hayflick L. The limited in vitro lifetime of human diploid cell strains. Exp Cell Res 1965;37: 614–636.

113. Hazard GW, Ganz RN, Nevin RW, et al. Rocky Mountain spotted fever in the eastern United States: thirteen cases from the Cape Cod area of Massachusetts. N Engl J Med 1969;280:57–62.

114. Hechemy KE, Anacker RL, Philip RN, et al. Detection of Rocky Mountain spotted fever antibodies by a latex agglutination test. J Clin Microbiol 1980;12:144–150.

115. Hechemy KE, Stevens RW, Sasowski S, Michaelson EE, Casper EA, Philip RN. Discrepancies in Weil-Felix and microimmunofluorescence test results for Rocky Mountain spotted fever. J Clin Microbiol 1979;9:292–293.

116. Hendrickson DA, Krenz MM: Reagents and stains. In Balows A, Hausler WJ Jr, Herrmann KL, Isenberg HD, Shadomy HJ, eds. Manual of clinical microbiology. 5th ed. Washington, DC, American Society for Microbiology, 1991.

117. Hendry RM, McIntosh K. Enzyme-linked immunosorbent assay for detection of respiratory syncytial virus infection: development and description. J Clin Microbiol 1982;16:324–328.

118. Hersh T, Melnick JL, Goyal RK, Hollinger FB. Nonparenteral transmission of viral hepatitis type B (Australia antigen-associated serum hepatitis). N Engl J Med 1971;285:1363–1364.

119. Higgins PG, Ellis EM. The isolation of influenza viruses. J Clin Pathol 1972;25:521–524.

120. Hirsch MS, Curran J. Human immunodeficiency virus: biology and medical aspects. In: Fields BN, Knipe DM, Chanock RM, et al, eds. Virology. 2nd ed. New York, Raven Press, 1990.

121. Ho DD, Moudgil T, Alam M. Quantitation of human immunodeficiency virus type 1 in the blood of infected persons. N Engl J Med 1989; 321:1621–1625.

122. Ho M, Suwansirikul S, Dowling JN, Youngblood LA, Armstrong JA. The transplanted kidney as a source of cytomegalovirus infection. N Engl J Med 1975;293:1109–1112.

123. Hochberg FH, Miller G, Schooley RT, Hirsch MS, Feorino P, Henle W. Central nervous system lymphoma related to Epstein-Barr virus. N Engl J Med 1983;309:745–748.

124. Hollinger FB. Non-A, non-B hepatitis viruses. In: Fields BN, Knipe DM, Chanock RM, et al, eds. Virology. 2nd ed. New York, Raven Press, 1990.

125. Hollinger FB, Ticehurst J. Hepatitis A virus. In: Fields BN, Knipe DM, Chanock RM, et al, eds. Virology. 2nd ed. New York, Raven Press, 1990.

126. Hondo R, Kurata T, Sato S, Oda A, Aoyama Y. Enzymatic treatment of formalin-fixed and paraffin-embedded specimens for detection of antigens of herpes simplex, varicella-zoster and human cytomegaloviruses. Jpn J Exp Med 1982; 52:17–25.

127. Hoofnagle JH. Type D (delta) hepatitis. JAMA 1989;261:1321–1325.

128. Hornsleth A, Friis B, Andersen P, Brene E. Detection of respiratory syncytial virus in nasopharyngeal secretions by ELISA: comparison with fluorescent antibody technique. J Med Virol 1982;10:273–281.

129. Horsburgh CR Jr, Ou CY, Jason J, et al. Duration of human immunodeficiency virus infection before detection of antibody. Lancet 1989;2:637–639.

130. Horwitz CA, Henle W, Henle G, et al. Clinical and laboratory evaluation of infants and children with Epstein-Barr virus–induced infectious mononucleosis: report of 32 patients (aged 10–48 months). Blood 1981;57:933–938.

131. Horwitz CA, Henle W, Henle G, Polesky H, Leonardy J. Spurious rapid infections mononucleosis test results in non-infectious mononucleosis sera: the role of high-titer horse agglutinins. Am J Clin Pathol 1982;78:48–53.

132. Howard C, Friedman DL, Leete JK, Christensen ML. Correlation of the percent of positive *Chlamydia trachomatis* direct fluorescent antibody detection tests with the adequacy of specimen collection. Diagn Microbiol Infect Dis 1991;14: 233–237.

133. Howell CL, Miller MJ. Effect of sucrose phosphate and sorbitol on infectivity of enveloped viruses during storage. J Clin Microbiol 1983; 18:658–662.

134. Hsiung GD. Diagnostic virology illustrated by light and electron microscopy. 3rd ed. New Haven, CT, Yale University Press, 1982.

135. Jacobs JW, Peacock DB, Corner BD, Caul EO, Clarke SKR. Respiratory syncytial and other viruses associated with respiratory disease in infants. Lancet 1971;1:871–876

136. Jansen RW, Newbold JE, Lemon SM. Combined immunoaffinity cDNA-RNA hybridization assay

for detection of hepatitis A virus in clinical specimens. J Clin Microbiol 1985;22:984–989.

137. Johnson FB. Transport of viral specimens. Clin Microbiol Rev 1990;3:120–131.

138. Johnson FB, Leavitt RW, Richards DF. Evaluation of the virocult transport tube for isolation of herpes simplex virus from clinical specimens. J Clin Microbiol 1984;20:120–122.

139. Jones MF, Smith TF, Houglum AJ, Herrmann JE. Detection of *Chlamydia trachomatis* in genital specimens by the Chlamydiazyme test. J Clin Microbiol 1984;20:465–467.

140. Judson BA, Lambert PP. Improved Syva Micro-Trak *Chlamydia trachomatis* direct test method. J Clin Microbiol 1988;26:2657–2658.

141. Kahlon J, Chatterjee S, Lakeman FD, Lee F, Nahmias AJ, Whitley RJ. Detection of antibodies to herpes simplex virus in the cerebrospinal fluid of patients with herpes simplex encephalitis. J Infect Dis 1987;155:38–44.

142. Kao CL, McIntosh K, Fernie B, Talis A, Pierik L, Anderson L. Monoclonal antibodies for the rapid diagnosis of respiratory syncytial virus infection by immunofluorescence. Diagn Microbiol Infect Dis 1984;2:199–206.

143. Kapikian AZ, ChanocK RM. Rotaviruses. In: Fields BN, Knipe DM, Chanock RM, et al, eds. Virology. 2nd ed. New York, Raven Press, 1990.

144. Kapikian AZ, Wyatt RG, Dolin R, Thornhill TS, Kalica AR, Chanock RM. Visualization by immune electron microscopy of a 27-nm particle associated with acute infectious nonbacterial gastroenteritis. J Virol 1972;10:1075–1081.

145. Kaplan JE, Schonberger LB.:The sensitivity of various serologic tests in the diagnosis of Rocky Mountain spotted fever. Am J Trop Med Hyg 1986;35:840–844.

146. Kaplan JE, Spira TJ, Fishbein DB, Bozeman LH, Pinsky PF, Schonberger LB. A six-year follow-up of HIV-infected homosexual men with lymphadenopathy: evidence for an increased risk for developing AIDS after the third year of lymphadenopathy. JAMA 1988;260:2694–2697.

147. Kessler HA, Blaauw B, Spear J, Paul DA, Falk LA, Landay A. Diagnosis of human immunodeficiency virus infection in seronegative homosexuals presenting with an acute viral syndrome. JAMA 1987;258:1196–1199.

148. Kluytmans JAJW, Niesters HGM, Mouton JW, et al. Performance of a nonisotopic DNA probe for detection of *Chlamydia trachomatis* in urogenital specimens. J Clin Microbiol 1991;29:2685–2689.

149. Koenig S, Gendelman HE, Orenstein JM, et al. Detection of AIDS virus in macrophages in brain tissue from AIDS patients with encephalopathy. Science 1986;233:1089–1093.

150. Koff RS, Grady GF, Chalmers TC, Mosley JW, Swartz BL, the Boston Inter-Hospital Liver Group. Viral hepatitis in a group of Boston hospitals: III. Importance of exposure to shellfish in a nonepidemic period. N Engl J Med 1967;276:703–710.

151. Komaroff AL, Aronson MD, Schachter J. *Chlamydia trachomatis* infection in adults with community-acquired pneumonia. JAMA 1981;245:1319–1322.

152. Koneman EW, Allen SP, Janda WM, Schreckenberger PC, Winn WC, Jr. Color atlas and textbook of diagnostic microbiology, ed 4. Philadelphia, JB Lippincott, 1992.

153. Lafferty WE, Coombs RW, Benedetti J, Critchlow C, Corey L. Recurrences after oral and genital herpes simplex virus infection. Influence of site of infection and viral type. N Engl J Med 1987;316:1444–1449.

154. Lafferty WE, Krofft S, Remington M, et al. Diagnosis of herpes simplex virus by direct immunofluorescence and viral isolation from samples of external genital lesions in a high-prevalence population. J Clin Microbiol 1987;25:323–326.

155. Landry ML, Fong CK. Nucleic acid hybridization in the diagnosis of viral infections. Clin Lab Med 1985;5:513–529.

156. Lane HC, Depper JM, Greene WC, Whalen G, Waldmann TA, Fauci AS. Qualitative analysis of immune function in patients with the acquired immunodeficiency syndrome. N Engl J Med 1965;313:79–84.

157. Lane HC, Masur H, Edgar LC, Whalen G, Rook AH, Fauci AS. Abnormalities of B-cell activation and immunoregulation in patients with the acquired immunodeficiency syndrome. N Engl J Med 1983;309:453–458.

158. Lauer BA. Comparison of virus culturing and immunofluorescence for rapid detection of respiratory syncytial virus in nasopharyngeal secretions: sensitivity and specificity. J Clin Microbiol 1982;16:411–412.

159. Lennette EH, Schmidt NJ. Diagnostic procedures for viral, rickettsial and chlamydial infections. 5th ed. Washington, DC, American Public Health Association, 1979.

160. Levin MJ, Leventhal S, Masters HA. Factors influencing quantitative isolation of varicella-zoster virus. J Clin Microbiol 1984;19:880–883.

161. Levy RA, Warford AL. Evaluation of the modified Chlamydiazyme immunoassay for the detection of chlamydial antigen. Am J Clin Pathol 1986;86:330–335.

162. Liang TJ, Hasegawa K, Rimon N, Wands JR, Ben-Porath E. A hepatitis B virus mutant associ-

ated with an epidemic of fulminant hepatitis. N Engl J Med 1991;324:1705–1709.

163. Lipkin ES, Moncada JV, Shafer MA, Wilson TE, Schachter J. Comparison of monoclonal antibody staining and culture in diagnosing cervical chlamydial infection. J Clin Microbiol 1986;23:114–117.

164. Livengood CH III, Schmitt JW, Addison WA, Wrenn JW, Magruder Habib K. Direct fluorescent antibody testing for endocervical *Chlamydia trachomatis*: factors affecting accuracy. Obstet Gynecol 1988;72:803–809.

165. MacDonald NE, Hall CB, Suffin SC, Alexson C, Harris PJ, Manning JA. Respiratory syncytial viral infection in infants with congenital heart disease. N Engl J Med 1982;307:397–400.

166. Magder LS, Klontz KC, Bush LH, Barnes RC. Effect of patient characteristics on performance of an enzyme immunoassay for detecting cervical *Chlamydia trachomatis* infection. J Clin Microbiol 1990;28:781–784.

167. Marcus R, CDC Cooperative Needlestick Surveillance Group: surveillance of health care workers exposed to blood from patients infected with the human immunodeficiency virus. N Engl J Med 1988;319:1118–1123.

168. Masur H, Michelis MA, Greene JB, et al. An outbreak of community-acquired *Pneumocystis carinii* pneumonia: initial manifestation of cellular immune dysfunction. N Engl J Med 1981;305:1431–1438.

169. McCutchan JA. Epidemiology of venereal urethritis: comparison of gonorrhea and nongonococcal urethritis. Rev Infect Dis 1984;6:669–688.

170. McIntosh K. Diagnostic virology. In: Fields BN, Knipe DM, Chanock RM, et al, eds. Virology. 2nd ed. New York, Raven Press, 1990.

171. Miller G. Epstein-Barr virus: biology, pathogenesis, and medical aspects. In: Fields BN, Knipe DM, Chanock RM, et al, eds. Virology. 2nd ed. New York, Raven Press, 1990.

172. Minnich LL, Goodenough F, Ray CG. Use of immunofluorescence to identify measles virus infections. J Clin Microbiol 1991;29:1148–1150.

173. Morton HJ. A survey of commercially available tissue culture media. In Vitro 1970;6:89–108.

174. Mowat NAG, Albert-Recht F, Brunt PW, Walker W. Outbreak of serum hepatitis associated with tatooing. Lancet 1973;1:33–34.

175. Mufson MA, Belshe RB, Orvell C, Norrby E. Respiratory syncytial virus epidemics: variable dominance of subgroups A and B strains among children, 1981–1986. J Infect Dis 1988;157:143–148.

176. Mulley AG, Silverstein MD, Dienstag JL. Indications for use of hepatitis B vaccine, based on cost-effectiveness analysis. N Engl J Med 1982;307:644–652.

177. Murphy D, Todd JK, Chao RK, Orr I, McIntosh K. The use of gowns and masks to control respiratory illness in pediatric hospital personnel. J Pediatr 1981;99:746–750.

178. Murphy FA, Kingsbury DW. Virus taxonomy. In: Fields BN, Knipe DM, Chanock RM, et al, eds. Virology. 2nd ed. New York, Raven Press, 1990.

179. Mushahwar IK, McGrath LC, Drnec J, Overby LR. Radioimmunoassay for detection of hepatitis B e antigen and its antibody: results of clinical evaluation. Am J Clin Pathol 1981;76:692–697.

180. N'Galy B, Ryder RW, Bila K, et al. Human immunodeficiency virus infection among employees in an African hospital. N Engl J Med 1988;319:1123–1127.

181. Nahmias AJ, Josey WE, Naib ZM, Freeman MG, Fernandez RJ, Wheeler JH. Perinatal risk associated with maternal genital herpes simplex virus infection. Am J Obstet Gynecol 1971;110:825–837.

182. Nahmias AJ, Whitley RJ, Visintine AN, Takei Y, Alford CAJ. Herpes simplex virus encephalitis: laboratory evaluations and their diagnostic significance. J Infect Dis 1982;145:829–836.

183. Newhouse VF, Shepard CC, Redus MD, Tzianabos T, McDade JE. A comparison of the complement fixation, indirect fluorescent antibody, and microagglutination tests for the serological diagnosis of rickettsial diseases. Am J Trop Med Hyg 1979;28:387–395.

184. Niederman JC, Evans AS, Subrahmanyan L, McCollum RW. Prevalence, incidence and persistence of EB virus antibody in young adults. N Engl J Med 1970;282:361–365.

185. Niederman JC, Miller G, Pearson HA, Pagano JS, Dowaliby JM. Infectious mononucleosis: Epstein-Barr-virus shedding in saliva and oropharynx. N Engl J Med 1976;294:1356–1359.

186. Niel C, Gomes SA, Leite JPG, Pereira HG. Direct detection and differentiation of fastidious and nonfastidious adenoviruses in stools by using a specific nonradioactive probe. J Clin Microbiol 1986;24:785–789.

187. Nurminen M, Leinonen M, Saikku P, Makela PH. The genus-specific antigen of *Chlamydia*: resemblance to the lipopolysaccharide of enteric bacteria. Science 1983;220:1279–1281.

188. Okada K, Kamiyama I, Inomata M, Imai M, Miyakawa Y, Mayumi M: e antigen and anti-e in the serum of asymptomatic carrier mothers as indicators of positive and negative transmission of hepatitis B virus to their infants. N Engl J Med 1976;294:746–749.

189. Omata M, Ehata T, Yokosuka O, Hosoda K,

Ohto M. Mutations in the precore region of hepatitis B virus DNA in patients with fulminant and severe hepatitis. N Engl J Med 1991;324:1699–1704.

190. Oxtoby MJ. Human immunodeficiency virus and other viruses in human milk: Placing the issues in broader perspective. Pediatr Infect Dis J 1988;7:825–835.

191. Palva A, Ranki M. Microbial diagnosis by nucleic acid sandwich hybridization. Clin Lab Med 1985;5:475–490.

192. Patel JM, Rizzolo E, Hinshaw JR. Spontaneous subcapsular splenic hematoma as the only clinical manifestation of infectious mononucleosis. JAMA 1982;247:3243–3244.

193. Pattengale PK, Smith RW, Perlin E. Atypical lymphocytes in acute infectious mononucleosis: identification by multiple T and B lymphocyte markers. N Engl J Med 1974;291:1145–1148.

194. Pereira L, Dondero DV, Gallo D, Devlin V, Woodie JD. Serological analysis of herpes simplex virus types 1 and 2 with monoclonal antibodies. Infect Immun 1982;35:363–367.

195. Peterson EM, Oda R, Alexander R, Greenwood JR, De la Maza LM. Molecular techniques for the detection of *Chlamydia trachomatis*. J Clin Microbiol 1989;27:2359–2363.

196. Philip RN, Casper EA, Ormsbee RA, Peacock MG, Burgdorfer W. Microimmunofluorescence test for the serological study of Rocky Mountain spotted fever and typhus. J Clin Microbiol 1976;3:51–61.

197. Phillips RS, Hanff PA, Holmes MD, Wertheimer A, Aronson MD. *Chlamydia trachomatis* cervical infection in women seeking routine gynecologic care: criteria for selective testing. Am J Med 1989;86:515–520.

198. Phillips RS, Hanff PA, Kauffman RS, Aronson MD. Use of a direct fluorescent antibody test for detecting *Chlamydia trachomatis* cervical infection in women seeking routine gynecologic care. J Infect Dis 1987;156:575–581.

199. Pothier P, Nicolas JC, De Saint Maur GP, Ghim S, Kazmierczak A, Bricout F. Monoclonal antibodies against respiratory syncytial virus and their use for rapid detection of virus in nasopharyngeal secretions. J Clin Microbiol 1985;21:286–287.

200. Prince AM, Metselaar D, Kafuko GW, Mukwaya LG, Ling CM, Overby LR. Hepatitis B antigen in wild-caught mosquitoes in Africa. Lancet 1972;2:247–250.

201. Rabinowitz M, Hallak A, Grunberg J, Levy Y, Gilat T. A modified, solid phase radioimmunoassay for the differential diagnosis of acute and convalescent phases of hepatitis A infection. Am J Clin Pathol 1987;88:738–742.

202. Raga J, Chrystal V, Coovadia HM. Usefulness of clinical features and liver biopsy in diagnosis of disseminated herpes simplex infection. Arch Dis Child 1984;59:820–824.

203. Ramsey PG, Fife KH, Hackman RC, Meyers JD, Corey L. Herpes simplex virus pneumonia: clinical, virologic, and pathologic features in 20 patients. Ann Intern Med 1982;97:813–820.

204. Rapoza PA, Quinn TC, Kiessling LA, Green WR, Taylor HR. Assessment of neonatal conjunctivitis with a direct immunofluorescent monoclonal antibody stain for *Chlamydia*. JAMA 1986;255:3369–3373.

205. Ray CG, Minnich LL. Regional diagnostic virology services: are satellite laboratories necessary? JAMA 1982;247:1309–1310.

206. Redfield DC, Richman DD, Albanil S, Oxman MN, Wahl GM. Detection of herpes simplex virus in clinical specimens by DNA hybridization. Diagn Microbiol Infect Dis 1983;1:117–128.

207. Reeves WC, Corey L, Adams HG, Vontver LA, Holmes KK. Risk of recurrence after first episodes of genital herpes: relation to HSV type and antibody response. N Engl J Med 1981;305:315–319.

208. Reyes GR, Purdy MA, Kim JP, et al. Isolation of a cDNA from the virus responsible for enterically transmitted non-A, non-B hepatitis. Science 1990;247:1335–1338.

209. Richman D, Schmidt N, Plotkin S, et al. Summary of a workshop on new and useful methods in rapid viral diagnosis. J Infect Dis 1984;150:941–951.

210. Richman DD, Cleveland PH, Redfield DC, Oxman MN, Wahl GM. Rapid viral diagnosis. J Infect Dis 1984;149:298–310.

211. Richtsmeier WJ, Wittels EG, Mazur EM. Epstein-Barr virus–associated malignancies. Crit Rev Clin Lab Sci 1987;25:105–136.

212. Rose NR, Friedman H, Fahey JL, eds. Manual of clinical laboratory immunology. 3rd ed. Washington, DC, American Society for Microbiology, 1986.

213. Royston I, Sullivan JL, Periman PO, Perlin E. Cell-mediated immunity to Epstein-Barr virus–transformed lymphoblastoid cells in acute infectious mononucleosis. N Engl J Med 1975;293:1159–1163.

214. Saag MS, Hahn BH, Gibbons J, et al. Extensive variation of human immunodeficiency virus type-1 in vivo. Nature 1988;334:440–444.

215. Salmon VC, Turner RB, Speranza MJ, Overall JCJ. Rapid detection of herpes simplex virus in

Color Plates

Presumptive Bacterial Identification Based on Observing Microscopic Cellular Morphology in Stained Smear Preparations

Gram stain of bacteria, in addition to other staining techniques, is one of the more important determinations in the presumptive identification of microorganisms. The morphology of the bacterial cells, their arrangement, and their staining characteristics are often distinctive enough to allow a presumptive identification in a Gram-stained smear. The microscopic characteristics suggestive of several groups of bacteria are included in this plate.

A

Relatively slender, gram-positive bacilli arranged in Chinese letter pattern suggesting one of the coryneform (diphtheroids) bacteria.

B

Gram-positive, spore-forming bacilli. The aerobic spore formers belong to the genus *Bacillus*; the anaerobic spore formers belong to the genus *Clostridium*. Illustrated here are spore-forming cells of *Bacillus sphaericus*.

C

Direct Gram stain of a purulent exudate illustrating gram-positive cocci arranged in small clusters, characteristic of *Staphylococcus* species.

D

Direct smear of a necrotic exudate from a case of myonecrosis. The tiny, gram-positive cocci seen in this photomicrograph are streptococci.

E

Direct Gram stain of a smear of purulent sputum demonstrating gram-positive diplococci, characteristic of *Streptococcus pneumoniae*.

F

Purulent exudate from the chest wall of a patient with acute, suppurative empyema. Against the background of segmented neutrophils are numerous gram-positive, branching bacilli. *Actinomyces* species and *Nocardia* species can produce a picture similar to this; however, in this case, a pure culture of *Bifidobacterium* species was recovered in anaerobic culture.

G

Gram-stained preparation of a direct smear of urine sediment from a case of acute cystitis. Note the several gram-negative bacilli amid the background segmented neutrophils. *Escherichia coli* was recovered in pure culture.

H

Gram-stained preparation of a direct smear prepared from a purulent urethral exudate of a sexually active male, illustrating the intracellular, gram-negative, diplococci characteristic of *Neisseria gonorrhoeae*. The bacterial cells are paler staining in this photograph than normally seen by direct microscopic examination.

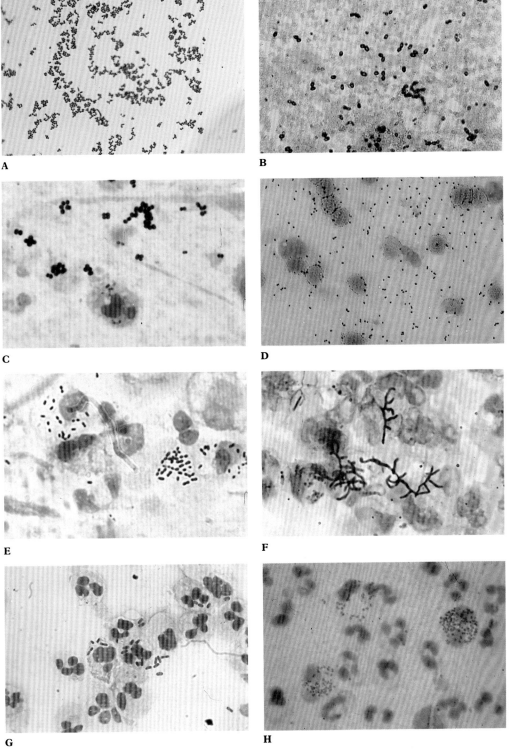

Color Plate 1-1

Miscellaneous Stains Used in Microbiology

Because many of the microbes of medical importance have refractive indices near that of water, stains are needed to make possible their detection and study. A variety of stains have been developed over the years, each designed to highlight internal organelles or specific components of the cell wall. Following are illustrations of selected stains and some of their applications.

A

Gram. The most common stain used in the microbiology laboratory is designed to differentiate between those bacteria that can retain crystal violet dye and appear deep blue-black after decolorization (gram-positive) from those that cannot and stain red (gram-negative). Illustrated here is a Gram-stained preparation revealing red-staining, gram-negative bacilli.

B

Acid-fast. This stain is commonly used to demonstrate a variety of acid-fast organisms, including *Nocardia* species in sputum specimens and *Cryptosporidium* oocysts in fecal samples. Shown here are clusters of red-staining, acid-fast bacilli in a liver biopsy specimen of a patient with the acquired immunodeficiency syndrome. The organisms stain red with the acid-fast stain, and those shown here were identified as belonging to the *Mycobacterium avium-intracellulare* complex.

C

Direct fluorescence. Fluorescent dyes (rhodamine and auramine) react directly with the cell wall of mycobacteria. Fluorescein-conjugated antibodies are also available to demonstrate a variety of microbial agents using the direct fluorescent antibody test. Shown here are yellow-green fluorescing mycobacteria in a sputum concentrate from a patient with pulmonary tuberculosis.

D

Acridine orange. This rapid fluorescent stain is used to demonstrate bacterial forms in direct smears and mounts of biologic fluids. It is particularly useful in detecting gram-negative bacteria in positive blood culture broths, which may be missed in Gram stains because of the deep red–staining debris in the background. Shown here is a long, rod-shaped bacterium with a characteristic orange glow when microscopically observed with a fluorescence microscope.

E

Methylene blue. This nonspecific, rapid stain is used to demonstrate bacteria and other microbes in direct smears. Illustrated here are bacilli that have taken the blue stain. One important application is in the detection of bacteria in direct smears of cerebrospinal fluid in cases of suspected acute meningitis, particularly gram-negative species, that may be obscured by the red background staining of the proteinaceous material.

F

Calcofluor white. This autofluorescent whitening agent has the property of coupling with carbohydrate moieties in the cell walls of fungi. Shown here are brilliant yellow-green staining hyphae in a direct calcofluor white-stained mount as observed with a fluorescence microscope.

G

Wright-Giemsa. This stain is commonly used to demonstrate the cellular elements in peripheral blood and bone marrow smears. In microbiology, the stain is most commonly used to detect intraerythrocytic (plasmodia, babesiae) and exoerythrocytic (trypanosomes, microfilaria) parasites, chlamydial inclusions, and, as shown here, the intracellular yeast forms of *Histoplasma capsulatum*.

H

Periodic acid–Schiff. This general stain is used to demonstrate polysaccharide-rich cell walls. It has specific applications in detecting fungi in tissue sections and smears. Recognized here is the fruiting body of *Aspergillus* species in an aspirate of a fungus ball lesion of the lung surrounded by red-staining *Aspergillus* spores.

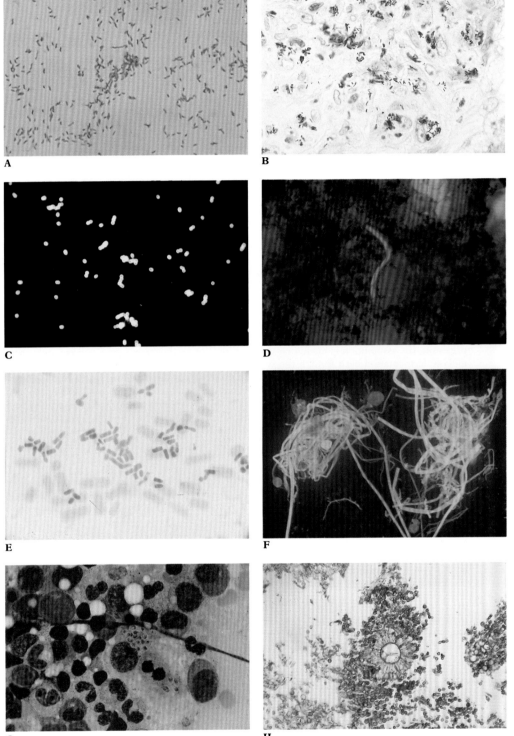

A

B

C

D

E

F

G

H

Presumptive Identification of the Enterobacteriaceae

Presumptive identification of the Enterobacteriaceae is based on the appearance of colonies growing on primary isolation media and on an assessment of certain biochemical reactions. By definition, for an organism to be classified within the Enterobacteriaceae, it must ferment glucose, producing acid or acid and gas; reduce nitrates to nitrites; and exhibit no cytochrome oxidase activity.

A

A blood agar plate showing 24-hour growth of gray-white, opaque, watery colonies consistent with one of the members of the Enterobacteriaceae.

B

Mixed culture showing 24-hour growth on blood agar of several relatively large, mucoid, nonpigmented colonies of *Klebsiella* species compared with the smaller, yellow-pigmented colonies of *Staphylococcus aureus*.

C

Blood agar plate illustrating a wavelike swarming pattern highly suggestive of a motile strain of *Proteus* species.

D

Swarming pattern of a motile strain of *Proteus* species on Endo agar.

E

Series of Kligler iron agar (KIA) slants illustrating several reaction patterns. Tube on the far left illustrates an alkaline (red) slant indicating a lack of lactose fermentation; the black deep indicates hydrogen sulfide (H_2S) production. When this type of reaction is seen with an oxidase-negative organism, the assumption is made that the deep portion of the tube is acid (yellow), indicating glucose fermentation even though the yellow color is masked from the H_2S production. The second tube from the left illustrates an alkaline slant (red)/acid deep (yellow) reaction characteristic of a non-lactose fermenter, in contrast to the acid/acid reactions seen in tubes 3 and 4 produced by lactose fermenters. The reaction pattern in the third tube from the left indicates both lactose fermentation and gas (CO_2) production (note split in agar near the bottom), a reaction that is commonly produced by strains of the *Klebsiella/Enterobacter* group. The fourth tube shows lactose fermentation with no gas.

F

Three tubes of purple broth media containing Durham tubes to demonstrate gas formation. The right and center tubes illustrate acid from glucose (yellow) compared with the negative control on the left; the center tube shows the collection of gas within the Durham tube characteristic of an organism that produces both acid and gas from glucose.

G

Nitrate test medium showing a positive reaction after addition of α-naphthylamine and sulfanilic acid. The test organism had reduced the nitrites in the medium to nitrates, which reacted with the reagents to form the red pigment *p*-sulfobenzene-azo-α-naphthylamine.

H

Cytochrome oxidase test revealing a positive purple color reaction (*left*) compared with a negative reaction (no blue color within 10 seconds). An organisms giving a positive reaction can be excluded from the family Enterobacteriaceae.

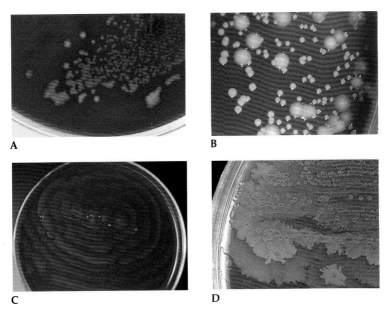

A

B

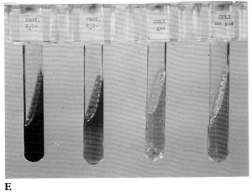

C

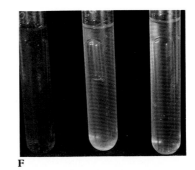

D

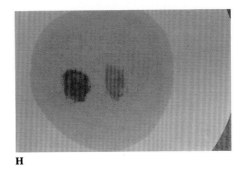

E

F

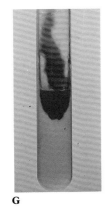

G

H

Appearance of the Enterobacteriaceae Colonies on MacConkey and EMB Agars

MacConkey and eosin methylene blue (EMB) agars are two commonly used selective primary isolation media for presumptive differentiation of lactose-fermenting from non–lactose-fermenting members of the Enterobacteriaceae. On MacConkey agar, lactose-fermenting colonies appear red because of the acid conversion of the indicator, neutral red. On EMB, a green metallic sheen is produced by avid lactose fermenters when production of acid is sufficient to lower the *p*H to approximately 4.5 or below.

A

Surface of MacConkey agar with 24-hour growth of red, lactose-fermenting colonies. The diffuse red color in the agar surrounding the colonies is produced by organisms that avidly ferment lactose, producing large quantities of mixed acids, and cause precipitation of the bile salts in the medium surrounding the colonies (*eg, Escherichia coli*).

B

Surface of MacConkey agar illustrating both red, lactose-fermenting colonies and smaller, clear non–lactose-fermenting colonies.

C and D

Surface of EMB agar plates illustrating the green sheen produced by avoid lactose- (or sucrose-) fermenting members of the Enterobacteriaceae. Most strains of *E. coli* produce colonies with this appearance on EMB agar, and since *E. coli* is among the most frequent isolates from clinical specimens, the appearance of such colonies can often serve as presumptive identification of *E. coli*. However, characteristics other than the production of a green sheen on EMB must be assessed before an organism can be definitively identified as *E. coli*, since other lactose-fermenting Enterobacteriaceae can have a similar appearance.

E and F

Surface of EMB agar plates illustrating a mixed culture of *E. coli* (green sheen colonies) and *Shigella* species. Most *Shigella* species do not ferment lactose and, thus produce nonpigmented, semitranslucent colonies on EMB agar. Other species incapable of fermenting lactose produce colonies that appear similar to those illustrated in these photographs.

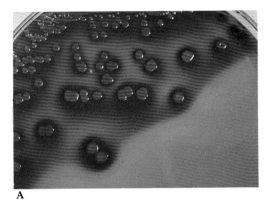

A

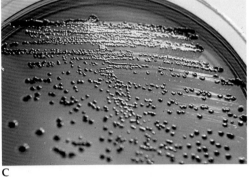

B

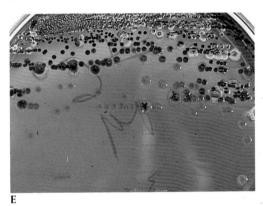

C

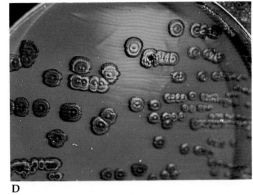

D

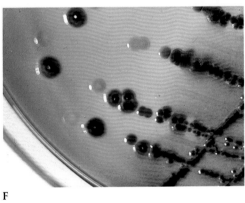

E

F

Color Plate 2-2

Appearance of the Enterobacteriaceae Colonies on XLD and HE Agar Plates

Several types of media more selective than MacConkey or EMB agars are commonly used in clinical microbiology laboratories for recovering select members of the Enterobacteriaceae. Xylose-lysine-deoxycholate (XLD) and Hektoen enteric (HE) agars are most commonly used; highly selected media such as bismuth sulfate agar are used only for special applications. These media not only have the capability of separating lactose fermenters from non–lactose fermenters but can detect hydrogen sulfide (H₂S)-producing microorganisms as well.

A

Surface of XLD agar illustrating yellow conversion of the medium from acid-producing colonies of *E. coli*.

B

Non-lactose-fermenting colonies (no acid conversion of the medium) of *Salmonella* species growing on the surface of XLD agar. Note the black pigmentation of some of the colonies, indicating H₂S production.

C

Photograph illustrating an XLD agar plate inoculated with a 50/50 mixture of *E. coli* and *Salmonella* species. Note the preponderant growth of the *Salmonella* species (red colonies) compared with the few yellow, lactose-fermenting colonies of *E. coli* that have been effectively inhibited. The distinct pink halo around the *Salmonella* colonies indicates the decarboxylation of lysine, a helpful feature in differentiating *Salmonella* species (positive) from H₂S-producing colonies of *Proteus* species.

D

XLD agar plate inoculated with an H₂S-producing strain of a *Proteus* species. Note the lack of a light pink halo around the colonies, indicating the lack of lysine decarboxylation (compare with the colonies shown in **C**).

E

Surface of HE agar illustrating yellow acid production by colonies of *E. coli*.

F

Surface of HE agar illustrating the faint green (colorless) colonies of non–lactose-fermenting members of the Enterobacteriaceae family.

A

B

C

D

E

F

Important Characteristics for Distinguishing Nonfermentative Gram-Negative Bacilli

A

No acid production in Kliger iron agar (KIA) or in triple sugar iron (TSI) agar, indicating the inability of nonfermenting bacteria to utilize the lactose or the dextrose in KIA (or the sucrose in TSI). The KIA tube on the left shows an alkaline slant/alkaline deep reaction characteristic of a nonfermenting organism; the tube on the right shows an acid slant/acid deep reaction indicating fermentation of dextrose and lactose (characteristic of many species of the Enterobacteriaceae).

B

Cytochrome oxidase test strips. The formation of a blue color within 10 seconds after smearing a test colony on the strip indicates cytochrome oxidase activity, a characteristic helpful in identifying many species of nonfermentative bacilli. All members of the Enterobacteriaceae are cytochrome oxidase negative.

C

Failure to grow on MacConkey agar or inhibited growth on MacConkey agar is a clue that a gram-negative rod may be a nonfermenter. Although many species of the nonfermentative bacilli are capable of growing on MacConkey agar, the lack of growth on this medium as illustrated on the right side of this split frame excludes the Enterobacteriaceae, all members of which show growth.

D

Oxidative utilization of glucose. Illustrated here are two tubes of Hugh-Leifson oxidative-fermentative (OF) medium. The tube on the left is open to the atmosphere; in the tube on the right the medium is covered with mineral oil to exclude exposure to atmospheric oxygen. Acid (yellow) is seen only in the open tube, characteristic of a glucose oxidizer.

E

Tubes of Motility B medium containing 2,3,5-triphenyltetrazolium chloride (TTC). Motility is often difficulty to observe with nonfermentative bacteria since the organisms tend to grow only in the upper (most aerobic) portion of the tube. The addiction of tetrazolium aids in detecting motility because organisms capable of reducing TTC will appear red along the stab line as well as in the area into which the cells have migrated, making it easier to differentiate between motile and nonmotile bacteria.

F

Plate of trypticase soy agar inoculated with a yellow, pigment-producing bacterium. Pigment production is an important differential characteristic in identifying nonfermentative gram-negative bacilli.

G

Tubes of Flo and Tech agar inoculated with *Pseudomonas aeruginosa* viewed under visible light. These media are used to enhance the production of two pigments: pyoverdin (fluorescein), which appears as a yellow diffusible pigment on Flo agar, and pyocyanin, which appears as a turquoise-blue pigment on Tech agar. Although three species of nonfermentative bacilli produce pyoverdin (*P. aeruginosa, P. fluorescens,* and *P. putida*), only one species (*P. aeruginosa*) produces pyocyanin.

H

Tubes of Flo and Tech agar inoculated with *Pseudomonas aeruginosa* viewed under ultraviolet (UV) light using a Wood's lamp. Note that the Flo agar tube (*left*) fluoresces while the Tech agar tube (*right*) does not fluoresce under UV light. Only the pyoverdin pigment, which is enhanced by growing the organism on Flo agar, fluoresces under UV light.

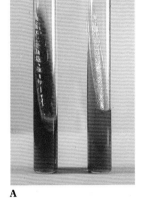

A

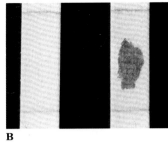

B

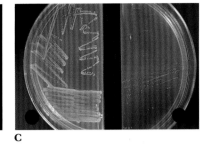

C

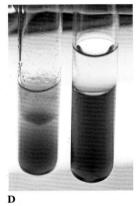

D

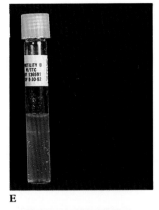

E

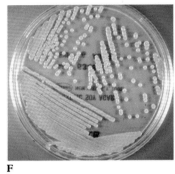

F

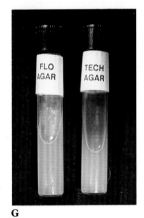

G

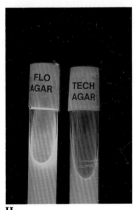

H

Color Plate 3-1

Laboratory Identification of Vibrio cholerae *and Other* Vibrio *Species*

A

Appearance of *Vibrio cholerae* on thiosulfate citrate bile sucrose (TCBS) agar. The yellow colonies result from citrate utilization and the formation of acid from utilization of the sucrose in the medium. The appearance of yellow colonies on this medium is virtually diagnostic of *V. cholerae.*

B

Colonies of *V. parahaemolyticus* growing on TCBS agar illustrating the characteristic semitranslucent, green-gray appearance.

C

Gelatin agar with white, opaque colonies of *V. cholerae*. Note the opalescence of the agar adjacent to the colonies, indicating hydrolysis and denaturation of the gelatin.

D

Gram stain of *V. vulnificus* illustrating gram-negative bacterial cells with the curved, rod-shaped morphology typical of *Vibrio* species.

E

Positive string test with *V. cholerae*. When colonies of *V. cholerae* are mixed in a drop of 0.5% sodium deoxycholate, they produce a viscous suspension that can be drawn into a string when the inoculating loop is slowly raised from the side.

F

Positive slide agglutination test for *V. cholerae* using polyvalent O antiserum.

G

Blood agar plate illustrating the relatively large, intensely β-hemolytic colonies of the El Tor biotype of *V. cholerae.*

H

Chicken erythrocyte agglutination test. Classic strains of *V. cholerae* do not agglutinate chicken erythrocytes (*top*), in contrast to the El Tor biotype (*bottom*), which is capable of agglutinating the erythrocytes.

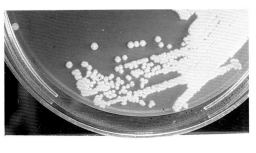

V. cholerae
TCBS

A

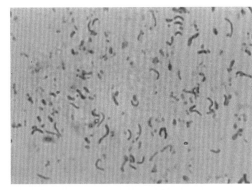

V. parahaemolyticus
TCBS AGAR

B

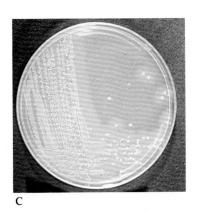

C

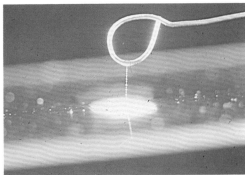

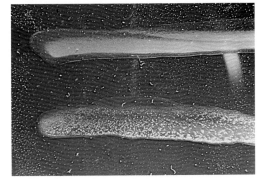

E

F

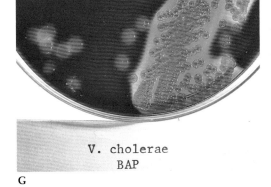

V. cholerae
BAP

G

H

Color Plate 4-1

Identification of Haemophilus *Species*

A

Gram stain of cerebrospinal fluid showing polymorphonuclear cells and scattered gram-negative bacilli of *Haemophilus influenzae*. These organisms characteristically appear as small, poorly staining coccobacilli on Gram stains of clinical specimens.

B

Growth of the moist, smooth, gray colonies of *H. influenzae* type b on chocolate agar. This medium contains hemoglobin (X factor) and is enriched with other cofactors, such as nicotinamide adenine dinucleotide (NAD, V factor) that allow the growth of *Haemophilus* and other fastidious microorganisms.

C

Satellite growth of *Haemophilus* species around streaks of *Staphylococcus aureus*. X-factor, or hemin, is provided by the lysed sheep erythrocytes surrounding the *Staphylococcus* streak, while the staphylococci themselves provide the V-factor, or NAD. These factors enable the tiny, dew-drop colonies of *Haemophilus* to grow adjacent to the *Staphylococcus* streak.

D

Growth factor test for identification of *H. influenzae*. The organism is inoculated onto a plate of brain-heart infusion or trypticase-soy agar, and disks containing X factor and V factor are placed in proximity to one another on the inoculum. After incubation in a CO_2-enriched atmosphere, factor requirements are determined by observing organism growth relative to the disks. In this picture, growth is observed between the X and V factor disks, indicating that the organism requires both exogenous X and V factors for growth.

E

ALA-porphyrin disk test. This test is an alternative method for detecting X-factor requirements of *Haemophilus* isolates. The disk is moistened with water, and a portion of the colonial growth is rubbed on the disk. After 2 hours of incubation, the disk is observed under a Woods light (ultraviolet light). If a brick-red fluorescence is observed, the organism is able to synthesize heme compounds from δ-aminolevulinic acid (ALA) and, therefore, does not require exogenous X factor. This photograph shows both a positive (*left*) and a negative (*right*) ALA-porphyrin disk test.

F

Biotyping of *Haemophilus* species. Both *H. influenzae* and *H. parainfluenzae* can be grouped into distinct biotypes based on their reactions in three biochemical tests: urease, ornithine decarboxylase, and production of indole. This plate shows these reactions for *H. influenzae* biotype I. Tests shown (*left to right*) are production of urease (positive), Moeller's decarboxylase broth base (negative), Moeller's ornithine decarboxylase broth (positive), and indole production in tryptone broth (positive).

G

The Vitek *Neisseria-Haemophilus* Identification (NHI) Card (Vitek Systems, Inc., Hazelwood, MO). The card is inoculated with the filling module of the Vitek instrument and is then incubated for 4 hours at 35°C. Biochemical reactions are read manually, and the results are entered into the Vitek computer module, along with the results of a catalase test, a spot indole test, and, for *Neisseria* species, the ability to grow on modified Thayer-Martin agar (see Chapter 7). The data base of the system then provides an identification. (Photo courtesy of bioMérieux Vitek)

H

The Microscan *Haemophilus-Neisseria* Identification (HNID) panel (American MicroScan, Sacramento, CA). This manual microtiter tray system identifies both *Haemophilus* and *Neisseria* species and provides biotype designations for *H. influenzae* and *H. parainfluenzae*. This slide shows the reactions for *H. influenzae* biotype I (urease-positive, ornithine decarboxylase-positive, and indole-positive). (Photo courtesy of American MicroScan)

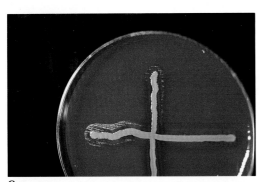

A

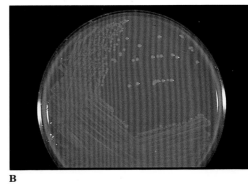

B

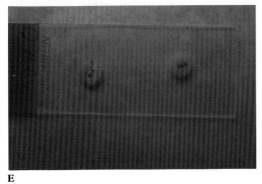

C

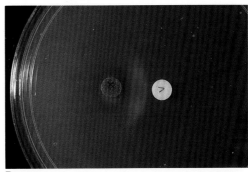

D

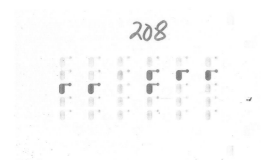

E

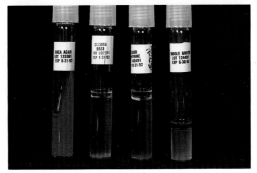

F

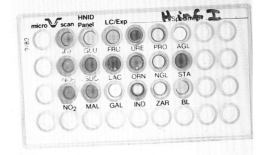

G

H

A
Colonies of *Haemophilus aphrophilus* on chocolate agar after 48 hours of growth. These colonies are small and have a slight yellow pigment. This species will also grow on sheep blood agar since X and V factors are not required for growth.

B
Gram stain of *H. aphrophilus* from culture media. This organism appears as short, pale-staining gram-negative coccobacilli, a characteristic that is shared with many of the other HACEK group bacteria.

C
Colonies of *Actinobacillus actinomycetemcomitans* on chocolate agar after 72 hours of growth. These colonies are small, are variable in size, have irregular edges, and are usually adherent to the growth media on primary isolation. This organism, like *H. aphrophilus*, does not require X or V factors and grows on sheep blood agar.

D
Gram stain of *A. actinomycetemcomitans* from agar media. The bacteria appear as small, gram-negative coccobacilli. After repeated subculture, longer cells are frequently noted.

E
Gram stain of *Cardiobacterium hominis*. These organisms are often gram variable but are staining uniformly gram negative in this photomicrograph. The cells of *C. hominis* are generally longer than other HACEK bacteria and show pleomorphism (ie, cells with pointed or swollen ends, teardrop-shaped and dumbell-shaped cells). The characteristic palisading of the cells in "picket fence" arrangements and the clustering of cells to form compact rosettes are also evident in this picture.

F
Growth of *C. hominis* on sheep blood agar after 72 hours of incubation. The colonies are small, opaque, and glistening. Some strains may also pit the agar similar to *Eikenella corrodens* (see *H*).

G
Biochemical tests for the identification of *C. hominis*. The Kligler iron agar (KIA) slant on the far left illustrates the faint orange-yellow conversion of the medium that is characteristic of a slow fermentative organism. Although difficult to see in this picture, there is a faint tinge of hydrogen sulfide precipitate on the lead acetate strip draped under the cap of the KIA slant. The fermentative nature of *C. hominis* is further illustrated in both the open and sealed OF-dextrose tubes. The organism also fermented sucrose, maltose, and mannitol, as shown by the next three tubes. The urease test (*seventh tube from the left*) was negative. The next tube shows the indole test, which is an important identification characteristic of this organism. The positive indole reaction was obtained only after growing the organism for 48 hours in tryptone broth, extracting the medium with xylene, and adding Erhlich's indole reagent. Generally, this organism produces very small amounts of indole that will not be detected with Kovac's or with the spot indole (*p*-dimethyl-aminocinnamaldehyde) reagents. The second tube from the right illustrates the organism's negative nitrate reduction test. The last tube, showing the same reaction after the addition of zinc dust, confirms that nitrate was not reduced by the organism.

H
Growth of *E. corrodens* on sheep blood agar. Although frequently difficulty to photograph, the incident light on the plate in this photograph demonstrates the pitting of the agar surface that is characteristic of many strains of *E. corrodens*. Nonpitting strains may also be identified.

I
Capnocytophaga species on sheep blood agar. This photograph shows the characteristic colonial morphology of these organisms, illustrating the fringe of "gliding" bacteria at the periphery of the growth. Toward the center of the areas of growth, the colonies become more mottled and rough appearing.

J
Gram stain of *Capnocytophaga* species. These organisms characteristically appear as gram-negative, slightly curved, fusiform bacteria with pointed ends, resembling the obligate anaerobe *Fusobacterium nucleatum*.

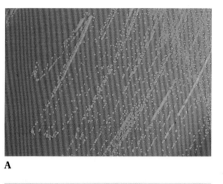

A

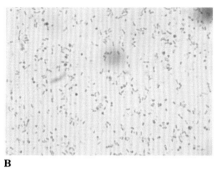

B

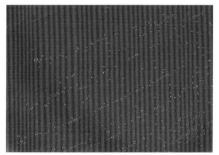

C

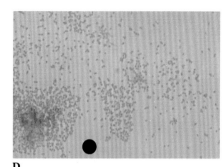

D

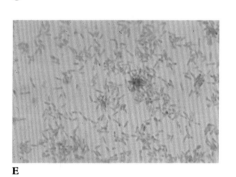

E

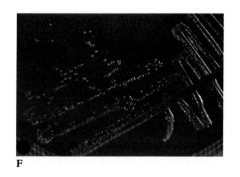

F

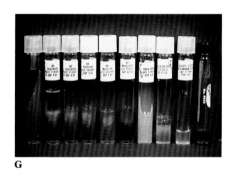

G

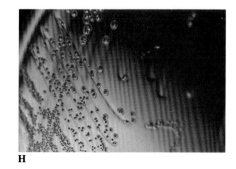

H

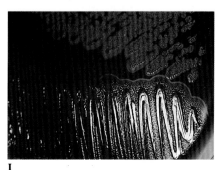

I

J

A
Gram stain of a urethral discharge from a male with gonococcal urethritis, showing intracellular gram-negative diplococci within pale-staining segmented neutrophils.

B
Typical colonies of *N. gonorrhoeae* on modified Thayer-Martin (MTM) medium. Pathogenic *Neisseria* species, notably *N. gonorrhoeae* and *N. meningitidis*, grow well on MTM medium.

C
This photograph shows the typical battery of carbohydrates used for identification of *Neisseria* species: (*left to right*) CTA-glucose, CTA-maltose, CTA-sucrose, and CTA-lactose. A color change from red to yellow indicates the production of acid. Acid has been produced from glucose only, identifying this organism as *N. gonorrhoeae*.

D
API QuadFERM + system (Analytab Products, Inc, Plainview, NY) for identification of *Neisseria* species and *M. catarrhalis*. The series of wells are (*from left to right*) a carbohydrate-free control reagent (CTRL) and reagents for glucose (GLU), maltose (MAL), lactose (LAC), and sucrose (SUC). Wells for acidometric detection of deoxyribonuclease (DNase) for confirmation of *M. catarrhalis*, and for detection of β-lactamase (β-LAC) are also included on the strip. Shown here is a β-lactamase negative strain of *N. gonorrhoeae*.

E
Gonochek II tube (DuPont deNemours, Wilmington, DE). Thee chromogenic substrates are included in a single plastic tube to detect glycosidase and aminopeptidase enzymes. The identifying patterns are blue (*upper left*)—*N. lactamica* (β-galactoside hydrolysis); yellow (*upper right*)—*N. meningitidis* (γ-glutamyl-*p*-nitroanilide hydrolysis); red (*lower left*)—*N. gonorrhoeae* (prolyl-β-naphthylamide hydrolysis). Lack of a color reaction (*lower right*) presumptively identified *M. catarrhalis*. (Courtesy of DuPont deNemours Co.)

F
Fluorescent antibody (FA) test for confirmation of *N. gonorrhoeae* (Syva Co., Palo Alto, CA). In a positive test, apple-green fluorescent diplococci are observed.

G
Meritec coagglutination test for identification of *N. gonorrhoeae* (Meridian Diagnostics, Cincinnati, OH). Shown are two isolates of *N. gonorrhoeae*; in circles 1 and 2, and in circles 3 and 4. Circles 1 and 3 contain the control reagent, while circles 2 and 4 contain the test reagent. The expected reactions (control circles—no agglutination; test circles—positive agglutination) are demonstrated by both isolates.

H
Typical gray-yellow, entire, semitranslucent colonies of *N. meningitidis* growing on trypticase-soy agar with 5% sheep blood.

I
M. CAT CONFIRM test for identification of *Moraxella catarrhalis* (Adam Scientific, West Warwick, RI). The small cuvette contains a disk saturated with tributyrin. Change in the color of the indicator from red (*left*) to yellow (*right*) during incubation indicates hydrolysis of tributyrin.

J
Nitrocefin filter paper disks (Cefinase, Becton Dickinson Microbiology Systems, Cockeysville, MD) for the detection of β-lactamase. Material from a bacterial colony growing on solid medium is rubbed on the moistened disk. If the test organism produces β-lactamase, the cephalosporin reagent is hydrolyzed and changes from yellow (*left*) to red (*right*).

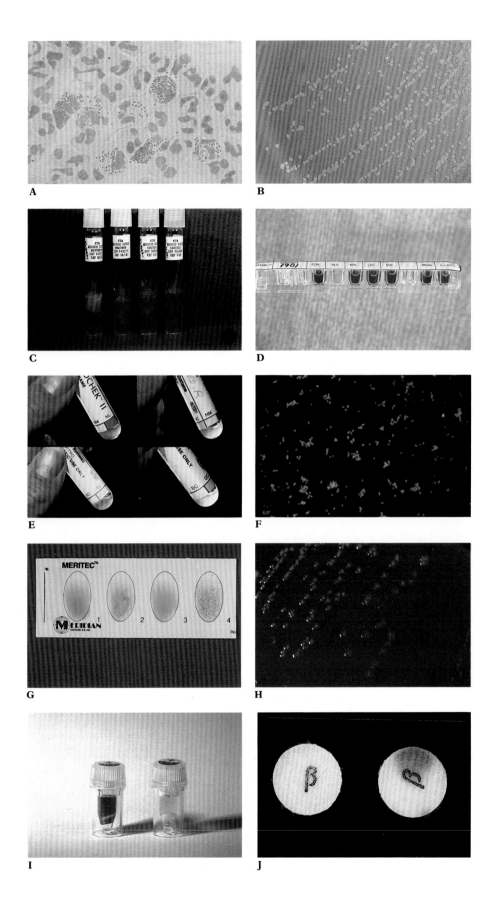

Identification of Staphylococci

A
Gram stain of staphylococcal cellulitis, showing small clusters of extracellular gram-positive cocci amid pink-staining polymorphonuclear leukocytes. (Courtesy of Schering Corp, Kenilworth, NJ)

B
Pale yellow colonies of *S. aureus* on sheep blood agar after 24 hours of incubation.

C
Positive catalase test. The test is performed by placing material from a colony onto a glass slide and adding a drop of 3% hydrogen peroxide to the inoculum. Immediate and vigorous bubbling is due to the production of oxygen gas. Micrococci and staphylococci are catalase-positive, while streptococci and enterococci are catalase-negative.

D
Susceptibility to furazolidone. Staphylococci are inhibited by furazolidone and show a zone of inhibition, as shown in the photograph, while micrococci are resistant and grow to the edge of the disk.

E
Slide coagulase test. Most strains of *S. aureus* produce a cell-bound coagulase or "clumping factor" that is detected by mixing a suspension of the organism with EDTA-rabbit plasma. A saline control (*left*) must be included to assess autoagglutination.

F
Tube coagulase test. Extracellular coagulase produced by *S. aureus* complexes with a component in plasma called coagulase reacting factor, which reacts with fibrinogen to form fibrin and, consequently, a visible clot (tube below compared with negative control above).

G
Latex agglutination test for identification of *S. aureus*. Latex spheres are coated with plasma to detect clumping factor and protein A on the surface of the staphylococci. Mixing of colonial material of *S. aureus* with the latex reagent results in rapid agglutination (*left*). A coagulase-negative staphylococcus is also shown (*right*). (Courtesy of Wellcome Diagnostics, Research Triangle Park, NC)

H
Mannitol salt agar. The high concentration of sodium chloride in the medium (7.5%) discourages the growth of other organisms. *S. aureus* strains are detected by the fermentation of mannitol, resulting in acid production and a change in the phenol red indicator from red to yellow (*lower half of plate*).

I
Disk tests for identification of staphylococci. Susceptibility to novobiocin is useful for presumptive identification of *S. saprophyticus*. In this figure, furazolidone, bacitracin, and novobiocin disks are shown on an isolate of *S. saprophyticus*. Susceptibility to furazolidone (FX, 100 μg) and resistance to bacitracin (A disk, 0.04 unit) indicate that the organism is a *Staphylococcus* species rather than a *Micrococcus* species. Resistance to novobiocin (C−, 5 μg) identifies this isolate as *S. saprophyticus*.

J
Staph-TRAC for identification of staphylococci and micrococci (Analytab Products, Inc, Plainview, NY). The strip is inoculated with an organism suspension and is incubated overnight. Interpretation of the reactions generates a biotype number that is used along with a computer-assisted data base to identify the organism.

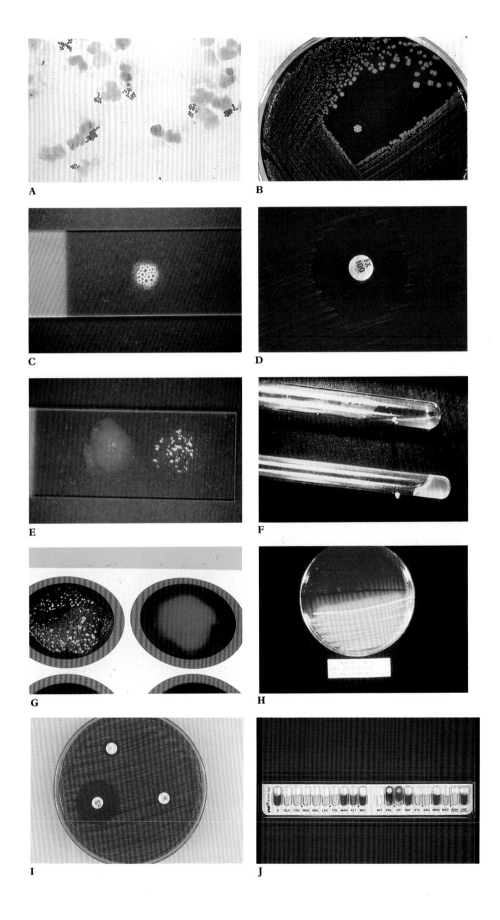

A

B

C

D

E

F

G

H

I

J

Identification of Aerobic and Facultatively Anaerobic Gram-Positive Bacilli

A

Gram stain of a broth culture of *Bacillus* species, illustrating short gram-positive bacilli containing distinct spores. This Gram stain morphology is interesting by demonstrating that not all *Bacillus* species produce the longer, characteristic "boxcar" cells and that the deep blue gram-positive staining of the cells may be lost in older cultures.

B

Blood agar plate on which is growing a subculture of *Bacillus subtilis*. Colonies of *Bacillus cereus* often appear similar, and biochemical differentiation is usually necessary. Note the dry, somewhat wrinkled nature of the colonies and the distinct β-hemolysis. The β-hemolysis is a valuable feature in ruling out *Bacillus anthracis*, which is not hemolytic.

C

Gram stain of *Listeria monocytogenes* grown in trypticase-soy broth at 35°C for 24 hours. The bacterial cells are short, gram-positive bacilli that may lie singly, lie in small clusters at times with a diphtheroid arrangement, or form short chains.

D

Sheep blood agar plate on which are growing tiny colonies producing a "soft" β-hemolysis. This picture is consistent with one of the β-hemolytic streptococci; however, shown here is a 48-hour growth of *Listeria monocytogenes*. Gram stains must always be performed on any β-hemolytic, *Streptococcus*-like colonies that are recovered from blood cultures, cerebrospinal fluid, and genital cultures.

E

Semisolid agar motility test medium illustrating the subsurface umbrella-like motility pattern characteristic of *Listeria monocytogenes*. This pattern of motility is best seen when the culture is incubated at room temperature.

F

Surface of a sheep blood agar plate on which are growing colonies of *Erysipelothrix rhusiopathiae* after 24 hours of incubation at 35°C. This culture represents the smaller, convex, circular, and transparent colony type. Larger, rough colonies with a matte surface and a fimbriated edge may be formed by other strains.

G

Gram stain of a smear prepared from a 24-hour broth culture of *E. rhusiopathiae* illustrating short, slender, straight, and curved gram-positive bacilli. There is a tendency for the cells to form long filaments, a feature only minimally evident in this photograph.

H

Split frame of subcultures of *E. rhusiopathiae* on Kligler iron agar (*left*) and soft gelatin agar (*right*). The KIA tube reveals an alk/alk reaction with production of a small amount of hydrogen sulfide in the deep of the medium along the course of the stab line. In soft gelatin agar, *E. rhusiopathiae* characteristically produces a "bottle brush" extension laterally from the streak line.

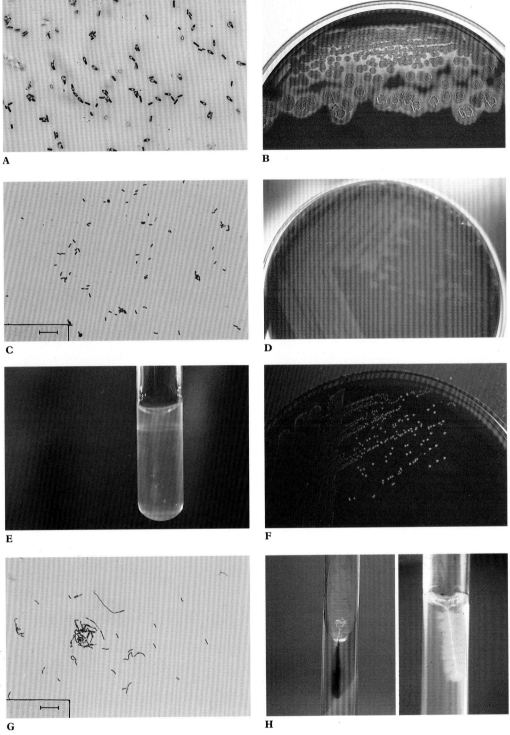

A

B

C

D

E

F

G

H

Identification of Anaerobic Bacteria: Bacteroides *and* Fusobacterium *Species*

A
Bacteroides fragilis. Gram stain of cells in 48-hour thioglycollate broth culture.

B
B. fragilis. Colonies on anaerobe blood agar after 48 hours of incubation at 35°C.

C
Prevotella melaninogenica. Gram stains of cells from a 48-hour colony on blood agar.

D
P. melaninogenica. Black colonies on blood agar after 5 days of incubation at 35°C. Note hemolysis.

E
Fusobacterium nucleatum. Gram stain of cells from a 48-hour colony on anaerobe blood agar. Note long, gram-negative bacilli with pointed ends.

F
F. nucleatum. Characteristic colonies on anaerobe blood agar after 48 hours of incubation at 35°C, illustrating the opalescent effect.

G
F. necrophorum. Gram stain of cells from a 48-hour colony on anaerobe blood agar. Note pleomorphism.

H
F. necrophorum. Colonies on anaerobe blood agar after 48 hours of incubation at 35°C.

Color Plate 11-1

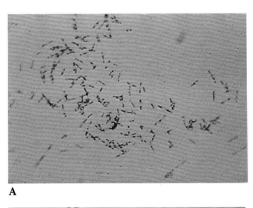

A

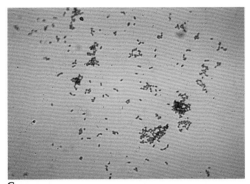

C

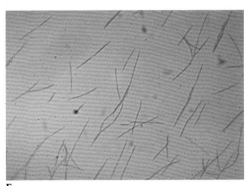

E

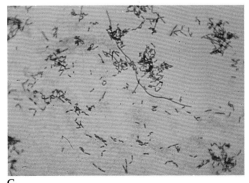

G

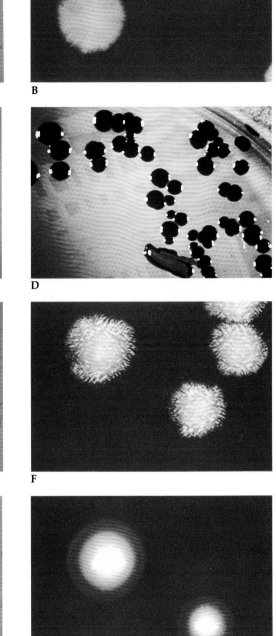

B

D

F

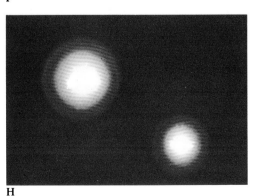

H

A
Gram-stained direct smear of a purulent exudate showing degenerated neutrophils and a mixture of gram-negative rods of different sizes. The tiniest coccobacilli suggest one of the pigmented *Prevotella-Porphyromonas* species; the larger, pleomorphic rods suggest a member of the *Bacteroides fragilis* group.

B
Gram-stained direct smear of a purulent exudate from an intraabdominal abscess showing segmented neutrophils, gram-positive cocci in pairs and short chains, and tiny gram-negative coccoid rods. Anaerobic infections usually contain a mixed bacterial flora.

C
Dissecting microscope view of actinomycotic "sulfur granules" (× 10). (Exudate from an abdominal wound infection was photographed within a Petri dish.)

D
Appearance of a Gram-stained smear from the same specimen as in **C**, showing sulfur granule with thin, branching filaments of an *Actinomyces* species (× 800).

E
Actinomyces israelii. Gram-stained preparation of growth from a colony on blood agar. Note branching of cells.

F
A. israelii. Characteristic "molar tooth" colonies produced on brain–heart infusion agar after 7 days of anaerobic incubation at 35°C.

G
Eubacterium alactolyticum. Gram stain of cells from growth in enriched thioglycollate broth after 48 hours of incubation at 35°C.

H
E. alactolyticum. Forty-eight-hour colonies on anaerobic blood agar.

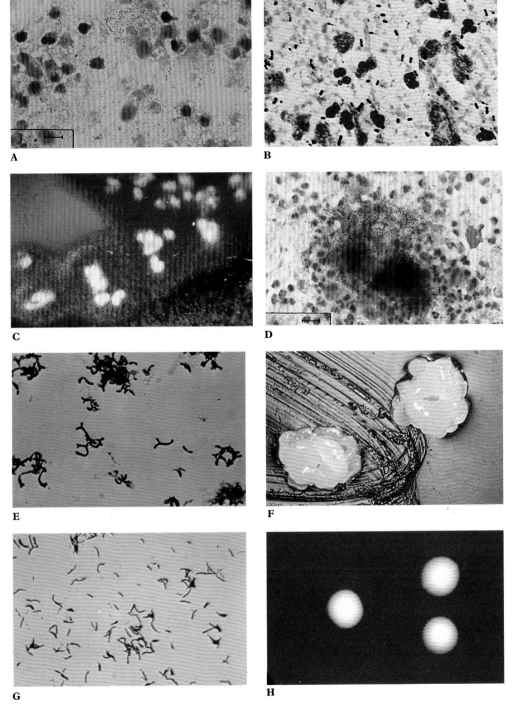

A

B

C

D

E

F

G

H

Identification of Anaerobic Bacteria: Clostridium *Species*

A

Clostridium perfringens. Gram stain of cells from a 24-hour colony on blood agar. Note lack of spores and of some cells that tend to stain red (gram-negative).

B

C. perfringens. Gram stain of cells from a 24-hour thioglycollate broth culture. Note lack of spores and presence of a few filamentous forms.

C

Typical appearance of *C. perfringens* on blood agar after a 24-hour incubation at 35°C. Note the double zone of hemolysis. The inner zone of complete hemolysis is due to t-toxin and the outer zone of incomplete hemolysis to α-toxin (lecithinase activity).

D

C. perfringens. Direct Gram stain of a muscle tissue aspirate from a patient with gas gangrene–myonecrosis. There is a necrotic background, without intact inflammatory cells or muscle cells, and relatively large boxcar-shaped gram-positive rods and a gram-negative rod that is either a gram-variable *C. perfringens* cell or another organism.

E

Colonies of *C. perfringens* on modified McClung egg yolk agar. The precipitate surrounding the colonies indicates lecithinase activity of α-toxin produced by the organism.

F

Lipase production on egg yolk agar. A few clostridia, such as *C. botulinum*, *C. sporogenes*, and *C. novyi* type A, exhibit lipase activity on egg yolk agar, as shown here. Note the iridescent pearly layer on the surface of the colonies extending onto the surface of the medium immediately surrounding them.

G

C. septicum. Rough, irregular, flat, rhizoid, spreading colony on a 48-hour anaerobe blood agar plate.

H

Direct Gram-stained smear of a positive blood culture that contained *C. septicum.* Numerous ovoid or citron-shaped, subterminal spores are present.

I

Colonies of *C. tetani* on stiff blood agar (4% agar), which is used to inhibit the swarming of the microorganism so that it can be isolated from other bacteria present in mixed cultures.

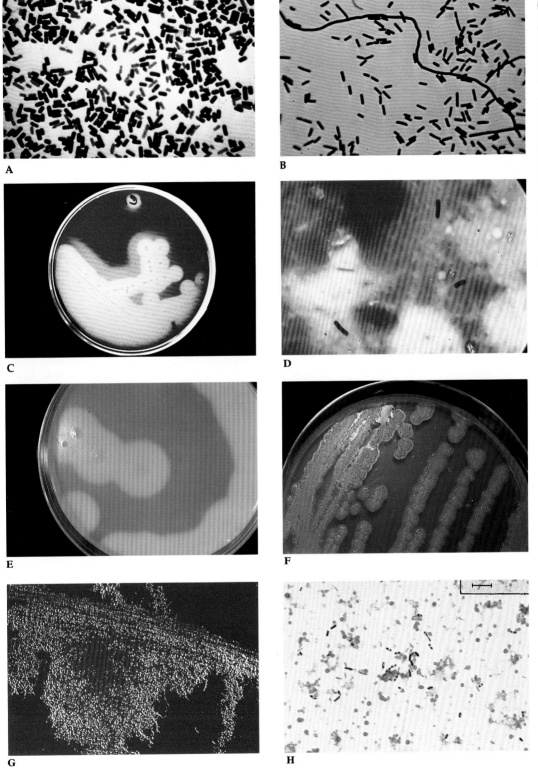

A

B

C

D

E

F

G

H

Colony Characteristics of Mycobacteria Helpful in Making Identifications

A
Two Middlebrook 7H10 agar plates illustrating the phenomenon of photoreactivity. Both plates were inoculated with the same culture of *M. kansasii.* Both plates had been shielded from light during incubation; however, the plate on the right had been exposed to light for a few hours. Note the yellow pigment of the colonies grown in the plate on the right.

B
Two plates of Middlebrook 7H10 agar, both growing yellow colonies. Both plates were shielded from the light during incubation and were pigmented as shown here immediately on examination. This is an example of the phenomenon of scotochromogenicity, characteristic of *M. scrofulaceum.*

C
Two Middlebrook 7H10 agar plates inoculated with subcultures of *Mycobacterium szulgai.* Both plates were shielded from light during incubation; the plate on the left, however, had been incubated at 37°C and shows a distinct yellow pigmentation. *M. szulgai* has the property of being scotochromogenic only when incubated at 35°C. At room temperature, however, the colonies remain unpigmented or are slightly photochromogenic.

D
Yellow pigmented colonies of *M. gordonii*, one of the more commonly recovered mycobacteria in clinical laboratories.

E
Isolated colonies of light yellow–pigmented colonies of *M. avium-intracellulare* complex. This group of organisms was previously assigned to the group III nonchromogens in the archaic Runyon classification of "atypical" mycobacteria.

F
Colonies of *M. avium-intracellulare* complex of an isolate recovered from a patient with the acquired immunodeficiency syndrome. Many of these strains develop a yellow pigmentation after prolonged incubation.

G *and* **H**
Middlebrook 7H10 agar plates showing a 3-day growth of the rapidly growing *Mycobacterium fortuitum.* The colonies shown in **G** are one of the smooth variants. Isolated colonies are nonpigmented, entire, and convex and have a smooth consistency. The colonies in **H** are similar to those seen in **G**, except they are rougher in consistency.

A

B

C

D

E

F

G

H

clinical specimens by centrifugation and immunoperoxidase staining. J Clin Microbiol 1986; 23:683–686.

216. Schachter J. Chlamydial infections. N Engl J Med 1978;298:428–434.

217. Schachter J, Grossman M, Sweet RL, Holt J, Jordan C, Bishop E. Prospective study of perinatal transmission of *Chlamydia trachomatis*. JAMA 1986;255:3374–3377.

218. Schaffner W, Drutz DJ, Duncan GW, Koenig MG. The clinical spectrum of endemic psittacosis. Arch Intern Med 1967;119:433–443.

219. Schmidt NJ. Cell culture techniques for diagnostic virology. In: Lennette EH, Schmidt NJ, eds. Diagnostic procedures for viral, rickettsial and chlamydial infections. 5th ed. Washington, DC, American Public Health Association, 1979.

220. Sellors J, Mahony J, Jang D, et al. Rapid, on-site diagnosis of chlamydial urethritis in men by detection of antigens in urethral swabs and urine. J Clin Microbiol 1991;29:407–409.

221. Shafritz DA, Shouval D, Sherman HI, Hadziyannis SJ, Kew MC. Integration of hepatitis B virus DNA into the genome of liver cells in chronic liver disease and hepatocellular carcinoma: studies in percutaneous liver biopsies and post-mortem tissue specimens. N Engl J Med 1981;305:1067–1073.

222. Sharpe AH, Fields BN. Pathogenesis of viral infections: basic concepts derived from the reovirus model. N Engl J Med 1985;312:486–497.

223. Shepard CC, Redus MA, Tzianabos T, Warfield DT. Recent experience with the complement fixation test in the laboratory diagnosis of rickettsial diseases in the United States. J Clin Microbiol 1976;4:277–283.

224. Sherry MK, Klainer AS, Wolff M, Gerhard H. Herpetic tracheobronchitis. Ann Intern Med 1988;109:229–233.

225. Shibata D, Martin WJ, Appleman MD, Causey DM, Leedom JM, Arnheim N. Detection of cytomegalovirus DNA in peripheral blood of patients infected with human immunodeficiency virus. J Infect Dis 1988;158:1185–1192.

226. Sixbey JW, Nedrud JG, Raab-Traub N, Hanes RA, Pagano JS. Epstein-Barr virus replication in oropharyngeal epithelial cells. N Engl J Med 1984;310:1225–1230.

227. Smith DW, Frankel LR, Mathers LH, Tang ATS, Ariagno RL, Prober CG. A controlled trial of aerosolized ribavirin in infants receiving mechanical ventilation for severe respiratory syncytial virus infection. N Engl J Med 1991;325:24–29.

228. Smith TF, Brown SD, Weed LA. Diagnosis of

Chlamydia trachomatis infections by cell cultures and serology. Lab Med 1982;13:92–100.

229. Smith TF, Martin WJ, Washington JA II. Isolation of viruses from single throat swabs processed for diagnosis of group A beta-hemolytic streptococci by fluorescent antibody technic. Am J Clin Pathol 1973;60:707–710.

230. Snydman DR, Dienstag JL, Stedt B, Brink EW, Ryan DM, Fawaz KA. Use of IgM-hepatitis A antibody testing: investigating a common-source, food borne outbreak. JAMA 1981;245:827–830.

231. Solomon AR, Rasmussen JE, Weiss JS. A comparison of the Tzanck smear and viral isolation in varicella and herpes zoster. Arch Dermatol 1986; 122:282–285.

232. Specter S, Lancz GJ, eds. Clinical virology manual. New York, Elsevier Science, 1986

233. Sperber SJ, Hayden FG. Antiviral chemotherapy and prophylaxis of viral respiratory disease. Clin Lab Med 1987;7:869–896.

234. Stamm WE, Handsfield HH, Rompalo AM, Ashley RL, Roberts PL, Corey L. The association between genital ulcer disease and acquisition of HIV infection in homosexual men. JAMA 1988; 260:1429–1433.

235. Stamm WE, Harrison HR, Alexander ER, Cles LD, Spence MR, Quinn TC. Diagnosis of *Chlamydia trachomatis* infections by direct immunofluorescence staining of genital secretions: a multicenter trial. Ann Intern Med 1984;101:638–641.

236. Stamm WE, Tam M, Koester M, Cles L. Detection of *Chlamydia trachomatis* inclusions in McCoy cell cultures with fluorescein-conjugated monoclonal antibodies. J Clin Microbiol 1983; 17:666–668.

237. Strand CL. Role of the microbiology laboratory in the diagnosis of opportunistic infections in persons infected with human immunodeficiency virus. Arch Pathol Lab Med 1990;114:277–283.

238. Strano AJ. Light microscopy of selected viral diseases (morphology of viral inclusion bodies). Pathol Annu 1976;11:53–75.

239. Straus SE, Rooney JF, Sever JL, Seidlin M, Nusinoff LS, Cremer K. NIH conference: herpes simplex virus infection: biology, treatment, and prevention. Ann Intern Med 1985; 103:404–419.

240. Sullivan BJZ, Hull HF, Wilson C, Smith AL, Corey L. Presentation of neonatal herpes simplex virus infections: implications for a change in therapeutic strategy. Pediatr Infect Dis 1986;5:309–314.

241. Supran EM, Craske J, Hart RJ, et al. Report of a joint DMRQC/Organon field trial to detect hep-

atitis A IgM by ELISA. J Clin Pathol 1983;36: 1111–1115.

242. Sweet RL, Blankfort-Doyle M, Robbie MO, Schacter J. The occurrence of chlamydial and gonococcal salpingitis during the menstrual cycle. JAMA 1986;255:2062–2064.

243. Swenson PD, Kaplan MH. Rapid detection of respiratory syncytial virus in nasopharyngeal aspirates by a commercial enzyme immunoassay. J Clin Microbiol 1986;23:485–488.

244. Swierkosz EM, Arens MQ, Schmidt RR, Armstrong T. Evaluation of two immunofluorescence assays with monoclonal antibodies for typing of herpes simplex virus. J Clin Microbiol 1985;21: 643–644.

245. Tam MR, Stamm WE, Handsfield HH et al. Culture-independent diagnosis of *Chlamydia trachomatis* using monoclonal antibodies. N Engl J Med 1984;310:1146–1150.

246. Tedder RS, O'Connor T, Hughes A, N'Jie H, Corrah T, Whittle H. Envelope cross-reactivity in Western blot for HIV-1 and HIV-2 may not indicate dual infection. Lancet 1988;2:927–930.

247. Terni M, Caccialanza P, Cassai E, Kieff E. Aseptic meningitis in association with herpes progenitalis. N Engl J Med 1971;285:503–504.

248. Thomas EE, Puterman ML, Kawano E, Curran M. Evaluation of seven immunoassays for detection of rotavirus in pediatric stool samples. J Clin Microbiol 1988;26:1189–1193.

249. Virtanen M, Palva A, Laaksonen M, Halonen P, Soderlund H, Ranki M. Novel test for rapid viral diagnosis: detection of adenovirus in nasopharyngeal mucus aspirates by means of nucleic-acid sandwich hybridisation. Lancet 1983;1:381–383.

250. Walker DH. Rocky Mountain spotted fever: a disease in need of microbiological concern. Clin Microbiol Rev 1989;2:227–240.

251. Walker DH, Burday MS, Folds JD. Laboratory diagnosis of Rocky Mountain spotted fever. South Med J 1980;73:1443–1449.

252. Waner JL. Isolation and identification of viruses from respiratory specimens. Newsl Pan Am Group Rapid Viral Diagn 1986;12:1–4.

253. Ward RL, Knowlton DR, Pierce MJ. Efficiency of human rotavirus propagation in cell culture. J Clin Microbiol 1984;19:748–753.

254. Warford AL, Levy RA, Rekrut KA. Evaluation of a commercial enzyme-linked immunosorbent assay for detection of herpes simplex virus antigen. J Clin Microbiol 1984;20:490–493.

255. Warford AL, Levy RA, Strong CA, Rekrut KA. Comparison of two commercial enzyme-linked immunosorbent assays for detection of herpes simplex virus antigen. Am J Clin Pathol 1986;85: 229–232.

256. Warford AL, Rekrut KA, Levy RA, Drill AE. Sucrose phosphate glutamate for combined transport of chlamydial and viral specimens. Am J Clin Pathol 1984;81:762–764.

257. Waris M. Pattern of respiratory syncytial virus epidemics in Finland: two-year cycles with alternating prevalence of groups A and B. J Infect Dis 1991;163:464–469.

258. Weiland TL, Noller KL, Smith TF, Ory SJ. Comparison of Dacron-tipped applicator and cytobrush for detection of chlamydial infections. J Clin Microbiol 1988;26:2437–2438.

259. White NJ, Juel JBE. Infectious mononucleosis hepatitis. Semin Liver Dis 1984;4:301–306.

260. Whitley R, Arvin A, Prober C, et al. Predictors of morbidity and mortality in neonates with herpes simplex virus infections. N Engl J Med 1991;324: 450–454.

261. Whitley RJ. Herpes simplex viruses. In: Fields BN, Knipe DM, Chanock RM, et al, eds. Virology. 2nd ed. New York, Raven Press, 1990.

262. Whitley RJ, Alford CA, Hirsch MS, et al. Vidarabine versus acyclovir therapy in herpes simplex encephalitis. N Engl J Med 1986;314:144–149.

263. Whitley RJ, Soong S, Linneman C, et al. Herpes simplex encephalitis: clinical assessment. JAMA 1982;247:317–320.

264. Williams T, Maniar AC, Brunham RC, Hammond GW. Identification of *Chlamydia trachomatis* by direct immunofluorescence applied in specimens originating in remote areas. J Clin Microbiol 1985;22:1053–1054.

265. Winn WC, Jr, Degrove K, Reardon D, Weisburgh S. Evaluation of Gen Probe *Chlamydia* Assay. J Clin Microbiol 1991.

266. Woods GL, Young A, Scott JC Jr, Blair TM, Johnson AM. Evaluation of a nonisotopic probe for detection of *Chlamydia trachomatis* in endocervical specimens. J Clin Microbiol 1990;28: 370–372.

267. Yolken RH. Use of monoclonal antibodies for viral diagnosis. Curr Top Microbiol Immunol 1983;104:177–195.

268. Zagury D, Bernard J, Leibowitch J, et al. HTLV-III in cells cultured from semen of two patients with AIDS. Science 1984;226:449–451.

19

New and Emerging Technologies: Rapid Bacterial Identification and Detection Methods

The future of diagnostic microbiology may well lie with several new and emerging technologies directed toward the detection of specific outer membrane, cell wall and protoplasmic markers and the demonstration of certain nucleic acid sequences within the genome used either to identify the microorganism or to demonstrate key virulence factors that indicate an infectious disease process. The following is a brief summary of selected nonculture procedures and techniques to make more rapid bacterial identifications, either for culture confirmation of important isolates or by directly identifying microbes and their telltale markers in clinical specimens.

CHROMOGENIC ENZYME SUBSTRATE TESTS

In contrast to employing conventional, growth-dependent procedures for making bacterial identifications, the use of chromogenic enzyme substrates allows for the rapid identification of many species of microorganisms. Chromogenic substrates can rapidly detect a spectrum of preformed enzymes that often allow organism identifications when taken in context with other observations, such as morphology, Gram stain reactivity, and other direct biochemical tests. The most commonly used enzymatic substrates for bacterial identification are those for glycosidase and aminopeptidase enzymes. Substrates for glycosidases are usually various types of monosaccharides and disaccharides that are linked to *ortho*- or *para*-nitrophenol. On hydrolysis by glycosidases that are specific for individual sugars of groups of sugars, the yellow nitrophenol moiety is released. Aminopeptidase substrates are generally *p*-nitroanilide or β-naphthylamide derivatives of amino acids. Hydrolysis of nitroanilide substrates releases nitroaniline, a yellow compound that is detected directly. The β-naphthylamine that is released by enzymatic hydrolysis of the naphthylamide amino acid analogs is detected by the addition of a colorless diazo-dye coupler such as *p*-dimethylaminocinnamaldehyde, which results in the formation of a pink or red end product.

By using such substrates, researchers have developed rapid tests for specific bacterial identifications that are in use in many laboratories. Chromogenic substrate tests and modified conventional tests have been combined into kit systems that are able to identify a variety of bacterial species, and these state-of-the-art systems are in common use in clinical laboratories the world over. The RapID NH system (Innovative Diagnostic Systems, Atlanta, GA), the Vitek NHI card (bioMérieux Vitek, Hazelwood, MO), and the HNID panel (American Microscan, Sacramento, CA) provide 4-hour identification for *Neisseria* species, *Haemophilus* species, and a variety of other fastidious gram-negative bacilli.[9,10] Reliable identification of the clinically significant anaerobic bacteria can be achieved with the RapID ANA II (Innovative Diagnostic Systems, Atlanta, GA), the Vitek ANI card (bioMérieux Vitek, Hazelwood, MO), and the An-IDENT system (Analytab Products, Inc, Plainview, NY).[3,22] All of these systems use an expanded battery of glycosidase and aminopeptidase enzyme substrates to obtain a characteristic enzyme profile. Comparison of the profile of an individual isolate to reactions for a large number of strains in a computerized data base allows specific identifications to be made.

GAS–LIQUID CHROMATOGRAPHY

The principle of chromatography is to achieve an absorption equilibrium between two phases, one mobile and the other stationary. In gas–liquid chromatography (GLC), an inert carrier gas (eg, nitrogen, helium, or argon) is the mobile phase, into which the sample for analysis is injected. The stationary phase consists of an inert solid matrix (eg, silica or celite) coated with an inert, easily volatilized liquid, such as carbowax or methyl silicone. These materials are coated onto the inner surface of a coiled, capillary glass tube (column) that is enclosed in a heating unit. The sample to be analyzed is volatilized by heat at the port of injection into the column, where it immediately mixes with the stream of carrier gas. Compounds present in the sample become distributed between the inert and mobile phases of the column by their relative affinities for the phase coated onto the column. Those compounds with low affinity pass through the column most rapidly and are detected first; those with higher affinity move through the column more slowly and emerge last. The time between injection of a given material into the column and its appearance in the detection system is called the retention time. The identification of an unknown material can be made by comparing its retention time with that of a known standard.

The basic components of a gas–liquid chromatograph include an oven containing the packed column through which a regulated flow of carrier gas is passed, a heated port where the sample to be analyzed is injected and immediately volatilized, and a detector system to measure the unknown components as they emerge from the distal end of the column. The retention times of materials in the analyte are compared with retention times of similarly prepared controls, allowing the identification of unknown metabolites. The heights of "peaks" on the tracing are directly related to the amount of a given metabolite in a specimen.

GLC has found its greatest application in anaerobic bacteriology. These bacteria produce a variety of short-chain fatty acids, alcohols, and amines that can be extracted from broth media by aqueous or organic solvents. GLC can also be used to assist in the identification of a wide variety of other bacterial species as well.[16,17,24]

IMMUNOLOGIC DIAGNOSES OF INFECTIOUS DISEASES

The diagnosis of infectious diseases can often be made by directly detecting free or bound antigens in biologic fluids. An antigen is a material that evokes the formation of antibodies in an animal that is immunized or infected with that antigen. An antigen is generally immunogenic, that is, it has the capability to stimulate antibody formation and is also able to specifically combine with the antibodies that are formed against it. Those parts of the molecule that interact with and are most often recognized by antibodies are called immunodominant antigenic determinants or epitopes. The unique characteristics of each antigen depend on the types, sequences, and configurations of amino acids in proteins and on the structural and chemical composition of polysaccharides, glycoproteins, and nucleic acids. All of these are genetically determined.

In clinical microbiology, antibody molecules, primarily of the IgG class, can be used to detect specific bacterial antigens. These IgG molecules may be polyclonal or monoclonal. Polyclonal antibodies are generally purified from animals that are immunized with the antigen of interest. Consequently, the antibodies produced against a complex antigen are reactive with a variety of different immunogenic determinants or epitopes. Monoclonal antibodies are antibodies that are produced against specific epitopes of an antigen; these antibodies, therefore, are highly specific.

Antigen–Antibody Reactions

Antigens are detected by one of several methods in the clinical microbiology laboratory.

Precipitin Reaction

The precipitin reaction is found in test systems that allow the free diffusion of antigen and antibody fronts toward one another. At a critical point of interface, at which place the concentrations of antigens and antibody are optimal for a reaction to occur, a visible precipitate composed of combined antigens and antibodies forms. In a single diffusion system, antibody is incorporated into an agar gel into which antigen is allowed to diffuse. In the tube method, antigen is overlaid onto agar containing antisera and one or more precipitin lines form at zones of equivalence (Fig. 19-1). In radial immunodiffusion, antibody is contained in agar that is coated onto a glass slide. Material containing antigen is then placed into circular wells cut into the agar. During incubation, the antigen diffuses into the agar and a ring of precipitate forms. The diameter of the ring is directly proportional to the amount of antigen present in the material. Semiquantitation of the antigen can be obtained by comparing the diameter of the precipitin reaction with those of material containing known quantities of antigen (Fig. 19-2). In double diffusion tests, both antigen and antibody are placed in wells adjacent to one another and the materials diffuse out toward one another. A line of precipitate then forms between the lines when concentrations of equivalence are reached (Fig. 19-3).

Agglutination Reactions

Agglutination reactions can be defined as the immunochemical-specific aggregation of particles (bacteria, erythrocytes, synthetic latex particles) coated with antigen or antibody that can be used to

Figure 19-1. Principles of single and double immunodiffusion in Oudin tubes. In the single diffusion system (*left*), antiserum is incorporated into the agar in the lower portion of the tube. A liquid sample, containing the antigen or antigens to be detected, is placed on the surface of the agar. As the antigens diffuse into the agar, precipitin lines form at zones where conditions for specific antigen–antibody reactions are optimal. The double diffusion system (*right*) is similar, except that the antigen and the antibody are separated by a plug of neutral agar into which each diffuses. Again, precipitin lines form at points where conditions for antigen–antibody interaction are optimal.

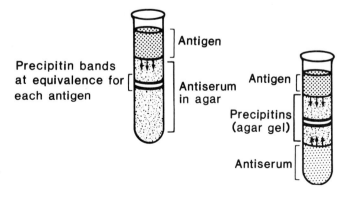

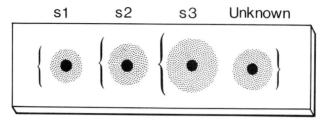

Figure 19-2. Antigen quantitation by single radial immunodiffusion. Illustrated is a glass slide supporting a thin layer of antibody-containing agar. The sample containing the complementary antigen to be measured (unknown) is placed into a small well and allowed to diffuse into the agar. A precipitin ring is formed around the sample well, the diameter of which is directly proportional to the concentration of antigen contained. Exact quantitation of antigen in the sample can be calculated by comparing its diameter with the sizes of a series of antigen standards of known concentrations (s1, s2, s3, etc).

detect either soluble antibodies or antigens, respectively.[8] Antigens or antibodies are attached to the particulate surfaces either by intramolecular electrical forces or by covalent bonds. Clumping of the carrier particles occurs as an indicator of the antigen–antibody interactions occurring on the surface of the carriers. Either antigens or antibodies can be detected by agglutination reactions, depending on the reactant that is bound to the carrier. Agglutination reactions are more sensitive than precipitin reactions because fewer reactions are required before the secondary agglutination reaction becomes visible. This property to react at high dilutions allows test systems to be devised by which semiquantitative measurements of antigens or antibodies can be carried out by determining the degree of dilution (titer) that will still produce a reaction.

Solid-Phase Immunoassays

Solid-phase immunoassay, an extension of the basic principles discussed earlier, refers to the binding of either antigen or antibody to a variety of solid-phase substances, such as polystyrene microtube wells, plastic beads, and ferrous metal beads. For example, solid-phase systems designed for the detection of antibody in an unknown sample have antigen covalently bound to the inner lining of plastic microtubes or on polystyrene beads. The initial reaction occurs when the specimen to be tested is incubated for a prescribed time with a solid-phase substance where the type-specific antibody reacts. After the reaction mixture is washed to remove any excess or extraneous protein, an antiglobulin conjugated with a fluorescent, radioactive tag or other label is added to the reaction mixture.

In radioimmunoassay procedures, the label is a radioactive isotope; in enzyme-linked immunosorbent assay (ELISA) methods, the tag is an enzyme. Horseradish peroxidase and alkaline phosphatase are the enzymes most commonly used. If the initial antigen–antibody reaction has occurred, the antiglobulin (with its radioactive or enzyme tag) binds to the antibody. The final step in the assay is to detect the presence of radioactive or enzyme activ-

Top View

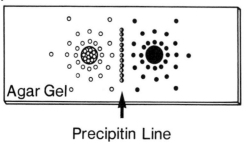

Agar Gel

Precipitin Line

Figure 19-3. Illustration of double immunodiffusion of an agar-coated microscope slide. Wells are cut into the agar in close proximity to one another. One well contains antibody (*open circles*); the other contains the complementary antigen (*solid circles*). A line of precipitation forms where antigen and antibody are in optimal concentrations where their zones of diffusion overlap. With this system, unknown samples containing either antigen or antibody can be tested by placing the complementary reactant in the opposite well.

ity; a positive reaction indicates that antibody was present in the original sample. The intensity of the final reaction is proportional to the concentration of antibody present. To circumvent the use of radioactive materials, enzyme immunoassays (EIA and ELISA procedures) using chemiluminescent or biotin-avidin reactive (biotinylated) probes as the final detector have found widespread use in diagnostic microbiology laboratories. ELISA techniques have been adapted to detect a wide variety of bacterial, fungal, and parasite antigens in various types of clinical specimens. The direct detection of the capsular antigens of *Streptococcus pneumoniae*, *Haemophilus influenzae* type b, *Neisseria meningitidis* and the cell wall antigens of group A streptococci and the detection of *Giardia lamblia*–specific antigen in stool specimens are examples of the application of this technology.[1,2,15,23]

Immunofluorescence Technology

Immunofluorescence provides an alternative to immunoabsorbent assays as a means for detecting and localizing antigens in making the diagnosis of bacterial, fungal, parasitic, and viral diseases. With this technique, specific antibody is conjugated with fluorescent compounds, resulting in a sensitive tracer with unaltered immunologic reactivity. The conjugated antiserum is added to cells or tissues on a slide and becomes fixed to antigens, forming a stable immune complex. Nonreacting materials are removed by washing, and the preparation is then dried and observed with a fluorescence microscope. Antigens bound specifically to fluorescent antibody can be detected as bright apple-green or orange yellow objects against a dark background, depending on the fluorochrome being used. This test is particularly useful in the identification of organisms that may be difficult or delayed in recovery in culture, including bacteria such as *Legionella* species and *Bordetella pertussis*, *Chlamydia trachomatis*, and a variety of viral agents such as the herpes simplex, varicella-zoster, and respiratory syncytial viruses and cytomegaloviruses. Additional information on this test is provided in other texts.[12]

Direct immunofluorescence techniques involve direct application of the conjugate to the material being examined, followed by a 30- to 45-minute period of incubation in a humid environment at 35° to 37°C to allow the antigen–antibody reaction to come to completion. After a series of steps to wash the preparation free of background interference, the preparation is stained, air dried, and mounted for observation under a microscope fitted with an appropriate fluorescent light source. In the indirect procedure, the material to be examined is first overlaid with an excess of immune serum directed at the antigen and allowed to react for 30 to 45 minutes at 35° to 37°C. The specimen is washed with phosphate-buffered saline solution and then allowed to react with a fluorescent-tagged antiserum against the species of immunoglobulin used in the initial reaction. After washing the background free, the presence of microscopic fluorescence indicates the presence of antigen.

The direct method is simple and rapid to perform with fewer nonspecific reactions but is less sensitive. The indirect method is more sensitive and gives brighter fluorescence, but it is less specific and subject to increased cross-reactivity.

NUCLEIC ACID PROBES

In broad terms, a nucleic acid probe is a sequence of single-stranded nucleic acid that can hybridize specifically with its complementary strand by way of nucleic acid base-pairing. A probe may be constructed to detect either single-stranded DNA or RNA (ssDNA or ssRNA). Many of the commercially available nucleic acid probes are directed against sequences found in the ssRNA that, along with ribosomal proteins, comprise the ribosome (the site of protein synthesis in both procaryotic and eucaryotic cells). The commercial availability of an increasing number of nucleic acid probe systems is making it more and more possible for clinical microbiology laboratories to make rapid diagnoses of various bacterial, mycobacterial, fungal, and viral infections.[4,6,7,13,14,19,20] A discussion of the underlying principles of this technology is beyond the scope of this book. Further general information can be found in other texts.[12]

POLYMERASE CHAIN REACTION

Polymerase chain reaction (PCR) and gene amplification refers to a highly sensitive technique by which minute quantities of specific DNA or RNA sequences can be enzymatically amplified to the extent that a sufficient quantity of material is available to reach a threshold signal for detection using a specific probe.[18] The technique is used specifically to detect trace amounts of nucleic acid material directly in clinical specimens, where bacterial, viral, or fungal agents are believed to play a causative role. The fundamental basis of this technology is that each infectious disease agent possesses a unique signature sequence in its DNA or RNA composition by which it can be identified. PCR is carried out by using a thermocycler, which produces a series of heat–cool cycles whereby double-stranded DNA is dissociated into single strands that in turn are allowed to anneal in the presence of specific primers on cooling. Through the successive heat–cool cycles, the DNA sequence to be detected is amplified a hundredfold or more. PCR technology is finding an increasingly wider use in clinical laboratories[11,12,21] but is currently limited to laboratories where the environment and techniques are under strict control to prevent the introduction of contaminating nucleic acids into the reaction mixture.[5,25]

REFERENCES

1. Addiss DG, Mathews HM, Stewart JM, et al. Evaluation of a commercially available enzyme-linked immunosorbent assay for *Giardia lamblia* antigen in stool. J Clin Microbiol 1991;29:1137–1142.

2. Brown SL, Bibb WE, McKinney RM. Retrospective examination of lung tissue specimens for the presence of *Legionella* organisms: comparison of indirect fluorescent antibody system with direct fluorescent antibody testing. J Clin Microbiol 1984;19:468–472.

3. Celig DM, Schreckenberger PC. Clinical evaluation of the RapID-ANA II panel for identification of anaerobic bacteria. J Clin Microbiol 1991;29:457–462.

4. Daly JA, Clifton NI, Seskin KC, Kooch WM III. Use of rapid, nonradioactive DNA probes in culture confirmation tests to detect *Streptococcus agalactiae*, *Haemophilus influenzae* and *Enterococcus* spp. from pediatric patients with significant infections. J Clin Microbiol 1991;29:80–82.

5. Ehrlich GK. Caveats of PCR. Clin Microbiol Newsletter 1991;13:149–151.

6. Grimont PA, Grimont F, Desplaces N, et al. DNA probe specific for *Legionella pneumophila*. J Clin Microbiol 1985;21:431–437.

7. Hammond G, Hannan C, Yeh T, et al. DNA hybridization for diagnosis of enteric adenovirus infection from directly spotted human fecal specimens. J Clin Microbiol 1987;25:1881–1885.

8. Ingram DL, Pearson AW, Occhiuti AR. Detection of bacterial antigens in body fluids with the Wellcogen *Haemophilus influenzae* b, *Streptococcus pneumonia* and *Neisseria meningitidis* (ACYUW135) latex agglutination tests. J Clin Microbiol 1983;18:1119–1121

9. Janda WM, Malloy PJ, Schreckenberger PC. Clinical evaluation of the Vitek *Haemophilus–Neisseria* identification card. J Clin Microbiol 1987;25:37–41

10. Janda WM, Bradna JJ, Ruther P. Identification of *Neisseria* spp, *Haemophilus* spp. and other fastidious gram-negative bacteria with the MicroScan *Haemophilus–Neisseria* identification panel. J Clin Microbiol 1989;27:869–873.

11. Kato N, Ou C, Kato H, et al. Identification of toxigenic *Clostridium difficile* by the polymerase chain reaction. J Clin Microbiol 1991;29:33–37.

12. Koneman EW, Allen SD, Janda WM, Schreckenberger PC, Winn WC Jr. Color Atlas and textbook of diagnostic microbiology, 4th ed. Philadelphia, JB Lippincott, 1992.

13. Lewis JS, Kranig-Brown D, Trainor DA. DNA probe confirmatory test for *Neisseria gonorrhoeae*. J Clin Microbiol 1990;28:2349–2350, 1990

14. Lim SD, Todd J, Lopez J et al. Genotypic identification of pathogenic *Mycobacterium* species by using a nonradioactive oligonucleotide probe. J Clin Microbiol 1991;29:1276–1278.

15. Macone AB, Arakere G, Letourneau JM, et al. Comparison of a new rapid enzyme-linked immunosorbent assay with latex particle agglutination for the detection of *Haemophilus influenzae* type b infections. J Clin Microbiol 1985;21:711–714.

16. Moss CW. Gas–liquid chromatography as an analytical tool in microbiology. J Chromatogr 1981;203:337–347.

17. Moss CW. Uses of gas-liquid chromatography and high-pressure liquid chromatography in clinical microbiology. In: Lennette EH, Balows A, Hausler WJ Jr, Shadomy HJ, eds. Manual of clinical microbiology. 4th ed. Washington, DC, American Society for Microbiology, 1985:1029–1036.

18. Mullis KB, Faloona FA, Scharf S, et al. Specific enzymatic amplification of DNA in vitro: the polymerase chain reaction. Cold Spring Harbor Symp Quant Biol 1986;L1:263–272.

19. Musial CE, Tice LS, Stockman L, Roberts GD. Identification of mycobacteria from culture by using the Gen-Probe rapid diagnostic system for *Mycobacterium avium* complex and *Mycobacterium tuberculosis* complex. J Clin Microbiol 1988;26:2120–2123.

20. Pasculle AW, Veto GE, Krystofiak S, et al. Laboratory and clinical evaluation of a commercial DNA probe for the detection of *Legionella* species. J Clin Microbiol 1989;27:2350–2358.

21. Pershing DH. Polymerase chain reaction: trenches to benches. J Clin Microbiol 1991;29:1281–1285.

22. Quentin C, Desailly-Chanson ME, Bebear C. Evaluation of AN-Ident. J Clin Microbiol 1991;29:231–235.

23. Sippel JE, Hider PA, Controni G. Use of directigen latex agglutination test for detection of *Haemophilus influenzae*, *Streptococcus pneumoniae*, and *Neisseria meningitidis* antigens in cerebrospinal fluid from meningitis patients. J Clin Microbiol 1984;20:884–886.

24. Taylor AJ, Skinner PR. Gas–liquid chromatography in medical microbiology. Med Lab Sci 1983;40:375–385,

25. Wright PA, Wynford-Thomas. The polymerase chain reaction: Miracle or mirage? A critical review of its uses and limitations in diagnosis and research. J Pathol 1990;162:99–117.

Index

Page numbers followed by *f* indicate illustrations; *t* following a page number indicates tabular material.